KU-776-642

OXFORD MEDICAL PUBLICATIONS

Oxford Handbook of
Ophthalmology

SECOND EDITION

Published and forthcoming Oxford Handbooks

Oxford Handbook of
Ophthalmology

SECOND EDITION

Alastair K.O. Denniston

MRC Clinical Research Fellow
University of Birmingham, UK

Philip I. Murray

Professor of Ophthalmology
University of Birmingham, UK

OXFORD
UNIVERSITY PRESS

OXFORD
UNIVERSITY PRESS

Great Clarendon Street, Oxford OX2 6DP

Oxford University Press is a department of the University of Oxford.
It furthers the University's objective of excellence in research, scholarship,
and education by publishing worldwide in

Oxford New York

Auckland Cape Town Dar es Salaam Hong Kong Karachi
Kuala Lumpur Madrid Melbourne Mexico City Nairobi
New Delhi Shanghai Taipei Toronto

With offices in

Argentina Austria Brazil Chile Czech Republic France Greece
Guatemala Hungary Italy Japan Poland Portugal Singapore
South Korea Switzerland Thailand Turkey Ukraine Vietnam

Oxford is a registered trade mark of Oxford University Press
in the UK and in certain other countries

Published in the United States
by Oxford University Press Inc., New York

British Library Cataloguing in Publication Data
Data available

Library of Congress Cataloging-in-Publication-Data
Data available

Typeset by Cepha Imaging Private Ltd., Bangalore, India
Printed in China
on acid-free paper by
Asia Pacific Offset

ISBN 978–0–19–955264–1

10 9 8 7 6 5 4 3 2

Foreword

Three years ago I wrote the foreword for the first edition of the *Oxford Handbook of Ophthalmology* by Alastair Denniston and Philip Murray. I am now delighted to write the foreword for the second edition. As expected, it has very rapidly become one of the most popular books for ophthalmology trainees in the UK with three UK printings, two international printings, three translations in progress, and an American edition in the pipeline. The pocket book format continues to be very popular, even in these days of the ubiquitous personal digital assistant.

The first edition covered all the standard topics and included other useful chapters not often found in a handbook including clinical skills, investigations, aids to diagnosis, vision in context, perioperative care, therapeutics, and a rather nice miscellaneous chapter on eponymous syndromes. Further chapters on the all-important evidence-based ophthalmology have now been included as well as a refractive ophthalmology chapter, useful not just in examinations but when asked at dinner parties. The new anti-VEGF therapies are also covered.

I hope this second edition of the handbook will continue to help you to improve the care of your patients. Lists are more than just a way to pass examinations—they help to make us think around diagnoses and management, and they will help to ensure we do not miss something that may be sight or even life threatening to our patients. The *Oxford Handbook of Ophthalmology* has now proved itself as an essential addition to the books that help us all learn, enjoy, and deliver the wonderful specialty that is ophthalmology.

Peng Tee Khaw
Professor and Consultant Ophthalmic Surgeon
Director, National Institute for Health Research
Biomedical Research Centre
Moorfields Eye Hospital and UCL Institute of Ophthalmology
London
2009

Preface to the second edition

Since the first edition of the *Oxford Handbook of Ophthalmology* emerged three years ago, it has—to our delight—rapidly established itself as one of the most popular ophthalmic handbooks in the UK, and with a significant impact further afield. We wrote the first edition because neither of us could find a handbook that would meet the needs of ophthalmic trainees (and other health care professionals in ophthalmology) in covering emergency and out-patient ophthalmology, that had both a UK and international focus and that tried as far as possible to be evidence and guideline based. We weren't sure that anybody other than our immediate families (and possibly sympathetic colleagues) would see things the same way, and we recognized the possibility that this small book, representing an unbelievable amount of our own and our colleagues' time, would gather dust in the Oxford University Press cellars.

The response, however, has been unbelievable: three UK printings, two international printings, three translations in progress, and an American edition planned. More important to us has been the very positive and helpful feedback from ophthalmologists of all levels of experience throughout the world. Many of their suggestions have been incorporated into this edition.

Fully revised and updated throughout, this second edition of the *Oxford Handbook of Ophthalmology* reflects a number of important changes, such as the wide-ranging impact of anti-VEGF therapy, and emerging therapies including stem cell transplantation. Additionally, there are new pages on a diversity of important topics ranging from amniotic membrane transplantation to the treatment of low vision.

New for this edition are chapters on 'Evidence-based ophthalmology', a helpful introduction to critical appraisal, levels of evidence, and medical statistics as relevant to ophthalmology, and 'Refractive ophthalmology' that contains practical advice on the correction of refractive error by spectacles, contact lenses, and refractive surgery.

Whilst this handbook is broader in scope than the first edition, we have tried to ensure that at its core it remains true to its original purpose: to give you the information you need, when and where you need it. So, recycle your first edition and get this one—you won't be disappointed!

Alastair K.O. Denniston, Philip I. Murray
2009

Preface to the first edition

Welcome to the first edition of the *Oxford Handbook of Ophthalmology*.

The aspiration of the *OHO* is to be your portable repository of knowledge, accessible in emergencies and easily dipped in and out of between examining patients. It provides immediate access to the detailed clinical information you need—in casualty, clinic, theatre, and on the wards. It is also highly suitable for revision for postgraduate examinations. It is not exhaustive and we would expect it to complement, rather than replace, your collection of desktop ophthalmology heavyweights.

The core of the book comprises a systematic synopsis of ophthalmic disease directed towards diagnosis, interim assessment, and ongoing management. Assessment boxes for common clinical conditions, and algorithms for important clinical presentations illustrate this practical approach. The information is easily accessed, being presented in standard format with areas of importance being highlighted. Key sections for the trainee include: clinical skills, aids to diagnosis, and investigations and their interpretation. Basic perioperative care and advanced life support protocols are included as specialists often find that their general medical knowledge somewhat hazy at times of crisis.

Primarily intended for ophthalmologists, this handbook is a valuable resource for anyone working with ophthalmic patients, whether optometrists, orthoptists, ophthalmic nurses or other health professions in ophthalmology. While the earlier pages may be thumbed mainly by the trainee, it is envisaged that even the experienced Consultant will find the *OHO* useful. We have tried to include information that you would not easily find elsewhere: vision in context (low vision, registration and benefits, driving requirements), management of systemic disease (diabetes, thyroid disorders, systemic immunosuppression), a glossary of eponymous syndromes, and NICE and RCOphth guidelines.

Although we have endeavoured to provide up-to-date, accurate, evidence-based information any comments would be gratefully received so that we can make future editions even better. Point your web browser to: www.oup.co.uk/academic/medicine/handbooks/ where you will be able to have your say and to download any updates.

We hope the *OHO* will be an essential addition to your personal library of ophthalmology textbooks, and be an invaluable companion to you in your practice of ophthalmology.

Alastair K.O. Denniston, Philip I. Murray
2006

Consultant advisers

Clinical skills
Mr Andrew Jacks
Prof. Philip Murray

Trauma
Mr Malcolm Woodcock
Miss Saaeha Rauz
Mr Aidan Murray

Lacrimal
Mr Aidan Murray

Cornea
Miss Saaeha Rauz

Lens
Mr Paul Chell

Uveitis
Prof. Philip Murray

Medical retina
Miss Hope-Ross

Intraocular tumours
Prof. Ian Rennie
Mr Manoj Parulekar

Strabismus
Mr Tim Matthews
Miss Fiona Dean

Refractive ophthalmology
Prof. Sunil Shah
Mrs Waheeda Illahi (Optometrist)

Vision in context
Mr Mike Burdon
Mr Sonal Rughani (RNIB)

Therapeutics
Mrs Lucy Titcomb (Pharmacist)

Investigations
Prof. Philip Murray
Dr Peter Good
Dr Angela Luck (Radiologist)

Lids
Mr Aidan Murray

Conjunctiva
Miss Saaeha Rauz

Sclera
Prof. Philip Murray

Glaucoma
Prof. Peter Shah
Miss Rosemary Robinson

Vitreoretinal
Mr Graham Kirkby

Orbit
Mr Omar Durrani

Neuro-ophthalmology
Mr Andrew Jacks

Paediatric ophthalmology
Miss Lucy Butler

Aids to diagnosis
Mr Mike Burdon

Perioperative care
Dr Shashi Vohra (Anaesthetist)

Evidence-based ophthalmology
Dr Merrick Moseley

Acknowledgements

We would like to thank the many colleagues who contributed to the writing of this book. We are grateful to all the junior ophthalmologists who made significant contributions to specific chapters, in particular: Susie Mollan for her outstanding efforts with Ophthalmic Investigations and Neuro-ophthalmology for which she was rewarded by having her name mis-spelt in the first edition; also to the faculty of Arun Reginald (Trauma, Cornea), Geraint Williams (Conjunctiva), Anil Arilakatti (Cornea), Vijay Savant (Lens), Sumit Dhingra (Glaucoma), Paul Tomlins (Vitreoretinal), Rajen Gupta (Medical Retina), Joseph Abbott (Paediatric Ophthalmology), James iDoc Cameron (web resources), James Flint and Rosie Auld (Orthoptics), Tahir Masoud and David Lockington (contributions to the first edition) and Graham Brack (independent drug scrutineer). We particularly want to thank Saaeha Rauz both for her contributions and her continued support during the writing of this second edition. We also thank Rizwana Siddiqui and Dr Peter Good for images, and the many people world-wide who have enthusiastically contributed to this second edition.

We especially thank the senior ophthalmologists (listed on p. xi) who gave generously of their time to advise on each chapter and to critically review the recent developments in their field. The success of this book is in very large measure due to the contributions of consultants who are not only at the forefront of their specialties, but are also passionate about passing this wisdom on to the rest of us.

We are grateful to Angela Luck for yet more beautiful anatomical illustrations and her ongoing appreciation of the artistic merits of the slit lamp (despite being a radiologist).

It has been a great pleasure to work with the staff of OUP throughout. We thank Alison Langton, Elizabeth Reeve, Beth Womack, Anna Winstanley, and Kate Wanwimolruk for their enthusiasm and practical assistance.

AD wishes to thank his wife (Sarah) for her inspiration and patience, and his two boys (Arran and Ewan) for their critical assessment of the manuscript. He also wishes to thank his clinical mentors (Marie Tsaloumas, Tim Matthews, Saaeha Rauz, Phil Murray) for their advice and encouragement.

PM wishes to thank his family (Tricia, Hannah, Ella, and Ford the cat) for trying to keep out of his way while attempting to write this book. He is grateful to Out of the Blue Jazz Orchestra for almost keeping him sane on Friday nights, and now acknowledges his mid-life crisis by buying his third sports car, when he should have just gone for a Skoda Estate.

Alastair K.O. Denniston, Philip I. Murray
2009

Additional acknowledgements

We are indebted to a number of colleagues from across the UK and the rest of the world who have given us invaluable feedback which has helped direct the development of this second edition. We thank: Mr Ajay Tyagi, Mr Sam Elsherbiny, Mr Sam Mirza, Mr Sung, Dr Zakaria, Dr Hannah Baker, Mr Maged Nessim, Dr Imran Khan, Dr Kwesi Amissah-Arthur, Dr Anna Gao, Dr Lei Liu, Mr Nachiketa Acharya, Mr James Denniston, Dr Ed Moran, Miss Vaneeta Sood, Dr Y.C. Yap, Miss Anne Williams, and Miss Katya Tambe.

Contents

Symbols and abbreviations

📖	cross reference
↑	increased
↓	decreased
Δ	prism dioptre
5-FU	5-fluorouracil
AACG	acute angle closure glaucoma
AAU	acute anterior uveitis
AC	anterior chamber
AC:A	accommodative convergence to accommodation ratio
ACE	angiotensin converting enzyme
Ach	acetylcholine
AD	autosomal dominant
AIDS	acquired immunodeficiency syndrome
AION	anterior ischaemic optic neuropathy
ALT	argon laser trabeculoplasty
AMD	age-related macular degeneration
AMG	amniotic membrane graft
ANA	anti-nuclear antibody
ANCA	anti-neutrophil cytoplasmic antibody
APMPPE	acute posterior multifocal placoid pigment epitheliopathy
APTT	activated partial thromboplastin time
AqH	aqueous humour
AR	autosomal recessive
ARC	abnormal retinal correspondence
AMD	age-related macular degeneration
ARN	acute retinal necrosis
AS	anterior segment
asb	apostilbs
ASD	atrial septal defect
AVM	arteriovenous malformation
Ax	allergies
AZOOR	acute zonal occult outer retinopathy
BCL	bandage contact lens
BCVA	best-corrected visual acuity
BDR	background diabetic retinopathy
BDUMP	bilateral diffuse uveal melanocytic proliferation
BM	finger-prick blood glucose testing (from Boehringer Mannheim test)

BNF	British National Formulary
BP	blood pressure
BRAO	branch retinal artery occlusion
BRVO	branch retinal vein occlusion
BSV	binocular single vision
BUT	break-up time (of tear film)
C/D	cup disc ratio
C3F8	perfluoropropane
CCF	carotid-cavernous (sinus) fistula
CCT	central corneal thickness
CCTV	closed circuit television
CF	counting fingers
CFEOM	chronic fibrosis of extraocular muscles
CHED	congenital hereditary endothelial dystrophy
CHRPE	congenital hypertrophy of retinal pigment epithelium
CHSD	congenital hereditary stromal dystrophy
CL	contact lens
CMO	cystoid macular oedema
CMV	cytomegalovirus
CNS	central nervous system
CNV	choroidal neovascular membrane
COPD	chronic obstructive pulmonary disease
CPEO	chronic progressive external ophthalmoplegia
CPSD	corrected pattern standard deviation
CRAO	central retinal artery occlusion
CRP	C-reactive protein
CRVO	central retinal vein occlusion
CSF	cerebrospinal fluid
CSNB	congenital stationary night blindness
CSR	central serous (chorio) retinopathy
CT	computer tomography
CVA	cerebrovascular accident
CVS	cardiovascular system
CWS	cotton wool spot
CXR	chest X-ray
d	day
D	dioptre
dB	decibels
DC	dioptre cylinder
DCG	dacryocystogram

DCR	dacryocystorhinostomy
DD	disc diameter
DIC	disseminated intravascular coagulopathy
DNA	deoxyribonucleic acid
ds	double-stranded (of nucleic acids)
DS	dioptre sphere
DVLA	Driver and Vehicle Licensing Agency
Dx	drug history
EBV	Epstein–Barr virus
ECCE	extracapsular cataract extraction
ECG	electrocardiogram
EDT	electrodiagnostic tests
EEG	electroencephalogram
ELISA	enzyme-linked immunosorbent assay
EMG	electromyogram
ENT	ear, nose and throat specialist (otorhinolaryngologist)
EOG	electro-oculogram
ERD	exudative retinal detachment
ERG	electroretinogram
ESR	erythrocyte sedimentation rate
EUA	examination under anaesthesia
E-W	Edinger–Westphal (nucleus)
FB	foreign body
FBC	full blood count
FEF	frontal eye fields
FFA	fundus fluorescein angiography
FH	family history
FNA	fine-needle aspiration
g	guttae (drops)
GA	general anaesthesia
GCA	giant cell arteritis
GEN	gaze evoked nystagmus
GI	gastrointestinal system
GU	genitourinary system
GVHD	graft versus host disease
h	hour
HHV8	human herpes virus 8
HIV	human immunodeficiency virus
HLA	human leucocyte antigen
HM	hand movements

HPC	history of presenting complaints
HPV	human papillomavirus
HRT	Heidelberg retinal tomography
HSV	herpes simplex virus
HTLV-1	human T-cell lymphotropic virus type 1
H	History
HZO	herpes zoster ophthalmicus
IBD	inflammatory bowel disease
ICA	internal carotid artery
ICCE	intracapsular cataract extraction
ICE	iridocorneal endothelial syndrome
ICG	indocyanine green angiography
ICP	intracranial pressure
IIIn	oculomotor nerve
IIn	optic nerve
IM	intramuscular
INO	internuclear ophthalmoplegia
IO	inferior oblique
IOFB	intraocular foreign body
IOL	intraocular lens
IOP	intraocular pressure
IPCV	idiopathic polypoidal choroidal vasculopathy
IR	inferior rectus
IV	intravenous
IVC	inferior vena cava
IVn	trochlear nerve
I	investigations
JIA	juvenile idiopathic arthritis
KP	keratic precipitate
LASEK	laser subepithelial keratomileusis
LASIK	laser stromal in-situ keratomileusis
LFT	liver function tests
LGN	lateral geniculate nucleus
LHON	Leber's hereditary optic neuropathy
LogMAR	logarithm of the minimum angle of resolution
LP	lumbar puncture
LPS	levator palpebrae superioris
LR	lateral rectus
LVA	low vision aid
MC&S	microscopy, culture and sensitivities

MD	mean deviation
MEWDS	multiple evanescent white dot syndrome
MG	myasthenia gravis
min	minute
M:F	male:female ratio
MLF	medial longitudinal fasciculus
MMC	mitomycin C
MR	medial rectus
MRI	magnetic resonance imaging
MS	multiple sclerosis
mth	month
n	refractive index
NBM	nil by mouth
Nd-YAG	neodymium-yttrium-aluminium-garnet laser
NFI,II	neurofibromatosis types I and II
NFL	nerve fibre layer
nocte	at night
NorA	noradrenaline
NPL	no perception of light
NRR	neuroretinal rim
NSAID	non-steroidal anti-inflammatory drug
NVD	new vessels of the optic disc
NVE	new vessels elsewhere
NVG	neovascular glaucoma
Oc	ointment
OCT	optical coherence tomography
OD	right eye
O/E	on examination
OHT	ocular hypertension
OS	left eye
OVD	ophthalmic viscosurgical devices
PAS	peripheral anterior synechiae
PC	presenting complaint
PCO	posterior capsular opacification
PCIOL	posterior chamber intraocular lens
PCR	polymerase chain reaction
PDR	proliferative diabetic retinopathy
PDS	pigment dispersion syndrome
PDT	photodynamic therapy
PERG	pattern electroretinogram

PF	preservative free
PI	peripheral iridotomy
PIC	punctate inner choroidopathy
PK	penetrating keratoplasty
PL	perception of light
plt	platelets
PMH	past medical history
PMMA	poly (methyl methacrylate)
PNS	peripheral nervous system
PO	per os (by mouth)
POAG	primary open angle glaucoma
POH	past ophthalmic history
POHS	presumed ocular histoplasmosis syndrome
PORN	progressive outer retinal necrosis
PPD	posterior polymorphous dystrophy
PPDR	preproliferative diabetic retinopathy
PPRF	paramedian pontine reticular formation
PRK	photorefractive keratectomy
PRP	pan retinal photocoagulation
PS	posterior synechiae
PSD	pattern standard deviation
PTT	prothrombin time
PUK	peripheral ulcerative keratitis
PVD	posterior vitreous detachment
PXF	pseudoexfoliation syndrome
q	every (e.g. q 1 hour = every 1 hour)
RA	rheumatoid arthritis
RAPD	relative afferent pupillary defect
RCES	recurrent corneal erosion syndrome
RCOphth	Royal College of Ophthalmologists
RF	rheumatoid factor
RGP	rigid gas permeable (of contact lenses)
RNA	ribonucleic acid
RNFL	retinal nerve fibre layer
ROP	retinopathy of prematurity
RP	retinitis pigmentosa
RPE	retinal pigment epithelium
RRD	rhegmatogenous retinal detachment
RS	respiratory system
s	second

SBS	shaken baby syndrome
SC	subcutaneous
SF6	sulphur hexafluoride
SH	social history
Si	silicone (of oil)
SITA	Swedish interactive threshold algorithm
SLE	systemic lupus erythematosus
SO	superior oblique
SR	superior rectus
SVC	superior vena cava
SVP	spontaneous venous pulsation
TB	tuberculosis
TED	thyroid eye disease
TEN	toxic epidermal necrolysis
TFT	thyroid function tests
TI	trans-illumination
TINU	tubulo-interstitial nephritis with uveitis
TNF	tumour necrosis factor
TPHA	*Treponema pallidum* haemagglutination assay
TRD	tractional retinal detachment
U+E	urea and electrolytes
UGH	uveitis-glaucoma-hyphaema syndrome
US	ultrasound
UV	ultraviolet
VA	visual acuity
Vn	trigeminal nerve
Va,b,c	ophthalmic, maxillary, and mandibular divisions of Vn
VDRL	venereal disease research laboratory test
VEGF	vascular endothelial growth factor
VEP	visual evoked potential
VHL	von Hippel–Lindau syndrome
VIIn	facial nerve
VIn	abducens nerve
VKC	vernal keratoconjunctivitis
VKH	Vogt–Koyanagi–Harada syndrome
VR	vitreoretinal
VSD	ventricular septal defect
VZV	varicella zoster virus
WHO	World Health Organization
yr	year

Orthoptic abbreviations

ACS	alternating convergent strabismus
ADS	alternating divergent strabismus
AHP	abnormal head posture
ARC	abnormal retinal correspondence
BD	base down (of prism)
BI	base in (of prism)
BO	base out (of prism)
BU	base up (of prism)
BSV	binocular single vision
CC	Cardiff cards
CI	convergence insufficiency
Conv XS	convergence excess
CSM	central steady maintained (of fixation)
CT	cover test
DVD	dissociated vertical deviation
DVM	delayed visual maturation
Ecc fix	eccentric fixation
EP	esophoria
ET	esotropia
E(T)	intermittent esotropia
FCPL	forced choice preferential looking
FL/FLE	fixing with left eye
FR/FRE	fixing with right eye
HP	hyperphoria
HT	hypertropia
Hypo	hypophoria
HypoT	hypotropia
KP	Kay's pictures
LCS	left convergent strabismus
LDS	left divergent strabismus
MLN	manifest latent nystagmus
MR	Maddox rod
MW	Maddox wing
NPA	near point of accommodation
NPC	near point of convergence
NRC	normal retinal correspondence

o/a	overaction
Obj	objection
Occ	occlusion
OKN	optokinetic nystagmus
PCT	prism cover test
PFR	prism fusion range
PRT	prism reflection test
RCS	right convergent strabismus
RDS	right divergent strabismus
Rec	recovery
SG	Sheridan Gardiner test
Sn	Snellen chart
SP	simultaneous perception
Supp	suppression
u/a	underaction
VOR	vestibulo-ocular reflex
XP	exophoria
XT	exotropia
X(T)	intermittent exotropia

More complex variations for intermittent strabismus include:

R(E)T	intermittent right esotropia predominantly controlled
RE(T)	intermittent right esotropia predominantly manifest

Adjust according to whether:
R (right), L (left), or A (alternating)
ET (esotropia), XT (exotropia), HT (hypertropia), or hypoT (hypotropia).

These abbreviations are in common usage and are approved by the British and Irish Orthoptic Society.

Detailed contents

10   Glaucoma   301

11 Uveitis   **353**

14 Orbit

19 Refractive ophthamology   **737**

Chapter 1

Clinical skills

Taking an ophthalmic history

One of the first and most vital skills acquired by those involved in eye care is the accurate and efficient taking of an ophthalmic history. In ophthalmology clinical examination is very rewarding, probably more so than in any other specialty. However, this is additional to, rather than instead of, the history. Apart from the information gained, a rapport is established that should help the patient to tolerate the relatively 'invasive' ophthalmic examination. The patient is also more likely to accept any subsequent explanation of diagnosis and ongoing management if they know they have been heard.

Presenting complaint
Why are they here? Have they got a problem at all?
Routine optometric review has a valuable role in screening for asymptomatic disease (notably glaucoma) but may generate unnecessary referrals for benign variants (e.g. anomalous discs, early lens opacities). Consider who has the problem—the patient or the referring practitioner? Also consider what anxieties and expectations they bring with them.

History of presenting complaint
The analysis of most ophthalmic complaints centre on general questions regarding onset, precipitants, associated features (e.g. pain, redness, discharge, photophobia, etc.), duration, relieving factors, recovery, and specific questions directed by the presentation. Even after clinical examination further information may be needed to 'rule-in' or 'rule-out' diagnoses. Although some of these processes can be formalized as algorithms, their limitations should be recognized—they cannot emulate the multivariate processing, recognition of exceptions, and calculation of diagnostic probabilities subconsciously practised by an experienced clinician.

Past ophthalmic history
The background for each presentation is important. Ask about previous surgery/trauma, previous/concurrent eye disease, and refractive error. The differential diagnosis of an acute red eye will be affected by knowing that they had complicated cataract surgery 2d previously, or that they have a 10yr history of recurrent acute anterior uveitis or even that they wear contact lenses.

Past medical history
Similarly, consider the whole patient. Ask generally about any medical problems. In addition ask specifically about relevant conditions that they may have omitted to mention. The patient presenting with recurrently itchy eyes may not mention that they have eczema or asthma. Similarly, if presenting with a vascular event ask specifically about diabetes, hypertension and hypercholesterolaemia.

Family history
This is relevant both to diseases with a significant genetic component (e.g. retinitis pigmentosa, some corneal dystrophies; there may be consanguinity) and to infective conditions (e.g. conjunctivitis, TB, etc.).

Social history

Ask about smoking, alcohol intake if relevant to the ophthalmic disease (e.g. vascular event or unexplained optic neuropathy respectively). Consider the social context of the patient. Will they manage hourly drops? Can they even get the top off the bottle?

Drugs and allergies

Ask about concurrent medication and any allergies to previous medications (e.g. drops) as these may limit your therapeutic options. In addition to actual allergies consider contraindications (e.g. asthma/COPD and β-blockers).

Box 1.1 Taking the history of the presenting complaint (HPC)—an example

Patient presenting with loss of vision

Did it happen suddenly or gradually? Sudden loss of vision is commonly due to a vascular occlusion (e.g. AION, CRAO, CRVO) or bleed (e.g. vitreous haemorrhage, 'wet' macular degeneration). Gradual loss of vision is commonly associated with degenerations/depositions (e.g. cataract, macular dystrophies or 'dry' macular degeneration, corneal dystrophies).

Is it painful? Painful blurring of vision is most commonly associated with anterior ocular processes (e.g. keratitis, anterior uveitis), although orbital disease, optic neuritis, and GCA may also cause painful loss of vision.

Is the problem transient or persistent? Transient loss of vision is commonly due to temporary/subcritical vascular insufficiency (e.g. GCA, amaurosis fugax, vertebrobasilar artery insufficiency), whereas persistent loss of vision suggests structural or irreversible damage (e.g. vitreous haemorrhage, macular degeneration).

Does it affect one or both eyes? Unilateral disease may suggest a local (or ipsilateral) cause. Bilateral disease may suggest a more widespread or systemic process.

Is the vision blurred, dimmed, or distorted? Blurring or dimming may arise due to pathology anywhere in the visual pathway from cornea to cortex; common problems include refractive error, cataract, and macular disease. Distortion is commonly associated with macular pathology, but again may arise due to high refractive error (high ametropia/astigmatism) or other ocular disease.

Where is the problem with their vision? A superior or inferior hemispheric field loss suggests a corresponding inferior or superior vascular event involving retina (e.g. retinal vein occlusion) or disc (e.g. segmental AION). Peripheral field loss may indicate retinal detachment (usually rapidly evolving from far periphery), optic nerve disease, chiasmal compression (typically bitemporal loss) or cortical pathology (homonymous hemianopic defects). Central blurring of vision suggests disease of the macula (positive scotoma: a 'seen' spot) or optic nerve (negative scotoma: an unseen defect).

When is there a problem? For example, glare from headlights or bright sunlight is commonly due to posterior subcapsular lens opacities.

Assessment of vision: acuity (1)

Measuring visual acuity

Box 1.2 An approach to measuring visual acuity

Select (and document) appropriate test:	consider age, language, literacy, general faculties of patient
Check distance acuity (for each eye):	unaided with distance prescription with pinhole (if <6/9)
Check near acuity (for each eye): (where appropriate)	unaided with near prescription

Selecting the appropriate clinical test

Table 1.1 Tests of visual acuity

Patient	Distance	Near
Adult: literate	Snellen LogMAR	Test type N chart
Adult: illiterate	Illiterate E Landholt ring Sheridan–Gardiner (single optotype)	Reduced Sheridan–Gardiner
Children: age ≥3yrs	Sheridan–Gardiner (single optotype) Sonsken–Silver (multiple optotype)	
Children: age ≥2yrs	Kay picture test (single optotype) Multiple Picture Test	Reduced Kay picture test
Babies/infants	Clinical tests: fixing and following, objection to occlusion, picking up fine objects Preferential looking tests: Keeler, Teller, Cardiff cards Electrodiagnostic tests: VEP response to alternating chequerboard of varying frequency	

Distance acuity

Snellen charts

The optotypes (letters) subtend 5min of arc if read at the distance ascribed to that line, with each component of the letter subtending just 1min. This is the denominator. The actual distance at which it is used (usually 6m; 20ft in the USA) is the numerator. Thus if the top (60m) line can only be read at 2m, the Snellen acuity is 2/60. Normal VA is 1min of arc 6/6, although Vernier acuity may be up to 5s of arc. A change of 2 lines should be regarded as significant.

Fig.1.1 Schematic example of Snellen chart.

Assessment of vision: acuity (2)

Distance acuity *(continued)*

LogMAR charts

This records the logarithm of the Minimum Angle of Resolution. Based on the Bailey–Lovie LogMAR chart, the actual chart in common usage is the Ferris modification known as the 'ETDRS' chart. LogMAR testing has marked advantages over Snellen, notably that: (1) all letters are equally legible; (2) it controls the crowding phenomenon with 5 letters on each line and appropriate separation; and (3) there is a logical geometric progression of resolution. Starting with the LogMAR 1.0 line (Snellen 6/60) each letter is read. It is usually read at 4m. Each correct line (worth 0.1 units) or each correct letter (worth 0.02 units) is subtracted from 1.0 to give the final score.

Table 1.2 Distance acuity scoring systems

Snellen (UK; in m)	LogMAR	Decimal	Snellen (USA; in feet)
6/60	1.0	0.1	20/200
6/24	0.6	0.25	20/80
6/12	0.3	0.5	20/40
6/6	0	1.0	20/20
6/3	−0.3	2.0	20/10

Crowding is a phenomenon by which neighbouring targets interfere as proximity increases. Patients who are amblyopic are particularly susceptible and may score better with single optotype tests (e.g. Sheridan–Gardiner), than on a multiple test (e.g. Snellen). This has led to the use of multiple optotype forms of letter matching or picture tests.

Although other tests may approximate to a Snellen acuity reading, they are not exactly equivalent. It is, therefore, important to document which test has been used.

Pinhole acuity

A pinhole (stenopaeic aperture, 1.2mm diameter) can neutralize up to 3DS of refractive error.

Near (reading) acuity

Various charts are available. Most have paragraphs of text that are read by the patient at their usual reading distance (usually about 30cm). The notation used is N, which corresponds to the point size of the text being read. The range of the booklets is from N5 to N48.

Testing low visual acuity

If the vision is less then 6/60 walk the patient metre by metre to the chart (or chart to patient). If less than 1/60, try counting fingers (scores CF), then hand movements (scores HM). If less than this, light perception (PL) is tested with a bright light. If PL is present try all four quadrants and ask the patient to point at which side the light is perceived (accurate projection).

Fig.1.2 Schematic example of LogMAR chart

Assessment of vision: clinical tests in children and tests of binocular status

Behavioural tests for babies/infants

Fixing and following

From 3mths of age a baby should be able to fix and follow a target. Note whether fixation is central, steady, and maintained when the target is moved. The use of different size targets can give an estimation of acuity.

Further information can be gained by observation of behaviour. Do they respond to fine stimuli ('hundreds and thousands test')? Do they object to occlusion of one eye more than the other?

Preferential looking tests

These tests depend on the normal preference to look at the more visually interesting target, i.e. patterned rather than blank.

- **Keeler (Fig. 1.3) and Teller acuity cards** comprise a series of cards each of which have a black and white grating on a grey background of matching luminance. The spatial frequency of the grating (i.e. the thinness of the lines) approximates to different acuity levels. The cards are presented so that the observer has to decide which direction the child has looked before knowing whether this corresponds to the position of the grating, i.e. it is 'forced choice'.
- **Cardiff acuity cards** have 'vanishing optotypes'. These are a series of pictures with increasingly fine outlines that are correspondingly difficult to see. These can either be used as a preferential looking test or as a picture test (if verbal).

Recognition tests for older children

Picture tests

These include Cardiff acuity cards, Kay picture cards (single picture opto-types: optotypes vary in size), and Multiple Picture Test cards (similar but multiple optotypes on each card). The patient then selects the matching optotype on a hand-held card or identifies the object verbally.

Sheridan–Gardiner test

This test has five booklets with single letter optotypes that are pre-sented at a distance of 6m (or if necessary 3m). The patient then selects the matching optotype on a hand-held card. This is useful for children or others unable to use a Snellen or LogMAR chart.

Sonsken–Silver test

This is similar to the Sheridan–Gardiner test but has multiple letter opto-types. Multiple optotype tests are generally only suitable for older children than the equivalent test using single optotypes.

Tests of binocular status (Table 1.3)

Binocular vision may be graded from simultaneous perception, to fusion and finally to steropsis (a '3-dimensional' perception). These can be dem-onstrated on a synoptophore ranging from the simultaneous perception of two images (e.g. bird + cage → bird in a cage), to the fusion of two images (e.g. rabbit with tail + rabbit with flowers → rabbit with tail and flowers) and, finally, to the perception of depth in a fused image (e.g. two disparate images of a bucket → 3-dimensional bucket). Normal disparity perceived is 60s of arc but may be up to 15s.

Table 1.3 Tests of binocular status

Test	Icon	Mechanism	Monocular clues	Disparity
Titmus		Polaroid glasses	Yes	40–3000s of arc
TNO		Red–green glasses	No	15–480s of arc
Lang	☆	Intrinsic cylinder lenses	Yes if not held perpendicular	550–1200s of arc
Frisby		Intrinsic plate thickness	Yes if not held perpendicular	15–600s of arc
Synoptophore		Separate eye-pieces	No	90–720s of arc

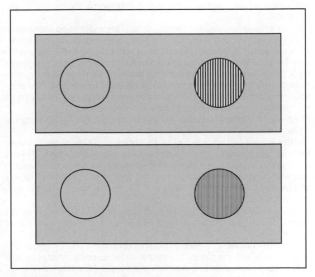

Fig.1.3 Schematic example of Keeler acuity cards.

Assessment of vision: contrast and colour

Contrast sensitivity

While VA charts (e.g. Snellen) test high contrast (black letters on a white background), most daily visual tasks require resolution of low/medium contrast. Contrast sensitivity may be reduced in the presence of normal Snellen acuity. It may be measured by a number of charts, all of which score the minimum contrast detectable for a specified target size. The Vistech chart employs rows of broken circles that decrease in contrast across the row, and diminish in size from row to row. Identification of target orientation is plotted on a template to give a graph of contrast vs spatial frequency. Charts are available for use at 45cm and 3m. Alternative charts maintaining a constant target size include the Pelli–Robson chart (triplets of capital letters, usually read at 1m, read until 2 or 3 mistakes in 1 triplet) (Fig. 1.4), or Cambridge chart (square wave gratings, usually read at 6m, forced choice as to which of 2 luminance matched pages the grating is on).

Colour vision

Red desaturation: compare the perception of 'redness' (e.g. of a red pin) between eyes, occluding one at a time. This can be done for both central vision (reduced in an optic neuropathy) or peripheral field (bitemporally reduced in a chiasmal lesion). An approximate score can be assigned by the patient to the 'washed-out' image in relation to the normal image, e.g. 5/10.

Ishihara pseudo-isochromatic plates: use at 2/3m under good illumination in patients with VA ≥6/18. The first test plate (seen even by achromats with sufficient acuity) is followed by a series of plates testing red–green confusion. Some of the plates differentiate whether the defect is of the protan (red) or deutan (green) system. It does not test the tritan (blue) system. Patients with congenital red–green colour blindness (protanopia, deuteranopia) tend to make predictable mistakes, whereas in acquired disease (optic neuropathy) the mistakes do not follow a specific pattern.

Hardy–Rand–Rittler plates: less commonly used, but has the advantage of testing tritan as well as protan and deutan discrimination.

Holmes Wright lantern: a test of binary choice of two or three coloured spots of light viewed at 6m. Colours are red, green, and white. This is a more practical assessment that aims to predict red–green discrimination in a work situation, e.g. distinguishing red and green lights on a runway. Used in conjunction with Ishihara plates for testing colour vision in military personnel.

Farnsworth-D15 test: a test of confusion giving limited information on the protan, deutan, and tritan systems. It may be used as a screening test of colour vision.

Farnsworth–Munsell 100-Hue test: a time-consuming test of colour discrimination where the patient attempts to order 85 coloured caps by hue. When this is plotted on to a dedicated chart it provides detailed information on protan, deutan, and tritan systems. This test is often used as the final arbiter for colour vision requiring professions.

Fig.1.4 Schematic example of a Pelli–Robson chart.

Biomicroscopy: slit-lamp overview

The slit-lamp (biomicroscope) provides excellent visualization of both the anterior segment and, with the help of additional lenses, the posterior segment of the eye. Advantages of the slit-lamp view are that it is magnified (6–40×) and stereoscopic. Although basic slit-lamp skills are quickly gained, mastering its finer points enables one to use it to its full potential. Careful preparation of the slit-lamp and patient is essential to optimize both quality of view and patient/clinician comfort.

Optical and mechanical features

The slit-lamp consists of a binocular compound microscope and an adjustable illumination system. As it has a fixed focal plane, objects are brought into focus by moving the slit-lamp forward or back. Movement of the slit-lamp laterally (adjusted with the joystick) and vertically (a dial often attached to the joystick) permits visualization of each eye without having to adjust patient position.

Magnification

Fig.1.5 Eye-pieces.

Most conventional slit-lamps have two objective settings (1× and 1.6×) and two eye-piece options (10× and 16×). The total magnification thus ranges from 10× to 25×).

Others have a series of Galilean telescopes that can be dialled into position to give magnifications ranging from 6.3× to 40×. Less commonly a zoom system is used.

Illumination: filters

Fig.1.6 Illumination filters.

The illumination can be adjusted by a series of filters. Options are unfiltered, heat-absorbing filter, 10% grey filter, red-free filter, and cobalt blue filter (commonly from left to right). In practice the heat-absorbing filter is generally used for high illumination and the grey filter for lower illumination. The red-free and cobalt blue filters are used in specific situations. The red-free filter increases visualization of the vitreous and retinal nerve fibre layer/vasculature. The cobalt blue filter is mainly used to visualize fluorescein but also assists detection of iron lines.

The beam height and width are adjusted by apertures; the beam height is recorded (in mm) and may be useful in measurement (e.g. disc size, corneal ulcer, etc.).

Illumination: orientation and angulation

Fig.1.7 Illumination arm.

The orientation of the beam may be adjusted from vertical to horizontal (or any other angle) by swinging the superior aspect of the illumination arm to left or right (useful for gonioscopy or in measuring lesions). Angulation of the beam is achieved by swinging the whole illumination arm to the side (horizontal) or tilting the illumination arm upward (vertical). The alternative techniques of direct illumination, retroillumination, scleral scatter, specular reflection (see Additional techniques for anterior segment examination 📖 p.17) require different angulations of the illumination arm and some require the illumination arm to be 'unlocked' to displace the beam from the centre of the field of view. Tilting the beam vertically may reduce troublesome reflections when using hand-held lenses.

Illumination: mirrors

Fig.1.8 Mirror.

In certain situations, such as when using small angulations (3–10°), the standard long mirror may partially obscure the view. If this is troublesome it can be replaced by the short mirror.

Fixation lamp
Many slit-lamps have a fixation target, either a standard fixation lamp or an annular target with a focusing range of −15 to +10. This is adjusted to the patient's refractive error enabling them to see the target clearly.

Stereovariator
Some slit-lamps have a stereovariator, which changes the angle of convergence from 13° to 4.5°. The conventional 13° provides better stereopsis but the 4.5° provides a larger binocular field of view and thus improved acuity (binocular acuity > monocular acuity). This means that the 4.5° setting may be advantageous for detailed examination of certain ocular surfaces (e.g. corneal endothelium).

Biomicroscopy: use of the slit-lamp

Box 1.3 Outline of slit-lamp examination

Set-up
- Adjust patient chair, slit-lamp, and your chair so that you can both be comfortable during the examination.
- Adjust chin rest until patient's eyes are at level of marker (on the side of the head rest).
- Adjust the eye-pieces: (1) dial in your refraction: use the nearer scale for the 10× eye-pieces and the further scale for the 16× eye-pieces); (2) fine-tune eye-pieces: focus each eye in turn on a focusing rod placed in the central column (requires removal of the tonometer plate); this may be more 'minus' than expected due to induced accommodation.
- Adjust the interpupillary distance.

Examination
- Start examination with lowest magnification (1× setting and 10× eye-pieces) and low illumination. Rather than inadvertently dazzling your patient first test brightness, e.g. on your hand.
- Start examination with direct illumination (usually fairly thin beam, angled 30–60°).
- Examine in a methodical manner from 'outside-in' i.e. orbit/adnexae, lids, anterior segment (see Anterior segment examination 📖 p.16), posterior segment (see Posterior segment examination 📖 p.22).
- Throughout examination: (1) Adjust illumination: adjust filter, orientation and angulation and illumination technique (direct illumination, retroillumination, scleral scatter, specular reflection) to optimize visualization; (2) Adjust magnification: to optimize visualization (e.g. of cells in the AC).
- At the end of the examination do not leave your patient stranded on the slit-lamp. Switch the slit-lamp off (for the sake of the patient and the bulb) and encourage the patient to sit back.

Additional techniques
- **Tonometry**: Goldmann tonometer used with fluorescein and blue light.
- **Gonioscopy and indirect fundoscopy**: performed with appropriate hand-held lenses.

1	Indicator for beam height	9	Head band
2	Lever for selecting filters	10	Height marker (patient eye level)
3	Control for beam height	11	Lever for selecting magnification
4	Mirror	12	Chin rest
5	Control for chin rest height	13	Tonometer plate
6	Centring screw	14	Control for beam width
7	5° stops	15	Joystick
8	Latch for vertically tilting beam		

Fig 1.9 Slit-lamp with key features identified.

Anterior segment examination (1)

Table 1.4 An approach to examining the anterior segment

Observe	Habitus, face, orbits
Examine **lashes**	Loss, colour, position, crusting
Examine **lid margins**	Position, contour, skin folds, defects, inflammation, lumps
Examine **palbebral conjunctiva** • Explain then gently evert the lids	Papillae, follicles, exudate, membrane, pseudomembrane
Examine **fornices**	Loss of fornices, symblepharon, Ankyloblepharon
Examine bulbar **conjunctiva/episclera**	Hyperaemia, haemorrhage, lumps, degenerations, FBs/deposits
Examine **sclera**	Hyperaemia, thinning, perforation
Examine **cornea** • Use diffuse/direct illumination/scleral scatter/specular reflection as required	Diameter, thickness, shape; pre-corneal tear film, epithelium, Bowman's layer, stroma, Descemet's membrane, endothelium;
Examine **anterior chamber**	Grade flare/cells/depth; fibrin, pigment, level
Examine **iris** • Use direct/retroillumination	Colour, structure, movement, transillumination defects,
Examine lens • Use direct/retroillumination	Opacity (pattern and maturity), size, shape, position, stability, capsule (anterior and posterior)
Examine **anterior vitreous**	Cells, flare, lens-vitreous interface, degenerations
Stain cornea • Use fluorescein ± Rose Bengal[1] Check corneal sensation • Use topical anaesthetic Perform applanation **tonometry**	Tear film break-up time (BUT), Seidel's test

Consider: gonioscopy, pachymetry, Schirmer's test;

1. Rose Bengal availability has decreased in recent years. Lissamine green is an alternative.

Additional techniques for anterior segment examination

Illumination techniques

Although **direct illumination** is most commonly used, additional pathology may be revealed by the following techniques:

- **Scleral scatter**: unlock the light source so that the slit beam can be displaced laterally to fall on the limbus while the microscope remains focused on the central cornea. Total internal reflection results in a generalized glow around the limbus and the highlighting of subtle opacities within the cornea, e.g. early oedema, deposits, etc.
- **Retroillumination**: direct the light source at a relatively posterior reflecting surface (e.g. iris or retina) and focus on the structure of interest (e.g. cornea, or iris and lens). View undilated for iris transillumination defects, dilated for lens opacities.
- **Specular reflection**: focus on the area of interest and change the angle of illumination to highlight discontinuities in an otherwise smooth reflecting surface, e.g. examining the endothelium for guttata.

Tear film break-up time (BUT)

Place a drop of fluorescein into the lower fornix. Ask the patient to blink once, and then not to blink (or hold lids open if necessary). Observe with blue light time taken until the tear film breaks up. A result less than 10s is abnormal.

Seidel's test

Place a drop of 2% fluorescein over the area of concern and observe with the cobalt blue light. The test is positive if there is a luminous green flow of aqueous. This results from local dilution of the stain by aqueous leaking from a surgical wound, penetrating injury, or bleb.

Schirmer's test

Whatman test paper is folded 5mm from the end, and inserted in the temporal fornix of both lower lids. After 5min the strips are removed and the length wetted is measured. This result is an indication of basic and reflex tearing. It is normal if >10mm, borderline 5–10mm, and abnormal if <5mm. Repeating the test after the addition of a topical anaesthetic gives an indication of basic secretion alone.

Applanation tonometry

Place a drop of combination of local anaesthetic and fluorescein into the lower fornix. Rotate the tonometer dial and record the pressure at which the inner aspect of the two luminous green circles just touch. Usually the white line on the prism is aligned with the horizontal meridian; however, in high astigmatism the red line should be aligned with the minor axis. This is also affected by corneal thickness 📖 Ocular hypotension p.306.

Tonometer checks and calibration: Goldmann tonometers may be checked by using the metal bar and control weight supplied. With the weight exactly midway along the bar (central stop) the tonometer should read 0mmHg. The next two stops correspond to 20 and 60mmHg respectively. Significant deviation from this indicates a need for formal recalibration by the supplier.

Anterior segment examination (2)

Anterior chamber depth measurement

Peripheral AC depth can be estimated using the Van Herick method: set the slit beam at 60° and directed just anterior to the limbus. If the AC depth is less than one-quarter of the corneal thickness, the angle is narrow and should be assessed on gonioscopy. A more central AC depth can be measured with a pachymeter. Alternatively, use a horizontal beam set at 60° to the viewing arm, and measure the length of beam at which the image on the cornea just abuts the image on the iris. Multiply this by 1.4 to get the depth in mm.

Anterior chamber activity

In the presence of AC inflammation grade both the flare (visible as haze illuminated by the slit-lamp beam) and cells (seen as particles slowly moving through the beam). This is important both in detecting intraocular inflammation and in monitoring the response to treatment.

Table 1.5 Grading of anterior chamber flare

Grade	Description
0	None
1+	Faint
2+	Moderate (iris + lens clear)
3+	Marked (iris + lens hazy)
4+	Intense (fibrin or plastic aqueous)

SUN 2005 *Am J Ophthalmol* 2005; **140**: 509

Table 1.6 Grading of anterior chamber cells (counted with 1 × 1mm slit)

Activity	Cells
0	<1
0.5+	1–5
1+	6–15
2+	16–25
3+	26–50
4+	>50

SUN 2005 *Am J Ophthalmol* 2005; **140**: 509

Gonioscopy

Use an indirect (Goldmann, Zeiss) or direct (Koeppe) goniolens to assess the iridocorneal angle, including the iris insertion, the iris curvature and the angle approach. If angle is closed, indent (with a Zeiss lens) to see if it can be opened ('appositional closure') or is zipped shut ('synechial closure'). Describe according to Shaffer or Spaeth and record which classification used, or a limited key (e.g. '4 = wide open' if using Shaffer).

Shaffer classification (see also ☐ Fig. 1.10)

Table 1.7 Shaffer classification

Shaffer grade	Grade 4	Grade 3	Grade 2	Grade 1	Grade 0
Angular approach	40°	30°	20°	10°	0
Most posterior structure clearly visualized	Ciliary body	Scleral spur	Trabeculum	Schwalbe's line	Cornea
Risk of closure	Closure not possible	Closure not possible	Closure possible	Closure probable	Closed
Summary	Wide open	Moderately open	Moderately open	Very narrow	Closed

Spaeth classification

Categorize according to iris insertion, angular approach, and iris curvature, e.g. D40R

Box 1.4 Spaeth classification

Iris insertion	A	B	C	D	E
	Above Schwalbe's line	Below Schwalbe's line	Below scleral spur	Deep	Extremely deep
Angular approach	°				
	Estimate in degrees °				
Iris curvature	R	S		Q	
	Regular convex	Steep convex		Queer, i.e. concave	

Fig. 1.10 Anterior chamber angle with gonioscopic views. See Table 1.7 (Shaffer classification) for details.

| Shaffer grade: | Grade 4 | Grade 3 | Grade 2 | Grade 1 | Grade 0 |
| Most posterior structure seen: | Ciliary body | Scleral spur | Trabeculum | Schwalbe's line | Cornea |

Ciliary body
Scleral spur
Trabeculum
Schwalbe's line

Posterior segment examination (1)

Table 1.8 An approach to examining the posterior segment

Pre-dilation perform RAPD, consider:	Amsler testing
Observe	Habitus, face, orbits
Examine **iris**	Adequate dilation, aniridia, albinism
Examine **lens**	Clarity, position, a/pseudophakia
Examine **vitreous**	Cells, flare, pigment, haemorrhage,
● *Use conventional/red-free illumination*	opacities, PVD, optical emptiness
Examine **disc**	Size, vertical cup:disc ratio, colour, flat/elevated/tilted, neuroretinal rim (inc contour, notches, haemorrhages), pits/colobomata
Examine **disc margin**	Oedema, capillaries, drusen
Examine **disc vessels**	Baring, bayonetting, anomalous vasculature, presence of spontaneous venous pulsation
Examine **peripapillary area** ● *Use conventional/red free illumination*	Haemorrhages, atrophy, pigmentation, retinal nerve fibre layer defects
Examine **macula**	Position, flat/elevated, fluid/haemorrhage/exudate, drusen/atrophy/gliosis, angioid streaks/lacquer cracks, retinal striae/choroidal folds, cherry-red spot
Examine *retinal vessels*	Attenuation/dilation, tortuosity, sheathing, emboli, IRMA/neovascularization/telangiectasia/shunt vessels
Examine **peripheral fundus**	Degenerations/breaks/retinal detachments/dialysis/retinoschisis fluid/haemorrhage/exudate pigmentary retinopathy, chorioretinal scars, tumours, laser/cryotherapy/buckles

At the **slit-lamp** consider: choice of lens, Watzke–Allen test

With the **indirect ophthalmoscope** consider choice of lens, scleral indentation

Instruments used in posterior segment examination

Slit-lamp

Most ophthalmologists examining the posterior segment use the slit-lamp with a hand-held lens (e.g. 90D or equivalent).

- **Optical features**: the choice of lens balances the advantages of greater magnification (e.g. 66D lens) against a wider field of view (e.g. 90D lens). Some (e.g. superfield/super66) attempt to combine both these qualities. Contact lenses provide the highest clarity and may be useful in assessing detail (e.g. area centralis for macular pathology) or where the view is poor (e.g. media opacities). The retinal view using these lenses is inverted. Three-mirror contact lens (e.g. Goldmann) facilitate examination of the periphery; the views are mirror image rather than fully inverted.
- **Method**: ideally the patient is dilated; the fundal view obtained without dilation is usually limited both in extent and in stereropsis. Adjust the slit-lamp so that it is coaxial and focused on the centre of the cornea. Interpose the lens 1cm in front of the eye and draw the slit-lamp back until a clear fundal view is obtained. To view the peripheral retina ask the patient to look in the direction of the area you wish to examine (i.e. down to view inferior retina). Troublesome reflections can be reduced by moving the illumination beam slightly off axis.

Indirect ophthalmoscope and scleral indentor

The indirect ophthalmoscope (assisted by scleral indentation) is the instrument of choice for examination of the peripheral fundus.

- **Optical features**: the choice of lens depends on the need for greater magnification (e.g. 3-fold with 20D lens but smaller field of view) vs wider field of view (e.g. larger field of view with 28D lens but only 2-fold magnification). The retinal view is inverted.
- **Method**: ensure patient is well-dilated, positioned flat and looking straight up at the ceiling. Have lens, indenter, and retinal chart/paper (for recording findings) available. Align eye-pieces and illumination by viewing your outstretched thumb. Ensure that the headband is sufficiently tight that the ophthalmoscope will remain secure as you move around. Illumination brightness is adjusted according to quality of view and patient comfort.

  View from above, with the ophthalmoscope directed downwards towards the pupil and with the lens held directly in the line of illumination. Resting this hand lightly against the patient's face helps steady the lens at an appropriate focal distance for a clear fundal view. To view the peripheral retina change the angulation by asking the patient to look in the direction of the area to be examined (i.e. down to view inferior retina) while angling your head and lens in the opposite direction.
- **Scleral indentation**: to view, for example, the inferior ora: ask the patient to look straight up and place the indenter on the outside of the lower lid, resting tangentially against the area to be indented; then ask the patient to look straight down, moving the indenter with the globe. Observe the area of interest, while gently exerting pressure over it. Continue for 360°. Warn the patient that the procedure may be uncomfortable.

Posterior segment examination (2)

Instruments used in posterior segment examination (cont.)

Direct ophthalmoscope

For those who see ophthalmic patients in the community this may be the only option available for fundal examination. Ophthalmologists may also choose to use it where access to a slit-lamp is not possible (e.g. on ITU).

- **Optical features**: there is high magnification (15×) but only a small field of view. The retinal view is not inverted.
- **Method**: optimize your view with adequate dilation, dimmed room, and a fully charged ophthalmoscope. The field of view should be maximized by coming very near to the eye. Optimal view of the optic disc is achieved by approaching from 15 to 20° temporally while on the same horizontal level as the patient.

Additional examination techniques for posterior segment examination

Amsler grid (Table 1.9)

View at 1/3m. Ask the patient to fixate one eye at a time on the central dot, and comment on whether any of the small squares are missing or distorted. There are seven charts of which chart 1 is suitable for most patients. It consists of a 20 × 20 grid of 5mm squares each representing 1° of central field (if viewed at 1/3m).

Table 1.9 Amsler charts

Chart	Design	Colour	Use
1	Standard grid	White on black	Most patients
2	Standard grid with diagonals	White on black	Helps fixation
3	Standard grid	Red on black	Tests colour scotoma, e.g. optic neuropathy, toxicity of chloroquines
4	Random dots	White on black	Tests scotoma only (no lines to become distorted)
5	Horizontal lines	White on black	Tests in one meridian (standard horizontal lines)
6	Horizontal lines	Black on white	Tests in one meridian (standard/fine horizontal lines)
7	Standard/fine central grid	White on black	High sensitivity for central lesions

Watzke–Allen test

While using the slit-lamp and hand-held lens to view the macula, project a thin strip of light across the fovea. Ask the patient whether the line they see is broken, narrowed, or complete. A clear gap (Watzke–Allen positive) suggests a full-thickness macular defect/hole.

Goldmann 3-mirror lens

This contact lens is used with the slit-lamp to examine the central and peripheral fundus. Note that this is a mirror image rather than a rotated image of the peripheral fundus (cf. standard indirect ophthalmoscopy). It comprises four parts: central (view central 30°); equatorial mirror (largest; views 30° to equator); peripheral mirror (intermediate; views equator to ora); and gonioscopic mirror (smallest; views ora, pars plana, and angle).

Retinal charts (Table 1.10)

One standardized representation of vitreo-retinal pathology uses the following code:

Table 1.10 Retinal chart key

Structure	Colour
Detached retina	Blue
Flat retina	Red
Retinal veins	Blue
Retinal breaks	Red within a blue outline
Retinal thinning	Red hatching within a blue outline
Lattice degeneration	Blue hatching within a blue outline
Pigment	Black
Exudate	Yellow
Vitreous opacities	Green

Table 1.11 Optical properties of commonly used lenses

Lens	Field of view	Magnification of image	Magnification of laser spot
With indirect ophthalmoscope			
20D	46°/60°	3.1	0.3
28D	53°/69°	2.3	0.4
Non-contact lens with slit-lamp			
60D	81°	1.2	0.9
Super 66	96°	1.0	1.0
78D	73°/97°	0.9	1.1
90D	69°/89°	0.8	1.3
Superfield NC	116°	0.8	1.3
Super VitreoFundus	124°	0.6	1.8
Contact lens with slit-lamp			
Area centralis	84°	1.1	0.9
3Mirror		0.9	1.1
Transequator	132°	0.7	1.4
QuadrAspheric	144°	0.5	2.0

When using lenses with the slit-lamp the overall magnification seen = lens magnification (listed above) × slit-lamp magnification (varies from 10 to 25x).

Pupils examination

Clinical examination

Box 1.5 An approach to examining the pupils

Observe   Check lids, iris colour
- Ask patient to look at a distant target

Measure pupil diameters in ambient **bright** light

Measure pupil diameters in ambient **dim** light

Check **direct** and **consensual** pupillary response for each side

Check for **RAPD**
- Ask patient to look at a near target   Check near response

For an approach to diagnosing anisocoria, see Anisocoria 🕮 p.662.

Anatomy and physiology

Parasympathetic pathway (light response)

IIn → **Pretectal** → **E-W** → IIIn → **ciliary** → short → CONSTRICT
      nucleus   **nuclei**   (inf)   **ganglion**   ciliary n
                (bilateral)

Known synapses are marked in **bold**.

Parasympathetic pathway (near response)

VACx → FEF → III/E-W → ciliary → short   →   CONSTRICT
(area 19)   nuclei   ganglion   ciliary n   ACCOMMODATE
                ↓
                → medial rectus   →   CONVERGE

- **Light–near dissociation**: this is where dorsal midbrain pathology selectively reduces the response to light while preserving the response to near. This is thought to be due to the fact that the near pathway is placed ventral to the more dorsal pretectal nucleus serving the light pathway.

Sympathetic pathway

Posterior hypothalamus   Long ciliary n   → DILATE
      ↓   ↑
      ↓   Va(nasociliary branch)
      ↓   ↑
      ↓   Internal carotid artery
      ↓   ↑
T1 (ciliospinal   → white rami   → **superior cervical**
centre of Budge)   communicantes   **ganglion**

Pharmacological testing

The diagnosis of anisocoria (see Anisocoria, 📖 p.620) may in some cases be assisted by pharmacological testing. These tests depend on comparing the response of the abnormal and the normal pupils; therefore, the agent should be instilled in both eyes and the response measured.

Diagnostic agents for an abnormally large pupil (e.g. for diagnosing Adie's pupil)

Pharmacology

Pilocarpine is a direct muscarinic agonist. A normal pupil will constrict in response to 1% pilocarpine. A response to 0.125% indicates denervation hypersensitivity as occurs in an Adie's pupil.

Method

Administer a drop of 0.125% pilocarpine to both eyes. At 0 and 30min measure pupil size when fixing on a distant target in identical dim lighting conditions. In Adie's the affected eye shows a significantly greater response.

Diagnostic agents for an abnormally small pupil (e.g. for diagnosing Horner pupil)

Pharmacology

- **Cocaine** inhibits NorA reuptake at the neuromuscular junction of the dilator pupillae so increasing sympathetic tone. In the presence of a normal sympathetic pathway cocaine results in dilation. In Horner syndrome the abnormal pupil does not dilate.
- **Hydroxyamphetamine** stimulates the release of preformed NorA. In a 1st or 2nd order Horner the post-ganglionic neurone is intact and thus the pupil will dilate in response to hydroxyamphetamine. In a 3rd order Horner the pupil will not dilate.

Method

- **Diagnose Horner pupil:** administer 4% cocaine to both eyes. Repeat at 1min. At 0 and 60min measure pupil sizes when fixing on a distant target in identical ambient (bright and dim) lighting conditions. The test is positive for Horner if there is no/poor dilation to cocaine.
- **Identify level:** this is primarily a research tool. Administer 1% hydroxyamphetamine to both eyes. Measure pupil sizes to distinguish between a 1st or 2nd order neuron lesion (normal dilation) and a 3rd order neuron lesion (no/poor dilation). This test is not reliable if performed within 48h of a cocaine test.

Ocular motility examination (1)

Table 1.12 An approach to examining ocular motility

Note VA	
Observe head posture	Face turn, head tilt, chin up/down
Hirschberg test	Manifest deviation
Cover/uncover + alternate cover test • with/without glasses targets: near (1/3m), distance (6m), non-accommodative	Manifest or latent deviation
Examine **versions** into 9 positions of gaze • Ask patient to follow target (usually a pentorch) • Perform cover test in each position • Ask patient to report any diplopia in primary position or during test	Any abnormality: under/overaction Paresis/restriction alphabet patterns Lid/head movements
Examine horizontal and vertical **saccades** • Ask patient to look rapidly between targets positioned at 30° on either side of the midline	Normal/slow Hypo/hypermetric
Examine **convergence** • Assess to both an accommodative and non-accommodative target	Normal/reduced
Examine horizontal/vertical **doll's eye movements**	Normal/absent
Examine horizontal/vertical **OKN** • Slowly rotate an OKN drum in horizontal and vertical direction	Normal/absent/Convergence retraction nystagmus
Consider: prism cover test, Krimsky test, caloric tests	

General approach

Once a deviation has been detected try to identify it as:
- Manifest or latent.
- Concomitant (constant in all positions of gaze 📖 p.658) or incomitant (varying 📖 p.662).

For incomitant deviations identify:
- Direction of maximum separation.
- Pattern typical of neurogenic 📖 p.612-617, mechanical 📖 p.622 or other (supranuclear 📖 p.608, myaesthenic 📖 p.634, myopathic 📖 p.638 etc.) pathology.

It is common practice to use a pen-torch as a target when examining versions and vergences as the positions of the eyes are highlighted by the corneal reflexes and it is a non-accommodative target. However, try to ensure that the pen-torch is not too bright since dazzling the patient is counter-productive.

Corneal reflection tests

Hirschberg test

To detect/estimate the size of a manifest deviation. Ask the patient to fix on a pen-torch at 1/3m, and note the corneal reflections. The normal position is just nasal to the centre of the cornea. Every 1mm deviation represents 7° or 15Δ. If the reflection is deflected nasally the eye is divergent (i.e. exotropic); if deflected temporally the eye is convergent (i.e. esotropic).

Krimsky test

In the Krimsky test this deviation is measured by placing a prism bar in front of the deviating eye and finding the prism strength at which the corneal reflexes are symmetrical. The prism should be orientated to 'point' in the direction of deviation, i.e. base-out for an esotropia, base-in for an exotropia.

Cover tests

Cover–uncover test

The cover test reveals a manifest deviation. Ask the patient to fix on a target (near, distance, non-accommodative, and sometimes far-distance). Occlude each eye in turn (starting with the fixing eye), and observe any movement of the uncovered eye. For example, inward movement indicates that the eye was previously divergent (i.e. exotropic) and downward movement that it was previously elevated (i.e. hypertropic).

The uncover test may reveal a latent deviation. Occlude the first eye again for a few seconds. Look for any movement of the covered eye as the occluder is removed. Repeat for the other eye. For example, inward movement indicates that the occluded eye has drifted out (i.e. exophoric).

Perform the cover test in the nine positions of gaze to (1) identify the direction of maximum separation (indicates the direction of paretic muscle's action/maximum restriction), and (2) compare ductions and versions.

Ocular motility examination (2)

Cover tests (continued)

Alternate cover test

This detects the total deviation (latent + manifest) by causing dissociation of binocular single vision (BSV). Ask the patient to fix on a target (near/distance/non-accommodative). Repeatedly cover each eye in turn for 2–3s, so that one eye is always covered. Note the direction and amplitude of any deviation elicited. Once BSV is broken down, remove the occluder and note the speed of recovery of each eye in turn. Also look for dissociated vertical deviation (DVD) and manifest latent nystagmus (MLN), which are common in infantile esotropia.

Prism cover test

This measures the angle of deviation. Repeat the alternate cover test but with a prism bar placed in front of one eye, adjusting the prism strength until first neutralization and then reversal of the corrective movement occurs. The prism should be orientated to 'point' in the direction of deviation, i.e. base-out for an esotropia.

Maddox tests

In these dissociative tests different images are presented to each eye. They are generally used for assessing symptomatic phorias: whether for distance (Maddox rod), for near (Maddox wing), or torsional (two Maddox rods).

Maddox rod

For distance a single Maddox rod (series of red cylinders) is placed horizontally in front of the right eye and the patient (with distance correction) fixates on a distant spot of white light. The patient will see a vertical red line and a white spot. If there is no phoria the line will pass straight through the spot. If the image is crossed (i.e. the line is to the left of the light) there is an exophoria; if the line is to the right there is an esophoria. The phoria is then quantified by finding the prism required to neutralize it. The Maddox rod is then orientated vertically and the procedure repeated to identify any vertical phoria. If the line appears below the light there is a right hyperphoria; if below there is a left hyperphoria. This is again quantified by neutralizing with prisms.

Maddox wing

For near a Maddox wing is used. The patient (wearing their usual reading correction) looks through the apertures to view a vertical and horizontal arrow (with the right eye) and corresponding vertical and horizontal scales (with the left eye). The numbers indicated by the arrows (as seen by the patient) indicates the direction and size of the near phoria.

Two Maddox rod test

For torsion a horizontally orientated Maddox rod is placed in front of each eye (one red, one white). The colour of the tilted line is identified by the patient. The corresponding Maddox rod is rotated until the patient reports that it is vertical. The rotation required indicates the size of torsion. The two lines will fuse if there is no residual non-torsional deviation.

Parks–Bielschewsky 3-step test (Box 1.6, Table 1.13)

This is used to identify a single underacting muscle in vertical/torsional deviations. It is particularly useful in superior oblique palsies.

1. Perform cover test in primary position: identify higher eye.
2. Perform cover test with gaze to right then left: identify where separation (and diplopia) is greatest.
   This stage is based on the eye-position where greatest vertical action occurs: for the obliques this is when the eye is adducted vs for the vertical recti this is when the eye is abducted.
3. Perform cover test with head tilt to right then left shoulder: identify where separation (and diplopia) is greatest.
   This stage is based on the fact that the superior muscles intort the eyes, whereas the inferior muscles extort.

Box 1.6 Parks–Bielschowksy 3-step test: example of right SO underaction

Step 1
Right eye is the higher eye
in the primary position

Step 2
Disparity is greatest
on gaze to the left

Step 3
Disparity is greatest
on head tilt to the right

Table 1.13 Theoretical manifestations of single muscle underactions

Step 1	Step 2	Step 3	Conclusions
Higher eye	Worst with gaze to	Worst with head tilt to	Underaction
RE	Right	Left	RIR
		Right	LIO
	Left	Left	LSR
		Right	RSO
LE	Right	Left	LSO
		Right	RSR
	Left	Left	RIO
		Right	LIR

Caloric tests

This tests the vestibular/nuclear/infranuclear pathways, and can be useful in patients with decreased consciousness. Ideally, position the patient with the head inclined backwards at 60°. Water placed in either ear, causes nystagmus with fast-phase as follows: Cold–Opposite, Warm–Same (COWS).

Visual fields examination

Table 1.14 An approach to examining visual fields

Note VA	Adjust target size if necessary
Observe	Features of stroke, acromegaly, etc.
• *Patient with both eyes open and looking at the bridge of your nose.* Ask if any part of your face appears to be missing.	Gross homonymous defects
• *Patient with non-testing eye occluded.* *Check they can see the white pin.* Map out right/left **visual field with the white pin** (coming from unseen to seen, asking the patient to identify when they first see the pin).	Peripheral defects
• **Repeat with the red pin** to map right/left central 30° (asking the patient to identify when the pin appears red).	Central defects
• Use red pin to map out right/left **physiological blind spots**	Enlarged/part of centrocaecal scotoma

Any visual field abnormality should be confirmed on formal perimetry, see 📖 p.48–57.

Consider:

• simultaneous presentation of gross targets to elicit inattention (this may occur in the context of stroke syndromes);
• simultaneous presentation of red targets across vertical and horizontal midlines (e.g. present across the vertical midline to elicit the temporal depression of red perception of early chiasmal disease—ask patient to report any difference in red colour between targets).

Additional clinical examinations may include pupils, discs, ocular motility, cranial nerves, peripheral nervous system

Lids/ptosis examination

Table 1.15 An approach to examining the lids

Shake hands	Check for myotonia (note slow release of grip)
Observe Measure **palpebral aperture**	Face, brow, globes, pupils
Measure **upper margin reflex distance**	
Measure **position of upper lid crease**	
Measure **levator function** • *Inhibit frontalis by placing a thumb on the brow*	
Measure any **lagophthalmos** • *Ask patient to close eyes, gently at first and then to squeeze eyes shut*	
Assess **orbicularis function** and **Bell's phenomenon** • *Try to open patient's eyes against resistance*	
Assess **fatiguability** over 1 min • *Ask patient to keep looking upward at a target held superiorly*	Any worsening of ptosis
Examine for **Cogan's twitch** • *Ask patient to look rapidly from downgaze to a target held in primary position*	Any overshoot
Assess for **jaw-winking** • *Ask patient to simulate chewing and to move jaw from side to side*	Any change in ptosis
Check **corneal sensation**	Implications for surgery
Examine **ocular motility**	Motility abnormality, change in ptosis
Examine **pupils**	Anisocoria, hypochromia
Consider: examination of fundus, systemic review (myopathy, fatiguability)	

Special tests

Fatiguability

The ability to sustain lid elevation is assessed in upgaze. Hold a target superiorly and ask the patient to maintain fixation on it for a minute. Note if either lid drifts down over that time, and reassess palpebral aperture in the primary position at the end of this period. If fatiguability is demonstrated examine for associated fatiguability of ocular motility and general musculature. This is usually a sign of myasthenia.

Cogan's twitch

Cogan's twitch is an overshoot of the eyelid which occurs on rapid elevation of the eyes from downgaze to the primary position. Ask the patient to look down and then to look at a target held directly in front of them. Cogan's twitch may be seen in myasthenia.

Jaw-winking

Synkinesis ('miswiring') may result in a ptosis that varies with use of other facial muscles (pterygoids). This may be seen as jaw-winking where the lid can be elevated by movement of the jaw (e.g. chewing, side to side movement of the jaw) (📖 p.144).

Normal lid measurements

Table 1.16 Normal lid measurements

Palpebral aperture	8–11mm (female>male)
Upper margin reflex distance	4–5mm
Upper lid excursion (levator function)	13–16mm
Upper lid crease position	8–10mm from margin (female>male)

Orbital examination

Table 1.17 An approach to examining the orbit

Vision	VA, colour
Observe	Behaviour, habitus, face, lids
Observe from above	Globe position
Palpate orbital margins	Notches, instability, soft tissue signs
Palpate globe (gentle **retropulsion**)	Pulsation, resistance, pain
Check **infraorbital sensation**	Hyposthesia
Perform **exophthalmometry** • Document which model used (e.g. Hertel, Rodenstock)	Globe position
If proptosis assess whether axial or non-axial • Use two clear rulers, one horizontally over the bridge of the nose and one vertically to detect whether axial or non-axial	
Auscultate the globe/temporal region	Bruit
Assess any effect of the **Valsalva** manoeuvre • Use stethoscope bell	Increased proptosis
Check **corneal sensation**	Hyposthesia
Proceed to **full ophthalmic examination**, including:	
Pupils	RAPD, anisocoria
Visual fields	
Ocular motility (± forced duction test)	Restriction, paresis
Cranial nerves	
Conjunctiva	Chemosis, injection
Cornea/sclera	Vessels, integrity
Tonometry	Change in upgaze, wide pulse pressure
Optic disc	Oedema, pallor, abnormal vessels
Fundus	Choroidal folds
Consider: refraction, neurological, and general systemic examination as indicated.	

Special tests

Exophthalmometry

Using the Hertel exophthalmometer, place it level with the orbits and adjust the separation so that the foot plates rest on the lateral orbital rims at the level of the lateral canthi. Close your right eye and ask the patient to fix on your open (left) eye, while you align the parallax markers (usually red) and read off where the patient's right corneal apex appears on the scale. Repeat with your right eye and the patient's left eye. Measurements >20mm or a difference of >2mm between globes is suggestive of proptosis. Beware of patient variables (racial differences, lateral orbitotomy), instrument variability (try to use the same exophthalmometer each time), and operator inconsistency.

Two-ruler test

Horizontal and vertical displacement of the globe may be demonstrated by using two clear plastic rulers. One is placed horizontally over the bridge of the nose at the level of the lateral canthi. Look for horizontal displacement by comparing the distance from the centre of the nasal bridge with equivalent points on the globe (e.g. nasal limbus). Look for vertical displacement by measuring vertically (second ruler) to compare the distance from the horizontal meridian (i.e. the first ruler) with equivalent points on the globe (e.g. the inferior limbus).

Nasolacrimal system examination

Table 1.18 An approach to examining the nasolacrimal system

Observe face	Asymmetry, scars, nasal bridge
Observe/palpate **lacrimal sac**	Mass, inflammation
• Check for regurgitation from canaliculi on pressing sac	
Observe **lids**	Contour, position, chronic lid disease
• Assess with eyes open and closed	
Assess **lid laxity**	
• Draw lid laterally, medially, and anteriorly	
Examine **puncta**	Position, calibre, discharge
• Assess with eyes open and closed	
Examine **conjunctiva/cornea**	Inflammation
Measure **tear meniscus**	
• Instil 2% fluorescein in lower fornix	
Assess **dye disappearance**	
Check **dye recovery** from nose	
• Use nasendoscope or cotton bud	
Cannulate and **probe** puncta/canaliculi	Patency of puncta, hard or soft stop
• Use lacrimal cannula attached to a syringe of saline (+ fluorescein)	
Irrigate with saline to estimate flow/regurgitation	Upper/lower systems
Consider: nasendoscopy, formal Jones testing	

Dye disappearance test

Instil a drop of fluorescein 2% into each lower fornix. Reassess at 2min, by which time (almost) complete clearance should have occurred. Prolonged retention indicates inadequate drainage.

Probing (Table 1.19)

Under topical anaesthesia insert a straight lacrimal cannula into the lower canaliculus, and guide it towards the medial wall of the lacrimal sac while exerting gentle lateral traction on the lower lid. Assess whether there is:
• a hard (abrupt) stop—indicates a patent system as far as the lacrimal sac, or
• a soft (spongy) stop—indicates a canalicular block.

Irrigation (Table 1.19)

Under topical anaesthesia insert a lacrimal cannula into the lower canaliculus, and place a finger against the lacrimal sac. Irrigate with saline and assess: (1) flow (estimate flow (e.g. in %) conducted (i.e. down nose/back of the throat) vs regurgitated—if regurgitated note from which canaliculus; (2) quality of regurgitated fluid—clear or purulent; (3) lacrimal sac distension.

Table 1.19 Interpretation of probing and irrigation tests

Level of block	Probing	Irrigation
Punctum	Cannot cannulate	Not possible
Canaliculus (upper/lower)	Soft stop	Regurgitates through same canaliculus only (high pressure)
Common canaliculus	Soft stop	May regurgitate through either canaliculus
Nasolacrimal duct	Hard stop	Lacrimal sac dilates; may regurgitate (± mucus) through either canaliculus

Jones testing (Table 1.20)

This may be considered in cases of partial obstruction to ascertain the level of block.

- **Primary test:** instil fluorescein 2% into the lower fornix. After 5min assess for dye recovery with a cotton-bud (can be moistened with 4% cocaine) placed at the nasolacrimal duct opening (below the inferior turbinate) or with a nasendoscope; an alternative way of looking for dye recovery is to ask the patient to blow one nostril at a time on to a tissue.
- **Secondary test:** wash out the fluorescein from the lower fornix. Under topical anaesthesia insert a lacrimal cannula into the lower canaliculus and irrigate. Assess dye recovery from the nose as before.

Table 1.20 Interpretation of Jones test

	Result	Interpretation
Primary test		
Dye recovered	Positive	Normal patency
Dye not recovered	Negative	Partial obstruction or lacrimal pump failure
Secondary test		
Dye recovered	Positive	Partial obstruction of nasolacrimal duct
Dye not recovered	Negative	Partial obstruction above the lacrimal sac

Refraction: outline

History

Box 1.7 **Essential history**

Age; profession; driver; special requirements; VDU use
Visual symptoms
Past ophthalmic history
Family ophthalmic history
Past medical history
Drugs/allergies
Previous spectacle/CL use

Examination

Box 1.8 **Preparation**

Focimetry on current spectacles 📖 p.44   ROOM LIGHTS ON

VA—unaided + with PH
Cover/uncover test

Measure IPD (distance) → set up trial frame

Box 1.9 **Retinoscopy**

ROOM LIGHTS OFF
Ask patient to look at a non-accommodative target (e.g. green duochrome).
Correct for working distance (e.g. if you work at 2/3m put in +1.5D DS).
Fog fellow eye with a high PLUS DS lens to prevent accommodation.

Check retinoscopy reflex
• Identify axis of astigmatism
• Neutralize reflex in one meridian with DS lenses
• If reflex is 'with' then add PLUS, if 'against' then add MINUS
• When point of reversal is reached in one meridian, add cylindrical
  lenses to neutralize in the other meridian

Box 1.10 **Subjective refraction**

Remove 'working distance' lenses   ROOM LIGHTS ON
Occlude eye not being tested
Check VA

Verify sphere
- Ask patient to look at the smallest line that they can see clearly
- Verify sphere by offering ±DS (usually ±0.25DS to fine-tune, but may need ±0.5DS if poor VA)
- Ask, 'Is the line clearer and easier to read with lens 1 or 2?'

Verify cylinder axis
- Ask patient to look at a round target/easily readable 'O'
- Use cross-cylinder (0.50D cross-cylinder cf. 1.00D if poor VA)
- Align handle with axis of trial cylinder
- Ask, 'Is the circle rounder and clearer with lens 1 or 2?'
- Rotate trial cylinder towards the preferred cross-cylinder position respecting its sign, i.e. a plus trial cylinder is rotated towards the plus sign of the cross-cylinder.

Verify cylinder power
- Repeat the procedure but with the handle at 45° to axis of trial cylinder. This will in effect offer ±0.25D cyl (if using the 0.50 cross-cylinder).
- Add 0.25DS for every 0.5DC lost.

Refine best sphere
- Plus 1 blur test (should reduce VA by 2 lines)
- Duochrome test (monocular and binocular; aim for no preference/slight red preference)

Measure and record back vertex distance; most important if >5DS
Check near requirement—at usual reading/working distance

Box 1.11 **Muscle balance, accommodation, and convergence**

Maddox rod (distance muscle balance): place in front of RE in horizontal then vertical orientation; neutralize with prisms until patient reports that the red line passes through white spot.

Maddox wing (near muscle balance): ask patient where arrows point.

RAF rule (perform 3 times for each test)
- accommodation amplitude: distance at where text blurs
- near point of convergence: distance where line becomes double

Refraction: practical hints

Hints on retinoscopy

Positioning yourself

Aim to be as close to the patient's visual axis without obscuring their fixation target. If your head gets in the way they are likely to look at it and start accommodating.

Plus or minus cylinders

Be consistent: either work with **plus** or with **minus** cylindrical lenses.
- If using **plus** cylindrical lenses you will wish to correct the most **minus** meridian first. This is identified by:
  - If both reflexes are *against* then it is the *slower* reflex
  - If one is *with* and one *against* then it is the *against* reflex
  - If both reflexes are *with* then it is the *faster* reflex.
- If using **minus** cylindrical lenses you will wish to correct the most **plus** meridian first. This is identified similarly:
  - If both reflexes are *against* then it is the *faster* reflex
  - If one is *with* and one *against* then it is the *with* reflex
  - If both reflexes are *with* then it is the *slower* reflex

Poor reflex

- Consider media opacity: optimize illumination, check that they are not accommodating on your head.
- Consider high refractive error: use large steps, e.g. 5DS, 10DS.
- Consider keratoconus if swirling reflex or oil-drop sign.

Hints on subjective refraction

Avoiding 'too much minus'

When verifying/refining sphere check that they find it 'clearer and easier to read' and not just 'smaller and blacker' due to the minification effect.

Higher refractive errors

- Put higher power lenses at back of trial frame.
- Measure and document back vertex distance especially if >5.0DS.

Prescribing 'reading add'

Estimate requirement based on age and lens status (Table 1.21). However this should be tailored to the individual and their needs.

Table 1.21 Estimated near corrections

Age 45–50yrs	+1.0DS
Age 50–55yrs	+1.5DS
Age 55–60yrs	+2.0DS
Age >60yrs or pseudophake	+2.5DS

The role of muscle balance tests

- These tests depend on binocular vision and are dissociative. They are, therefore, particularly useful for detecting and quantifying phorias (latent squints).

- If the patient has a manifest squint but no diplopia then there is no point in doing the muscle balance tests.
- Do not prescribe prisms unless symptomatic, and first consider whether further investigation (including orthoptic referral) is necessary.

Causes of spectacle intolerance

The following may lead to asthenopia (refractive discomfort or 'eyestrain'):

- Significant change in axis or size of cylinder.
- Change of lens form.
- Overcorrection, especially of myopes who will end up permanently accommodating.
- Excessive near correction resulting in an uncomfortably near and narrow reading distance.
- Unsuitable bifocal or progressive lenses—consider occupation, requirements, and general faculties of the patient.

Focimetry

The focimeter (Fig. 1.11) or lensometer measures the axis and power of spectacles and CL. The instrument can also be used to find the optical centre, and the power and base direction of any prism in unknown lenses.

Manual focimetry

The vertex power of the lens is measured by taking the inverse of the focal length of the unknown lens. Green light is used to eliminate chromatic aberration.

Components
- Moveable illumination target
- Viewing telescope
- Fixed collimating lens (renders light parallel).

Method

Ensure the eye-piece is focused and target seen sharply focused. Insert unknown lens (spectacles mounted with the back surface of the lens against the rest to measure back vertex power).

For simple spherical lenses
Dial (this moves the target backwards or forwards) until the graticules are sharp and read off the power.

For cylindrical power
The target is rotated, as well as dialled until one set of lines is sharp. The reading is noted. The target is then dialled again until the other lines are sharp. The difference in these two readings is the cylindrical power. The axis of the cylinder is then read from the dialling wheel.

Bifocal addition
Turn the spectacles around to measure the front vertex power. The difference between the front vertex power of the distance and near portions is the bifocal add.

Automated focimetry

In principle four parallel beams of light pass through the unknown lens and strike a photosensitive surface. The deflection of the beams from their original path is measured and used to compute the lens power.

There is a support frame for the spectacles; changing the lever on the unit above the support frame will automatically read either the right or the left lens as required.

The graticules are sharp at two positions

Position 1: the graticules are sharp at an angle of 150° and a power of +1.0D

Position 2: the graticules are sharp at an angle of 60° and a power of +4.0D

Result: the lens prescription is therefore +1.0/+3.0 × 060.

Fig. 1.11 View through the focimeter.

Investigations and their interpretation

Visual field testing: general

The visual field is 'an island of vision surrounded by a sea of darkness' (Traquair's analogy). It is a 3-dimensional hill: the peak of the hill being the fovea and at ground level it extends approximately 50° superiorly, 60° nasally, 70° inferiorly, and 90° temporally.

Indications

Aids diagnosis and monitors certain ophthalmic (e.g. glaucoma) and neurological disease.

Definitions

- A *scotoma* is an area of visual loss or depression surrounded by an area of normal or less depressed vision. An absolute scotoma represents a total loss of vision, where no light can be perceived. A relative scotoma is an area of partial visual loss, where bright lights or larger targets are seen, whereas smaller and dimmer ones cannot be seen.
- **Homonymous**: this is where the defects are in the corresponding region of the visual field in both eyes. For example, in a right homonymous hemianopia there is a defect to the right of the midline in both visual fields.
- **Congruousness** describes the degree to which the field defects match between the two eyes. Generally, the more congruous the field defect the more posterior along the visual pathway the lesion is located.
- **Isopter**: this is a threshold line joining points of equal sensitivity on a visual field chart.

Caution

Interpretation problems of all visual fields can include refractive status (overcorrection by 1D will cause a reduction in sensitivity of 3.6dB). To compare serial visual fields background luminance, stimulus size, intensity, and exposure times need to be standardized.

Confrontational visual fields (see Visual fields examination 📖 p.32)

This is a simple qualitative method for gross detection of defects in the peripheral visual field. The use of hat pins (white and red) enables more subtle defects to be plotted. Results should be recorded the way the patient sees them; however, there can be inter-examiner variability.

Amsler grid (see Posterior segment examination 📖 p.24)

This assesses the central 10° of the visual field. Easy to perform and portable, it is used to detect central and paracentral scotomas. Held at a testing distance of 33cm, each square subtends 1° of visual field.

Kinetic perimetry

This presents a moving stimulus of known luminance from a non-seeing area to a seeing area. The target is then presented at various points around the clock and marked when recognized; these points are then joined producing a line of equal threshold sensitivity, which is named the isopter.

Tangent screen

The tangent screen (Bjerrum screen) is not commonly used in clinical practice.

Indication

Examining the central 30° of visual field usually at 2m, although a 1m chart is available.

Method

Patient sits 2m (2000mm) away from the screen, wears corrective lens for distance, if required. The non-tested eye is occluded in turn. The patient fixates at a central spot and informs the operator when they see the target. White (w) or red (r) disc targets are used, either 1 or 2mm in diameter.

Results

The results are plotted on charts as the patient sees them. The target size and colour is the numerator (1w, 2w, 1r or 2r) and the denominator is the distance (mm) of the patient from the chart (e.g. 1r/2000).

Goldmann perimetry

This is the commonest type of kinetic perimetry in clinical practice (see Goldmann perimetry, 📖 p.50).

Static perimetry

Most automated perimetry is based on static on–off stimuli of variable luminance presented throughout the potential field (see Automated perimetry, 📖 p.52).

Goldmann perimetry

Outline
- Usually kinetic (static perimetry is used for the central field).
- Skilled operators are required for the manual Goldmann Perimeter.
- Newer software packages on automated machines simulate full field Goldmann kinetic perimetry (e.g. OCTOPUS 900™).
- Useful for neuro-ophthalmic patients and those need significant supervision to produce a visual field.

Method

The Goldmann Perimeter should be calibrated at the start of each session. Distance and near add with wide aperture lenses should be used (to prevent ring scotoma). Aphakic eyes should, where possible, be corrected with contact lenses. Seat patient with chin on chin-rest and forehead against rest; occlude non-test eye; ask patient to fix on central target and to press the buzzer whenever they see the light stimulus.

From the opposite side of the Goldmann the examiner directs the stimulus to map out their field of vision to successive stimuli (isopters). Move the stimulus slowly and steadily from unseen to seen, i.e. inward for periphery and outward for mapping the blind spot/central scotomas. To move the stimulus arm from one side to the other it must be swung around the bottom of the chart. Once the peripheral isopters are plotted, the central area is examined for scotoma. The examiner should monitor patient fixation via the viewing telescope. The central 20° with an extension to the nasal 30° is appropriate to pick up early glaucomatous scotomas. Points either side of the vertical meridian are explored in suspected chiasmal and post-chiasmal disease. The physiological blind-spot should be mapped.

Results

Isopters are contours of visual sensitivity. Common isopters plotted are:
- I-4e (0.25mm^2, 1000asb stimulus)
- I-2e (0.25mm^2, 100asb stimulus)
- II-4e (1.0mm^2, 1000asb stimulus)
- IV-4e if smaller targets not seen (16mm^2, 1000asb stimulus).

Interpretation

The target sizes are indicated by Roman numerals (0–V), representing the size of the target in square millimetres, each successive number being equivalent to a 4-fold increase in area.

The intensity of the light is represented by an Arabic numeral (1–4), each successive number being 3.15 times brighter (0.5 log unit steps). It is measured in Apostilbs (asb).

A lower case letter indicates additional minor filters progressing from 'a', the darkest, to 'e' being the brightest. Each progressive letter is an increase of 0.1 log unit.

Caution

Potential sources of error/artefact include miosis, media opacities, uncorrected refractive error, rim of the trial frame, ptosis or dermatochalasis, incomprehension of the test, tremor, or inadequate retinal adaptation.

Calibrating the Goldmann Perimeter

Set-up
- Insert standard test paper, making sure aligned.
- Lock stylus (at 70° on right-hand side), using the knob on the pointer arm.

Stimulus calibration
- All levers to the right (i.e. V-4e).
- Turn stimulus (or test) light to permanently on.
- Move the 'white flag' (photometer screen; located on left-hand side of machine) to the up position.
- Adjust the stimulus rheostat (knob furthest from examiner on left-hand side) until the light meter reads 1000asb. NB: if it does not reach 1000asb the bulb may need to be rotated or changed.

Background calibration
- Return 'white flag' to down position.
- Set levers to V-1e (stimulus intensity of 32.5asb).
- Adjust the background illumination to match this stimulus intensity; this is achieved by adjusting the lampshade while looking through the notch on one side of the hemisphere to the photometer screen opposite.
- The photometer can be removed and the pointer handle unlocked.

Intensity	dB	Intensity	dB		Object	mm²
1	0.0315	15	a	0.40	4		0	1/16
2	0.100	10	b	0.50	3		II	¼
3	0.315	5	c	0.63	2		II	1
4	1.00	0	d	0.80	1		III	4
			e	1.00	0		IV	16
							V	64

Fig. 2.1 Normal Goldmann visual field of the right eye.

Automated perimetry: performance and interpretation (1)

The majority of these machines are configured to test static perimetry. The stimulus in this case is stationary but changes its intensity until the sensitivity of the eye at that point is found. It is measured at pre-selected locations in the visual field. Program selection includes the central 30°, 24°, 10°, or full field.

- **Suprathreshold** tests are quickest to perform and are screening tests. They calculate the threshold adjusted for age by testing a few pre-defined spots using a 4–6dB step. They may miss subtle variations in the scotoma's contour as they do not go on to map defects. They should not be used to monitor glaucoma.
- **Threshold testing** steps of 4dB are used until detected then re-tested at this point in 2db steps. This is the gold standard for monitoring glaucoma and requires patient cooperation and concentration. Appreciably, there is a subject learning curve seen in the first few tests.

Humphrey perimetry

- Sensitive and reproducible, but difficult to perform.
- Fixation monitoring (by tracking gaze and retesting the blind spot).

Method

The machine automatically calibrates itself on start up. Selection of programs includes:

- Threshold (full threshold or SITA central 30-2, 24-2, 10-2).
- Suprathreshold testing (Screening central 76 point, full field 120 point, and Esterman (DVLA Visual driving standard test)).
- Coloured stimuli can also be used.

Interpretation of Humphrey perimetry (Tables 2.1–2.4)

When analysing the results of automated perimetry consider reliability indices, absolute retinal thresholds, comparison with age-matched controls and overall performance indices (global indices).

Table 2.1 Reliability indices (subject reliability)

Fixation losses	Fixation plotted, if patient moves and the machine re-tests and patient sees spot then a fixation loss is recorded Fixation losses above 20% may significantly compromise the test
False positives	Patient responds to the normal whirr of the computer noise when it sounds as if it is about to present a light, but does not. A high false positive occurs in 'trigger happy' patients
False negatives	A brighter light is presented in an area in which the threshold has already been determined and the patient does not see it. A high false negative score occurs in fatigued or inattentive patients

Table 2.2 Common visual field abnormalities

Altitudinal field defects	Ischaemic optic neuropathy
	Hemibranch retinal artery or vein occlusion
	Glaucoma
	Optic nerve or chiasmal lesions
	Optic nerve coloboma
Arcuate scotoma	Glaucoma
	Ischaemic optic neuropathy
	Optic disc drusen
Binasal field defect	Glaucoma
	Bitemporal retinal disease (e.g. RP)
	Bilateral occipital disease
	Compressive lesion of both optic nerves or chiasm
	Functional visual loss
Bitemporal hemianopia	Chiasmal lesions
	Tilted optic discs
	Sectoral RP
Central scotoma	Macular lesions
	Optic neuritis
	Optic atrophy
	Occipital cortex lesions
Homonymous hemianopia	Optic tract or lateral geniculate lesions
	Temporal, parietal, or occipital lobe lesions
Constriction of peripheral fields	Glaucoma
	Retinal disease (e.g. RP)
	Bilateral panretinal photocoagulation
	Central retinal artery occlusion
	Bilateral occipital lobe lesions with macular sparing
	Papilloedema
	Functional visual loss (spiral visual fields)
Blind spot enlargement	Papilloedema
	Glaucoma
	Optic nerve drusen
	Optic nerve coloboma
	Myelinated nerve fibres
	Myopic discs
Pie in the sky	Temporal lobe lesion
Pie on the floor	Parietal lobe lesion

Automated perimetry: performance and interpretation (2)

Interpretation of Humphrey perimetry *(continued)*

Table 2.3 Typical graphical results from automated perimetry

The grey scale	Decreasing sensitivity is represented by the darker tones. Grey-scale tones correspond to 5dB change in threshold
Numerical display	Gives the threshold for all points checked (in decibel)
	Bracketed results show the initial test if the sensitivity was 5dB less sensitive than expected
Total deviation	Calculated by comparing the patient's measurements with age-matched controls. Upper chart is in dB and lower is in grey scale
Pattern deviation	Adjusted for any generalized depression in the overall field. This highlights focal depressions in the field, which might be masked by generalized depressions in sensitivity (e.g. cataract and corneal opacities)

Table 2.4 Global indices (a summary of the results as a single number used to monitor change)

Mean deviation (MD)	A measure of overall field loss
Pattern standard deviation	Measure of focal loss or variability within the field taking into account any generalized depression. An increased pattern standard deviation is more indicative of glaucomatous field loss than MD
Short-term fluctuation (SF)	An indication of the consistency of responses. It is assessed by measuring threshold twice at 10 pre-selected points and calculated on the difference between the 1st and 2nd measurements
Corrected pattern standard deviation	A measure of variability within the field after correcting for SF (intra-test variability)

Probability values (p)
Indicate the significance of the defect <5%, <2%, <1%, and <0.5%. The lower the *p* value the greater its clinical significance and the lesser the likelihood of the defect having occurred by chance.

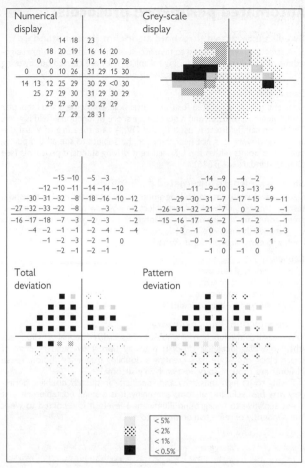

Fig. 2.2 Typical graphical results from automated perimetry of the right eye of a patient with glaucoma demonstrating nasal step and developing superior arcuate field defect.

Automated perimetry: protocols

Swedish interactive threshold algorithm (fast or standard)

SITA strategies were created to take 50% less time than conventional algorithms to perform, thus increasing reliability. They are carried out by using prior information and establishing threshold values more quickly.

Esterman grid

Different grids are available for the central field, whole field and binocular field. Subjects are tested and a percentage score of functional field is given. The binocular field test is used by the DVLA as a measure of visual disability for drivers. It is not necessary for the subject to see all the points, but to see points within the UK's current driving standard protocols (see Driving standard 🕮 p.816).

Short wavelength automated perimetry

Short wavelength automated perimetry uses standard static threshold testing strategies with a blue test object on a yellow background (red and green cones are desensitized by adapting the eye to yellow light). Results suggest that this is more sensitive than conventional white on white perimetry to early glaucomatous damage.[1]

Caution
• Increased total test time.
• Difficulty to set up test.
• High short-term fluctuation.
• Data affected by lens opacities.

Frequency doubling perimetry

This measures the function of a subset of specialized retinal ganglion cells (the large Magnocellular (M-cell) pathway fibres) by rapid reversal of broad black and white bars creating a doubling frequency illusion. These M-fibres are thought to be lost early in glaucoma.

Owing to its high sensitivity and specificity, frequency doubling perimetry may be useful in glaucoma screening. It is a small portable unit that is not sensitive to background illumination levels. It is reported to work independently of refractive errors up to ±7D.

---

1. Johnson CA et al. (1993). Progression of early glaucomatous visual field loss as detected by blue on yellow and standard white on white automated perimetry. Arch Ophthalmol **111**:651.

Glaucoma Progression Analysis

Identifying visual field progression using serial printout of stored field tests (as single charts) in consecutive order allows subjective comparison of charts to show change over time. Trend and event analysis allow quantitative assessment of progression in a visual field series.

Trend analysis

Measures rate of change of the visual field and the statistical significance. Can be measured point by point (point-wise linear regression) or on a cluster basis. *Examples*: PROGRESSOR software (Institute of Ophthalmology, London) and PeriData.

Event analysis

Designed to highlight any visual field changes from baseline that are larger than typical clinical variability. *Examples include*: the Glaucoma Progression Analysis for the Humphrey Field Analyser.

Glaucoma Progression Analysis

Glaucoma Progression Analysis is simple to interpret and corrects for media opacities (such as progressive cataracts that cause a generalized depression).

It defines visual progression according to the Early Manifest Glaucoma Trial (EMGT) criteria[1]: any patient who lost three or more test points in the same location on three consecutive field tests. The EMGT criteria has been shown to identify progression earlier and more often than the Advanced Glaucoma Intervention Study (AGIS) or the Collaborative Initial Glaucoma Treatment Study (CIGTS) criteria.[2]

Results

Glaucoma Progression Analysis can calculate the variability then adjusts for this to calculate the probability that a change at a specific point is indeed true change or not. The probability plot progression symbol key:

- *Open triangles*: when a point is a statistically significant from baseline fields at that location.
- *Half-black triangle*: if a point has changed on two consecutive fields (indicates possible progression).
- *Black triangle*: if three consecutive fields show change at that particular location (indicates likely progression).

Glaucoma Progression Analysis Alert™

- *Three half black triangles* in one analysis indicate 'possible progression'.
- *Three black triangles* in one analysis indicate 'likely progression'.

Caution

Full threshold strategy fields can only be used as baseline and not as follow-up tests (SITA standard or fast must be used).

---

1. Heijl A et al. (2002). Reduction of IOP and glaucoma progression: results from the early manifest glaucoma trial. *Arch Opthalmol* **120**:1268.

2. Heijl A et al. (2008). A comparison of visual field progression criteria of 3 major glaucoma trials in early manifest glaucoma trail patients *Ophthalmology* **115**:1157.

Anterior segment imaging (1)

Keratometry

Measurement of the anterior curvature of the central cornea (3mm diameter). Assesses the magnitude and axis of astigmatism.

Indications

- Fitting of contact lenses.
- Used in ocular biometry.
- Assessment of corneal curvature post-surgery.

Methods

Dim the room lights. Ensure the patient is comfortable and still. Occlude the other eye. Record both the 'k' (dioptres) and axis readings in both horizontal and vertical meridians.

The Javal–Schiotz keratometer

- Uses a fixed image and adjustable object (mire) size.
- A red rectangle and a green step-shaped mire are projected on to the anterior cornea (each step is equivalent to 1D).
- The mires are mounted on a side arm, so they can be rotated about any axis. The reflected image is doubled through a Wollaston prism.
- For both horizontal and vertical end points, mires should be just touching with no overlap and axis markings aligned.

The Bausch and Lomb type keratometers

- Uses a fixed object size (circle mires) and adjustable image size.
- Helmholtz design (uses vertical and horizontal moveable prisms).
- The horizontal axis is correct when plus signs just touch (read from the horizontal mark) and power is when they are superimposed.
- Vertical end points are read with the minus signs and from the top markings on the keratometer.

Corneal topography

Maps the entire cornea providing accurate measurement of corneal shape, refractive power, and thickness. Most systems designs use Placido reflected images.

Indications

- Assess the corneal curvature and postoperative corneal changes.
- Detection of macro-irregularities, such as astigmatism, keratoconus, and pellucid marginal degeneration.
- Monitoring contact lens warpage on the cornea, and disease progression.

Methods

Multiple light concentric rings are projected on to the anterior surface of the cornea. The reflected images are captured, computer software analyses the data and generates topographical colour-coded maps.

Results

Curvature is expressed as radii of curvature in mm or in keratometric dioptres. A colour scale is used representing the range of values. The maps are constructed by either comparing the data with itself (relative or normalized scales) or to set ranges (absolute scale). Consequently, different colour maps cannot be directly compared and have to be interpreted based on their actual numerical values.

Interpretation

Normal corneas are usually classified as (1) round, (2) oval, (3) symmetric bow-tie, (4) asymmetric bow-tie and (5) irregular. The average adult cornea is steeper in the vertical meridian compared with the horizontal. ie. has with-the-rule astigmatism.

Scanning-slit videokeratography (Orbscan™ corneal analyser)

A highly accurate and reproducible corneal topography system that uses optical scanning-slit topography, combining Placido reflections and direct triangulation.

Indications

- Assessment of anterior and posterior corneal surface elevations (useful for wavefront-guided surgery).
- Indirect measurement of corneal thickness.

Methods

A high-resolution video-camera projects numerous light slits at the anterior segment; it captures and analyses the light reflected using a triangulation system.

Results

The software calculates elevation, i.e. the points per half-slit from both the anterior and posterior surfaces. It then indirectly calculates the corneal thickness.

Caution

Inability to detect interfaces (e.g. post-LASIK flap).

In vivo confocal microscopy

Non-invasive technique that images the cornea and conjunctiva *in vivo*.

Indications

- Detection of corneal pathology, including dystrophies, degenerations, deposits, and infections (e.g. fungi elements and acanthamoeba).
- Post-surgical analysis (e.g. refractive surgery, collagen cross-linking, filtering blebs post-trabeculectomy).

Methods

Light passes through an aperture and is focused by a condenser. Reflected light then passes through an observation system that has the same focal length as the condenser. Systems included tandem-scanning, scanning-slit and laser-scanning confocal microscopes.

Results

Axial resolution of 5–10μm and lateral resolution 1–2μm allowing magnification of up to ×600.

Anterior segment imaging (2)

Scheimpflug imaging

In a normal camera the object, image and lens planes are perpendicular to the lens axis. Scheimpflug images are produced by altering the object and image planes. This results in high-quality images that are corrected for eye movements. This investigation is not widely available.

Indications

AC depth, angle estimation, and measurement of corneal thickness.

Methods

A 3-dimensional mathematical model of the anterior segment is generated from 50 slit images, evaluating 500 measured points from each image, in 2s taken with the non-contact rotating Scheimpflug camera (e.g. Pentacam).

Results

Corneal topography (anterior/posterior; elevation maps), corneal pachymetry, 3-dimensional AC imaging (including chamber angle, volume analysis), lens density.

Anterior segment optical coherence tomography

The slit-lamp adapted OCT (SL-OCT) and Visante™ OCT are high-resolution, non-contact OCT customized for anterior segment examinations.

Indications

- AC depth, angle estimation and visualization.
- Corneal thickness measurements.
- Imaging of filtering blebs.

Methods

Scan with the patient in the sitting position (📖 p.70)

Results

Direct angle visualization includes anatomical details such as the iris root, angle recess, anterior ciliary body, scleral spur, and canal of Schlemm.

Ophthalmic ultrasonography: A-scan

An inexpensive, reliable diagnostic imaging technique that uses relatively high-frequency ultrasound waves: ocular 8–10MHz; orbital 4–5MHz; anterior segment 50–100MHz.

Indications
- Measurement of axial length (biometry).
- Assessment of orbital tumours.
- Assessment of orbital disease (thyroid eye disease, measurement of muscles).
- Evaluation of the anterior or posterior segments with opaque ocular media (i.e. cataract or vitreous haemorrhage).
- Location of intraocular FBs.

Method
Suitable electrical stimulation of a piezoelectric crystal results in emitted ultrasound waves. Ultrasound waves reflected back re-stimulate the crystal, which then produces an electric current that then can be converted to a display. Imaging is effectively 1-dimensional (A-scan) or 2-dimensional (B-scan).

A-scans

These are curves of the amplitude of reflectivity of ocular structures and are used to obtain accurate measurements within the eye. They are mainly used in biometry.

Indications
- Measurement of axial length most commonly for intraocular lens power calculation (biometry).
- Measurement of AC depth or other intraocular distances.
- Measurement of intraocular mass thickness and characterization of acoustic properties.

Method
A transducer with coupling medium is placed on anaesthetized cornea. The ultrasonic beam is emitted and deflections from the ocular tissues are recorded and displayed on a computer. Non-axial scans are rejected.

Interpretation
This is a 1-dimensional time–amplitude display. Corrections need to be made for different mediums, such as silicone oil in the eye, as the speed of sound varies in different media (slower in oil compared with vitreous media). Artefactually, low axial lengths may occur in conditions such as ateroid hyalosis and with inappropriate application.

Ophthalmic ultrasonography: B-scan

B-scans

Cross-sectional images of ocular or orbital tissues are obtained. The acoustic echoes are represented as a 2-dimensional image with their x–y coordinates determined by the echo origin and their brightness by the echo amplitude.

Indications
- Identification of posterior segment pathology in the presence of media opacity preventing fundal view, e.g. identifying retinal break/detachment obscured by vitreous haemorrhage.
- Characterization of intraocular masses.

Method
Ocular (static) (Table 2.5, Figs. 2.3–2.8)
- 8–10MHz transducer
  - Lubrication agent applied to closed eyelids.
  - The marker on the probe shows one side of the display screen. When the marker is lined horizontally with the lids, it shows a horizontal plane. Vertical placement (line to eyebrows) provides a vertical cross-section.
  - Scans are captured with the patient's eye in primary position and then sequentially in all four quadrants, horizontally and vertically.

Note: if the probe is moved temporally from the primary position the scan shows the nasal retina. If the patient moves their left eye nasally while probe is moved temporally, the nasal retina anterior to the equator can be scanned.

Ocular (dynamic)
Scanning during eye movements can help differentiate between posterior vitreous detachments and retinal detachments.

Orbital
- 3–5MHz transducer
  - Vertical scan planes used to measure extraocular muscle thickness.
  - Horizontal and vertical for orbital masses.
  - Eyelids closed and lubricating agent.

Anterior segment (syn high-frequency or ultrasound biomicroscopy) (Figs. 2.9–2.10)
- 50–100MHz transducer
  - *Indications*: corneal thickness, plateau iris syndrome, pigment dispersion syndrome, iris tumours/masses, position of intraocular lens haptics, assessment of the anterior segment in cases of corneal opacification (e.g. Peter's anomaly and sclerocornea).
  - *Method*: anaesthetized cornea and eyelids open with an immersion bath (water or methylcellulose) as coupling agent. High-frequency scans are taken radial and parallel to the limbus at various predetermined positions.
  - *Results*: a 2-dimensional cross-sectional display of the globe and orbit is seen.

Table 2.5 Diagnostic features on ultrasound

Posterior vitreous detachment	Faintly reflective posterior hyaloid face may appear incomplete except on eye movement
	Eye movement induces staccato movement with 1s after-movement
	No blood demonstrated on colour flow mapping
RRD	Highly reflective irregular convex membrane
	Eye movement induces undulating after-movement (unless proliferative vitreoretinopathy)
	Blood demonstrated on colour flow mapping
Tractional retinal detachment	Highly reflective concave membrane tented into vitreous
	Eye movement induces no after-movement of membrane
	Blood demonstrated on colour flow mapping
Choroidal detachment	Highly reflective regular dome-shaped membrane
	Attached to the vortex ampulla/vein
	Blood demonstrated on colour flow mapping both in retina (6–8cm/s) and choroid (8–10cm/s)
Vitreous haemorrhage	Reflective particulate matter within the vitreous space (indistinguishable from vitritis)
Vitreous inflammation	Reflective particulate matter within the vitreous space (indistinguishable from haemorrhage)
Choroidal effusion	Acoustically empty suprachoroidal space
Suprachoroidal haemorrhage	Reflective acoustically heterogeneous suprachoroidal space
Posterior scleritis	Scleral thickness >2.0mm
	Fluid in Tenon's space and optic nerve sheath ('T-sign')

Ophthalmic ultrasonography: images (1)

Fig. 2.3 Ultrasound (B-scan) of posterior vitreous detachment. *Note*: posterior hyaloid face is only faintly reflective and appears incomplete on a static image.

Fig. 2.4 Ultrasound (B-scan + A-scan) of retinal detachment. *Note*: retina appears as a highly reflective convex membrane which is complete but irregular.

Fig. 2.5 Ultrasound (B-scan + A-scan) of choroidal detachment. *Note*: retina/choroid appears as a highly reflective regular dome-shaped membrane.

Fig. 2.6 Ultrasound (B-scan, vector A-scan and standard A-scan) of choroidal melanoma. *Note* dome-shaped membrane with low internal reflectivity on standard A-scan.

Ophthalmic ultrasonography: images (2)

Fig. 2.7 Ultrasound (B-scan) of buried drusen. *Note* highly reflective bodies overlying the optic nerve.

Fig. 2.8 Ultrasound (B-scan) of posterior scleritis. *Note* well-defined thickened sclera and fluid in Tenon's space.

Fig. 2.9 High-frequency ultrasound of the anterior segment in a patient with pha-komorphic glaucoma. *Note* anteriorly displaced iris with secondary narrowing of the angles.

Fig. 2.10 High-frequency ultrasound of the anterior segment in a patient with ciliary body melanoma.

Ophthalmic ultrasonography: Doppler and pachymetry

Doppler ultrasound

A duplex scanner combines real-time B-scan images with pulsed Doppler images. Vessel patency and flow velocity can be assessed. Venous and arterial flows can be distinguished by colour Doppler flow mapping. Caution should be taken as distinguishing severe stenosis from complete occlusion is difficult.

Indications

- Assessment of blood flow in central retinal artery, posterior ciliary arteries, ophthalmic artery, and central retinal vein.
- Carotid-cavernous fistulas.
- Vascular lesions.

Corneal ultrasonic pachymetry

Measurement of the thickness of the cornea using a contact 20Hz ultrasonic probe.

Indications

- Assess the appropriateness of refractive surgery (in particular LASIK, to prevent postoperative corneal ectasia).
- Assessment of accurate applanation IOP (important in normotension glaucoma and ocular hypertension).

Methods

Instil topical local anaesthetic. Hold the ultrasonic probe at 90° to the corneal surface. No coupling agent is required. Pachymetry should be measured centrally, infero-nasaly and infero-temporaly.

Results

Average central corneal thickness is approximately 490–560µm.

Interpretation

A simple, portable, and low-cost reproducible method; however, inaccurate positioning of the probe may result in erroneous results.

Optical coherence tomography

OCT (see also Figs. 2.11–2.14) uses light in the near-infrared spectrum (810nm) from a superluminescent diode to create high-resolution cross-sectional images of the retina. A partially reflective mirror is used to split the coherent light beam into a measuring beam and a reference beam. The measuring beam is directed into the eye where succeeding optical interfaces (e.g. retinal layers, RPE, choriocapillaris) reflect the beam to a variable extent. The reference beam is directed to a reference mirror that is adjusted to synchronize the reflected reference beam with the reflected measuring beam returning from the retinal surface. This results in constructive interference. Reflections from deeper structures will be out of phase and cause variable degree of destructive interference. The interference is interpreted as depth and amplitude of reflection as brightness.

Indications
- Detection and monitoring of macular pathology, e.g. macular oedema, macular hole, etc.
- Detection of glaucomatous retinal nerve fibre layer changes.
- Detection of glaucomatous optic disc change.

Method
- A large pupil and clear media ensure accurate measurement.
- Choose appropriate OCT program for the area to be imaged.
- An 810nm diode laser measuring beam is directed at the area of interest.
- A series of cross-sectional images is automatically generated from a sequence of 100 (OCT1,2) or 500 (OCT3) axial scans.

Results
The cross-section indicates layers within the retina that are represented in artificial colour: highly reflective (red → white) and poorly reflective (blue → black). Resolution is about 8µm (OCT3).

The distribution percentages are colour coded: *green*, 95% of the normal population falls in or below this band; *yellow*, represents 5% of the normal population; and *red* represents 1% of the normal population.

Interpretation
OCT imaging provides high-resolution images and may be supported by additional analysis software (e.g. for optic disc and retinal nerve fibre analysis).

Fig. 2.11 OCT of a normal patient.

Fig. 2.12 OCT of cystoid macular oedema.

Fig. 2.13 OCT of a full-thickness macular hole.

Fig. 2.14 OCT of chronic serous chorioretinopathy.

Imaging the retinal nerve fibre layer

Scanning laser ophthalmoscopy

The Heidelberg Retinal Tomographer (HRT) is a type of confocal scanning laser ophthalmoscope. It is designed for 3-dimensional imaging of the posterior segment of the eye. It requires an experienced operator.

Indications
- Detection of glaucomatous optic disc damage.
- Longitudinal or progressive change detection.

Contraindications
- Advanced cataract.
- Corneal opacities.
- Nystagmus.

Method
- A large pupil and clear media ensure accurate measurements.
- A 670nm diode laser images a series of 2-dimensional sections of the optic nerve head and the peripapillary retina.
- A 3-dimensional topographic image is then built from a series of 16–64 serial optical sections using algorithms to find the surface at each of 256 × 256 (HRT 1) or 384 × 384 (HRT II) pixels over a 10° or 15° field of view. The HRT II automatically captures three consecutive 15° images and generates a mean topographic image.

Results
Laser polarimetry can measure RNFL thickness by measuring a change in the rotation of a polarized beam of laser light reflected from the retinal surface. The transverse resolution is about 10µm, but axial resolution is only about 300µm. The in-built Moorfields regression analysis compares the actual measured rim area with that predicted for an optic disc of a particular size, age, and ethnicity.

Interpretation
Pupil size, media opacities, and ability of patient to fixate can all affect the quality and variability of the results. Measurements are also influenced by acute changes in IOP and possibly the cardiac cycle.

Scanning laser polarimetry

The GDx nerve fibre analyser is a scanning laser polarimeter that utilizes the birefringent properties of the retinal nerve fibre layer. This birefringence arises due to the parallel architecture of the axonal microtubules. The change in polarization, called retardation, can be quantified by determining the phase shift between polarization of light returning from the eye with that of the illumination laser beam. The degree of retardation is linearly related to the retinal nerve fibre thickness. The nerve fibre analyser thus estimates the thickness of the peripapillary RNFL based on the retardation of polarized light.

Indications
- Glaucoma detection.

Contraindications
- Nystagmus.
- Dense cataracts.
- Large amounts of peripapillary atrophy.
- Corneal refractive surgery.

Method
A polarized laser beam (820nm) scans the peripapillary retina circumferentially around the scleral canal opening to acquire an image. The backscattered light is captured and analysed. Does not require pupillary dilation.

Results
- RNFL thickness values are compared to an age- and race-matched normal population.
- A neural network within the GDx analyses more than 200 parameters from the image. It then assigns a number between zero and 100 (zero means normal and 100 means glaucoma) indicating the likelihood of glaucoma.
- The symmetry analysis evaluates the ratio of the average of the 1500 thickest points in the superior quadrant over the average of the 1500 thickest points in the inferior quadrant. The closer this number is to 1.0, the more symmetry is present, and the higher the chance of the scan being normal.
- Max modulation is an indication of the difference between the thickest part of the RNFL and the thinnest part. The higher the number, the greater the difference. In a normal eye in which the superior and inferior region is thicker than the nasal or temporal region, the modulation number will usually be greater than 1.0. Lower numbers are associated with loss of thickness of the RNFL and are characteristic of glaucoma.

Interpretation
Cornea, lens, and sclera also demonstrate birefringent properties. This must be neutralized to isolate the RNFL retardation. There is a high incidence of artefacts, with erroneous measurements in areas of peripapillary atrophy or chorioretinal scarring. Note: mild to moderate cataracts do not degrade the result.

Fundus fluorescein angiography

FFA is fundal photography performed in rapid sequence following IV injection sodium fluorescein ($C_{20}H_{10}O_5Na_2$), an organic water-soluble dye, to image the choroidal and retinal vasculature using spectrally appropriate blue excitation and yellow–green barrier filters.

Sodium fluorescein (wt 376Da) is 70–85% bound to plasma albumin. Metabolized by the liver and excreted by the kidneys in 24h, it has a peak absorption at 490nm (blue visible spectrum) and emits at 530nm (yellow visible spectrum). Good visualization requires clear media and dilated pupils.

Indications
- Diagnostic test directly assessing the retinal and choroidal vessels (functional integrity and flow), but indirectly providing information about other retinal structures and pathological features. It is an adjunct to the clinical history and examination findings.
- Planning of retinal laser procedures.

Contra-indications
- Renal impairment.
- Known allergy to fluorescein.

Side-effects
- Skin discoloration.
- Nausea and vomiting.
- Pruritis.
- Urine discoloration (orange).
- Vasovagal syncope (1 in 340).
- Severe anaphylaxis (1 in 1900).
- Fatal anaphylaxis (1 in 220 000).

Method
- *Prepare patient*: explain procedure, risks, and benefits, and take formal consent; dilate; check BP; cannulate (medium/large bore vein); ensure resuscitation facilities (including 'crash' trolley) are readily available.
- Seat patient at camera and adjust height for patient comfort and camera alignment. Ask patient to fix on the fixation target.
- Take colour and 'red-free' fundal photographs.
- Inject fluorescein (5ml 10% IV) and take early rapid sequence photographs (at about 1s intervals) for 25–30s. Continue less frequent shots alternating between eyes for up to 5–10min. Late images may be taken at 10–20min.
- *The early shots are critical*: it is generally only possible to get a good series of early shots from one eye due to the time it takes to move between eyes. It is therefore important that the photographer is informed which eye takes priority.

Interpretation

FFAs should be read sequentially according to their phases: choroidal (pre-arterial), arterial, capillary, venous, and late. This test should be reported in conjunction with patient history and examination.

Reporting

Box 2.1 Reporting an FFA

1. Report the red-free photo
2. Specify the phase
3. Note hyper- and hypofluorescence and any delay in filling (see Box 2.2)
4. Note distinctive features (petalloid, smoke stack etc.)
5. Note any change in area, intensity, or the fluorescence over time

Box 2.2 Morphological analysis of FFA features

Feature	Common causes
Hyperfluorescence	
Window defect	RPE defect (e.g. RPE atrophy, macular hole)
Leakage of dye	*At macula*: cystoid macular oedema (petalloid appearance), other macular oedema
	At disc: papilloedema, ischaemic optic neuropathy, inflammation
	Elsewhere: new retinal vessels, vasculitis, CNV
Pooling of dye	Detachment of the neural retina or RPE (e.g. CSR, AMD)
Staining of dye	Drusen, disc, disciform scars sclera (seen if overlying chorioretinal atrophy/thinning)
Abnormal vessels	Tumours (haemangiomas, melanomas, etc.)
Autofluorescence (visible without dye)	Disc drusen, large lipofuscin deposits
Hypofluorescence	
Transmission defect	*Pre-retinal* (blocks view of retinal and choroidal circulations): media opacity especially vitreous opacities (inflammation, haemorrhage, degenerative), pre-retinal haemorrhage
	Inner retinal (blocks view of capillary circulation but larger retinal vessels seen): dot and blot haemorrhages (e.g. vein occlusion), intraretinal lipid (e.g. diabetic retinopathy)
	Pre-choroidal (blocks view of choroidal circulation, but retinal circulation seen): subretinal haemorrhage, pigment (e.g. choroidal naevi, CHRPE, melanoma), lipid, lipofuscin
Filling defects (circulation abnormalities)	Retinal arteriolar non-perfusion (e.g. arterial occlusion)
	Retinal capillary non-perfusion (e.g. ischaemia secondary to diabetes, vein occlusion)
	Choroidal non-perfusion (e.g. infarcts secondary to accelerated hypertension, etc.)
	Disc non-perfusion (e.g. ischaemic optic neuropathy)

Indocyanine green angiography

ICG is a useful way of studying the choroidal circulation, and is usually performed in association with FFA. The contrast agent is indocyanine green, which is 98% bound to serum proteins that do not pass through the fenestrations of the choriocapillaris. With an excitation peak at 810nm and emission of 830nm, the dye is excited by infrared radiation.

Indications
- Suspected CNV not clearly visualized on FFA (particularly occult-type).
- Recurrence of CNV after treatment.
- Consideration of feeder vessel treatment in CNV.
- Suspected IPCV.
- Suspected RPE detachments.
- Can be helpful in the assessment of choroidal tumours, inflammatory disease, or other diseases of the choroidal vasculature.

Method
- ICG powder is mixed with aqueous solvent to make a solution of 40mg in 2ml. A red-free photo is taken and the bolus IV injection is given. Frequent images are taken over the first 3min and then later images at, for example, 5, 10, 15, 20, and 30min.

Contra-indications
- Pregnancy.
- Renal impairment.
- Iodine allergy (ICG contains 5% iodine).

Side-effects
- Nausea and vomiting.
- Sneezing and pruritus.
- Backache.
- Staining of stool.
- Vasovagal syncope.
- Severe anaphylaxis (1 in 1900).

Interpretation
The angiogram is split into early phase (2–60s), early mid-phase (1–3min), late mid-phase (3–15min), and late phase (15–30min).

Box 2.3 Morphological analysis of ICG features

Feature	Common causes
Hyperfluorescence	
Window defect	RPE defect
Leakage of dye	Choroidal: CNV, IPCV; also leakage from other structures (retina, disc)
Abnormal blood vessels	Choroidal haemangioma
Hypofluorescence	
Transmission defect	RPE detachment (hypofluorescent centrally); blood, pigment, and exudate cause less blockage than in FFA
Filling defects (circulation abnormalities)	Choroidal infarcts secondary to accelerated hypertension, SLE, etc.
	Choroidal atrophy (e.g. atrophic AMD, some chorioretinal scars, choroideraemia)

Electrodiagnostic tests (1)

All electrodiagnostic tests should be performed to the International Society for Clinical Electrophysiology of Vision (ISCEV) Standard, as the responses and normal values can still differ between centres due to variation in equipment and technique.

The results of each test are interpreted by the polarity and amplitude of the electrophysical deflections and their latency (implicit time).

Electroretinography

ERG is a record of the mass electrical activity from the retina when stimulated by an intense flash of light.

Indications

- Diagnosis of generalized retinal degenerations (such as RP, Leber's congenital amaurosis, choroideraemia, gyrate atrophy, achromatopsia, CSNB, and cone dystrophies).
- Investigating family members for known hereditary retinal degenerations (such as RP).
- Determining visual function (paediatric cases).
- Assessing generalized retinal function in opaque media.
- Evaluation of functional visual loss.

Method

A Ganzfeld or full-field stimulation is created by a bowl perimeter. Electrodes are embedded in a contact lens on the cornea with a reference electrode on forehead.

The scotopic rod-response ERG is measured in dark-adapted eyes (after 30min in the dark) with a dim white flash 2.5 log units below the standard flash. The maximal response ERG is obtained in dark-adapted eyes using the standard flash. The photopic single-flash cone response ERG is in light-adapted eyes (after 10min in the light). The cone-derived flicker response is obtained using a 30Hz white light flicker stimulus; the rods are unable to respond due to poor temporal resolution.

Results

A single flash stimulus is followed by an initial negative 'a wave' and then a positive 'b wave', superimposed on oscillatory potentials. This usually takes less than 250ms. Amplitude (microvolts) and implicit time (milliseconds) of these waves are the 2 major parameters that are used to evaluate the ERG response.

- a wave arises from the photoreceptors.
- b wave arises from the bipolar and Muller cells.
- c wave is an additional waveform that is seen only in the dark-adapted eye, which reflects RPE activity.

Example: ERG can be useful in CRVO distinguishing between non-ischaemic and ischaemic CRVO. The b wave is affected by large areas of ischaemia. This produces a reduced b wave amplitude, reduced b:a wave ratio, and/or a prolonged b wave implicit time.

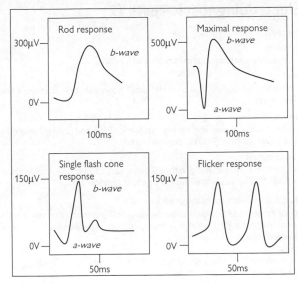

Fig. 2.15 Typical ERG in a normal patient.

Interpretation

Table 2.6 Interpreting ERG results

Reduced *a* and *b* waves	RP
	Ophthalmic artery occlusion
	Neuroretinitis
	Metallosis
	Total retinal detachment
	Drugs (phenothiazines, chloroquine)
	Cancer and melanoma associated retinopathy (CAR and MAR)
Normal *a* wave and reduced *b* wave	CSNB
	X-linked juvenile retinoschisis
	Central retinal vein or artery occlusion (ischaemic)
	Myotonic dystrophy
	Oguchi's disease
	Quinine toxicity
Abnormal phototopic and normal scotopic ERGs	Achromatopsia
	Cone dystrophy
Reduced oscillatory potentials	In diabetic patients can correlate with an increased risk of developing severe proliferative diabetic retinopathy

Electrodiagnostic tests (2)

Pattern electroretinogram

Indication
- Objective assessment of central retinal function.

Method
A reverse chequerboard evokes the small potentials that arise from the inner retina.

Results
A prominent positive component at 50ms (P50) and a larger negative component at 95ms (N95) is demonstrated.

Interpretation
P50 is driven by macular photoreceptors and can be a key to macular function. N95 appears to identify the retinal ganglion cells.

Multifocal electroretinogram

Unlike standard ERG, which sums the electrical potentials from the whole retina, multifocal ERG creates a topographical map of visual function of the whole retina.

Indication
- Can be used in almost any retinal disorder; especially useful where retinal dysfunction is localized or patchy.

Method
Multiple small areas of the retina (100µm in diameter) are stimulated with appropriately scaled stimuli. Fourier transformation of the responses result in topographical localization of visual function as it varies across the retina.

Results
A 2-dimensional map demonstrates the topographical variation in ERG responses across the retina.

Interpretation
The multifocal ERG can be transformed into a 3-dimensional map of vision that resembles the hill of vision. A further transformation showing the differences between the recorded mfERG and a reference mfERG (from normal subjects) can be used to highlight areas of visual loss.

Electro-oculography

This indirectly measures the standing potential of the eye (approximately 6mV). It reflects the activity of the RPE and photoreceptors of the entire retina.

Indications
- Diagnosis of certain macular dystrophies (Best's disease).
- Aid diagnosis of CSNB and X-linked retinoschisis.
- Early detection/screening of individuals at risk (e.g. Best's disease).

Method

Electrodes are attached to the medial and lateral canthi. Patients fixate target lights that move from right to left over 30° horizontal distance. The cornea makes the nearest electrode positive to the other. The potential difference between the two electrodes is amplified and recorded. The test is performed in the dark and light adapted states.

Results

Results are expressed: light peak/dark trough × 100 = Arden index.

Interpretation

Normally the potential doubles from the dark-adapted to the light-adapted eye: >185% is considered to be normal, <165% abnormal.

Visual evoked potentials

VEP is a gross electrical response recorded from the visual cortex in response to a changing visual stimulus, such as multiple flash or chequerboard pattern stimuli. It can be thought of as a limited EEG. Useful in uncooperative or unconscious patients.

Indications

- Optic nerve disease, particularly subclinical demyelination.
- Chiasmal and retro-chiasmal dysfunction.
- Detection of non-organic visual loss.

Method

A reversing black and white chequerboard or grating is used. The voltage changes vary with time and are plotted as waveforms. As it reflects the central 6–10° of the visual field it corresponds to cone activity.

Results

A positive deflection occurs at about 100ms (P100). Negative deflections occur at N75 and N135.

Interpretation

Decreased amplitude and increased latency of P100 in optic nerve dysfunction. However, delays are also common in macular dysfunction; therefore, a delayed VEP should not be considered pathognomonic of optic nerve disease.

Fig. 2.16 Typical PERG and VEP in a normal patient.

Electrodiagnostic tests (3)

Dark adaptometry

This measures the absolute threshold of photoreceptor activity with time in the dark adapted eye. It is used in conjunction with the EOG and ERG.

Goldmann–Weekers adaptometry

Indications

- Retinal disorders causing night blindness.
- Cone dysfunction.
- Evaluation of drugs affecting dark adaption (vitamin A analogues such as isoretinoin).

Method

Subjects are totally light bleached by a bright background light, which is then extinguished. In the dark they are then presented with a series of dim flashes. The threshold value for which the light is perceived is then plotted against time.

Results

A biphasic curve is plotted. The first curve represents the cone threshold (reached at 5–10min), the next represents the rod threshold, which is reached at 30min. Rhodopsin has now fully regenerated and retinal sensitivity has reached its peak.

Interpretation

Defects in rod metabolism that produce abnormally high threshold (higher than 10^2 log units) at 30min.

Ophthalmic radiology: X-ray, DCG, and DSG

X-ray orbits

Indications

Although plain X-rays have been largely superseded by CT and MRI, plain films may be useful in excluding a radio-opaque FB (which may preclude an MRI). Other pathology (e.g. orbital fractures) may be identifiable on plain X-ray, but generally require further characterization by CT or MRI.

Method

Commonly used views include occipitomental (Water's view), overtilted occipitomental and lateral. If an IOFB is suspected upgaze and downgaze views may show a change in position of a radio-opaque IOFB.

Dacryocystography

Requires the injection of radio-opaque contrast medium (oil-based) into the lacrimal drainage system. The technique is similar to syringing the tear ducts. A DCG causes a typical effective dose of X-ray irradiation equal to 6–12mths of natural atmospheric radiation.

Indications

- Aid diagnosis of epiphora.
- Plan surgical procedures.

Method

The puncta are intubated with polyethylene tubing, a plain film X-ray is taken. With the patient supine, a radio-opaque contrast is then injected simultaneously into both lacrimal systems and further series of X-ray films is taken.

Results

Contrast is seen in the fornices, canaliculi, common canaliculi, and nasolacrimal ducts if bilateral systems are patent. Can identify the level of obstruction and distinguish masses, stenosis, or fistulae.

Interpretation

A blockage or filling defect at any level will be seen if pathology is present. Reflux of contrast is nearly always pathological.

Dacryoscintigraphy

This lacrimal drainage scintigraphic technique is useful as a physiological test of tear flow through the lacrimal system.

Indications

- Aid diagnosis of 'functional' epiphora.
- Helps plan surgical procedures.

Method
The patient is sitting upright in front of a pinhole collimator and camera. A drop of a radioactive tracer isotope (usually technetium-99m) is placed in the inferior fornix of both eyes. The patient remains still and blinks normally. The distribution of the tracer is imaged every 10s for the first 2–3min, then at 5, 10, 15, and 20min.

Results
Time–activity curves for asymptomatic normals have a large variation. Abnormal tests are split into 'presac', 'preductal', or 'intraductal' delay. Failure for the tracer to reach the lacrimal sac by the end of the study is termed pre-sac delay. Preductal delay with early filling of the lacrimal sac, but no sign of sac emptying at 5min. Intraductal delay is defined as tracer in the upper part of the lacrimal system, but no further drainage over 15min.[1]

Interpretation
DSG is useful for proximal obstruction, which may be masked in the DCG by overvigorous injection of dye into the lacrimal system.

1. Wearne MJ et al. Comparision of dacryocystography and lacrimal seintigraphy in the diagnosis of functional nasolacrimal duct obstruction Br J Ophthalmol 1999; **83**:1032.

Ophthalmic radiology: CT and CTA

Computerized tomography (CT)

CT is useful for detecting a wide range of orbital and intracranial pathology. A CT head causes a typical effective dose of X-ray irradiation equal to 10mths of natural background radiation.

Indications
- Orbital cellulitis
- Orbital lesions
- Orbital trauma
- Intracranial lesions
- Detection of FB
- Cerebrovascular accidents
- Contraindication to MRI.

Method
CT involves the rotation of a tightly collimated X-ray beam and detector around the patient. From the data gained in different projections an image of a single plane ('slice') is reconstructed. A series of slices are recorded through the area of interest.

Interpretation
Visualization of the bony orbit and lesions with calcification makes this a good technique for the orbit and globe. The planes that CT can image in are limited; however, additional projections can be reconfigured by computer.

Caution
Diabetic patients with normal renal function should have metformin stopped 48h after radio-opaque contrast media to reduce risk of developing metformin associated lactic acidosis. In addition, IV contrast may aggravate pre-existing renal disease. Both renal function and use of metformin should be highlighted to the radiology team.

Computerized tomography angiography (CTA)

Indications
- Intracranial aneurysms
- Vascular lesions
- Neurosurgical planning.

Method
High-resolution thin cut CT scan combined with IV contrast media injection.

Results
Excellent vasculature anatomy in 3 dimensions combined with adjacent bony structure. Helps delineate borders of aneurysms in relation to the subarachnoid space to help surgical approach planning. Useful in small aneurysms of the circle of Willis.

Ophthalmic radiology: MRI and MRA/V

Magnetic resonance imaging

Tissue exposed to a short electromagnetic pulse undergoes rearrangement of its hydrogen nuclei. When the pulse subsides, the nuclei return to their normal resting state, re-radiating some energy they have absorbed. Sensitive receivers pick up this EM echo. T1 and T2 times are two complex parameters that depend on proton density, tissue components and their magnetic properties.

Indications

- Optic nerve disease such as glioma, intracranial extension of orbital tumours, and suspected compressive optic neuropathy.
- In retrobulbar neuritis the presence of multiple white matter plaques is predictive of the development of clinical MS.
- Suspected lesions of the chiasm such as pituitary tumours.
- Intracranial aneurysms.

Method

Conventional sequences are T1- and T2-weighted tests determined by the examining radiologist based on the clinical situation. In addition orbital imaging uses specialized fat suppression techniques, which is useful for optic nerve visualization, usually masked by the high signals from orbital fat.

Diffusion weighted, or diffusion tensor, MRI sequences (image Brownian motion within tissues) were initially found to be useful in acute strokes. More recently the technique has been shown to be useful for intracranial abscesses and distinguishing an epidermoid from an arachnoid cyst.

IV paramagnetic gadolinium is used as 'contrast'. Gadolinium enhanced scans are useful in the detection of blood–brain barrier abnormalities, inflammatory changes, and increased vascularity.

Results

Box 2.4 Characteristics of T1- and T2-weighted scans

T1	T2
Excellent anatomical detail	More pathological detail seen
CSF and vitreous low intensity signal (black)	CSF and vitreous have high intensity signal (white)
White matter (light grey)	White matter (dark grey)
Grey matter (grey)	Grey matter (grey)

Interpretation

Always review your own scans in conjunction with the radiology team. It is also important to consider the quality of the scan (e.g. adequate slices, appropriate use of contrast/processing), especially when unexpectedly 'normal'.

Caution

Gadolinium-based contrast medium (Gd-CM) can precipitate nephrogenic systemic fibrosis. It can be delayed, progressive and fatal. It is mandatory to screen for renal dysfunction before Gd-CM are used.[1]

Box 2.5 Advantages and disadvantages of MRI (compared with CT)

Advantages	Disadvantages
No ionizing radiation	Contraindicated in patients with pacemakers,
More sensitive than CT for	metallic FBs, magnetic aneurysm clips, cochlear
early tumours	implants, and transcutaneous neural stimulators.
Excellent for surgical planning	Recent haemorrhage not imaged
Excellent anatomical views	Requires patient cooperation (steady fixation to
High contrast sensitivity	prevent ocular movement degrading image)
Multiplanar imaging capability	Noise and claustrophobia
	Not approved for the first trimester of pregnancy

Magnetic resonance angiography

MRA is a non-invasive method of imaging the intra- and extracranial carotid and vertebrobasilar circulations. The principle of the computerized image construction is based on the haemodynamic properties of flowing blood, rather than on vessel anatomy.

Indications

Demonstrates abnormalities such as stenosis, occlusion, arteriovenous malformations, and aneurysms.

Methods

MRA is usually a static evaluation; however, time resolved MRA can be useful as it highlights the separate arterial and venous supplies to an intracranial AVM.

Disadvantages

Cannot detect aneurysms less than 5mm in diameter. Long acquisition time. Unable to detect intravascular calcifications. Unable to image vessels and bone together. Conventional intra-arterial angiography remains the gold standard for accurate diagnosis and surgical planning for berry aneurysms.

Magnetic resonance venography

MRV is similar to MRA but the imaging is 'gated' to the speed of venous flow. It is useful in identifying venous thromboses (e.g. sagittal sinus thrombosis). It is, therefore, commonly performed in cases of idiopathic intracranial hypertension.

1. BFCR (07)14 The Royal College of Radiologists, Nov 07. Available at http:// www.rcr.ac.uk

Ophthalmic radiology: MRI of the normal brain

Fig. 2.17 MRI of a normal brain (sagittal section).

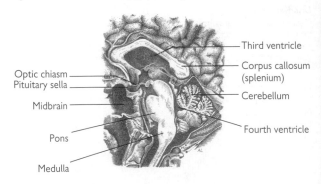

Fig. 2.18 Illustration corresponding to Fig 2.17 with key structures identified.

Trauma

Ocular trauma: assessment

Box 3.1 An approach to assessing ocular trauma

Incident	Date, time, place, witness history (if assault or paediatric case), mechanism of injury, associated head injury (loss of consciousness, nausea, vomiting, fits), other injuries
Symptoms	↓VA (sudden/gradual), floaters, flashes, field defects, diplopia, pain
POH	Previous/current eye disease
PMH	Any systemic disease, tetanus status
SH	Family support, alcohol/drug abuse
FH	Family history of eye disease
Dx	Drugs
Ax	Allergies
GCS	Conscious level
Visual function	VA, RAPD, colour vision, visual fields to confrontation ± formal perimetry
Orbits	Continuity of orbital rim, infraorbital sensation
Soft tissues	Periorbital bruising/oedema/surgical emphysema, lid lacerations
Globes	Proptosis/enophthalmos/hypoglobus, pulsatility
Motility	Mechanical restriction or paretic muscle
Conjunctiva	Diffuse/defined subconjunctival haemorrhage, laceration, ischaemia
Cornea	Abrasion or full thickness laceration (sealed/leaking), FB, rust-ring, infiltrate, oedema, limbitis
AC	Depth, flare, cells (erythrocytes, leucocytes), pigment
Gonioscopy	(may need to be deferred) angle recession/dialysis, FB in angle
Iris	Anisocoria, traumatic mydriasis, iridodialysis, iridodonesis, transillumination defect, FB
Lens	Cataract, FB, phacodonesis, subluxation, Vossius ring (iris pigment imprinted on anterior capsule)
Tonometry	Applanation (may need to be deferred); if IOP consider penetrating injury, retinal detachment
Vitreous	Haemorrhage, pigment, posterior vitreous detachment
Fundus	Retinal oedema (commotio retinae), haemorrhage, tear, detachment, dialysis; choroidal rupture; exit wound; optic nerve avulsion
Indirect ophthalmoscopy	(indentation may need to be deferred)

Documentation

Careful assessment and accurate documentation is critical. Legal proceedings often follow trauma cases. Clinical photographs can be very helpful.

Investigations

- If the eye cannot be examined due to soft tissue swelling or no fundal view is possible due to opaque media consider B-scan US (use water bath) ± CT scan to identify gross intraocular/orbital pathology.
- CT orbits/face/head is also valuable in IOFBs, orbital/maxillofacial fractures and associated cerebral injuries. Ask for 2mm slices to reduce the risk of missing a small IOFB. MRI should be avoided in cases where a ferromagnetic IOFB is suspected. Facial X-rays may assist in diagnosing radio-opaque IOFB (upgaze/downgaze views) and orbital fractures; it has largely been replaced by CT.
- If there is suspected globe rupture, manipulation must be kept to a minimum. This includes deferring gonioscopy, scleral indentation, and even tonometry.

Tetanus status and prophylaxis

Current immunization protocol

Tetanus vaccines

- *For children*: adsorbed tetanus vaccine is given as part of DTPer at 2mths, 3mths, and 4mths of age followed by booster doses at school entry (DTPer) and school leaving (diphtheria (low dose) and tetanus).
- *For non-immune adolescents/adults*: three doses of 0.5ml IM diphtheria (low dose) and tetanus separated by 4wks with a booster after 10yrs.

Definitions

- *Immune*: primary immunization is complete (three doses) and within 10yrs of a booster dose, or if the patient has received a total of five doses.
- *Tetanus-prone wound*: wound is septic, devitalized, soil-contaminated, puncture wound or significant delay before surgery (>6h).
- *Very high-risk wound*: unusual in ophthalmology but would include injuries such as major facial trauma with soil contamination.

Treatment

Table 3.1 Treatment of open wounds

Patient	Wound	Action
Immune	Clean	Nil needed
	Tetanus-prone	Clean/debride wound as required
		Give tetanus immunoglobulin only if very high risk. Consider antibiotic prophylaxis (e.g. coamoxiclav)
Non-immune	Clean	Immediate dose of vaccine followed by completion of standard schedule (by GP)
	Tetanus-prone	Clean/debride wound as required
		Immediate dose of vaccine (as above) and tetanus immunoglobulin (at a different site), followed by completion of standard schedule (by GP). Consider antibiotic prophylaxis (e.g. coamoxiclav)
Uncertain of vaccination status	Clean	As for non-immune patients with clean wounds. Request GP to check medical records and complete standard schedule if necessary
	Tetanus-prone	As for non-immune patients with tetanus-prone wounds. Request GP to check medical records and complete standard schedule if necessary

If tetanus vaccine indicated it should be given immediately. Immunoglobulin should be given at a different site to vaccine.

Table 3.2 Summary of indications for tetanus prophylaxis

Risk		Treatment required		
Patient	Wound	Vaccine	Immunoglobulin	Completion of course by GP
Immune	Clean	No	No	No
	Tetanus-prone	No	Yes if very high risk	No
Non-immune	Clean	Yes	No	Yes
	Tetanus-prone	Yes	Yes	Yes
Uncertain of vaccination status	Clean	Yes	No	Yes if needed
	Tetanus-prone	Yes	Yes	Yes if needed

Chemical injury: assessment

For chemical injuries, treat first, ask questions later (see Chemical injury treatment, 📖 p.98).

Chemical injuries are among the most destructive of all traumatic insults suffered by the eye. They may occur in domestic, industrial, and military settings. Alkalis cause liquefactive necrosis and thus penetrate the eye to a greater extent than acids, which cause coagulative necrosis and so impede their own progress.

Prognostic factors

The severity of a chemical corneal injury is determined by the following:
- *pH*: alkaline agents generally cause more severe injuries than acids, although very acidic solutions may behave similarly; most domestic chemical agents are alkaline (or neutral) rather than acidic.
- *Duration of contact.*
- *Corneal involvement*: surface area, duration of contact.
- *Limbal involvement*: corneal re-epithelialization relies on migration of the limbal stem cells.
- *Conjunctival involvement*: blind ended sacs that may retain chemical and cause continuing ocular damage.
- *Associated non-chemical injury*: blunt trauma, thermal injury.

Clinical features

- Conjunctival injection or ischaemia (beware the 'white' eye) ± chemosis, haemorrhage, epithelial defects, ulceration, necrosis, or complete loss of conjunctiva; perilimbal ischaemia/limbitis (blanched vessels with no visible blood flow); corneal epitheliopathy (punctate to complete loss; **NB** may stain poorly with fluorescein); corneal oedema; corneal stromal necrosis; AC activity and fibrin; traumatic mydriasis, ↑IOP (consider Tonopen rather than Goldmann); rarely scleral necrosis, vitritis, necrotic retinopathy.

Classification of severity

The Roper-Hall classification (Table 3.3) assesses the state of the cornea and limbus, whereas the Dua classification (Table 3.4) assesses the limbus and conjunctiva (with a view to predicting prognosis from the extent of stem cell loss).

Table 3.3 Classification of severity of ocular surface burns (Roper-Hall classification[1])

Grade	Corneal appearance	Limbal ischaemia	Prognosis
Grade I	Clear cornea	Nil	Good
Grade II	Hazy cornea: Iris details visible	<1/3	Good
Grade III	Opaque cornea: Iris details obscured	1/3 to 1/2	Guarded
Grade IV	Opaque cornea: Iris details obscured	>1/2	Poor

1. Roper-Hall MJ. Thermal and chemical burns. *Trans Ophthalmol Soc UK* 1965; **85**:631.

Table 3.4 Alternative classification of ocular surface burns highlighting limbal involvement (Dua classification[2])

Grade	Limbal involvement	Conjunctival involvement	Prognosis
Grade I	0 clock hours	0%	Very good
Grade II	≤3 clock hours	≤30%	Good
Grade III	>3–6 clock hours	>30–50%	Good
Grade IV	>6–9 clock hours	>50–75%	Good–guarded
Grade V	>9–12 clock hours	>75–<100%	Guarded–poor
Grade VI	12 clock hours (total)	100% (total)	Very poor

The above information can also be presented in component form, e.g. 4.5/40 indicates 4.5 clock hours of limbus and 40% conjunctiva involved. Conjunctiva refers to bulbar conjunctiva up to and including the forncies.

2. Dua *et al. A* new classification of ocular surface burns. *Br J Ophthalmol* 2001;**85**:1379–83.

Complications
- *Conjunctival burns*: cicatrization (scarring), symblepharon formation, loss of goblet cells, keratinization.
- *Significant limbal ischaemia*: conjunctivalization, vascularization, and opacification of the cornea.
- *Full thickness burns*: scleritis, vitritis, retinitis, glaucomatous optic neuropathy or hypotony, iris, ciliary, and lenticular damage; may progress to phthisis bulbi; very poor prognosis.
- *Periorbital burns*: first/second/third degree chemical burns of periorbital tissues.

Chemical injury: treatment

Immediate

- Neutralization of pH by irrigation before full history and examination.

Immediate irrigation

This is probably the most important determinant of outcome.

- Test pH, then instil topical anaesthetic (e.g. proxymetacaine), insert a speculum and irrigate with water or normal saline through IV tubing and deliver a minimum of 2 litres or until normal pH is restored. Delay to obtain irrigants other than water is not warranted.

Inspection

Evert the lids (double evert the upper lid) and inspect the fornices. Remove retained particulate matter that may perpetuate alkalinity (e.g. lime, cement).

Indicator test

Test pH at end of irrigation and 5min after completion of irrigation.

- If pH neutral/near neutral (normal tears may be slightly alkaline), then you may begin examination and initiate further treatment. However, recheck pH after 20min.
- If pH abnormal, then repeat irrigation cycle (with another 2 litres) until pH normal.
- pH should be recorded on a daily basis until ocular surface is healed (to exclude release of chemical from inherent forniceal particles of chemical).

Acute: all injuries

- *Admit* if severe or any other concerns.
- *Topical antibiotics*: prophylaxis (e.g. preservative free chloramphenicol 0.5% 4×/d).
- *Topical cycloplegia* for comfort/AC activity (e.g. preservative-free cyclopentolate 1% 3×/d or atropine 1% once daily).
- *Topical lubricants*: (preservative free, e.g. carmellose (Celluvisc®) 1–4 hourly day and night + liquid paraffin nocte).
- *Oral analgesia*: (e.g. paracetamol ± codeine).

Topical medication should be preservative free where possible.

Acute: severe injuries

Admit and consider:

- Topical steroids (e.g. prednisolone 0.5–1% initially 4–8×/d for <10d).
- Topical ascorbic acid (e.g. sodium ascorbate 10% up to 2-hourly for <10d).
- Oral ascorbic acid (e.g. 1g 2×/day).
- Systemic tetracyclines, e.g. doxycycline 100mg 1×/d or oxytetracycline 500mg 4×/d for 3mths (tetracyclines contraindicated in children <12, in pregnant/breast-feeding women, and in hepatic and renal impairment).

Ascorbic acid is essential for collagen formation and is an effective scavenger of damaging free radicals; it should not be used in acid chemical burns. Doxycycline is a proteinase inhibitor and serves to not only prevent tissue necrosis and facilitate healing, but also has anti-inflammatory properties.

Less commonly used are topical sodium citrate 10% (reduces neutrophil chemotaxis and inhibits collagenases, but is painful). Paracentesis and replacement of aqueous with a buffered phosphate solution can help to normalize the AC pH more quickly.[1]

Acute: injuries with ↑IOP

Acetazolamide 250mg 4×/d ± topical β-blocker (e.g. preservative-free timolol 0.5% 2×/d).

Long-term: complicated cases

Poor corneal healing

Medical treatment as for persistent epithelial defects (📖 p.214). Surgical treatment includes techniques to assist epithelial migration (amniotic membrane transplantation) and re-epithelialization of the cornea (limbal stem cell transplantation; see Limbal stem cell deficiency, 📖 p.216).

Obliterated fornices and pseudopterygium formation

Consider

- pseudopterygium excision together with conjunctival autograft (if adequate host conjunctiva) or amniotic membrane facilitated by anti-proliferatives (intra-operative mitomycin C), and
- forniceal reconstructive surgery, including division of symblepharon and mucous membrane or amniotic membrane grafting.

Corneal opacification

Consider penetrating keratoplasty if adequate tear film and limbal stem cell population. In bilateral cases, keratoprosthesis remains a surgical option in severely damaged eyes.

Table 3.5 Strong acids and alkalis in common use

Substance	Chemical	pH
Common alkalis		
Oven cleaning fluid	Sodium hydroxide	14
Drain cleaning fluid	Sodium (or potassium) hydroxide	14
Plaster	Calcium hydroxide	14
Fertilizers (some)	Ammonium hydroxide	13
Common acids		
Battery fluid	Sulphuric acid	1
Lavatory cleaning fluid	Sulphuric acid	1
Bleach	Sodium hypochlorite	1
Pool cleaning fluid	Sodium (or calcium) hypochlorite	1

1. Paterson CA *et al.* Aqueous humor pH changes after experimental alkali burns. *Am J Ophthalmol* 1975;**79**: 414.

Thermal injury/burns (1)

It is vital to first assess the extent of the burns injury. If there is any suspicion from the history or examination that the mouth/airways may have been involved, immediate anaesthetic assistance is mandatory with a view to assessing and stabilizing the airway. Inhalational burns injuries can lead to airway oedema and fatal airways/respiratory compromise.

Assessment

Thermal injuries most commonly affect the lids, but cornea and conjunctiva may also be involved, They range from the mild and visually insignificant to the severe and blinding.

Assessment of burns to the lids is performed in the standard manner used for cutaneous burns elsewhere: superficial/partial thickness/full thickness. Assessment of burns to the globe requires careful slit-lamp examination in a similar manner to that used for chemical injuries (see Chemical injury assessment, 📖 p.96).

Assessment of the ocular thermal burns must be taken in context with whole body involvement, i.e. estimation of total body surface area involvement. *Proportion of each body area is dependent on age*: face is 19% total body surface area of child <1yr of age, 13% of a 5–9yrs old and only 7% of an adult.

Clinical features

Corneal and ocular surface

Direct contact thermal injury
- Keratopathy:
  - spectrum ranges from mild punctuate/confluent defects (e.g. most cigarette ash injuries), to severe limbitis and permanent opacification, stromal melting or perforation (e.g. from molten metal, which may form a complete cast between lid and globe);
  - associated features include conjunctival injection, ischaemia (the eye may be white), chemosis, necrosis and cataract (if severe).

Secondary exposure
- Exposure keratopathy may occur acutely if there is significant loss of lid tissue, or as a late complication of lid cicatrization.

Lids

- *Superficial (1st degree) burns*: commonly caused by sunburn or short-duration flash burns. Dry burns with oedema and no blistering; erythema and pain are common; heals in ≤1wk accompanied by superficial peeling, and no scar formation (although discoloration may occur).
- *Partial thickness (2nd degree) burns*: causes include longer duration scalds and flame injury. Blisters and weeping of the skin; intense erythema; significant pain and temperature sensitivity. Heals in 1–4wks with little scarring but pigmentary changes common.
- *Full thickness (3rd degree) burns*: commonly caused by chemical, electrical, flame, and scald injuries. Skin appears dry, inflexible and leathery with little/no pain. Heals with significant cicatrization and scarring.

Thermal injury/burns (2)

Management

Systemic

Liaise with a burns specialist to optimize systemic care, and preferably for admission to a specialist burns unit. Some general principles are included below:

Resuscitation with IV fluids

Fluid resuscitation is critical within the first 24h. The amount of fluid resuscitation can be determined from the percentage of body surface area (%BSA) involved.

- *Estimate %BSA by the 'Rule of 9's':*
  - Rule of 9's for adults: 9% for each arm, 18% for each leg, 9% for head,18% for front torso, 18% for back torso.
  - Rule of 9's for children: 9% for each arm, 14% for each leg, 18% for head, 18% for front torso, 18% for back torso.
- *Estimate fluid replacement by the Parkland Formula:*
  - Fluid for first 24h (ml) = 4 × patient's weight in kg × %BSA.
  - Give 50% of this fluid in the first 8h, and the remaining 50% in the next 16h.

General skin care

- Air-fluidized bed if large BSA involved.
- Reverse barrier nursing.
- Leave intact blisters and gently remove necrotic skin only.
- Simple emollients, e.g. 50:50 white soft paraffin:liquid paraffin applied to the burns.
- *Dressings*: non-adherent, e.g. Jelonet®/Mepitel® (daily changes) or Acticoat Silver® (change every 2–3d).
- Isotonic, sterile saline to irrigate mouth, nostrils, eyes, and anogenital areas frequently.

Management of corneal and ocular surface thermal injuries

Essentially as for chemical injuries (see Chemical injury treatment, 📖 p.98), but limited role for irrigation. In summary:

- *Topical antibiotics*: prophylaxis (e.g. preservative free chloramphenicol 0.5% 4×/d).
- *Topical cycloplegia* for comfort/AC activity (e.g. preservative-free cyclopentolate 1% 3×/d or atropine 1% 2×/d).
- *Topical lubricants* (preservative-free, e.g. carmellose (Celluvisc®) 1–4-hourly + liquid paraffin nocte).
- *Oral analgesia* (e.g. paracetamol ± codeine).

Topical medication should be preservative free where possible. In more severe cases consider similar strategies to those used for chemical injuries, including systemic ascorbic acid, tetracyclines, and ocular surface protection, including the use of amniotic membrane overlay (see Amniotic membrane transplantation, 📖 p.250).

NB Symblepharon formation can occur and early removal of pseudomembrane formation and surgical division of acute forniceal adhesions may be necessary.

Management of lid thermal injuries
- *Superficial burns*: cool compresses; lubrication; pain control.
- Partial thickness burns: topical antibiotic ointment; copious lubrication ± occlusion dressing or moisture chamber; trim eyelashes if singed (lash particles cause irritation); consider lid suture or temporary tarsorrhaphy if risk of corneal exposure.
- Full thickness burns: As above + debride dead tissue and eschar; protect the eye with lubrication, Jelonet and Geliperm® dressings, and tarsorrhaphy. Refer to oculoplastic team for specialist assessment, including skin grafting.

Complications
- *Loss of lid tissue*: leads to corneal exposure.
- *Lid cicatrization*: leads to entropion/ectropion, trichiasis, and corneal exposure.
- *Epiphora* from damage to the punctae/lacrimal ducts.
- *Conjunctival burns*: cicatricial changes, symblepharon, and severe dry eye (through damage to goblet cells, accessory lacrimal and meibomian glands).
- *Significant limbal ischaemia*: conjunctivalization, vascularization, and opacification of the cornea.

Orbital fractures: assessment

Assessment

Table 3.6 Specific features in assessment of potential orbital fractures

Hx	Mechanism of injury
	Diplopia, areas of numbness, epistaxis, visual symptoms (associated ocular injury)
O/E	Pain, periorbital bruising/oedema/haemorrhage, surgical emphysema, globe position, globe pulsation, ocular motility, subconjunctival haemorrhage, discontinuity of orbital rim
	Any associated ocular injury
	Any potential cervical or head injury (refer to trauma team); collapse may be due to oculocardiac reflex secondary to EOM entrapment
Ix	Facial X-rays: droplet sign (soft tissue prolapse in orbital floor fracture); fluid level in maxillary sinus; visible fracture.
	CT (2mm coronal slices): identify fractures (bony windows), prolapsed orbital fat/extraocular muscles and haemorrhage.
	Hess/Lees and Fields of Binocular vision tests show characteristic mechanical restrictive patterns and allow monitoring of recovery

Clinical features

Orbital floor (maxillary bone)

This is the commonest orbital fracture. It usually follows a blow from an object >5cm (e.g. tennis ball/fist). The force may be transmitted by hydraulic compression of globe/orbital structures ('blow-out') or may be directly transmitted along the orbital rim.

- Soft tissue: periorbital bruising/oedema/haemorrhage, surgical emphysema.
- Vertical diplopia due to mechanical restriction of upgaze. This may be secondary to tissue entrapment following prolapse through the bony defect (persistent) or soft tissue swelling tenting the extraocular muscle insertion (transient).
- Enophthalmos.
- Infraorbital anaesthesia due to nerve damage in infraorbital canal.

Medial wall (ethmoidal)

Medial wall fractures are rare as an isolated feature but they may accompany orbital floor fractures.

- Soft tissue signs as for orbital floor fractures but surgical emphysema may be prominent.
- Horizontal diplopia due to mechanical restriction from medial rectus entrapment.

Orbital roof (frontal)

Orbital roof fractures are very rare as an isolated feature. They are most commonly seen in children following brow trauma.

- Soft tissue signs as for orbital floor fractures but bruising may spread across midline.
- Superior subconjunctival haemorrhage with no distinct posterior limit.

- Inferior/axial globe displacement.
- May have bruit/pulsation due to communication with CSF; carry risk of meningitis.

Lateral wall (zygomatic arch)

The lateral wall is very robust and acts as a protective shield to the globe. Lateral wall fractures are usually only seen following major maxillofacial trauma.

Orbital fractures: treatment

All orbital fractures

- Advise patients to refrain from nose blowing, which may contribute to surgical emphysema and herniation.
- Consider antibiotic prophylaxis: commonly anaerobic cover is prescribed (e.g. co-amoxiclav) but limited evidence for any benefit.
- Refer to orbital or maxillofacial team for consideration of surgical repair.
- Arrange orthoptic follow-up to monitor recovery/postoperative course.

Fractures of the orbital floor

Table 3.7 Indications for surgical intervention in orbital floor fractures

Immediate	Persistent oculocardiac reflex
	Young patient with 'white-eyed' trap-door fracture (orbital floor buckling occurring in children)
	Significant facial asymmetry
Early (<2wks)	Persistent symptomatic diplopia
	Significant enophthalmos
	Hypoglobus
	Progressive infraorbital hyposthesia
Observation	Minimal diplopia (e.g. just in upgaze)
	Minimal restriction
	Minimal enophthalmos

Box 3.2 Outline of repair for orbital floor fractures

- Use a subciliary or transconjunctival incision to expose the inferior orbital rim.
- Incise the periosteum 2mm outside the orbital rim and dissect posteriorly, elevating the periorbita/periosteum off the orbital floor.
- Carefully release all herniated orbital contents taking care to separate from infraorbital nerve and vessels.
- Continue until the whole fracture has been exposed.
- Repair bony defect with an implant (e.g. Teflon, Supramyd) with an overlap of ≥5mm, which should be fixed in position.
- Close periosteum with absorbable suture (e.g. 4-0 vicryl).
- Close subciliary/transconjunctival incision.

Lid lacerations

Lacerations involving the eyelid are common, occurring in the context of both blunt and sharp injuries. They carry morbidity in their own right and may be associated with significant injuries of globe or orbit.

Lid lacerations require careful exploration and precise closure, particularly at the lid margin.

Assessment

Box 3.3	Specific features in assessment of lid lacerations
Hx	Mechanism of injury and likelihood of associated injuries (e.g. stab injuries), likely infective risk (e.g. bites)
O/E	Lid laceration (depth, length, tissue viability), lid position, orbicularis function, lagophthalmos, intercanthal distance
	Canalicular involvement, nasolacrimal drainage
	Beware: associated injury of globe or orbit
Ix	All stab injuries should have orbital X-ray and/or orbital and head CT (FBs, pneumocranium) and if associated globe/orbital injury suspected

Treatment

- *Prophylaxis*: protect cornea with generous lubrication; administer tetanus vaccine/immunoglobulin if indicated (see Tetanus status and prophylaxis, 🕮 p.94).
- *Surgery*: assess for surgical repair according to depth, extent of tissue loss, involvement of lid margin, and involvement of canaliculus.
- Complicated lid lacerations (e.g. involving lid margin or canaliculi) should be repaired in theatre by an experienced surgeon.

Table 3.8 Outline of repair for lid lacreations

Simple superficial not involving margin	Close with interrupted 6-0 sutures parallel to lid margin; absorbable (e.g. vicryl) are often preferred (especially for children) but non-absorbable (e.g. silk) may be used
Partial thickness	Small defect restricted to anterior lamella consider allowing repair by granulation
	Larger defect requires a reconstructive procedure
Full thickness with tissue loss	*Small defect (0–25% tissue loss):*
	Debride/freshen up wound edges; close with interrupted absorbable (e.g. 6-0 vicryl) sutures in 1 layer to tarsus and 1 layer to skin
	Large defect (25–60% tissue loss):
	Consider lateral canthotomy/cantholysis, Tenzel or McGregor myocutaneous flap
	Very large defect (>60% tissue loss):
	For lower lids consider Hughes tarsoconjunctival flap and skin graft or transposition skin flap or Mustarde myocutaneous flap
	For upper eyelids consider Cutler–Beard flap or Mustarde lid-switch (2-stage)
Involving margin	Debride/freshen up wound edges
	Place grey line suture (non-absorbable or absorbable e.g. 6-0 vicryl), leave long
	Close tarsus with interrupted absorbable suture (e.g. 6-0 vicryl)
	Place additional marginal suture (lash line) if required, leave long
	Close overlying skin with interrupted absorbable suture (e.g. 6-0 vicryl); these sutures should also catch the long ends of the marginal sutures to prevent corneal abrasion
Canalicular laceration	Internally splint the opened duct with silicone tubing, e.g. Mini Monoka stent .
	For upper and lower canalicular laceration consider bicanalicular intubation
	For lower lids consider reapposing medial edge of eyelid to posterior lacrimal crest
	Close laceration with 6-0 vicryl
	Leave silicone tubes *in situ* for 3mths
Postoperative	Topical antibiotic/lubrication (e.g. oc chloramphenicol 3×/d to wound and fornix for 1wk)
	Remove skin sutures at 5–7d

Blunt trauma: assessment

Traumatic eye injuries account for about 4500 admissions in the UK per year. They are commonly associated with more extensive injuries: ocular involvement occurs in about 10% of all non-fatal casualties. Most ocular trauma is blunt (80%) rather than penetrating (20%) with IOFBs occurring in 1%.

In the UK, legislation (notably the compulsory wearing of seatbelts and health and safety at work) has effectively reduced some sources of eye injuries, such that now most are related to sport or other leisure activities.

Assessment

Box 3.4 Specific features in assessment of blunt injury

Hx	Mechanism, associated injuries, tetanus status
O/E	*Globe*: look for anterior or posterior rupture *Cornea*: check fluorescein staining, clarity *AC*: check for cells/flare, and depth (compare with other eye) *Iris/ciliary body*: note abnormalities of pupil and examine iris root/angle by gonioscopy (if stable) *Lens*: opacity, position, stability *Vitreous*: PVD, haemorrhage *Fundus*: note commotio retinae (usually temporal); check macular pathology (e.g. hole); examine equator/periphery for retinal tears/dialysis; consider choroidal rupture (often masked by blood) *Optic nerve*: check function and disc appearance *IOP* *Beware*: 'occult' posterior rupture; check for associated orbital/adnexal injuries
Ix	Consider orbital/facial X-ray, B-scan US, CT orbits/brain (assess extent of damage particularly where clinical assessment limited)

Clinical features

Globe
- *Anterior rupture*: usually obvious with herniation of uveal tissue, lens and vitreous, and other signs of injury (e.g. severe subconjunctival haemorrhage, hyphaema, etc.).
- *Posterior rupture*: suspect if deep AC ± low IOP (compare with contralateral eye).

Anterior segment
- Corneal abrasion (epithelial defect, see Corneal foreign bodies and abrasions, 📖 p.118), corneal oedema (transient endothelial decompensation, spontaneously resolves).
- *Hyphaema*: red blood cells in the AC (see Hyphaema, 📖 p.120).
- *Iris*: miosis (usually transient), mydriasis (often permanent), and sphincter rupture (irregular pupil; permanent); iris root abnormalities include iridodialysis (dehiscence from ciliary body) and angle recession (late risk of glaucoma, see Other secondary open angle glaucoma, 📖 p.328).

- *Lens*: Vossius ring (imprint of iris pigment on anterior capsule), cataract (anterior or posterior subcapsular); subluxation/luxation of the lens.

Posterior segment
- *Vitreous*: posterior vitreous detachment, vitreous haemorrhage.
- *Commotio retinae*: grey–white retinal opaqueness as a result of fragmentation of the photoreceptor outer segments and intracellular oedema (photoreceptors and pigment epithelium); with increasing severity intraretinal haemorrhages.
  - In most cases commotio retinae completely resolves, but in a minority macular hole/pigmentary change ensues.
  - In extreme cases, such as where a projectile has grazed but not penetrated the globe, haemorrhagic necrosis of the choroid and retina may occur (chorioretinitis sclopetaria; *syn* chorioretinitis sclopteria).
- *Retinal dialysis*: full thickness circumferential break at the ora serrata; commonly superonasal (when traumatic). It is not related to PVD and thus progression to any retinal detachment is slow (several months); irregular retinal tear(s) may occur at the equator (*see* Retinal breaks, 📖 p.422).
- *Macular holes*: acute or late (*see* Macular hole, 📖 p.442).
- *Choroidal rupture*: rupture through choroid/Bruch's membrane/RPE but sclera intact; the rupture is usually concentric to the disk; it is usually obscured initially by overlying subretinal blood; later a white streak of sclera may be visible; CNV is a late complication.
- *Traumatic optic neuropathy*: acutely ↓optic nerve function (including RAPD) in presence of normal disc appearance; later disc pallor.
- *Optic nerve avulsion*: ↓/absent optic nerve function depending on completeness of avulsion; defect in place of optic disc; confirm on B-scan US if dense vitreous haemorrhage prevents clinical view.

Blunt trauma: treatment

Primary repair of globe rupture

- *Admit and prepare for GA*: nil by mouth, determine last meal/drink, liaise with anaesthetist, ECG/bloods (if indicated).
- *Prophylaxis*: protect globe with clear plastic shield systemic antibiotic (e.g. ciprofloxacin PO 750mg BD) ± preservative free topical antibiotic; administer tetanus vaccine/toxoid if indicated (see Tetanus status and prophylaxis, 📖 p.94).
- *Surgery*: assess and proceed with primary repair (Table 3.9).

Secondary repair

- *Iris*: most injuries involving the iris (other than herniation through a ruptured globe) do not require surgical intervention.
- *Lens*: significant lens injuries resulting in ↓VA (opacity, subluxation), ↑IOP (lens-related glaucoma, see 📖 p.326) or inflammation (breached capsule) warrant removal of the lens; some cases may require a vitreoretinal approach.
- *Vitreoretinal*: retinal tears or retinal dialysis require urgent referral for vitreoretinal assessment and repair; macular holes should also be referred but can generally be seen electively.

Other

- *Commotio retinae*: no treatment usually indicated as most spontaneously recover; some have persistent/late ↓VA due to macular hole/pigmentary change.
- *Choroidal rupture*: no treatment is indicated; however, if a CNV develops this can be treated in the conventional manner.
- *Traumatic optic neuropathy*: liaise with a neuro-ophthalmologist; 'megadose' systemic corticosteroids are sometimes given, which, while of proven benefit in spinal injuries, are unproven in traumatic optic neuropathy.

Penetrating trauma/IOFBs: assessment

Small (<2mm) FBs may leave a sealed wound and minimal clinical signs. Penetrating trauma should be excluded following injury from sharp objects and projectiles with high mass and/or velocity.

An IOFB must be excluded in all cases of penetration. Multiple IOFBs are not uncommon and some form of X-ray imaging should be carried out even in cases where an IOFB has been identified under direct vision.[1] Double perforation (through and through injury) should be considered even if IOFB is now within the globe. Posterior rupture following significant blunt trauma should always be considered.

Complications of IOFB injury (infection, retinal detachment, and toxicity) may have a more severe impact on visual outcome than the initial physical injury.[2] Occasionally iatrogenic penetrating injuries occur, e.g. in up to 1 in 1000 peribulbar injections.

Assessment

Box 3.5 Specific features in assessment of penetrating injury and IOFBs

Hx	*Source* (e.g. hammer on steel, machinery, explosive), probable IOFB material, likely toxicity and infective risk, tetanus status
O/E	*Entry site*: identify location and integrity (leak) of wound ↓ IOP
	Trajectory: look for iris hole (transillumination), focal cataract/lens tract, retinal haemorrhage
	Location: including gonioscopy and dilated fundoscopy
	Beware: occult IOFB in angle, ciliary body, pars plana
Ix	X-ray examination: orbital X-ray (in upgaze and downgaze) or CT with 2mm slices in all cases even if an IOFB is clearly visible
	US, VEP (chronic retained IOFB → reduced b wave)

Clinical features

Mechanical injury

- *Globe*: penetration, perforation or double perforation ('through and through') of corneosclera and uvea.
- *Anterior segment*: angle recession (late risk of glaucoma, *see* Other secondary open angle glaucoma, 📖 p.328; hyphaema, see 📖 p.120); lens capsule injury, cataract formation, zonular dehiscence, subluxation.
- *Posterior segment*: vitreous liquefaction, vitreous haemorrhage, abnormal vitreoretinal traction, retinal haemorrhage, retinal tear, retinal detachment.

Introduction of infection

Endophthalmitis, panophthalmitis.

Toxicity

Siderosis, chalcosis.

Siderosis (ferrous foreign body)

- Dissociated iron has a predilection for deposition in epithelial tissue (lens, RPE) causing metabolic toxicity and cellular death.
- RPE toxicity results in ↓VA, constricted VF and RAPD.
- Clinical features include injection, heterochromia (iris reddish brown), ↑IOP (secondary glaucoma), anterior capsular cataract, reddish ferrous deposits at lens epithelium, coarse degenerative pigment dispersion, retinal detachment. VEP shows b-wave attenuation.

Chalcosis (copper foreign body)

- Pure copper IOFBs result in rapid fulminant endophthalmitis.
- Chalcosis results from FB of alloys of copper (brass, bronze) and mirror the ocular signs of Wilson's disease: Kayser–Fleischer ring, anterior 'sunflower' cataract, yellow retinal plaques.

Box 3.6 Toxicity and IOFB

Inert ←- →Toxic			
Platinum	Aluminium	Iron	Copper
Silver	Zinc		Organic material
Gold	Nickel		Soil
Lead	Mercury		
Glass			
Plastic			
Stone			
Carbon			

1. Woodcock M *et al.* Mass and shape factors in intraocular foreign body injuries. *Ophthalmology* 2006;**113**:2262–9.

2. Roper-Hall MJ. Review of 555 cases of intra-ocular foreign body with special reference to prognosis. *Br J Ophthalmol* 1954;**38**:65–98.

Penetrating trauma/IOFBs: treatment

With penetrating injuries the urgent priority is to repair the integrity of the globe.

If present, IOFBs are ideally removed at the time of primary repair but closure of the globe should not be delayed if vitreoretinal expertise is not readily available. Similarly additional procedures (e.g. lensectomy, vitrectomy, retinal detachment repair) may be carried out at the time of primary repair, but are commonly deferred to a planned secondary rehabilitative procedure.[1,2]

General

- *Admit and prepare for GA*: nil by mouth, determine last meal/drink, liaise with anaesthetist, ECG/bloods (if indicated).
- *Prophylaxis*: protect globe with clear plastic shield systemic antibiotic (e.g. ciprofloxacin PO 750mg BD) ± preservative-free topical antibiotic; administer tetanus vaccine/toxoid if indicated (see Tetanus status and prophylaxis, 📖 p.94).
- *Surgery*: assess and proceed with primary repair, IOFB removal and any additional procedures required (Table 3.9).

Primary repair

Table 3.9 Primary repair

All wounds	Debride contaminated non-viable tissue Carefully maintain the AC to avoid expulsion of ocular contents
Small self-sealing corneal wound	Shelved corneal laceration with formed AC may not require formal closure Observe until healed; consider BCL and cover with adequate antibiotic cover
Corneal wound	May require AC deepening/stabilization with viscoelastic Return exposed viable iris tissue through perforation; abscise exposed tissue if non-viable Directly close corneal wound with perpendicular deep 10-0 nylon sutures and rotate sutures to bury knots Remove viscoelastic
Involving limbus	Expose adjacent sclera to determine full posterior extent of wound Start closure at limbus and proceed posteriorly
Scleral	Conjunctival peritomy, expose and explore sclera Return exposed viable uveal tissue through perforation Cut prolapsed vitreous flush to wound, taking care not to induce vitreous traction Direct scleral closure

IOFB removal

Table 3.10 IOFB removal

AC IOFB	Corneal approach; removal with fine forceps
Angle IOFB	Scleral trap-door approach
Lenticular IOFB	If in clear lens matter consider leaving *in situ* or remove with cautious cataract surgery (potential capsular and zonular instability)
Ciliary body IOFB	Cannot be directly visualized so consider using an electroacoustic locator and electromagnetic removal through scleral trap-door approach
Posterior segment IOFB	IOFB removal should be undertaken as soon as optimal surgical expertise and operating room conditions are available. Use an intraocular magnet or vitrectomy forceps. Reserve direct trans-scleral delivery for those IOFB that are easily accessible

Secondary procedures

Planned secondary repair of posterior segment trauma is usually performed 4–10d after initial injury after formation of PVD.

Secondary repair may be performed earlier in the presence of an IOFB (not removed at the primary repair), retinal detachment, or endophthalmitis. The timing of IOFB removal is a balance between the risk of infection and the ease of surgically inducing a PVD. However, in a recent large case-series, delayed IOFB removal was not found to be associated with increased presence of a PVD. It is, therefore, suggested that IOFB removal should be performed early. The risk of infection is significantly reduced by the use of systemic antibiotics.[1,2]

Secondary repair may include vitrectomy, membrane dissection (if proliferative vitreoretinopathy), encircling buckle (if breaks), lensectomy (if cataract; IOL commonly deferred), intravitreal antibiotics (if endophthalmitis), and tamponade (usually C3F8 or silicone oil).

Sympathetic ophthalmia

Sympathetic ophthalmia is a rare bilateral granulomatous panuveitis in which trauma to one eye may cause sight-threatening inflammation in the untraumatized 'sympathizing' eye. Its nature, clinical features, prophylaxis, and treatment are discussed elsewhere (see Sympathetic ophthalmia, 📖 p.390).

1. Woodcock M et al. Mass and shape factors in intraocular foreign body injuries. *Ophthalmology* 2006;**113**:2262–9.

2. Colyer MH et al. Delayed intraocular foreign body removal without endophthalmitis during Operations Iraqi Freedom and Enduring Freedom. *Ophthalmology* 2007;**114**:1439–47.

Corneal foreign bodies and abrasions

Corneal foreign bodies (FBs)

Most corneal FBs are metallic and only rarely cause infection. Microbial keratitis more commonly follows stone, ceramic, and organic FBs. Remember to exclude additional intraocular or subtarsal FB.

Clinical features

- Photophobia, pain, injection, lacrimation, blurred vision; history of projectile striking eye; failure to wear protective eye-wear while working, welding, hammering.
- FB ± rust ring (forms within 48h) or infiltrate; ± anterior uveitis.

Treatment

- *Removal*: explain what you are about to do and give them a target to stare at; instil topical anaesthetic (e.g. oxybuprocaine 0.4%); remove FB and rust ring under slit-lamp visualization (e.g. with 26-gauge needle).
- Topical antibiotic (e.g. chloramphenicol oc 1% 4×/d for 5d); consider short-term cycloplegic (for comfort/AC activity) and non-steroidal anti-inflammatory preparations.
- Warn the patient that their eye will be uncomfortable once the anaesthetic has worn off.

Corneal abrasions

Corneal abrasions are superficial corneal wounds. Corneal abrasions are common and often innocuous, but may cause severe pain and distress. Epithelial denuding exposes the stromal nocioreceptors triggering pain, photophobia, lacrimation, and increasing the risk of bacterial invasion.

Clinical features

- *Superficial/partial thickness corneal laceration*: differentiate from deeper partial/full thickness lacerations by careful oblique illumination of the wound tract and by the Seidel's test (identifies leaking full-thickness wounds); note depth + dimensions.
- *Complications*: microbial keratitis (see Microbial keratitis: assessment, 📖 p.194), recurrent erosions (especially if abrasion is large, ragged, involving the basement membrane, and in a predisposed patient) (see Recurrent corneal erosion syndrome, 📖 p.212).

Treatment

- Topical antibiotic (e.g. chloramphenicol oc 1% 4×/d for 3d); if there is associated infiltration treat as a microbial keratitis. Debride any rough devitalized (grey) tissue that may hamper re-epithelialization from ingrowth of neighbouring epithelium.
- *Supportive*: consider short-term topical cycloplegic (for comfort/ AC activity) and topical NSAIDs. Patching is not advisable for most abrasions as it has been shown to delay closure for abrasions <10mm. However, it may help make larger abrasions more comfortable.

Hyphaema

Blood in the anterior chamber (AC) is most commonly seen in the context of blunt trauma. It ranges from a relatively mild microhyphaema (erythrocytes suspended in the aqueous) to a total '8-ball' hyphaema where the AC fill is complete.

Box 3.7	Specific features in assessment of hyphaema
Hx	Mechanism of injury (potential for IOFB, globe rupture), ↓VA (stable, worsening may suggest rebleed), Sickle-cell status, risk factors, drug history (e.g. aspirin, NSAIDs, warfarin, etc.)
O/E	Measure/record depth/distribution of hyphaema, IOP, iris trauma/abnormality, (defer gonioscopy where possible)
	Dilated fundoscopy: rule out any posterior segment injury
Ix	Sickle-cell status;
	Consider B-scan US and CT to rule out additional globe/orbital injuries (particularly if adequate clinical assessment not possible)

Causes
- *Trauma*: blunt or penetrating.
- *Surgery*: e.g. trabeculectomy, iris manipulation procedures.
- *Spontaneous*: iris/angle neovascularization, haematological disease, tumour (e.g. juvenile xanthogranuloma), IOL erosion of iris (UGH syndrome).

Clinical features
- *Erythrocytes in the AC*: in minor bleeds most erythrocytes fail to settle and are only visible with the slit-lamp (microhyphaema); larger bleeds result in a macroscopically visible layer (hyphaema).
- *Complications*: rebleeds, corneal staining (especially if ↑IOP), red cell glaucoma.

Treatment
- Admit high-risk cases (Box 3.8).
- Strict bed-rest and globe protection (e.g. shield/glasses).
- Avoid aspirin/antiplatelet agents, NSAIDs, warfarin if possible (liaise with prescribing physician).
- Topical steroid (e.g. dexamethasone 0.1% 4×/d) and consider cycloplegia (e.g. atropine 1% 2×/d, but controversial).

Monitoring/follow-up
- Daily review (in-patient or out-patient) for IOP check and to rule-out rebleeds while hyphaema resolving; as improves can be discharged and follow-up become less frequent.
- From 2wks after resolution the patient can usually return to normal levels of activity and gonioscopy ± indented indirect ophthalmoscopy can be performed.
- Annual IOP checks (risk of angle recession glaucoma).

Red cell glaucoma

Hyphaema (usually traumatic) leads to blockage of the trabecular meshwork by red blood cells.

In 10% of cases a rebleed may occur, usually at about 5d. Patients with sickle-cell disease/trait do worse and are harder to treat (e.g. sickling may be worsened by the acidosis from carbonic anhydrase inhibitors).

Treatment

- *Of hyphaema*: as above.
- *Of IOP*: topical (e.g. β-blocker, $\alpha2$-agonist, carbonic anhydrase inhibitor) or systemic (e.g. acetazolamide) agents as required but avoid topical and systemic carbonic anhydrase inhibitors in sickle-cell disease/trait.

If medical treatment fails consider AC paracentesis ± AC wash out. If all else fails trabeculectomy is an effective treatment. Although a trabeculectomy's 'life-expectancy' in these circumstances is short, it usually works long enough for the blood to clear.

Box 3.8 High-risk features in hyphaema

Children and others with increased risk of non-compliance
Rebleed
Large hyphaema (>1/3)
Sickle-cell disease/trait
On antiplatelets (e.g. aspirin) or anticoagulants (e.g. warfarin)
Significant associated injury

Lids

Anatomy and physiology (1)

The eyelids are vital to the maintenance of ocular surface integrity. Their functions include a mechanical barrier to a variety of insults, a sweeping mechanism to remove debris from the cornea (e.g. blink reflex) and a vital contribution to the production and drainage of the tear film. They also contribute to facial expression, and even minor aberrations or asymmetry may affect cosmesis.

General

- At their simplest the lids comprise a layered structure of skin, orbicularis oculi, tarsal plates/septum, and conjunctiva.
- The orbital portion is more complex with preaponeurotic fat and retractors lying deep to the septum.
- The interpalpebral fissure is usually 30mm wide and 10mm high (slightly higher in females).
- The resting position of the upper lid is 2mm below the superior limbus (higher in children); for the lower lid the resting position is level with or just above the inferior limbus.

Skin and eyelashes

- The skin of eyelids is very thin, and has loose connective tissue but no subcutaneous fat.
- It contains eccrine sweat glands and sebaceous glands.
- The lashes are arranged in 2–3 rows along the lid margins with about 150 on the upper and 75 on the lower lid. They are replaced every 4–6mths but can grow back faster if cut. The lash follicles have apocrine sweat glands (of Moll) and modified sebaceous glands (of Zeis).

Orbicularis oculi

- This sheet of striated muscle is divided into orbital and palpebral portions; the latter is further divided into preseptal and pretarsal parts. Innervation is by temporal and zygomatic branches of VIIn for the orbicularis overlying the upper lid, and by the zygomatic branch alone for the lower lid.
- The *orbital* portion forms a ring of muscle arising from the medial canthal tendon and parts of the orbital rim.
- The *preseptal* part of each lid runs from the medial canthal tendon, arch over the anterior surface of the orbital septum and insert into the lateral horizontal raphe. Similarly, each *pretarsal* part arises from the medial canthal tendon, arches over the tarsal plates and inserts into the lateral canthal tendon and horizontal raphe.
- Horner muscle is formed by deep pretarsal fibres running medially to insert on to the lacrimal crest.
- Functions of the orbicularis oculi include lid closure and the lacrimal pump mechanism.

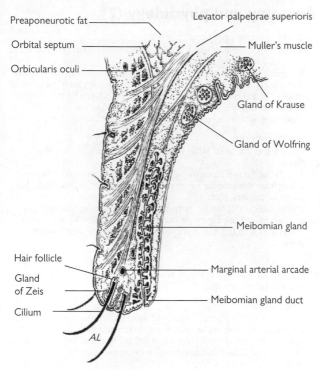

Preaponeurotic fat

Orbital septum

Orbicularis oculi

Levator palpebrae superioris

Muller's muscle

Gland of Krause

Gland of Wolfring

Meibomian gland

Hair follicle

Gland of Zeis

Cilium

Marginal arterial arcade

Meibomian gland duct

AL

Fig. 4.1 Anatomical section of the lid.

Anatomy and physiology (2)

Orbital septum and tarsal plates

The septum is a sheet of tissue that arises from the orbital rim where it is continuous with orbital fascia and periosteum.

Towards the palpebral margin it is thickened forming the tarsal plates that maintain the shape of the lid. These are 25mm long, 1mm thick, and of variable height: about 10mm high for the upper lid, 5mm for the lower lid. They also contain the Meibomian glands (about 35 in the upper lid, 25 in the lower lid) which secrete the lipid component of the tear film.

Canthal tendons

- At each end the tarsal plates are stabilized by a horizontal canthal tendon.
- The medial canthal tendon is well developed with an anterior limb arising from the anterior lacrimal crest, and a posterior limb from the posterior lacrimal crest.
- The lateral canthal tendon lies just posterior to the horizontal raphe and inserts into the zygomatic bone (Whitnall's tubercle), and merges posteriorly with the lateral check ligament (from the sheath of lateral rectus).

Fat pads

The preaponeurotic fat pads are extensions of orbital fat lying just posterior to the orbital septum.

Lid retractors

- The upper lid retractors comprise LPS and Muller's muscle. LPS originates from the orbital apex and runs forward over superior rectus to the orbital rim. At this point it is stabilized by the superior transverse ligament of Whitnall (a fascial bridge running between the trochlea and the lacrimal gland fascia) permitting the distal LPS to run steeply downward and insert as an aponeurosis into the septum, tarsus, and orbicularis.
- Innervation is by IIIn. Muller's muscle is an accessory retractor muscle supplied by the sympathetic system.
- Overaction is demonstrated in sympathetic overdrive and thyroid eye disease; underaction is seen in Horner syndrome.
- The lower lid retractors are more rudimentary but are similarly divided into voluntary and sympathetic groups.

Conjunctiva (see Anatomy and physiology 📖 p.158)

The conjunctiva is a mucous membrane comprising non-keratinized epithelium, basement membrane, and stroma. The epithelium of the palpebral conjunctiva is of stratified squamous form. It contains mucin-secreting goblet cells and crypts of Henle.

Nerves, arteries, veins, and lymphatics

Nerves

- *Sensation to the lower lid* is mainly by the infraorbital nerve (Vb), with infratrochlear branch of the nasociliary nerve (Va) innervating the medial canthal area.
- *Sensation to the upper lid* is by lacrimal, supraorbital, and supratrochlear nerve (all Va).
- Orbicularis oculi is innervated by VIIn, LPS by IIIn, and Muller's muscle by the sympathetic system.

Arteries

- Arterial supply is by 3 arcades that form anastamoses between the medial palpebral artery (from the terminal ophthalmic artery) and the lateral palpebral artery (from the lacrimal artery).
- *In the upper lid* there is a marginal arcade 2mm above the margin and a peripheral arcade at the top of the tarsal plate.
- *In the lower lid* the arcade lies 4mm below the margin.

Veins

Venous drainage is to superficial temporal vein laterally and to the ophthalmic and angular veins medially.

Lymphatics

Lymphatic drainage is to the parotid glands laterally, the submandibular glands inferiorly, and the anterior cervical chain inferomedially.

Eyelash disorders

Misdirected lashes

Misdirection of the eyelashes is a common source of ocular irritation. Corneal changes range from mild punctate epitheliopathy to ulceration, secondary infection, and scarring. *Treatment options include*: epilation, electrolysis, cryotherapy (double freeze–thaw technique), photoablation, and surgery. In pseudotrichiasis surgical correction of the entropion is curative. In other forms of misdirection, surgical excision is usually reserved for resistant cases.

Trichiasis

Lashes arise from their normal position but are posteriorly directed.

Distichiasis

Lashes arise from an abnormal position (e.g. from or slightly posterior to the Meibomian glands). It is an uncommon congenital abnormality that may be sporadic or autosomal dominant.

Metaplastic lashes

Lashes arise from an abnormal position secondary to chronic injury, e.g. cicatrizing conjunctivitis (*see* Cicatrizing conjunctivitis, 📖 p.172).

Pseudotrichiasis

Lashes arise from normal position but are posteriorly directed due to lid entropion.

Lash infestations

Infestation of the lashes by lice causes itching, blepharitis, and a follicular conjunctivitis. The lice and nits (eggs) are easily identified on slit-lamp examination.

Treatment options include mechanical removal or destruction (e.g. cryotherapy) for localized cases, and chemical for generalized cases. Chemical options (e.g. malathion or permethrin) require a 12h application to the whole body and repeated 7d later; aqueous malathion is effective in treating lash phthiriasis (unlicensed use), but ocular contact is contraindicated with all these agents.

Generalized infestation also requires laundry of all clothes and linen to >50°C.

Phthiriasis

Infestation by *Phthirus pubis* ('crab louse'). It is most commonly seen in adults in whom it is usually acquired as a sexually transmitted infection.

Pediculosis

Infestation by *Pediculus humanus corporis* or *capitis* ('head-louse'). If heavily infested the lice may spread to involve lashes.

Madarosis

This is partial or complete loss of lashes. It may be a purely local phenomenon, or associated with systemic disease (Table 4.1).

Table 4.1 Causes of madarosis

Local	Cicatrizing conjunctivitis (see 📖 p.172)
	Iatrogenic (cryotherapy/radiotherapy/surgery)
Systemic	Alopecia (patchy/totalis/universalis)
	Psoriasis
	Hypothyroidism
	Leprosy

Lash poliosis

This is whitening of the lashes. It may be associated with premature greying of the hair, a purely local phenomenon or be associated with systemic pathology (Table 4.2).

Table 4.2 Causes of poliosis

Local	Chronic lid margin disease
Systemic	Sympathetic ophthalmia
	Vogt–Koyanagi–Harada syndrome
	Waardenburg syndrome

Blepharitis

In general ophthalmology the term blepharitis is often used as shorthand for chronic lid margin disease. However, blepharitis refers to any inflammation of the lid, and thus includes a wide range of disease such as preseptal cellulitis, internal and external hordeola, HSV/VZV infections, etc. The diagnosis 'blepharitis' therefore lacks precision, but is often used due to the considerable overlap between the main causes of chronic lid margin inflammation discussed below. The descriptive terms anterior and posterior blepharitis are sometimes used to indicate the distribution of disease.

Unilateral blepharitis (and recurrent chalazia) should be treated with extreme suspicion as lid tumours (e.g. sebaceous cell carcinoma) may present in this way.

Bacterial blepharitis

This results in a mainly anterior blepharitis. It is usually due to lid commensals, most commonly *Staphylococci*, but may also arise from *Streptococci*, *Propionibacterium acnes*, and *Moraxella*.

Clinical features
- Burning, gritty, crusted.
- Injected lid margins, scales at lash bases ± external hordeolum (abscess of lash follicle and associated glands) ± preseptal cellulitis.

Treatment
- *Lid hygiene*: regular lid margin cleaning (e.g. by cotton bud dipped in dilute baby shampoo).
- *Ocular lubricants*: tear film instability is common.
- *Antibiotics*: topical antibiotics may be required for acute exacerbations; external hordeola and preseptal cellulitis also require oral antibiotics.
- *Topical steroids (weak)*: may be required in severe cases with corneal involvement.

Meibomianitis

This is a mainly posterior blepharitis arising from inflammation of the meibomian glands. It is often associated with facial rosacea.

Clinical features
- Burning, worse in mornings.
- Inflamed meibomian gland openings, thickened secretions, glands may become obstructed ± chalazia (lipogranulomatous inflammation within meibomian gland) ± internal hordeolum (acute abscess formation within meibomian gland).

Treatment
- Oral tetracyclines (e.g. oxytetracycline 500mg 2×/d for 12wks; tetracyclines are contraindicated in children under 12, in breast-feeding or pregnant women, or in hepatic or renal impairment).
- Consider lid hygiene, and topical therapies as for bacterial blepharitis.

Seborrhoeic blepharitis

This results in a mixed anterior/posterior blepharitis arising from excessive meibomian secretions. It is commonly associated with seborrhoeic dermatitis of the scalp.

Clinical features
- Burning, gritty, crusted.
- Lashes stuck together by soft scales, oily lid margin, foamy tear film.

Treatment
As for meibomianitis with tetracyclines, lid hygiene, and topical therapies as needed.

Lid lumps: cysts, abscesses, and others

Anterior lamella

External hordeolum (stye)

This is an acute abscess within a lash follicle and its associated glands of Zeis and Moll.

It results in a tender lump with associated inflammation.

Is usually staphylococcal in origin.

Treatment: warm compresses; if associated with preseptal cellulitis add in oral antibiotics (see Orbital and preseptal cellulitis, 📖 p.526, e.g. flucloxacillin 250–500mg 4×/d for 1wk).

Cyst of Moll

These chronic cysts (or apocrine hidrocystomas) are markedly translucent and arise from blockage of the apocrine duct of the gland of Moll. They may be incised under topical anaesthesia. Similar lesions may arise from blockage of the eccrine ducts of sweat glands of the eyelid skin.

Cyst of Zeis

These chronic cysts are poorly translucent and arise from blockage of the gland of Zeis. Similar sebaceous cysts may arise in the periorbital skin but rarely from the lids.

Xanthelasma

These common lesions result from the deposition of lipids within perivascular xanthoid cells and may be a sign of hyperlipidaemia. Clinically, they appear as yellowish subcutaneous deposits located on the medial aspect of the lids and periorbit.

Molluscum contagiosum

- These pearly, umbilicated nodules are common in children/young adults. They are caused by a dsDNA virus of the pox virus group; profuse lesions are seen with HIV infection.
- Transmission is by close contact. If at the lid margin, they may cause a persistent follicular conjunctivitis (see Viral conjunctivitis, 📖 p.166). A unilateral follicular conjunctivitis should lead the clinician to search the eyelid margins for such lesions.
- *Treatment*: if troublesome the lesions may be removed by cryotherapy, cauterization, shave excision or expression.

Posterior lamella

Internal hordeolum

- This is an acute abscess within a meibomian gland. It results in a tender lump with associated inflammation. It is usually staphylococcal in origin.
- *Treatment*: acute—warm compresses; acute with preseptal cellulitis—add in oral antibiotics (see Orbital and preseptal cellulitis, 📖 p.526); chronic (or large acute lesion)—also perform incision and curettage.

Chalazion

- This is the commonest of all lid lumps. They arise from chronic lipogranulomatous inflammation of blocked meibomian glands. They are usually located on the upper lid, and are commoner in patients with chronic marginal blepharitis, rosacea, or seborrhoeic dermatitis.
- *Treatment*: small chalazia are often ignored by the patient and resolve with time. Persistent or symptomatic lesions may be treated surgically by incision and curettage. Any recurrence of the lesion should be regarded as suspicious and a biopsy sent for histology.

Box 4.1 Outline of incision and curettage of a chalazion

- *Consent*: discuss what the procedure involves, likelihood of further chalazia/recurrence and risks including bruising, bleeding, and infection.
- Identify location of chalazion (it will be less obvious after instillation of anaesthetic)
- Instil topical anaesthesia (e.g. oxybuprocaine) in the fornix of the affected eye
- Prepare surgical area with 5% povidone iodine
- Inject local anaesthetic (e.g. 1–2% lidocaine with adrenaline 1 in 200 000) SC to the affected lid
- Evert lid with guarded lid clamp
- Incise chalazion vertically with surgical blade (e.g. no. 11) from the conjunctival surface
- Curette to remove the chalazion contents and to break down any loculations
- Instil topical antibiotic (e.g. oc chloramphenicol 1%)
- Remove clamp and apply pressure to ensure haemostasis
- Apply eye-patch; this can be removed before leaving the department
- Post-procedure: topical antibiotic (e.g. oc chloramphenicol 1% 4×/d for 1wk); if atypical or recurrent chalazion curettings/biopsy should be sent for histology

Lid lumps: benign and premalignant tumours

Benign tumours

Anterior lamella

Papillomas
- Skin papillomas are very common.
- They are derived from squamous cells.
- May be non-specific or related to human papillomavirus (viral wart or verruca vulgaris).
- They are either broad-based (sessile) or narrow-based (pedunculated) protrusions with irregular surfaces formed from finger-like extensions.

Seborrhoeic keratosis (basal cell papilloma)
- Common, especially in the elderly.
- Derived from basal cells.
- Are broad-based protrusions, usually brown in colour, with a greasy irregular surface.

Keratoacanthoma
- Uncommon tumours that grow rapidly for 2–6wks and then spontaneously involute over a few months.
- Are non-pigmented protrusions with a keratin-filled central crater.
- Some cases cannot be distinguished clinically from a squamous cell carcinoma. In these cases complete excision is necessary as an incomplete specimen may again be indistinguishable from a squamous cell carcinoma on histological examination.

Naevi
- Common cutaneous lesions that are classified according to depth.
- They arise from arrested epidermal melanocytes.
- *Junctional naevi* are flat, brown, and are located at the epidermis/dermis junction. *Dermal naevi* are elevated, may not be visibly pigmented and are located within the dermis. *Compound naevi* are slightly elevated and share features of junctional and dermal types.
- Overall, there is a low risk of transformation that is slightly higher for the more superficial naevi.

Vascular
Congenital vascular anomalies, such as capillary haemangiomas (strawberry naevi) and port wine stain, may involve the lids.

Posterior lamella

Pyogenic granuloma
This is an abnormal response to injury, such as trauma or, less commonly, inflammation. It is a red, highly vascular mass that appears to be a haemangioma with associated granulation tissue.

Premalignant tumours

Actinic keratosis

This common lesion of sun-exposed skin is relatively uncommon on the lids. Clinically, it is a flat, scaly lesion with hyperkeratosis and may have a keratin horn. Histologically, it shows parakeratosis and cellular atypia but no invasion.

Lid lumps: malignant tumours

Basal cell carcinoma

- This is the *commonest lid malignancy* (90% of lid malignancies).
- Preferentially affects the lower lid, followed by medial canthus, upper lid, and then lateral canthus.
- *Risk factors include*: increasing age, white skin, sun exposure, and some cutaneous syndromes (xeroderma pigmentosa, basal cell naevus syndrome).
- It is locally invasive but very rarely metastasizes.

Clinical features

- *Nodular type*: firm nodule, rolled pearly edges, fine telangiectasia, surface ulceration.
- *Morpheiform (sclerosing) type*: often minimal surface changes overlying extensive infiltration, so may mimic chronic inflammation/scarring (e.g. chronic marginal blepharitis).

Treatment

Wide local excision may be achieved by Mohs' micrographical technique (especially for morpheiform type) or by excisional biopsy ideally with histological (e.g. frozen section) control. A 3–4mm margin is recommended.

Squamous cell carcinoma

This is much less common (2–5% of lid malignancies), but has a much higher risk of malignant spread. It preferentially affects the lower lid.

Risk factors include: increasing age, white skin, sun exposure, and xeroderma pigmentosa.

Clinical features

- *Nodular type*: hyperkeratotic, with irregular margins; resemble BCC.
- *Plaque type*: erythematous, scaly, hyperkeratotic plaque.
- *Both types* may ulcerate, show lymphatic and perineural spread and metastasize.

Treatment

Wide local excision may be achieved by Mohs' micrographical technique or by excisional biopsy ideally with histological (e.g. frozen section) control. This is usually curative for early lesions. Orbital involvement may require exenteration.

Sebaceous gland carcinoma

This uncommon tumour (1–2% of lid malignancies) usually arises from the meibomian glands, or occasionally the glands of Zeis. It is aggressive and carries a significant mortality rate (10% overall mortality rate, but up to 67% 5yr mortality if metastasizes). It is commoner in the upper lid.

Risk factors include increasing age and female sex.

Clinical features

- *Nodular type*: firm nodule resembling chalazion (so biopsy 'recurrent chalazion')
- *Spreading type*: diffuse infiltration may involve the conjunctiva and resemble chronic blepharoconjunctivitis.

Treatment

Perform mapping biopsies of conjunctiva to assess extent of tumour, because of the risk of pagetoid spread, and confirm diagnosis with full thickness lid biopsy (warn histopathologist and send fresh tissue to assist with fat staining). Wide local excision is essential but may be difficult to achieve due to pagetoid and multicentric spread.

Regional lymph node clearance and exenteration may be performed depending on tumour extent.

Malignant melanoma

- Melanoma only rarely affects the lids (<1% lid malignancies). However, it must be considered when assessing pigmented lesions as it can be fatal.
- It has a non-invasive horizontal growth phase followed by an invasive vertical growth phase.
- *Risk factors include*: increasing age, white skin, sun exposure and sun burn, and some cutaneous syndromes (dysplastic naevus syndrome, xeroderma pigmentosa).

Clinical features

- *Lentigo maligna type*: initially flat pigmented lesion with well-defined margins (lentigo maligna) that starts to show elevation as it invades dermis (malignant transformation).
- *Superficial spreading type*: smaller pigmented lesion with irregular margins and mild elevation, ± nodules, induration; more aggressive.
- *Nodular type*: nodule (may not be visibly pigmented) with rapid growth, ulceration, and bleeding.

Treatment

Wide local excision with 10mm margins (confirmed on histology) is recommended, but not always possible. Some recommend regional lymph node dissection for tumours >1.5mm thick or with evidence of haematogenous or lymphatic spread.

Prognosis

Poor prognosis correlates with histological depth of invasion (by Clark's levels) and thickness (by the Breslow system). Thus 5yrs survival post-excision is 100% for tumours ≤0.75mm thick but only 50% for those >1.5mm thick.

Kaposi's sarcoma

This is a rare tumour arising from HHV8 in the general population but is relatively common in patients with AIDS. Clinically, it is a vascular purple-red nodule that may also affect the conjunctiva.

Treatment for symptomatic lesions is usually radiotherapy; it is not curative.

Merkel cell carcinoma

This is a very rare tumour that is more common in the elderly. It shows rapid growth and is highly malignant. Clinically, it is a non-tender purple nodule, usually on the upper lid.

Ectropion

Ectropion is the abnormal eversion of the eyelid (usually the lower) away from the globe. This disruption frequently causes irritation and may threaten the integrity of the ocular surface. It may occasionally be congenital, but is usually acquired as a result of involutional, cicatricial, mechanical, or paralytic processes.

Involutional ectropion

This is the commonest form and results from age-related tissue laxity.

Clinical features (non-specific)

These are present in most ectropia:
- Variable irritation, epiphora, recurrent infections.
- Everted lid (varies from slightly everted punctum to eversion of the whole lid), conjunctival irritation (keratinization).

Clinical features (specific)

- Test for lid laxity (pull away from globe; >10mm is abnormal), medial canthal tendon laxity (pull lid laterally; >2mm movement of punctum is abnormal. Although treatment is usually reserved for cases where the punctum can be distracted to the level of the centre of the pupil), lateral canthal tendon laxity (pull lid medially; >2mm movement of canthal angle is abnormal; lateral canthus also has rounded appearance), inferior retractor weakness.

Treatment

Surgery is directed towards the specific defect. Most commonly this requires lid shortening for horizontal laxity, but the procedure of choice will depend on the relative contribution of lid, tendons, canthal position, etc. (Table 4.3).

Cicatricial ectropion

This is uncommon. It occurs when scarring vertically shortens the anterior lamella. Causes include trauma, burns, radiotherapy, and dermatitis.

Clinical features (specific)

- Scarring, no skin laxity, tension lines in skin when lid put into position; features of underlying disease.

Treatment

Medical: the cicatrizing process should be controlled as best possible.
Surgical: skin-gaining procedures (Table 4.3).

Mechanical ectropion

This is uncommon. It occurs when masses (e.g. tumours) displace the lid away from the globe.

Clinical features (specific)

- Visible/palpable mass, e.g. tumour, cyst, oedema.

Treatment

Removal of the cause may lead to complete resolution; if residual lid laxity treat as for involutional (Table 4.3). However, occasionally, an autogenous fascia lata sling may be required.

Paralytic ectropion

This is uncommon. It occurs when VIIn palsy causes orbicularis weakness.

Clinical features (specific)

Weakness of orbicularis and other facial muscles; lagophthalmos, corneal exposure likely.

NB Corneal sensation may be compromised by underlying disease. These patients must be taught their only warning of exposure-related problems might be redness of the eye or ↓ VA.

Treatment

Topical: ocular lubricants, consider taping eye shut at night.
Surgical: depends on severity and associated laxity; options include medial canthoplasty, lateral tarsorrhaphy, lid-shortening procedures, and botulinum toxin to the upper lid.

Congenital

This is rare, but may be seen in Down syndrome and blepharophimosis syndrome. It may occur in both the lower and upper lids and is due to a shortage of skin.

Table 4.3 Overview of common ectropion operations

Operation	Indication	Procedure
Horizontal lid shortening		
Wedge excision	Lid laxity, no tendon laxity	Full thickness pentagon excised
Kuhnt–Symanowski	As above + excess skin	Wedge excision + lower lid blepharoplasty
Lateral tarsal strip	Lateral/generalized laxity	Lid shortened laterally and tightened elevated at lateral canthus
Medial canthal resection	Medial laxity only	Lid shortened laterally and tightened at medial canthus
Vertical lid shortening		
Diamond excision	Mild medial ectropion	Diamond of tarsoconjunctiva excised just inferior to punctum
Combined shortening procedures		
Lazy-T procedure	Medial ectropion with lid laxity	Diamond excision + wedge excision
Skin-gaining procedures		
Z-plasty	Focal scars	Z-incision with middle stroke excising scar gains vertical height
Skin flap/graft	Congenital/cicatricial skin loss	Transposition flap with pedicle or distant graft
Horizontal fissure shortening		
Lateral tarsorrhaphy and medial canthoplasty	Cornea threatened by lagophthalmos	Fuses the lids at lateral and medial aspect

Entropion

Entropion is abnormal inversion of the eyelid (usually the lower) toward the globe. Abrasion of the cornea by the inwardly directed lashes can result in ulceration and secondary infection.

Occasionally, it may be congenital, but is usually acquired as a result of involutional or cicatricial, processes.

Involutional entropion

This is the commonest form and results from inferior retractor dysfunction tissue laxity and possibly override of preseptal orbicularis over pretarsal orbicularis.

Clinical features (non-specific)

These are present in most entropia:

- FB sensation, photophobia, blepharospasm, epiphora.
- Inverted lid (transient/permanent), pseudotrichiasis, keratopathy, pannus formation.

Clinical features (specific)

- *Test for inferior retractor weakness/dehiscence* (reduced movement of lower lid in downgaze); *lid laxity* (pull away from globe; >10mm is abnormal); *medial canthal tendon laxity* (pull lid laterally; >2mm movement of punctum is abnormal); *lateral canthal tendon laxity* (pull lid medially; >2mm movement of canthal angle is abnormal; lateral canthus also has rounded appearance).

Treatment

Surgery is directed towards the specific defect. Most commonly this requires reattachment of the retractors and lid shortening for horizontal laxity (Table 4.4).

Procedures that are primarily directed against orbicularis (Wies) were previously popular but are no longer considered to be effective.

Cicatricial entropion

This is uncommon. It occurs when scarring vertically shortens the posterior lamella. It is caused by cicatrizing conjunctivitis most commonly due to trachoma, ocular cicatricial pemphigoid and other bullous diseases, chemical injuries, radiotherapy, and trauma (see Cicatricial conjunctivitis 🕮 p.172).

Clinical features (specific)

- *Chronic*: loss of plica semilunaris, loss of forniceal depth, formation of symblepharon/ankyloblepharon, dry eye signs.
- *Acute*: papillary conjunctivitis, subconjunctival vesicles, evolving picture.

Treatment

- *Medical*: the cicatrizing process should be optimally controlled, especially before surgical intervention (see Cicatricial conjunctivitis 🕮 p.172).
- *Surgical*: retractor reattachment may suffice in mild cases; transverse tarsotomy (tarsal fracture) or mucosal graft if moderate/severe loss of posterior lamella (Table 4.4). Recently, anterior lamellar excision has been proposed as a simple treatment that does not appear to aggravate the inflammatory process.

Congenital entropion

This is very rare, and often resolves with time without the need for intervention. Pretarsal orbicularis is hypertrophied forming a marked ridge. The lashes do not usually damage the cornea but recurrent infections are common.

Upper lid entropion

This is most commonly seen in cicatricial disease, notably trachoma. As with lower lid entropion it may threaten corneal integrity.

Treatment depends on the underlying disease and severity of entropion.

Table 4.4 Overview of common entropion operations

Operation	Indication	Procedure
Retractor reattachment		
Jones plication (modified)	Retractor dehiscence with no horizontal lid laxity	Reattachment/tightening of the retractors via subciliary incision
Horizontal lid shortening		
Wedge excision	Lid laxity, no tendon laxity	Full thickness pentagon excised
Kuhnt–Symanowski	As above + excess skin	Wedge excision + lower lid blepharoplasty
Lateral tarsal strip	Lateral/generalized laxity	Lid shortened laterally and tightened elevated at lateral canthus
Medial canthal resection	Medial laxity only	Lid shortened laterally and tightened at medial canthus
Posterior lamella reconstruction		
Transverse tarsotomy	Moderate loss of posterior lamella	Tarsal fracture and eversion of distal tarsus
Hard palate mucosal graft	Severe loss of posterior lamella	As above + limited separation of lamellae + graft to posterior lamella
Limitation of orbicularis override		
Quickert procedure	Lid laxity and retractor dehiscence	Everting sutures and full-thickness lid split + wedge excision to shorten lid

Ptosis: acquired

Ptosis is an abnormal low position of the upper lid. Normal lid position and, therefore, lid measurements vary slightly according to age, sex, and ethnicity. These are average values:

Table 4.5 Normal lid measurements

Palpebral aperture	8–11mm (female>male)
Upper margin reflex distance	4–5mm
Upper lid excursion (levator function)	13–16mm
Upper lid crease position	8–10mm from margin (female>male)

An appearance of ptosis may be simulated by a number of conditions (pseudoptosis). True ptosis may be congenital (either isolated or syndromic), but is most commonly acquired as an involutional degeneration.

Ptosis, however, may also be the presenting feature of a number of serious conditions.

Involutional ptosis

This very common condition arises from disinsertion of the LPS. It increases with age and is more common after ophthalmic surgery (occurs in 6% post-cataract extraction), trauma, or chronic contact lens use.

Clinical features
Uni/bilateral ptosis, high upper lid crease, compensatory brow lift, normal levator function, deep upper sulcus, low relative eyelid position in down-gaze.

Treatment
Surgery: anterior levator advancement (Box 4.2).

Neurogenic ptosis

- *Third nerve palsy:* ptosis may arise as part of a third nerve palsy, a potential ophthalmic emergency (see Third nerve disorders, 🕮 p.612). It is classically a complete ptosis due to loss of levator function, usually associated with ocular motility abnormalities and sometimes with mydriasis. Aberrant regeneration is common in chronic compressive lesions. *Surgery* (frontalis suspension) is delayed for at least 6mths (spontaneous improvement is common) and until any motility disturbance has been successfully corrected.
- *Horner syndrome:* causes a partial ptosis with preservation of levator function (see Anisocoria: sympathetic chain, 🕮 p.622). It may be associated with ipsilateral miosis, lower lid elevation, and in some cases anhydrosis. *Surgery* for persistent and significant ptosis is by anterior levator resection or less commonly by Fasanella–Servat procedure (posterior mullerectomy).

Myasthenic ptosis

Myasthenia gravis may cause variable and fatiguable uni/bilateral ptosis and ocular motility disturbance (see Myasthenia gravis, 🕮 p.634).

Surgical repair should be avoided except in refractory disease causing severe visual disability.

Myopathic ptosis

The chronic progressive external ophthalmoplegia group cause a bilateral, usually symmetric ptosis, associated with restricted ocular motility.

Surgical repair (usually frontalis suspension) requires caution as lid closure is also abnormal. It is, therefore, delayed until ptosis is visually significant.

Mechanical ptosis

Masses, infiltrations, or oedema of the upper lid may cause ptosis. The ptosis often resolves with correction of the underlying disease.

Pseudoptosis

- *Brow ptosis*: a lowering of the eyebrow due to frontalis dysfunction.
- *Dermatochalasis*: a common condition where upper eyelid skin hangs in folds from the lid; it is commoner in the elderly.
- *Blepharochalasis*: abnormal lid elastic tissue permits recurrent episodes of lid oedema that lead to abnormal redundant skin folds.

Other simulators of ptosis are listed in Table 4.6.

Table 4.6 Causes of pseudoptosis

Ipsilateral pathology	Excessive skin	Brow ptosis
		Dermatochalasis
	Inadequate globe size	Microphthalmos
		Phthisis bulbi
		Prosthesis
	Incorrect globe position	Enophthalmos
		Hypotropia
Contralateral pathology	Large globe	Contralateral lid retraction
		High myopia
		Contralateral proptosis

Ptosis: congenital

Isolated congenital ptosis

This is a developmental myopathy of the levator. It is usually unilateral, with absent skin crease, reduced levator function, and the lid fails to drop normally in downgaze.

Treatment

Surgery: if levator function is reasonable then anterior levator resection will suffice. For poor levator function, frontalis suspension should be performed. To optimize symmetry this should be bilateral with excision of the uninvolved levator.

Blepharophimosis syndrome

This autosomal dominant condition is characterized by horizontally shortened palpebral fissures, telecanthus, severe bilateral ptosis with poor levator function and commonly epicanthus inversus and ectropia.

Treatment

Surgery is first directed towards correcting the telecanthus and epicanthus. Bilateral frontalis slings are performed later.

Marcus Gunn jaw-winking syndrome

This is a synkinesis in which innervation of the ipsilateral pterygoids causes elevation of the ptotic lid during chewing.

Treatment

Surgery requires levator resection (mild) or bilateral levator excision with frontalis suspension (severe).

Box 4.2 Outline of anterior levator advancement

- Administer SC local anaesthetic (unless GA).
- Mark level of desired postoperative lid crease and make skin incision at this level.
- Divide orbicularis and septum and retract the preaponeurotic fat pads up to expose LPS.
- Free LPS both from any remaining attachments to the tarsus and from the underlying Muller muscle.
- Advance the aponeurosis and suture to tarsus (partial thickness—evert lid to check; e.g. 6-0 Mersilene).
- In the awake patient the resultant position should be observed and adjusted accordingly.
- Reform the lid crease by suturing the subcutaneous tissues/orbicularis to the tarsus (e.g. 7-0 Vicryl).
- Close skin incision (e.g. 7-0 polypropylene—remove at 1wk).

Miscellaneous lid disorders

Congenital

Epiblepharon
This is a common horizontal fold of skin running just below the lower lid. It may cause the lid to invert with pseudotrichiasis. It is rarely significant and usually resolves.

Epicanthic folds
These are common folds of skin that may arise in one of four patterns around the medial canthus:
- *Epicanthus palpebraris*: medial vertical fold between upper and lower lids; present in 20% normal children, usually resolves.
- *Epicanthus tarsalis*: primarily upper lid fold typical of oriental races.
- *Epicanthus inversus*: primarily lower lid fold seen in blepharophimosis and Down syndromes.
- *Epicanthus superciliaris*: fold arising above the brow; rare.

Telecanthus
This is wide separation of the medial canthi despite normally positioned orbits (i.e. normal interpupillary distance) in contrast to hypertelorism where the whole orbits are widely separated. It may be isolated or syndromic (e.g. blepharophimosis).

Cryptophthalmos
This is a failure of lid development so that the surface ectoderm remains continuous over the surface of an often poorly developed eye. Even with cosmetic improvement visual prognosis is often poor. It is sometimes autosomal dominantly inherited.

Ankyloblepharon
These are abnormal areas of upper and lower lid fusion and are of variable severity. They may be isolated or syndromic.

Coloboma
These are focal lid defects arising from failure of lid development or interference of amniotic bands. They are usually located medially in the upper lid and laterally in the lower lid.

Acquired

Floppy eyelid syndrome
In this uncommon condition an excessively lax upper lid can spontaneously evert during sleep, resulting in exposure and chronic papillary conjunctivitis.

It is more common in the obese and may be associated with sleep apnoea (with risk of pulmonary hypertension and other cardiovascular complications). Sleep studies are therefore recommended.

Severe lid disease may be cured by lid-shortening procedures.

Lid retraction

Table 4.7 Causes of lid retraction

Congenital		Isolated
		Down syndrome
		Duane syndrome
Acquired	Systemic	Thyroid eye disease
		Uraemia
	Neurological	VIIn palsy
		IIIn misdirection
		Marcus Gunn syndrome
		Parinaud syndrome
		Hydrocephalus
		Sympathetic drive (incl. medication)
	Mechanical	Cicatricial
		Surgical
		Globe (Buphthalmos/myopia/proptosis)

Lacrimal

Anatomy and physiology

The lacrimal system comprises a secretory component (tear production by the lacrimal gland) and an excretory component (tear drainage by the nasolacrimal system).

Anatomy

Lacrimal gland

- This almond-shaped bilobar gland is located in the shallow lacrimal fossa of the superolateral orbit. It is held in place by fascial septae and divided into palpebral (smaller superficial part) and orbital (larger deeper part) lobes by the levator palpebrae superioris aponeurosis.
- Approximately 12 ducts run from the orbital lobe through the aponeurosis and palpebral lobe to open into the superolateral fornix.
- The gland is of serous type, but also contains mucopolysaccharide granules.
- It is innervated by the parasympathetic system: superior salivary nucleus (pons) → greater petrosal n → synapse at pterygopalatine ganglion → zygomatic n (Vb) → lacrimal n (Va) → lacrimal gland.

Nasolacrimal system

Tear drainage starts with the upper and lower lacrimal puncta (0.3mm diameter) that are located about 6mm lateral to the medial canthus. These are angled backward and are located within the slightly elevated lacrimal papillae.

The superior and inferior canaliculi comprise a vertical part (the ampulla: 2mm long, up to 3mm wide) and a horizontal part (8mm long, up to 2mm wide). The terminal canaliculi usually fuse to form the common canaliculus, on average 2mm before entering the lacrimal sac. The sac is about 12mm in length and lies within the lacrimal fossa. The lacrimal fossa lies posterior to the medial canthal tendon and lateral to the ethmoid sinus (although this is variable).

The nasolacrimal duct is about 18mm long and runs parallel to the naso-jugal fold (i.e. inferolaterally). The first 12mm lies in the bony nasolacrimal canal and the last 6mm within the mucous membrane of the lateral wall of the nose. It opens into the inferior meatus via the ostium lacrimale just beneath the inferior turbinate.

There are a number of valves along the system of which the most important are the valves of Rosenmuller (entry into the lacrimal sac) and Hasner (exit from the nasolacrimal duct).

Physiology

Production (secretion) of tears may be basic or reflex.

Basic secretion

- *Lid*: meibomian glands (about 60) → outer lipid layer, which reduces evaporation.
- *Conjunctiva*: glands of Krause (about 28) and glands of Wolfring (about 3) → middle aqueous layer, which has washing and antimicrobial functions; and goblet cells → inner mucin layer, which helps stabilize the tear film.
- *Lacrimal gland*: may also contribute to basal secretion.

Reflex secretion
Lacrimal gland: innervated by the parasympathetic system.

Excretion
Tears flow along the marginal tear strips and are drained into the distensible ampullae. This is probably both passive (70% is drained via the inferior canaliculus vs 30% via the superior) and active (i.e. suction).

From the ampullae an active lacrimal pump then drives the tears first into the sac and then down the nasolacrimal duct into the nose. Contraction of the pretarsal orbicularis oculi (superficial and deep heads) compresses the loaded ampullae while contraction of the preseptal orbicularis (deep head that inserts on to lacrimal fascia) forcibly expand the sac creating a wave of suction towards the sac. With relaxation of the orbicularis, the ampullae reopen and the sac collapses expelling the tears down the nasolacrimal duct.

Lacrimal gland
Ampulla
Superior canaliculus
Common canaliculus
Lacrimal sac
Inferior canaliculus
Nasolacrimal duct
Valve of Hasner

Fig. 5.1 Anatomy of the nasolacrimal system.

The watery eye: assessment

This is a common complaint particularly in the elderly population. It ranges from the transient and trivial (e.g. associated with a local irritant) to the permanent and disabling. Objective quantification is difficult but the main issue is how much of a problem it is for the patient.

Box 5.1 An approach to assessing the watery eye

Symptoms	episodic/permanent, frequency of wiping eyes, exacerbating factors, site where tears spill over (laterally/medially)
POH	previous surgery/trauma; concurrent eye disease; herpes simplex blepharoconjunctivitis
PMH	previous ENT problems (e.g. sinusitis) surgery/nasal fracture
Dx	pro-secretory drugs (e.g. pilocarpine)
Ax	allergies or relevant drug contraindications
Visual acuity	best-corrected/pin-hole
Facies	scars (previous trauma/surgery), asymmetry, prominent nasal bridge
Lacrimal sac	swelling, any punctal regurgitation on palpation
Lids	position (ectropion/entropion/low lateral canthus), laxity (lid/canthal tendons)
Puncta	position, scarring, concretions, patency
Conjunctiva	irritation (e.g. chronic conjunctivitis)
Cornea	inflammation, chronic corneal disease
Tear film	meniscus high/low
Dye disappearance test	
Dye recovery	cotton bud or ideally nasendoscope
Cannulation	patency of puncta
Probing	hard/soft stop
Irrigation	flow, regurgitation

Perform nasendoscopy where possible. Consider formal Jones testing and imaging (contrast dacryocystography, lacrimal scintillography) if required.
For specific tests, see Nasolacrimal system examination, 📖 p.38.

Table 5.1 Causes of the watery eye (common causes in bold)

Increased production	Basal	Autonomic disturbance
		Pro-secretory drugs
	Reflex	Local irritant (e.g. FB, trichiasis)
		Systemic disease (e.g. TED)
		Chronic lid disease (e.g. blepharitis)
		Chronic conjunctival disease (e.g. ocular mucous membrane pemphigoid)
		Chronic corneal disease (e.g. keratoconjunctivitis sicca)
Lacrimal pump failure	Lid tone	**Lid laxity**
		Orbicularis weakness (e.g. VIIn palsy)
	Lid position	**Ectropion**
Decreased drainage	Punctal obstruction	Congenital: punctal atresia
		Idiopathic stenosis (elderly)
		HSV infection
		Post-irradiation
		Trachoma
		Cicatricial conjunctivitis
		Secondary to punctal eversion
	Canalicular obstruction	**Idiopathic fibrosis**
		HSV infection
		Chronic dacrocystitis
		Cicatricial conjunctivitis
		5-FU administration (systemic)
	Nasolacrimal duct obstruction	Congenital: **delayed canalization**
		Idiopathic stenosis
		Trauma (nasal/orbital fracture)
		Post-irradiation
		Wegener's granulomatosis
		Tumours (e.g. nasopharyngeal carcinoma)
		Nasal pathology (chronic inflammation polyps)

The watery eye: treatment

Increased production

This is usually due to reflex tearing in response to a chronic irritant or disease.

Treatment is directed towards controlling the disease process, e.g. ocular lubricants for keratoconjunctivitis sicca. It is important to explain this to the patient as it will seem counterintuitive to be treating a watery eye with drops.

Lacrimal pump failure

This is usually a function of lid laxity and ectropion causing punctal eversion. This often leads to secondary punctal stenosis. Treatment is directed towards restoring the position of lid and punctum, often with a lid-shortening procedure (Table 5.2 and see Ectropion, 🕮 p.138).

Decreased drainage

Obstruction may arise at the level of the punctum, canaliculi, sac, or nasolacrimal duct. The extent of surgery required will depend on the level of blockage, but most cases arising distal to the puncta require a DCR (Table 5.2).

Table 5.2 Overview of operations to improve nasolacrimal drainage

Operation	Indication	Procedure
Punctal position		
Ziegler cautery	Very mild medial ectropion	Cauterise tissue 5mm inferior to punctum causes scarring/inversion
Diamond excision	Mild medial ectropion	Diamond of tarsoconjunctiva excised just inferior to punctum
Lazy-T procedure	Medial ectropion with lid laxity	Diamond excision + wedge excision
Lateral tarsal strip	Ectropion with generalized laxity	Lid shortened laterally and tightened + elevated at lateral canthus
Punctal obstruction		
1- or 3-snip procedure	Isolated punctal stenosis	Vertical and small medial cut in the punctal ampulla enlarges opening
Canalicular obstruction		
Silastic tube insertion	Partial obstruction	Canaliculi intubated with silastic tube secured at nasal end; left for 6mths
DCR with Jones tube	Complete obstruction	DCR with a Jones (pyrex) tube from sac to medial canthus
Nasolacrimal duct obstruction		
DCR	Most nasolacrimal duct obstructions	The lacrimal sac is opened directly to nasal mucosa by a rhinostomy

Dacryocystorhinostomy (DCR)

A DCR aims to create an epithelium-lined tract from the lacrimal sac to the nasal mucosa. The conventional external route has a success rate of about 90%.

Endonasal DCR has the advantage of no external scar but may be less effective. It is also unsuitable for cases with canalicular obstruction.

Laser-assisted endonasal DCR has the lowest success rates, possibly due to the smaller ostium created.

Indication

Acquired nasolacrimal duct obstruction (± dacryocystorhinitis), congenital nasolacrimal obstruction in which a probe cannot be passed.

Method

Box 5.2 Outline of external dacryocystorhinostomy

1. Cutaneous incision on lateral aspect of nose and inferior to medial canthal tendon (about 8–10mm long).
2. Dissect down to bone, reflect periosteum from anterior lacrimal crest, and divide the superficial limb of the medial canthal tendon.
3. Reflect the lacrimal sac laterally.
4. Use Kerrison punches to create an opening through the bone of the sac fossa to the nasal cavity.
5. Divide the lacrimal sac and the exposed nasal mucosa vertically to form anterior and posterior flaps.
6. Anastamose mucosa of the sac and the nose by suturing the posterior and then the anterior flaps together.
7. Silastic tubes can be inserted to keep the ostium open if there is concern over premature closure by granulation tissue.
8. Close skin incision.

Postoperative care

If the nose has been packed at the end of the operation this can usually be removed on the first day after surgery. Prophylactic oral antibiotics are commonly prescribed.

Complications

Haemorrhage with epistaxis may occur early (within 24h) or late (4–7d) when clot retraction occurs. Treat with nasal packing (± thrombin soaked packs). If haemostasis still not achieved the vessel may need embolization.

Other complications include failure (closure of the ostium), scar formation, infection, and very rarely orbital haemorrhage.

Lacrimal system infections

Canaliculitis

This uncommon chronic condition usually arises from the Gram-positive bacteria *Actinomyces israelii* (streptothrix), but may be due to *Nocardia*, fungi (*Candidia*, *Aspergillus*), and viruses (HSV, VZV).

Clinical features

- Unilateral epiphora, recurrent 'nasal' conjunctivitis, inflammation of the punctum and canaliculus, expression of discharge, or concretions from the canaliculi.
- In *Actinomyces* infection these are bright yellow concretions ('sulphur granules'). The lacrimal sac is not swollen, and both sac and nasolacrimal duct are patent.

Investigation and treatment

Perform an extended one snip procedure and remove concretions with curette (send for microbiological analysis) and consider irrigation (e.g. with penicillin G 100 000u/ml or iodine 1%—ensure drainage out through nose, not nasopharynx) and topical antibiotics.

Acute dacryocystitis

This condition is relatively common in patients with complete or partial nasolacrimal duct obstruction. It is usually due to staphylococci or streptococci.

Acute dacryocystitis is easily identified and requires urgent treatment to prevent a spreading cellulitis.

Clinical features

- Pain around sac, worsening epiphora.
- Tender, erythematous lump just inferior to medial canthus, may express pus from puncta on palpation, + preseptal cellulitis.

Investigation and treatment

- Send discharge to microbiology.
- *Antibiotics*: systemic (e.g. co-amoxiclav 625mg 3×/d for 1 wk) and topical (e.g. chloramphenicol oc 4×/d for 1 wk).
- Consider warm compress, gentle massage (encourages expression), and incision and drainage if pointing (but may not heal until DCR performed).
- *Surgery*: most cases have associated nasolacrimal duct obstruction requiring DCR.

Chronic dacryocystitis

In chronic dacryocystitis there may be recurrent ipsilateral conjunctivitis, epiphora, and a mucocele. It may be identified by demonstration of nasolacrimal duct obstruction and expression of the contents of the mucocele. Surgical *treatment* is by DCR.

Conjunctiva

Anatomy and physiology

The conjunctiva is a mucous membrane that is essential for a healthy eye. At the histological level it comprises epithelium, basement membrane, and stroma. At the macroscopic clinical level it is divided into palpebral, forniceal, and bulbar parts.

Microscopic

Epithelium

This is a 2–5-layered, non-keratinized epithelium that may be stratified squamous (palpebral and limbal) or stratified columnar (bulbar conjunctiva).

The microvilli on the apical surface secrete glycoproteins that form a hydrophilic glycocalyx layer that helps stabilize the tear film. The epithelial layer also contains goblet cells (constituting about 10% of epithelial cells).

Epithelial basement membrane

The basement membrane consists mainly of type IV collagen, anchoring fibrils and hemidesmosomes linking to the conjunctival epithelial cells.

Stroma

This consists of a superficial lymphoid layer and a deeper fibrous layer. The superficial layer is attached to the epithelium via the basement membrane and contains lymphoid tissue. The deeper fibrous layer is attached to the episclera/Tenon's layer and comprises collagenous elastic tissue interspersed with neurovascular tissue.

Macroscopic

Palpebral

This is firmly adherent to the posterior lamella of the lid; contains the crypts of Henle and goblet cells (both secrete mucin).

Forniceal

This is loose and relatively mobile. It contains accessory lacrimal glands of Krause and Wolfring (secrete aqueous component of tears) and goblet cells.

Bulbar

This is loosely attached to Tenon's layer, but firmly attached at the limbus. It contains glands of Manz (secrete mucin) and goblet cells.

The tear film

Although conventionally described as a defined trilaminar structure it is becoming apparent that the tear film is rather more complex. The layers blend together forming a sponge-like material on the surface of the eye. (Fig. 6.1.)

Mucin layer

The mucin layer (secreted primarily by the goblet cells) abuts the surface epithelium and provides a smooth hydrophilic surface that stabilizes the aqueous against the otherwise hydrophobic epithelium.

Aqueous layer
The aqueous component (secreted by the lacrimal gland and the accessory glands) consists primarily of water but also proteins such as epidermal growth factor, lactoferrin, lysozyme, immunoglobulins, and cytokines.

Phospholipid layer
The aqueous layer is supported by a phospholipid layer (secreted primarily by the meibomian glands) that resists evaporative loss of aqueous and stabilizes the tear film by increasing surface tension.

	Phospholipid	Meibomian glands Glands of Zeis
	Aqueous	Lacrimal gland Glands of Krause Glands of Wolfring
	Mucin	Goblet cells Glands of Manz Crypts of Henle
	Epithelium	

Fig. 6.1 Tear film components and their origins.

Conjunctival signs

Table 6.1 Conjunctival signs and their pathophysiology

Sign	Pathology	Causes
Hyperaemia	Dilated blood vessels, non-specific sign of inflammation	• *Generalized*—e.g. conjunctivitis, dry eye, drop hypersensitivity, contact lens wear, scleritis • *Localized*—e.g. episcleritis, scleritis, marginal keratitis, superior limbic keratitis, corneal abrasion, FB • *Circumcorneal*—e.g. anterior uveitis, keratitis
Discharge	Inflammatory exudate	• *Purulent*—bacterial conjunctivitis • *Mucopurulent*—bacterial or chlamydial conjunctivitis • *Mucoid*—vernal conjunctivitis, atopic keratoconjunctivitis, dry eye syndrome • *Watery*—viral or allergic conjunctivitis
Papillae	Vascular response: projections of a core of vessels, surrounded by oedematous stroma and hyperplastic epithelium; also chronic inflammatory cells	• Bacterial conjunctivitis • Allergic conjunctivitis (perennial/seasonal) • Atopic keratoconjunctivitis • Vernal keratoconjunctivitis • Blepharitis • Floppy eyelid syndrome • Superior limbic keratoconjunctivitis • Contact lens
Giant papillae	Papillae, which due to chronic inflammation, have lost the normal fibrous septa that divide them	• Vernal keratoconjunctivitis • Atopic keratoconjunctivitis • Contact-lens-related giant papillary conjunctivitis • Exposed suture • Prosthesis • Floppy eyelid syndrome
Follicles	Lymphoid hyperplasia with each follicle comprising an active germinal centre	• Viral conjunctivitis • Chlamydial conjunctivitis • Drop hypersensitivity • Parinaud oculoglandular syndrome
Lymph-adenopathy	Temporal 2/3 drains to the preauricular nodes, nasal 1/3 to the submandibular nodes	• Viral conjunctivitis • Chlamydial conjunctivitis • Gonococcal conjunctivitis • Parinaud oculoglandular syndrome
Pseudo-membrane	Exudate of fibrin and cellular debris; loosely attached to the underlying epithelium; easily removed without bleeding	• Infective conjunctivitis adenovirus *Streptococcus pyogenes* *Corynebacterium diphtheriae* *Neisseria gonorrhoeae* • Stevens–Johnson syndrome (acute) • Graft-versus-host-disease • Vernal conjunctivitis • Ligneous conjunctivitis • Thermal burn

Table 6.1 Conjunctival signs and their pathophysiology (*continued*)

Sign	Pathology	Causes
Membrane	Exudate of fibrin and cellular debris; firmly attached to the underlying epithelium; attempted removal strips off the epithelium causing bleeding	• Infective conjunctivitis: adenovirus *Streptococcus pneumoniae* *Staphylococcus aureus* *Corynebacterium diphtheriae* • Stevens–Johnson syndrome (acute) • Ligneous conjunctivitis
Cicatrization	Scarring	• Topical medication • Chemical injury (acid/alkali) • Ocular mucous membrane pemphigoid) • Stevens–Johnson syndrome/TEN • Other immunobullous disease (e.g. linear IgA disease, epidermolysis bullosa) • Trachoma • Atopic keratoconjunctivitis • Sjögren syndrome • Trauma/surgery • Graft-versus-host-disease
Haemorrhagic conjunctivitis	Subconjunctival haemorrhages	• Infective conjunctivitis: adenovirus enterovirus 70 coxsackie virus A24 *Streptococcus pneumoniae* *Haemophilus aegyptius* • Neonatal chlamydial conjunctivitis

Bacterial conjunctivitis (1)

Acute bacterial conjunctivitis

This is one of the commonest ocular problems seen in the community and is usually successfully treated by GPs.

The commonest conjunctival bacterial pathogens are *Staphylococcus epidermidis*, *Staphylococcus aureus*, *Streptococcus pneumoniae*, *Haemophilus influenzae*, and *Moraxella lacunata*. There is some variation according to climate (*Haemophilus aegyptius* in warm climates, *H. influenzae* and *Streptococcus* in cool climates) and age (classically *H. influenzae* in children). Atypical bacteria may be seen in immunocompromised patients.

Bacteria have to overcome the protective mechanisms of the eye: lids (physical barrier, blink reflex), tears (flushing effect, lysozyme, β-lysin, lactoferrin, IgG, IgA), and conjunctiva (physical barrier, conjunctiva-associated lymphoid tissue).

Clinical features
- Acute, red, gritty, sticky eye; usually bilateral but may be sequential.
- Purulent discharge, crusted lids, diffusely injected conjunctiva with papillae; may have mild chemosis.

Investigation
Reserve microbiological investigation for cases that are severe, recurrent, resistant to treatment, atypical, or occur in the vulnerable (e.g. immunosuppressed, neonate). For these take conjunctival swabs for culture/sensitivities.

Treatment
- Topical antibiotics (e.g. chloramphenicol 1% oc 4×/d, sodium fusidate (e.g. Fucithalmic®) 1% 2×/d or trimethoprim/polymyxin B oc 4×/d for 1wk). Patients may find drops easier than ointment. For guttae more frequent administration is required (*BNF* recommends ≥q 2h), reducing frequency as the infection is controlled and continuing for 48h after healing.
- *Advise patient*: follow-up if condition worsens or persists after treatment; measures to reduce spread, such as frequent hand washing, minimal touching of eyes, not sharing towels/flannels, not shaking hands etc. **NB** wash hands and clean equipment before the next patient.

Chronic or recurrent bacterial conjunctivitis

Chronic or recurrent bacterial conjunctivitis usually reflects a neighbouring reservoir of infection. Such sites include the lids (staphyloccal blepharitis), lacrimal sac (chronic dacryocystitis), or the upper fornices of the elderly ('Giant fornix syndrome'). Giant fornix syndrome[1] occurs when there is sequestration of bacteria (including *Staph. aureus*) in a proteinaceous coagulum in a deep upper fornix. It is more common in the elderly and typically results in a chronic relapsing copiously purulent conjunctivitis.

---

1. Rose GE. The giant fornix syndrome. *Ophthalmology* 2004;**111**:1539–45

Table 6.2 Conjunctivitis: an outline of clinical features

Insult	Main symptom	Onset	Uni/bilateral	Visual acuity	History	Discharge	Chemosis	Tarsal conjunctiva	Preauricular lymphadeno-pathy
Bacterial	Red Sticky Gritty	Acute/hyperacute	Uni- or bilateral	Should be normal/near normal when discharge blinked away. Reduced acuity and photophobia suggests additional involvement, such as keratitis.	Known contact	Purulent	Mild	Papillae	Occasional
Viral	Red Watery Gritty	Acute	Uni- or bilateral		Known contact	Watery	Moderate	Follicles	Common
Chlamydial	Red Persistent discharge	Subacute	Unilateral		Sexual history	Mucopurulent	Mild	Follicles	Common
Allergic	Red Itchy Swelling	Acute/subacute/recurrent	Bilateral		Atopy; exposure to antigen	Watery	Severe	Papillae	No
Toxic (drops)	Discomfort + redness worse with drop instillation	Acute	Uni- or bilateral		Medication	Minimal	Mild	Follicles	No

Bacterial conjunctivitis (2)

Gonococcus (adult)

Now rare, this important Gram-negative diplococcus is found in adults (sexual transmission) and neonates (born to infected mothers). The incubation period is 3–5d in adults and 1–3d in neonates. Gonococcus (*Neisseria gonorrhoea*) may penetrate cornea in the absence of an epithelial defect.

Clinical features

- Hyperacute onset (<24h) with severe purulent discharge, marked lid swelling and chemosis, papillae, preauricular lymphadenopathy, pseudomembrane, ± keratitis.
- Keratitis. Marginal ulceration may progress rapidly resulting in a ring ulcer, perforation, and endophthalmitis.
- *Systemic*: history of (unprotected) sexual activity, urethritis, proctitis, vaginitis; although often asymptomatic in women it is a significant cause of infertility.

Investigation

- Conjunctival scrapings/swabs for immediate Gram stain, culture, and sensitivities.
- After appropriate explanation to the patient refer to a genitourinary clinic for assessment, treatment, and contact tracing.

Treatment

- Local microbiological/infectious disease advice is vital.
- Topical antibiotic (e.g. ofloxacin 0.3% 2 hourly), saline irrigation of discharge 4×/d.
- With keratitis: consider admission, ceftriaxone 1g IV 2×/d for 3d, topical antibiotic (e.g. ofloxacin 0.3% hourly), saline irrigation, treat chlamydial coinfection.
- Systemic treatment usually by GU physician may include ceftriaxone 1g IM stat and co-treatment for possible chlamydial coinfection (e.g. azithromycin 1g single dose).

Gonococcus (neonate)

See Ophthalmia neonatorum p.700.

Viral conjunctivitis

Adenovirus

Over 40 serotypes of this dsDNA virus have been identified. The incubation period is approximately 1wk, and virus shedding continues for a further 2wks during which it is highly contagious. The spectrum of presentation may be generalized into two distinct syndromes:

- *Pharyngoconjunctival fever*—serotypes 3, 7, and many others; aerosol transmission; common in children/young adults; systemic upset (typically upper respiratory tract infection) is common, keratitis is only present in up to 30% and is usually mild.
- *Epidemic keratoconjunctivitis*—serotypes 8, 19, 37; transmission by contact (fingers, instruments); keratitis may occur in up to 80% and can be severe; systemic features are rare. Epidemics may be nosocomial (e.g. arising from eye clinics/casualty) or generalized.

Clinical features

- Acute onset (7–10d), watering, burning, itching, ± photophobia/blurred vision (if keratitis).
- Watery discharge, lid oedema, moderate chemosis, follicles (inferior > superior), tender pre-auricular lymphadenopathy, ± subconjunctival petechial haemorrhage, ± pseudomembrane, ± symblepharon, keratitis.
- Keratitis: first diffuse epithelial keratitis (days 1–7; fluorescein staining), then focal epithelial keratitis (days 7–30; fluorescein staining) and finally subepithelial opacities (day 11 onwards, may last years; non-staining).

Investigation

Conjunctival swabs (viral transport medium) for viral antigen determination or PCR.

Treatment

- Supportive (cool compresses and artificial tears) ± topical antibiotics (supposedly to prevent secondary bacterial infection). Where subepithelial opacities significantly affect vision some authors advocate low-dose topical steroids. However, the opacities recur on cessation of steroids encouraging long-term steroid dependency.
- *Advise patient*: follow-up if condition worsens or persists after treatment; measures to reduce spread such as frequent hand washing, minimal touching of eyes, not sharing towels/flannels, not shaking hands, etc.
- Wash hands and clean equipment before the next patient.

Molluscum contagiosum

This dsDNA virus of the pox virus group is common in children/young adults; profuse lesions are seen with HIV infection or severe immunosuppression. Transmission is by close contact. The lesions may be missed if buried in the lash margin. Shedding of viral particles from the lesion may cause a persistent follicular conjunctivitis.

Clinical features

- Chronic history, pearly, umbilicated nodule at lid margin, mucoid discharge, follicles.

Treatment

Remove the lid lesion (e.g. cryotherapy, cauterization, shave excision, expression).

Herpes simplex (type 1)

Blepharokeratoconjunctivitis usually occurs as a primary infection of this dsDNA virus.

Clinical features

- Burning, FB sensation; unilateral follicular conjunctivitis, preauricular lymphadenopathy, ± lid vesicles, ± keratitis (e.g. dendritic ulcer). (*See* Herpes simplex keratitis, 📖 p.204.)

Treatment

Topical (e.g. aciclovir 3% oc 5×/d for 3wks; *BNF* recommend treatment until 3d after complete healing). If keratitis then treat accordingly. (*See* Fungal keratitis: treatment, 📖 p.180.)

Other viruses

Other viruses causing follicular conjunctivitis include other members of the herpes group, enterovirus 70, coxsackie A24. influenza A, and the Newcastle disease virus.

Chlamydial conjunctivitis

Chlamydiae are Gram-negative bacteria that exist in two forms:
- a spore-like infectious particle (elementary body), and
- the obligate intracellular reproductive stage (reticular body) that replicates within the host cell (seen as an inclusion body).

Adult inclusion conjunctivitis

This disease of *Chlamydia trachomatis* serotypes D–K is almost always sexually transmitted, although occasional eye-to-eye infection is reported. It is commonest in young adults (males > females). It may be associated with keratitis.

Clinical features
- Subacute onset (2–3wks), usually unilateral (but may be bilateral), mucopurulent discharge, lid oedema ± ptosis, follicles (papillae initially), non-tender lymphadenopathy, superior pannus (late sign); signs are usually most severe on the superior tarsus and the bulbar conjunctiva with relatively mild disease elsewhere.
- *Keratitis*: punctate epithelial erosions, subepithelial opacities, marginal infiltrates.
- *Systemic* (common, but often asymptomatic): cervicitis (females), urethritis (males).

Investigation
- Conjunctival swabs: firmly swab superior tarsus to remove sufficient cells for immunofluorescent staining; cell culture, PCR, and ELISA may also be used.
- After appropriate explanation to the patient refer to a genitourinary clinic for assessment, treatment, and contact tracing.

Treatment
First line: chloramphenicol oc 1% 4×/d (bacteriostatic for *Chlamydia*). Systemic (oral) treatment is usually best administered by the genitourinary clinic (after appropriate investigation). Options include oral azithromycin 1g stat or doxycycline 100mg 2×/d for 1wk; if pregnant erythromycin (e.g. 500mg 2×/d for 2wks) is usually given.

Neonatal chlamydial conjunctivitis

See Ophthalmia neonatorum 📖 p.700.

Trachoma

Trachoma accounts for 10–15% of global blindness, and is the leading preventable cause. It is caused by *Chlamydia trachomatis* serotypes A, B, Ba, and C, in conditions of crowding and poor hygiene in which the common fly acts as the vector. In endemic areas it may start in infancy; in non-endemic areas (such as the UK) patients usually present with the complications of chronic scarring.

The WHO is aiming to eliminate trachoma as a blinding disease by 2020. Party to this is the SAFE strategy-Surgery for in-turned eyelashes, Antibiotics for active disease, Face washing (or promotion of facial cleanliness), and Environmental improvement to reduce transmission.

Clinical features
- Distinctive follicular reaction (more marked in the upper, rather than lower lid), conjunctival scarring (with ensuing Arlt lines on the superior tarsus, trichiasis, entropion, dry eyes), limbal follicles (which may scar to form Herbert pits).
- *Keratitis*: superficial, subepithelial, ulceration, secondary microbial keratitis, pannus formation.

Investigation (if acute)
Swabs: usually for immunofluorescent staining, but cell culture, PCR, and ELISA may be used.

Treatment
- Azithromycin 1g PO stat.
- Ocular lubricants, surgical correction of lid/lashes position.

Table 6.3 World Health Organization (WHO) classification

TF	Trachomatous inflammation: follicular	>5 follicles on upper tarsus
TI	Trachomatous inflammation: intense	Tarsal inflammation sufficient to obscure >50% of the tarsal vessels
TS	Trachomatous scarring	Conjunctival scarring
TT	Trachomatous trichiasis	Trichiasis
CO	Corneal opacity	Corneal opacity involving at least part of the pupillary margin

Allergic conjunctivitis

Seasonal and perennial allergic rhinoconjunctivitis

These extremely common ocular disorders arise due to type I hypersensitivity reactions to air-borne allergens. These may be seasonal (grass, tree, weed pollens (UK), ragweed (US)), or perennial (animal dander, house dust mite).

Clinical features
- Itching, watery discharge; history of atopy.
- Chemosis, lid oedema, papillae, mild diffuse injection.

Investigation
Consider conjunctival swabs (microbiology), skin prick testing, serum IgE, radioallergosorbent test (RAST).

Treatment
- Identify and eliminate allergen where possible (e.g. change bedding, reduce pet contact, introduce air conditioning).
- If *mild*: artificial tears (dilutes allergen).
- If *moderate*: mast cell stabilizer (e.g. sodium cromoglicate 2% g 4×/d, lodoxamide 0.1% 4×/d) or topical antihistamine (azelastine 0.05% 2–4×/d for 6wks maximum, levocabastine 0.05% 2–4×/d); and oral antihistamine (e.g. chlorphenamine 4mg 3–6×/d or cetirizine 10mg 1×/d).
- If *severe*, add in short course of mild topical steroid (e.g. fluoromethotone 0.1% 4×/d for 1wk); consider referral to clinical immunologist in severe cases for consideration of desensitization therapy.

Vernal keratoconjunctivitis (VKC)

This is an uncommon but serious condition of children and young adults (onset age 5–15yrs; duration 5–10yrs). Before puberty it is commoner in males but subsequently shows no gender bias.

Although its incidence is decreasing among the white population it is increasing in Asians. Paler-skinned Caucasians more commonly exhibit the tarsal/palpebral form, whereas the limbal form is commoner in darker races; however, a mixed picture is often seen. It is commoner in warm climates and is usually seasonal (spring/summer).

Over 80% have an atopic history. There is both type I hypersensitivity and a cell-mediated role with a predominantly Th2 cell type. It has been proposed that the Th2 cytokines inhibit matrix metalloprotetinases resulting in build-up of conjunctival collagens.

Clinical features
- Itching, thick mucous discharge; typically young male, presenting in spring with history of atopy.
- Tarsal signs: flat-topped giant ('cobblestone') papillae on superior tarsus.
- Limbal signs: limbal papillae, white Trantas dots (eosinophil aggregates).
- Keratitis: superior punctate epithelial erosions, vernal ulcer with adherent mucus plaque (may result in subepithelial scar), pseudogerontoxon.

Treatment

- *Topical*: mast cell stabilizer (e.g. sodium cromoglicate 2% g 4×/d) ± topical steroid ± ciclosporin (either 2% g or 0.2% oc 3–4×/d); consider mucolytic (e.g. acetylcysteine 5% 4×/d).
- **NB** Acute exacerbations may require intensive treatment with topical steroids (e.g. dexamethasone 0.1% PF hourly) but then titrate down to the minimum potency/frequency required to control exacerbations, e.g. fluoromethalone 0.1% 1–2×/d). Topical ciclosporin may be used as an adjunct with a 'steroid-sparing' role. It is available in two preparations: 2% ciclosporin drops and 0.2% ciclosporin ointment. The latter is only licensed for veterinary use ('target species dog') but has been widely used in humans (off-label).
- *Systemic*: if severe consider systemic immunosuppression in conjunction with dermatologist/clinical immunologist; if using immunosuppressants consider antiviral (e.g. aciclovir 200mg 5×/d or 400mg 2×/d) as these patients are vulnerable to herpes simplex keratitis.
- *Surgical*: debridement or superficial lamellar keratectomy to remove plaques/shield ulcers.

Atopic keratoconjunctivitis

This is a rare but serious condition of adults (onset 25–30yrs). Patients are usually atopic, commonly with eczema of the lids and staphylococcal lid disease. Control of lid disease is an important aspect of treatment. This is a mixed type I and IV hypersensitivity response, but with a higher Th1 cell type component than in vernal disease.

Clinical features

- Itching, redness; photophobia ± blurred vision (if keratitis); history of atopy.
- Lid eczema (often severe), staphylococcal lid disease (anterior blepharitis), small tightly packed papillae, otherwise featureless tarsal conjunctiva (due to inflammation); chemosis + limbal hyperaemia (acute exacerbations); may cicatrize (chronic) with forniceal shortening.
- *Keratitis*: inferior punctate epithelial erosions, shield ulcers, pannus, corneal vascularization, herpes simplex, or microbial keratitis.
- *Associations*: keratoconus, cataract (anterior subcapsular type).

Treatment

- *Topical*: as for VKC, including preservative free ocular lubricants + mast cell stabilizer (usually less effective than in VKC) ± topical steroid (e.g. initially dexamethasone 0.1% PF hourly) ± ciclosporin (2% g or 0.2% oc 3–4×/d).
- *Systemic*: consider oral antihistamines (may help with itching) and for severe exacerbations corticosteroids/immunosuppressants; if using immunosuppressants consider antiviral (e.g. aciclovir 200mg 5×/d or 400mg 2×/d) as these patients are vulnerable to herpes simplex keratitis.
- *Surgical*: consider debridement or superficial lamellar keratectomy to remove plaques.
- *For lid disease*: consider topical (e.g. chloramphenicol 1% oc 4×/d) and oral (e.g. doxycycline 100mg 1×/d 3mths) antibiotics.
- *For secondary infective keratitis*: topical antivirals and antibiotics.
- *Skin disease*: liaise with dermatologist; consider topical tacrolimus.

Cicatricial conjunctivitis (1)

In this potentially blinding condition, conjunctival inflammation with scarring leads to the loss of conjunctival function (such as goblet cells) and architecture.

Onset may be insidious, delaying diagnosis. Some types of cicatrizing conjunctivitis are typically progressive (e.g. in OMMP), whereas others are usually non-progressive after the initial period (e.g. associated with trauma or acute infectious membranous conjunctivitis).

Although there are many causes, cicatrization has broadly similar ocular features and similar treatment modalities may be considered.

Get expert help early—it is very easy to underestimate these conditions.

Ocular mucous membrane pemphigoid (OMMP)

Mucous membrane pemphigoid is a chronic inflammatory subepithelial blistering disease of the mucus membranes. It usually occurs >60yrs of age, but may occur in adolescents, in whom the disease is more severe;[1] it is slightly more common in females.

There is an association with other autoimmune disease (e.g. rheumatoid arthritis and pernicious anaemia).

Mucous membrane pemphigoid is thought to be a type II hypersensitivity reaction with linear deposition of immunoglobulin and complement at the basement membrane zone of mucosal surfaces. Although the target antigens are known (the antibodies are specific to components of the basement membrane and hemidesmesomes), the initiating agents for the disease are not clear. The consequences are chronic inflammation, loss of adhesion and bulla formation and subsequent cicatrization; during severe active disease acute inflammation may be seen. Oral mucosa and conjunctiva are most commonly affected although skin and other mucous membranes may be involved. Involvement of the trachea or oesophagus is potentially life-threatening.

According to International Consensus[2] the diagnosis of mucous membrane pemphigoid requires direct immunopathological confirmation as well as typical clinical features. However in the context of OMMP (formerly known as ocular cicatricial pemphigoid), diagnosis is primarily clinical with immunopathology providing supporting evidence.

Clinical features
- Irritation.
- Chronic papillary conjunctivitis, subconjunctival vesicles → ulcerate, progressive cicatrization (loss of plica semilunaris and fornices, formation of symblepharon/ankyloblepharon), dry eye signs, secondary microbial keratitis, corneal neovascularization, corneal melt, perforation, limbal stem cell failure.

NB Be alert for secondary microbial keratitis: the eye with OMMP is vulnerable due to the combination of poor ocular surface and immunosuppression.

Treatment
Early diagnosis and treatment improves outcome.[3] Refer early for specialist help.

- *Topical*: tear substitutes, corticosteroids, and antibiotics (PF).
- *Systemic immunosuppression (for acute phase of disease)*: dapsone if mild, mycophenolate, methotrexate, or azathioprine for moderate disease and high-dose IV methylprednisolone ± cyclophosphamide if severe (liaise with a rheumatologist; all need monitoring); systemic immunosuppression is generally required for >1yr.[3] Emerging therapies include new biologics (e.g. anti-TNF therapies and rituximab). Progression, however, may occur in the apparent absence of clinical inflammation.
- *Consider* silicone hydrogel contact lenses and surgery (for correction of lid and lash position; punctal occlusion or tarsorrhaphy; botulinum toxin is of limited use due to mechanical restriction; corneal transplant or surface reconstruction procedures; keratoprosthesis).

1. Raiz S et al. Evaluation of mucous membrane pemphigoid with ocular involvement in young patients. *Ophthalmology* 2005;**112**:1268–74.

2. Chan LS et al. The first international consensus of mucous membrane pemphigoid—definition, diagnostic criteria, pathogenic factors, medical treatment, and prognostic indicators. *Arch Dermatol* 2002;**138**:370–9.

3. Saw V et al. Immunosuppressive therapy for ocular mucous membrane pemphigoid. *Ophthalmology* 2008;**115**(2):253–61.

Cicatricial conjunctivitis (2)

Other types of primary cicatricial conjunctivitis

Erythema muliforme, Stevens–Johnson syndrome, and toxic epidermal necrolysis (Lyell disease)

These are acute vasculitides of the mucous membranes and skin associated with drug hypersensitivity (sulphonamides, anticonvulsants, allopurinol) or infections (e.g. mycoplasma, HSV). They are thought to result from a type III hypersensitivity response (circulating immune complexes) and represent a continuum of disease with varying severities of epithelial detachment.

TEN is the most severe, characterized histologically by keratinocyte apoptosis and clinically by >30% body involvement, and a 30–40% mortality rate.

Clinical features

- Acute fever/malaise and skin rash (e.g. target lesions or bullae) ± haemorrhagic inflammation of mucous membranes (SJS and TEN).
- Sloughing of epidermal surfaces (seen in TEN) is called Nikolsky's sign.
- Papillary or pseudomembranous conjunctivitis → cicatrization (as for OMMP).[1,2]
- Ocular disease progression, including ocular surface failure can occur years after the acute illness.[1]

Treatment

Acute phase

- Expert multidisciplinary care is required; should be treated in regional burns unit where possible.
- *Topical*: tear substitutes, corticosteroids, and antibiotics (PF).
- *Systemic immunosuppression*: controversy surrounds the use of corticosteroids as they have a role for ocular disease, but may have a negative effect on general disease and prognosis. There is a possible role for IV immunoglobulin and IV ciclosporin.
- Consider surgical division of adhesions and removal of membranes (e.g. glass rodding by an experienced ophthalmologist), symblepharon rings, *gas-permeable scleral contact lenses (controversial: need expert fitting and risk of infection)*, and surgery (amniotic membrane grafting to protect ocular surfaces and lids).

Chronic phase

- Management of chronic sequelae are as outlined for OMMP.
- Other bullous diseases in which cicatricial conjunctivitis is common include linear IgA disease (linear IgA at the dermoepidermal junction) and epidermolysis bullosa.

Secondary cicatricial conjunctivitis

Injury

Thermal, radiation, chemical (especially alkali), and surgical injuries (a critical issue in glaucoma surgery) may all cause cicatrization.

Anterior blepharitis (staphylococcal)

Limited cicatrization and keratinization of the lid margin with reduced tear film quality may cause chronic irritation.

Infective conjunctivitis

Cicatrization is most common with *Chlamydia trachomatis*, but may also occur after membranous and pseudomembranous conjunctivitis.

Drugs

This may vary from mild irritation to drug-induced cicatrizing conjunctivitis, clinically indistinguishable from OMMP. Drugs implicated may be systemic (practolol, penicillamine) and topical (propine, pilocarpine, timolol, idoxuridine, gentamicin (particularly 1.5%), guanethidine).

Inherited

This includes ectodermal dysplasia (associated abnormalities of hair and teeth) and epidermolysis bullosa (inherited hemidesmosome disease).

Systemic

Consider rosacea, Sjögren syndrome, and GVHD.

Graft-versus-host-disease (GVHD)

GVHD occurs in some allogeneic bone marrow transplant patients where the donor's leucocytes attack the immunosuppressed recipient. GVHD most commonly affects the ocular surface, although rarely posterior segment features (e.g. posterior scleritis, choroidal thickening) during the acute stage.

- In the acute response there is TEN, which may include a pseudomembranous conjunctivitis. It may be graded stage I, hyperaemia; stage II, hyperaemia with serosanguineous chemosis; stage III, pseudomembranous conjunctivitis; and stage IV, pseudomembranous conjunctivitis with corneal epithelial sloughing[3]
- In chronic GVHD there are scleroderma-like changes of the skin and Sjögren-like changes of the glands to cause dry eye and cicatricial changes of the conjunctiva.

Neoplastic

Unilateral cicatrizing conjunctivitis may be due to sebaceous cell carcinoma, conjunctival intraepithelial neoplasia, or squamous cell carcinoma.

1. Da Rojas MV et al. The natural history of Stevens Johnson syndrome: patterns of chronic ocular disease and the role of systemic immunosuppressive therapy. Ophthalmology 2007;**91**:1048–53.

2. Sotozona C et al. New grading system for the evaluation of chronic ocular manifestations in patients with Stevens-Johnson syndrome. Ophthalmology 2007;**114**:1294–302.

3. Jabs DA et al. The eye in bone marrow transplantation. III. Conjunctival graft-vs-host disease. Arch Ophthalmol 1989;**107**:1343–8.

Dry eyes (1)

Although patients report 'dry eyes' extremely commonly, most often they are describing mild tear film instability associated with blepharitis.

While some symptomatic relief will be obtained from artificial tears, in these cases the blepharitis itself should be the focus of treatment. However, true dry eyes (syn keratoconjunctivitis sicca (KCS)) may be severe, very painful, and threaten vision.

Causes

The major causes of dry eyes (Table 6.5) may be classified according to the Dry Eye Workshop (known as the DEWS report).[1,2]

Clinical features

- Burning (may be very painful) ± blurred vision (corneal involvement).
- Mucus strands; small/absent concave tear meniscus; punctate epitheliopathy; filaments; mucus plaques; tear film break-up time <10s; Lissamine green or Rose Bengal <o> pattern; Schirmer test <5mm over 5min (without topical anaesthetic). (Rose Bengal is now widely unavailable; Lissamine Green is an alternative.)

Scoring severity

Table 6.4 Grading of severity in dry eye disease (DEWS report)

Level Feature	1	2	3	4
Discomfort (severity/ frequency)	Mild and/ or episodic; response to environment	Moderate episodic or chronic; stress or no stress	Severe frequent or constant without stress	Severe and/or disabling and constant
Visual symptoms	None or episodic mild fatigue	Annoying and/ or activity-limiting episodic	Annoying, chronic and/ or constant, limiting activity	Constant and/ or possibly disabling
Conjunctival injection	None to mild	None to mild	+/–	+/++
Conjunctival staining	None to mild	Variable	Moderate to marked	Marked
Corneal staining	None to mild	Variable	Marked central	Severe punctate erosions
Corneal/tear signs	None to mild	Mild debris, ↓ meniscus	Filamentary keratitis, mucus clumping, ↑ tear debris	As for (3) + ulceration
Lids/ meibomian gland disease	Meibomian gland disease variably present	Meibomian gland disease variably present	Frequent	Trichiasis, keratinization, symblepharon
TFBUT	Variable	≤10s	≤5s	Immediate
Schirmer score	Variable	≤10mm/5min	≤5mm/5min	≤2mm/5min

For level 4, symptoms and signs are required.

Table 6.5 Causes of dry eyes

Aqueous deficient		
Sjögren syndrome	Primary Sjögren syndrome	KCS with xerostomia (dry mouth)
	Secondary Sjögren syndrome	KCS with xerostomia associated with connective tissue disease such as rheumatoid arthritis, SLE, systemic sclerosis, graft-versus-host-disease
Lacrimal gland deficiencies	Primary	Age-related dry eye Congenital alacrima Familial dysautonomia
	Secondary	Lacrimal gland infiltration • Sarcoidosis • Lymphoma • AIDS • Graft-vs-host disease Lacrimal gland ablation Lacrimal gland denervation
Lacrimal gland duct obstruction		Trachoma OMMP Erythema multiforme Chemical and thermal burns
Reflex hyposecretion		Reflex sensory block Contact lens wear Diabetes Neurotrophic keratitis Reflex motor block VII cranial nerve damage Multiple neuromatosis
Systemic drugs		
Evaporative		
Intrinsic (direct effect on evaporation)		Meibomian oil deficiency Lid aperture problems Low blink rate Drugs
Extrinsic (indirect effect via changes to ocular surface)		Vitamin A deficiency Topical drugs/preservatives Contact lens wear Ocular surface disease (e.g. allergy)

1. International Dry Eye Workshop: The Ocular Surface 2007; 5(2) www.tearfilm.org/dewsreport

2. Behrens A et al. Dysfunctional tear syndrome. A Delphi approach to treatment recommendations. Cornea 2006:**25**:900–7.

Dry eyes (2)

Treatment

General

Treat ocular disease according to its severity[1,2] (Table 6.6) and ensure that any underlying systemic disease is optimally controlled.

Table 6.6 Treatment according to severity level

Level 1	Level 2	Level 3	Level 4
	If level 1 treatment inadequate add:	If level 2 treatment inadequate add:	If level 3 treatment inadequate add:
Education and environmental/ dietary modifications	Topical anti-inflammatories	Autologous serum	Systemic anti-inflammatory drugs
Elimination of offending systemic medications	Tetracyclines (for meibomianitis or rosacea)	Contact lenses	Surgery (lid surgery, tarsorrhaphy; salivary gland transposition, mucus membrane/amniotic membrane)
Artificial tear substitutes, gels/ointments	Punctal plugs	Permanent punctal occlusion	
Lid hygiene	Secretogogues		

Tear substitutes

- *Consider viscosity*: low viscosity drops require frequent administration (sometimes more than hourly) but have minimal effect on vision; more viscous gels will transiently blur the vision but are longer lasting and may be effective when used only 4–6×/d; highly viscous paraffin-based ointments significantly blur vision and may only be suitable for night use.
- *Consider preservative free preparations*: to reduce the risk of epithelial toxicity if frequent administration required.
- *Consider physiological tear substitutes*:
  - hyaluronic acid is a natural component of tears. Sodium hyaluronate preparations are now commercially available for topical application (e.g. Vismed®, Clinitas Soothe™, Oxyal™). It improves the symptoms of dry eye and is cytoprotective, promotes basement membrane hemidesmosome formation, and have improved surface retention in inflamed eyes due to specific ligand binding to exaggerated CD44 (a transmembrane cell surface adhesion molecule) expression on the ocular surface during inflammation (Box 7.6).
  - carboxymethylcellulose (carmellose) is a widely used agent that appears to provide cytoprotection (in addition to being a lubricant).
  - autologous serum: in severe cases autologous serum may be used (available on a named-patient basis from the National Blood Service (UK)).

Table 6.7 Commonly used artificial tears and lubricants (selected)

Viscosity	Frequency	Preserved-form examples	PF examples
Low Hypromellose/ polyvinyl alcohol	q 4h–q ½h	Hypromellose Hypotears® Sno Tears®	Liquifilm® (PF) Refresh®
Medium Carbomer/ cellulose	1–6×/d	Viscotears® GelTears®	Celluvisc® (0.5%/1%) Minims® artificial Tears Viscotears PF®
High Paraffins	1–4×/d		Lacri-Lube® Lubri-Tears® Simple eye ointment

Lid treatments
Treat any blepharitis: lid hygiene ± oral antibiotic (e.g. doxycycline 100mg 1×/d 3mths; doxycycline also has significant anti-inflammatory role and is a proteinase inhibitor; note contraindications).

Anti-inflammatories
Treat any active inflammation: consider topical corticosteroids; if responsive these patients may benefit from topical ciclosporin (e.g. Restasis®, a 0.05% preparation of ciclosporin licensed for dry eyes, currently only available on a named patient basis from international pharmacies).

Secretogogues
• *Increase secretion*: pilocarpine hydrochloride 2.5mg 1–4×/d (increase slowly from 5mg/d to try to reduce anticholinergic side-effects).
• Pilocarpine is licensed for dry mouth and dry eyes in Sjögren syndrome but only effective if some residual lacrimal gland function).

Interventional/surgical
• *Punctal occlusion*: plugs can be intracanalicular or punctal, and either temporary (collagen-based) or permanent.(silicone-based); permanent occlusion can also be achieved by cauterization of the puncta.
• *Therapeutic contact lenses*: consider silicone hydrogel or, less commonly, scleral contact lenses (scleral contact lenses require expert fitting) to retain a protective tear lake over the cornea.
• *Surgery*: occasionally salivary gland transposition (the parotid or submandibular glands—*beware* severe reflex gustatory epiphora).

Other therapeutic options
• *Mucolytic* (if filaments, mucus plaques): acetylcysteine 5% 4×/d (warn that it stings).
• *Environmental*: lower room temperature, moist chamber goggles, room humidifier (limited success).
• *Dietary*: intake of fish high in omega-3 fatty acids is associated with ↓dry eye symptoms in women.

1. International Dry Eye Workshop: *The Ocular Surface* 2007;**5**(2). www.tearfilm.org/dewsreport/.
2. Behrens A *et al.* Dysfunctional tear syndrome. A Delphi approch to treatment recommendations. Cornea 2006, **25**:900–7.

Miscellaneous conjunctivitis and conjunctival degenerations

Toxic conjunctivitis

Topical medication (e.g. aminoglycosides, antivirals, glaucoma treatments, preservatives, and contact lens solutions) may result in an inferior papillary reaction. With chronic usage topical medication (e.g. glaucoma treatments, antibiotics, and antivirals) may cause a follicular reaction and conjunctival cicatrization. Inferior punctate epitheliopathy may be seen.

Treatment: discontinue precipitating agent and consider preservative free ocular lubricant (e.g. Celluvisc®).

Parinaud oculoglandular syndrome

This is a rare unilateral conjunctivitis with granulomatous nodules (+ follicles) on the palpebral conjunctiva, ipsilateral lymphadenopathy (preauricular/submandibular), and systemic upset (malaise, fever). Most commonly due to cat-scratch disease (*Bartonella henselae*), but also consider tularaemia, mycobacteria (e.g. tuberculosis), sarcoid, syphilis, lymphoproliferative disorders, infectious mononucleosis, fungi, etc.

Investigations will be dictated by history but consider conjunctival biopsy, conjunctival swabs, FBC, VDRL, CXR, Mantoux testing, serology (cat-scratch, and tularaemia).

Ligneous conjunctivitis

This is a rare idiopathic chronic conjunctivitis of children (especially girls) characterized by recurrent pseudomembranes or membranes of the 'wood-like' tarsal conjunctiva, and often of other mucous membranes (e.g. oropharynx, trachea, etc.). Histologically, these comprise fibrin, albumin, IgG, T and B cells. Treat with topical ciclosporin A. It is available in two preparations: 2% ciclosporin drops and 0.2% ciclosporin ointment. The latter is only licensed for veterinary use ('target species dog') but has been widely used in humans (off-label).

Pinguecula

Extremely common, this yellow–white patch of interpalpebral bulbar conjunctiva is located just nasal or temporal to the limbus. It represents elastotic degeneration of collagen.

Reassurance and occasionally ocular lubrication is usually all that is required.

Pterygium

This triangular fibrovascular band is commonest in males exposed to dry climates and high UV light. It usually arises from the nasal limbus, grows slowly across the cornea, and ceases before causing any significant visual impact. Histologically, it is akin to pinguecula with elastotic degeneration of collagen, but with additional destruction of Bowman's layer. It is adherent to underlying tissue for the whole length cf. pseudopterygium, which is a fold of conjunctiva, only attached at the base and apex, usually resulting from corneal ulceration with adherence of local conjunctiva.

Clinical features
- Cosmetic issues, astigmatism, may encroach on visual axis, FB sensation.
- Triangular pink–white fibrovascular band.
  - *Signs of activity*: rapid growth, engorged vessels, inflammation, grey leading edge in the cornea, punctate epitheliopathy.
  - *Signs of stability*: iron line (Stocker line) just anterior to the margin.

Treatment
- Reserve for progressive, vision threatening lesions as recurrence is common and may be aggressive.
- Excise with conjunctival autograft. Amniotic membrane graft, or MMC may be used when removing recurrent or large pterygia/pseudopterygia); if the visual axis is involved lamellar keratoplasty may also be required.

Concretions

Common in the elderly and those with chronic blepharitis, these yellow–white deposits may erode through the palpebral conjunctiva causing a FB sensation. If troublesome they can be removed with a needle (at the slit-lamp under topical anaesthetic).

Retention cyst

Very common, this thin-walled fluid-filled conjunctival cyst occasionally causes symptoms if it disturbs the corneal tear film. It can be punctured with a needle (at the slit-lamp under topical anaesthetic) but may recur, in which case consider excision.

Pigmented conjunctival lesions

Benign

Congenital

Conjunctival epithelial melanosis

Common, racial, bilateral flat patchy freely moving brown pigmentation, which may be diffuse (usually denser around the limbus and anterior ciliary nerves) or focal, e.g. round and intrascleral nerve (Axenfeld loop).

Conjunctival freckle

Common, tiny flat freely moving pigmented area.

Melanocytoma

Rare, black pigmentation, fixed, slowly growing.

Acquired

Deposits, e.g. mascara in the inferior fornix, coal dust tattoos, adrenochrome on forniceal/palpebral conjunctiva (from chronic adrenaline administration).

Premalignant

Primary acquired melanosis

Uncommon; very rare in African-Caribbeans. Histological differentiation is vital as PAM without atypia is a benign melanocytic proliferation, whereas PAM with atypia has a 50% risk of transformation to melanoma by 5yrs.

Clinical

- Unilateral, single/multifocal flat freely moving area of irregular brown pigmentation. Pigmentation and size of lesion may increase, decrease, or remain constant over time.
- Nodules within PAM suggest malignant transformation to melanoma.

Treatment

For PAM with atypia: excision + cryotherapy/radiotherapy/antimetabolite.

Conjunctival naevus

Uncommon; very low risk of transformation.

Clinical

Single defined freely moving brown pigmentation ± cysts; most commonly at the limbus, followed by the caruncle/plica; may increase in pigmentation/size at puberty. Extension in to the cornea may indicate malignant transformation.

Congenital ocular melanocytosis

Uncommon. Oculodermal melanocytosis (naevus of Ota) is the most common variant, followed by the limited dermal and ocular forms. Oculodermal melanocytosis is more common in females and Orientals.

Clinical

Subconjunctival, flat, grey lesions; associated unilateral hyperpigmentation face (most commonly in a Va/b distribution; ipsilateral iris hyperchromia, iris mamillations, glaucoma (10%) associated with trabecular hyperpigmentation); melanoma (ocular, dermal, or CNS).

Malignant

Melanoma

Consider this first when confronted with abnormal conjunctival pigmentation. Although rare it may be fatal. Commoner in middle age. It most commonly arises from atypical primary acquired melanosis, but may arise from a naevus or de novo.

Clinical

- Solitary grey/black/non-pigmented, vascularized nodule fixed to episclera; most commonly at the limbus.
- May metastasize to draining lymph nodes, lung, liver, brain.

Prognosis

Five-year mortality is 13%. Poor prognostic factors include: multifocal lesion; caruncle, fornix, or palpebral location; thickness >1mm; recurrence; lymphatic or orbital spread.

Treatment

- Wide local excision + double freeze–thaw cryotherapy to excised margins. Consider adjunctive radiotherapy/antimetabolite if incomplete excision/diffuse.
- Exenteration may be necessary if unresectable.

Key points

- Congenital pigmented lesions that are stable, regular, flat, and asymptomatic (i.e. not bleeding, discharging, inflamed, or affecting vision) are likely to be benign.
- Acquired pigmented lesions that are growing, irregular, elevated, or symptomatic (e.g. bleeding, itchy, painful, inflamed) are more likely to be malignant.
- *Specialist advice should be sought for all potentially malignant/premalignant lesions.*

Non-pigmented conjunctival lesions

Benign

Papilloma

- *Pedunculated form*—common from teenage onwards, associated with HPV 6, 11, 16, and 18; most commonly arise from palpebral/forniceal/caruncular conjunctiva, and are often bilateral and multiple.
  - *Treatment*: they often resolve spontaneously, but surgery, cryotherapy, oral cimetidine, topical MMC or intralesional interferon may be used for large/persistent lesions.
- *Sessile form*—common in middle age; most commonly arise from bulbar/limbal conjunctiva, and are usually unilateral and solitary.
  - *Treatment*: excision.

Transmission may be vertical, through sexual contact or autoinfection from distant papillomas. There is an important association with HIV infection. The potential for malignant transformation is controversial.[1]

Epibulbar choristoma

- *Dermoids*: uncommon choristoma of childhood; associated with Goldenhar syndrome. A soft yellow limbal mass that is usually unilateral; it may encircle the lmbus.
  - *Treatment*: can be excised with lamellar graft if limbal but forniceal require CT scan to rule out intra-orbital/intracranial extension.
- *Lipodermoid*: uncommon choristoma of adults. This is a soft white mass at the lateral canthus.
- *Ectopic lashes*: rare choristomas seen as subconjunctival cilia.

Pyogenic granuloma

Typically a rapidly growing red vascular mass after previous trauma/surgery.

Premalignant

Conjunctival intra-epithelial neoplasia (carcinoma in-situ, dysplasia)

Rare; commoner over age 50yrs. It is usually conjunctival in origin, but may arise from the cornea. It may transform to squamous cell carcinoma (with breaching of the basement membrane).

- *Clinical features*: it appears as a fleshy freely moving mass with tufted vessels located at the limbus.
- *Treatment*: excision + MMC ± cryotherapy to affected limbus.

Malignant

Conjunctival squamous cell carcinoma

The commonest malignant conjunctival tumour worldwide but rare in temperate climates.

Commoner over 50yrs of age.

UV light and human papillomavirus are risk factors, and it may be associated with HIV in younger patients.

It may arise from intra-epithelial hyperplasia or *de novo*;[2] although usually conjunctival, it may also arise from corneal epithelium.

Clinical features
Persistent unilateral keratoconjunctivitis; ranges from atypical 'dysplastic' epithelium to limbal gelatinous mass, which may infiltrate cornea, sclera, and penetrate the globe; rarely metastasizes.

Treatment
Excision (2–3mm clear margins) + MMC, double freeze–thaw cryotherapy to margins or enucleation/exenteration (if very advanced).

Conjunctival Kaposi sarcoma
Typically a bright red mass, usually in the inferior fornix, which may mimic a persistent subconjunctival haemorrhage.
May be caused by HHV8 (commonly in the presence of HIV).
- *Treatment*: focal radiotherapy if large/aggressive.

Conjunctival lymphoma
Typically a salmon-pink subconjunctival infiltrate, often bilateral. They are usually located in the fornices.
Histology is essential as it may be benign or malignant.
Most commonly it represents extranodal B-cell non-Hodgkin's lymphoma, although it may also arise in the orbit (anterior spread) or in mucosal associated lymphoid tissue (MALToma).
Imaging and haematological/oncological referral are required in confirmed cases.
- *Treatment*: excision ± cryotherapy or subconjunctival interferon α-2b may be employed ± local radiotherapy.

Muco-epidermoid carcinoma
This is a very rare, aggressive tumour that may mimic a pterygium. It arises from conjunctival mucus-secreting cells and squamous cells.

Infiltration from lid tumours
Sebaceous cell carcinoma of the lid may spread to involve the conjunctiva, so presenting as a unilateral cicatrising conjunctivitis (see Lid lumps: malignant tumours p.136).

> Key point
> - *Specialist advice should be sought for all potentially malignant/ premalignant lesions*

1. Karcioglu ZA *et al.* Human papilloma virus in neoplastic and non-neoplastic conditions of the external eye. *Br J Ophthalmol* 1997;**81**:595–8.

2. Tulvatana W *et al.* Risk factors for conjunctival squamous cell neoplasia: a matched case-control study. *BJO* 2003;**87**:396–8.

3. Ross JJ *et al.* Systemic remission of non-Hodgkin's lymphoma after intralesional interferon α-2b to bilateral conjunctival lymphomas. *Am J Ophthalmol* 2004;**138**:672–3.

Cornea

Anatomy and physiology

The cornea acts as a clear refractive surface and a protective barrier to infection and trauma. Its anterior surface is elliptical (11.7mm horizontally, 10.6mm vertically), whereas its posterior surface is circular (11.7mm). It is thinnest centrally (520μm), and thicker peripherally (660μm). The tear-film is discussed in (Conjuctival anatomy and physiology 🔲 p.158).

Anatomy

The cornea consists of five layers. From anterior to posterior these are:

Epithelium

The corneal epithelium is divided into two areas: the limbus (containing the limbal epithelial stem cells) and the central cornea (containing the terminally differentiated cells).

Epithelium of the central cornea

This is a non-keratinized stratified squamous epithelium (5–7 cell layers thick), which accounts for about 10% of the thickness of the adult cornea. It is of ectodermal origin.

Cells are firmly adherent to the underlying basement membrane and corneal stroma, by highly specific molecular building blocks known as hemidesmosomes. More superficially the cells flatten to become wing cells, and apical cells are characterized by microvilli coated by a negatively charged glycoprotein facilitating tear film stability.

Limbal epithelial stem cells

The corneo-scleral limbus represents the corneal stem cell niche (higher density superiorly and inferiorly). Stem cells amplify, proliferate, and differentiate into corneal epithelium. Damage to this area results in the invasion of conjunctival epithelium on to the cornea.

Basement membrane zone

The basement membrane zone consists of the epithelial basement membrane and Bowman's layer. Bowman's layer is a strong but thin avascular superficial stromal layer of collagen fibrils. Hemidesmosomes link the corneal epithelium to the basement membrane It is also of ectodermal origin. It is unable to regenerate and therefore heals by scarring.

Stroma

The stroma accounts for about 90% of corneal thickness. Despite active deturgence its main component is water (75%). Of its dry weight, 70% is collagen (type I, IV, V, VI) and the remainder is proteogylcan ground substance (chrondroitin sulphate and keratan sulphate). Keratocytes are a resident population of modified fibroblasts involved in remodelling following injury. It is of mesodermal origin. Collagen fibres are arranged to confer transparency. The avascular cornea derives nutrition from the tear film and aqueous humour.

Descemet's membrane

Descemet's membrane consists of a fetal anterior banded zone (present at birth) and a posterior non-banded zone (produced later by the endothelium). It is of mesodermal origin. It is not capable of regeneration.

Endothelium

This is a monolayer of hexagonal epithelial cells (misnamed as 'endothelial') forming a continuous mosaic best seen with specular microscopy. It is of mesodermal origin with the apical border in direct contact with the aqueous humour and basolateral border with the Descemet's membrane. It is unable to regenerate. Cell loss with age is compensated by enlargement (polymegathism) and migration of neighbouring cells. The endothelial sodium transporting capacity is critical for corneal deturgescence.

Physiology

Corneal transparency

Corneal transparency is dependent on:
- *Active deturgence*: the *endothelium* is relatively permeable. A passive flow of water and nutrients from the aqueous is drawn across into the stroma ('stromal swelling pressure'). To prevent overload (oedema) and maintain its transparency the endothelium pumps Na^+ back out into the aqueous by active $Na^+K^+ATPase$, together with a passive movement of water. Water may also pass through hormonally mediated aquaporins. The *epithelium* is relatively impermeable due to the presence of apical tight junctions.
- *Regular orientation and spacing of stromal collagen fibres*: this reduces diffractive scatter of light. After injury, loss of architecture may result in opacity and scarring.

Refraction

The cornea accounts for 70% of the eye's total dioptric power. The radii of curvature of the anterior surface is 7.7mm, the posterior surface is 6.8mm. The cornea is a robust elastic surface. Its shape is maintained by structural rigidity and intraocular pressure.

Nutrition and nerve supply

The cornea is avascular and relies on diffusion from the limbus and aqueous for nutrition. Langerhans cells (antigen-presenting cells) are present in the epithelium, but are usually restricted to the outer third. The first division of the trigeminal nerve forms stromal and subepithelial plexi responsible for corneal sensation.

Corneal signs

Table 7.1 Epithelial signs and their pathophysiology

Sign	Pathology	Causes
Punctate epithelial erosions	Multiple fine areas of epithelial loss; stain well with F, poorly with RB	• *Superior*—e.g. vernal keratoconjunctivitis, superior limbic keratitis, floppy eyelid syndrome, poor CL fit • *Interpalpebral*—e.g. keratoconjunctivitis sicca, UV exposure, corneal anaesthesia • *Inferior*—e.g. blepharitis, exposure keratopathy, ectropion, poor blink, poor Bell's phenomenon, rosacea, drop toxicity
Corneal filaments	Mucus strands adherent to cornea with mobile free tails; stain poorly with F, well with RB	• Keratoconjunctivitis sicca, recurrent erosion syndrome, corneal anaesthesia, exposure keratopathy, HZO
Punctate epithelial keratitis	Tiny white spots of epithelial and inflammatory cells; stains poorly with F, well with RB	• Viral keratitis (adenovirus, HSV, Molluscum contagiosum) • Thygeson's superficial punctate Keratopathy
Epithelial oedema	Loss of lustre + translucency; microvesicles and bullae	• ↑IOP, postoperative, CL over wear, aphakic/pseudophakic bullous keratopathy, Fuchs' endothelial dystrophy, trauma, acute hydrops, herpetic keratitis, congenital corneal clouding

F, fluorescein; RB, Rose Bengal; Lissamine Green is an alternative.

Table 7.2 Iron lines (best visualized with cobalt blue light on the slit-lamp)

Line	Location	Causes
Ferry's	At trabeculectomy margin so usually superior	Trabeculectomy
Stocker's	At pterygium margin so usually lateral	Pterygium
Hudson–Stahli	Usually horizontal inferior 1/3 of cornea	Idiopathic (common in elderly)
Fleischer	Ring around base of cone so usually inferocentral	Keratoconus

Table 7.3 Stromal signs and their pathophysiology

Sign	Pathology	Causes
Pannus	Subepithelial fibrovascular ingrowth	• Trachoma, tight CL, phlycten, herpetic keratitis, rosacea keratitis, chemical keratopathy, marginal keratitis, vernal keratoconjunctivitis, atopic keratoconjunctivitis, superior limbal keratoconjunctivitis
Stromal infiltrate	Focal opacification due to leucocyte aggregations (sterile) or microbial colonization	• Sterile—marginal keratitis, CL related • Infective—bacteria, fungi, viruses, protozoa
Stromal oedema	Thickened, grey opaque stroma	• Postoperative, keratoconus, Fuchs' endothelial dystrophy, herpetic disciform keratitis
Cornea farinata	Deep stromal faint flour-like opacities	• Idiopathic (innocuous)
Crocodile Shagreen	Reticular polygonal network of stromal opacity	• Idiopathic (innocuous)

Table 7.4 Endothelial signs and their pathophysiology

Sign	Pathology	Causes
Descemet's folds	Folds in intact DM	• Postoperative, IOP, disciform keratitis, congenital syphilis
Descemet's breaks	Breaks through DM associated oedema of overlying stroma	• Birth trauma, keratoconus/keratoglobus (hydrops), infantile glaucoma (Haab's striae)
Guttata	Wart-like protuberances at endothelium	• *Peripheral*: Hassall–Henle bodies (physiological in the elderly) • *Central*: Fuchs' endothelial dystrophy
Pigment on endothelium	Dusting of pigment from iris on endothelium	• Pigment dispersion syndrome (Krukenberg spindle), postoperative, trauma
Keratic precipitates	Aggregates of inflammatory cells on endothelium	• Keratitis (e.g. disciform, microbial, marginal) • Anterior uveitis (e.g. idiopathic, HLA-B27, Fuchs' heterochromic cyclitis, sarcoidosis, etc.)

DM, Descemet's membrane.

Corneal diagrams

Accurate documentation of corneal disease is important for assessing disease progression and response to treatment. Pictorial representation is generally the easiest. Note height, width, and depth of any lesions and any areas of corneal thickening or thinning.

Using standardized shading schemes can be useful, but as a number of different schemes have been described[1] include additional identifying labels to prevent any misunderstanding.

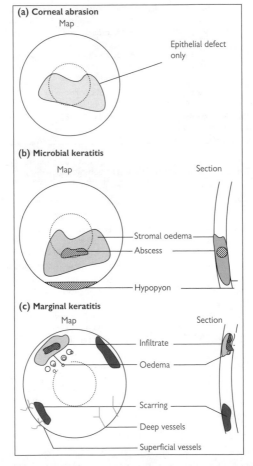

Fig. 7.1 (a) Corneal abrasion, (b) microbial keratitis, and (c) marginal keratitis.

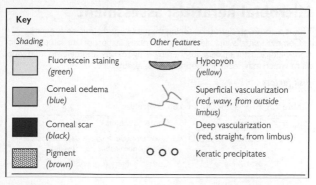

Fig. 7.1 *(Continued)*.

1. Bron AJ. A simple scheme for documenting corneal disease. *Br J Ophthalmol* 1973;**57**:629–34.

Microbial keratitis: assessment

This is a common sight-threatening treatable ophthalmic emergency.

Common pitfalls include delay in diagnosis, inappropriate sample collection, injudicious or inadequate therapy, drug toxicity, and delayed follow-up, all of which may result in suboptimal visual outcome.

Risk factors

Table 7.5 Risk factors for microbial keratitis

Ocular	Trauma	Corneal abrasion
	Contact lenses (CL)	Extended wear > soft > daily disposable > rigid gas permeable; poor hygiene
	Iatrogenic	Corneal surgery (e.g. LASIK) Removal of suture Loose suture Long-term topical steroids/antibiotics
	Ocular surface disease	Dry eyes Bullous keratopathy Chronic blepharoconjunctivitis Corneal anaesthesia Chronic keratitis (e.g. HSV) Cicatricial disease Neurotrophic keratitis (e.g. HSV, VZV, tumours of the cerebellopontine angle)
	Lid disease	Entropion Lagophthalmos Trichiasis
	Nasolacrimal disease	Chronic dacryocystitis
Systemic	Immunosuppression	Drugs Immunodeficiency syndromes Diabetes RA
	Nutritional	Vitamin A deficiency

Clinical features
- Pain, FB sensation, redness, photophobia, tearing, discharge (may be purulent), ↓VA.
- Circumlimbal/diffuse injection, single, or multiple foci of white opacity within stroma ± oedema, usually associated epithelial defect and anterior uveitis.
- *Complications*: limbal and scleral extension, corneal perforation, endophthalmitis (rare unless perforation or in the context of organisms, such as gonococcus or fungi, that can penetrate intact epithelia), panophthalmitis.

NB May present insidiously as infectious crystalline keratopathy (see Deposition keratopathies, 📖 p.240).

Investigations
- Perform early and adequate corneal scrapes (Box 7.1).
- If patient wears CL, send lenses, solutions, and cases for culture, but warn patient that they will be destroyed.
- Liaise with microbiologists especially with regards to length of incubation required, antibiotic sensitivities required, and if unusual clinical features.
- If herpetic disease is considered to be an underlying risk factor, take a swab for molecular diagnostics (PCR).

Box 7.1. How to perform a corneal scrape

- Instil PF topical anaesthesia (and perform scrape prior to use of fluorescein).
- Use a Kimura spatula, no. 15 blade or 25-gauge needle.
- Scrape both the base and leading edge of the ulcer (from uninvolved to involved cornea).
- Place material on to glass slide for microscopy and staining (Gram stain Ziehl–Neelson, methenamine silver, etc.).
- Plate on to blood agar (aerobes), chocolate agar (*Neisseria*, *Haemophilus*), Sabouraud agar (fungi), and consider non-nutrient *Escherichia coli* enriched agar (if Acanthamoeba suspected); when plating small samples, rows of 'C-streaks' are more effective than the traditional technique.
- Consider also culture in thioglycolate (anaerobes) and enrichment (bacteria) broths.

Table 7.6 Microbiological processing of corneal scrapes

Routine stains	Gram stain	B		F	A		
Additional stains	Giemsa stain	B		F	A		
	Gomori/Methenamine Silver			F	A		
	periodic acid Schiff			F	A		
	Calcofluor white			F	A		
	Ziehl–Neelson					M	N
Routine media	Blood agar	B					
	Chocolate agar	B					
	Sabouraud's dextrose agar			F			
	Thioglycolate broth	B(an)					
Additional media	Lowenstein–Jensen					M	N
	Non-nutrient *E. coli* enriched agar				A		

B, bacteria; B(an), anaerobic bacteria; F, fungi; A, acanthamoeba; M, mycobacteria; N, nocardia.

Microbial keratitis: treatment

The treatment of microbial keratitis can be divided into a sterilization phase followed by a healing phase. During the sterilization phase appropriate topical antibiotics are administered intensively for 48–72h. During the healing phase topical corticosteroids may be added and the topical antibiotics are reduced.

Initial treatment

- Stop contact lens wear.
- Admit patient if severe infection, poor compliance, or other concern.

Box 7.2 Indications for admission

- *Severe infection*: >1.5mm diameter infiltrate, hypopyon, purulent exudate, or complicated disease.
- *Poor compliance likely*: either with administering drops or returning for daily review.
- *Other concerns*: only eye, failing to improve, etc.

- *Intensive topical antibiotics*: initially use an hourly empirical broad spectrum regimen with either one or two topical antibiotics. If underlying ocular surface disease or immunocompromise then treatment should be dual therapy (e.g. cefuroxime + ofloxacin) and preservative free (PF).

Box 7.3 Dual therapy vs monotherapy in empirical treatment of microbial keratitis

Dual therapy
Commonly 'fortified' preparations of a cephalosporin (cefuroxime 5%) with a fluoroquinolone (e.g. ofloxacin). Penicillin 0.3% may be substituted for the cephalosporin if streptococcal infection suspected. Use aminoglycoside with caution (e.g. gentamicin 1.5%—beware toxicity and necrosis) particularly in patients with pre-existing ocular surface disease.

Monotherapy
Monotherapy with fluoroquinolones (e.g. ofloxacin) may be adequate for most cases of microbial keratitis, but is insufficient for resistant species of *Staphylococcus aureus* and *Pseudomonas aeruginosa*.

NB Always use PF therapy wherever possible in patients with existing ocular surface disease.

- *Consider oral antibiotics*: if limbal lesion or corneal perforation then add in systemic ciprofloxacin (e.g. oral 750mg 2×/d).
- *Cycloplegia* (e.g. cyclopentolate 1% 2×/d) for photophobia and ciliary spasm and oral analgesia if severe pain.
NB If stromal necrosis or threatened/actual perforation, consider oral tetracyclines and oral vitamin C (inhibit proteases and pro-inflammatory cytokines and ↓ toxic free radicals),

Ongoing treatment

- Monitor response/progression at daily review (in-patient and out-patient) by degree of injection, size of epithelial defect (measure on slit-lamp), size of infiltrate, extent of corneal oedema, and degree of anterior uveitis. Taper frequency and switch to non-fortified preparations with clinical improvement.
- If initial scrape results in no growth and current regimen proves clinically ineffective, consider withholding treatment for 12h before rescraping or performing a formal corneal biopsy. The original slides can be restained with a view to identifying less common organisms (e.g. mycobacteria, fungi, etc.).
- *Consider topical steroids*: use carefully following re-epithelialization, and in the presence of sterile culture, to reduce stromal scarring and possibly improve visual outcome. Initiation requires frequent (often inpatient) follow-up.

Treatment of complications

Persistent epithelial defect

If epithelial defect persists for >2wks then consider switching to PF preparations of topical medication (if not already PF), reducing frequency of topical medication, ocular lubrication, and assisting lid closure.

Resistant or progressive keratitis

Seek specialist advice. In threatened scleral extension consider oral ciprofloxacin that has high bioavailability at the limbus. In threatened corneal perforation consider oral ciprofloxacin, bandage CL (cyanoacrylate glue), or emergency penetrating keratoplasty. Emergency penetrating keratoplasty is usually only performed after a minimum of 2d intensive treatment.

Endophthalmitis

Perform diagnostic vitrectomy and administer intravitreal antibiotics (*see Postoperative endophthalmitis*, 🕮 p.292).

Table 7.7 Common bacterial causes of keratitis

		Frequency	Penetration of intact epithelium	Virulence
Gram +ve	Staphylococcus aureus	Common	–	+
	Staphylococcus epidermidis	Common	–	+/–
	Streptococcus pneumonia	Common	–	++
Gram –ve	Pseudomonas aeruginosa	↑ in CL wearers	–	+++
	Neisseria gonorrhoea	↑ in neonates	+	+++
	Haemophilus	↑ in children	+	+

Microbial keratitis: acanthamoeba

Isolated from soil, dust, sea, fresh, and chlorinated water, acanthamoeba are ubiquitous free-living protozoa. Capable of encystment in unfavourable conditions, the organisms can survive extremes of temperature, desiccation, and pH.

Acanthamoeba keratitis remains rare (0.14 per 1 000 000 UK population in 1996) but incidence is rising with increased contact lens (CL) use. Largely resistant to normal first-line broad-spectrum antibiotics, late suspicion/diagnosis can lead to devastating and irrevocable corneal scarring.

Risk factors

- *Contact lens wear:* especially with extended wear CL, poor CL hygiene (e.g. rinsing in tap water), or after swimming in CL (ponds, hot tubs, swimming pools).
- *Corneal trauma:* notably in a rural or agricultural setting.

Clinical features

- Variable: ranges from asymptomatic, FB sensation, ↓VA or tearing to a severe pain (disproportionate to often relatively mild clinical findings); may occasionally be bilateral.
- Epithelial ridges, pseudo and true dendrites; stromal infiltrates (may progress circumferentially to form a ring); perineural infiltrates; ↓corneal sensation.

NB Beware of missing this diagnosis—it is not uncommonly misdiagnosed as herpes simplex keratitis.

- *Complications:* limbal and scleral extension, corneal perforation, intractable scleritis.

Investigation

- If confocal microscopy available, direct visualization of cysts are diagnostic.
- Perform early and adequate corneal scrapes (Box 7.1). The epithelium is often fairly loose, and some practitioners deliberately debride all the affected epithelium.
- If patient wears CLs send lenses, solutions, and cases for culture, but warn patient that they will be destroyed.
  - *Stains:* Gram (stains organisms), Giemsa (stains the organism and cysts), Calcofluor white (stains cysts visualized under UV light); also send a sample to histology (in formalin).
  - *Culture:* non-nutrient agar with *E. coli* overlay, at 25 and 37°C, may require up to 14d.
- If strong clinical suspicion but negative investigations consider corneal biopsy and histological detection of acanthamoeba cysts. Consider electron microscopy, PCR, and immunofluorescent assay,

Treatment

Initial treatment

- Admit.
- Stop CL wear.
- Intensive topical anti-amoebic agents, commonly a biguanide (polyhexamethylene biguanide 0.02% or chlorhexidine 0.02%) and an aromatic diamidine (e.g. propamidine isethionate 0.1% or hexamidine 0.1%) administered hourly. Aminoglycosides or imidazoles (e.g. oral itraconazole or fluconazole may give additional benefit.
- Oral analgesia and cycloplegia.

Ongoing treatment

- Taper treatment according to clinical improvement. Relapse is common and may signify incomplete sterilization of active acanthoemba trophozites or reactivation of resistant intrastromal cysts. Treatment is prolonged (20–40wks).
- Consider cautious use of topical steroids (while continuing anti-amoebic agents) to reduce corneal scarring.

Treatment of complications

- *If scleritis*: consider immunosuppression with ciclosporin.
- *If poor visual outcome* consider penetrating keratoplasty once treatment is completed and cornea is sterile.
- *If severe*, intractable pain: patients may occasionally require enucleation for severe pain.

Prevention

Education: a known avoidable and predisposing practice is easily identified in more than 90% of cases of acanthamoeba keratitis.

Table 7.8 Anti-amoebic agents

Class	Mechanism	Examples
Aminoglycosides	Inhibit protein synthesis	Neomycin; paramonycin
Aromatic diamidines	Inhibit DNA synthesis	Propamidine isethionate (brolene); hexamidine
Biguanide	Inhibit function of membrane	Polyhexamethylene biguanide; chlorhexidine
Imidazoles	Destabilize cell wall	Clotrimazole; fluconazole; ketoconazoles

Fungal keratitis: assessment

Fungal infection of the cornea is rare.[1] It is usually seen only in the context of trauma (including contact with organic material), or where there is underlying susceptibility such as tissue devitalization or immunosuppression (including topical corticosteroid use).

Candida, *Fusarium*, and *Aspergillus* spp. are the most common infectious agents.

Risk factors

Risk factors include trauma (including LASIK), immunosuppression (e.g. topical corticosteroids, alcoholism, diabetes), ocular surface disease (e.g. dry eye, neurotrophic cornea), hot humid climate and contamination with organic matter (e.g. in the context of agricultural work).

Yeast vs filamentary fungal infections

The presentation of fungal keratitis and its treatment is dependent on the type of fungus responsible.
- *Yeast infection*: usually *Candida* species. Frequently associated with immunosuppression (topical or systemic), and those who have a compromised ocular surface, e.g. autoimmune cicatrizing conjunctivitis, neurotrophic corneas, and severe dry eye.
- *Filamentary fungal infection*: usually *Fusarium* and *Aspergillus* species.

Clinical features
- *General*: variable presentation with onset ranging from insidious to rapid; symptoms range from none to pain, photophobia, tearing, and ↓VA.
- *Yeast infection:* insidious or rapid; often localized with 'button' appearance, expanding stromal infiltrate, and a relatively small epithelial ulceration.
- *Filamentary fungal infection*: usually insidious. *Early*: may be asymptomatic, intact epithelium, minimal corneal stromal infiltrate and mild AC inflammation. *Later*: satellite lesions, feathery branching infiltrate, and immune ring. *In sever e infection*: ulceration, involvement of deeper corneal layers and Descemet's membrane, white plaque on the endothelium and severe AC inflammation (e.g. hypopyon).
- *Complications*: limbal and scleral extension, corneal perforation, endophthalmitis secondary bacterial infections, infectious crystalline keratopathy.

NB In late infection these distinctive patterns may be lost, and the clinical appearance may resemble an advanced bacterial keratitis.

Investigation
- Perform early and adequate corneal scrapes (Box 7.1).
- *Stains*: Gram (stains fungal walls), Giemsa (stains walls and cytoplasm); Gomori-Grocott methenamine silver (GMS), periodic acid Schiff (PAS), and Calcofluor white may also be used.
- *Culture*: Sabouraud's dextrose agar (for most fungi) and blood agar (for Fusarium); may require up to 14d; *in vitro* sensitivities are poorly predictive of *in vivo* sensitivity and so is little used clinically.

If strong clinical suspicion but negative investigations, consider confocal microscopy or corneal biopsy for histopathology and PCR for fungal DNA

---

1. Tuft SJ et al. Fungal keratitis in the United Kingdom. *Eye*. 2008; Oct 3. Epub ahead of print.

Fungal keratitis: treatment

Effective eradication of fungi is frequently difficult because of the deeply invasive nature of the infectious process. Identification of the organism (see Fungal Keratitis: assessment, 📖 p.200) must be a priority so as to ensure the optimal choice of therapy.

Treatment

Initial treatment

- Admit.
- Intensive topical broad-spectrum antifungal agents such as preservative free econazole 1% or natamycin 5% hourly (or voriconazole 10 mg/ml if available), day and night for the first 72h; econazole is the preferred agent for suspected/proven candidal infection, natamycin for filamentary fungal infection. For severe or unresponsive disease add a second agent (e.g. preservative free amphotericin 0.15% hourly day and night for first 24h, then reducing to day only).
- Avoid corticosteroids (reduce/stop them if already on them); may cautiously be used during healing phase (see below).
- Oral analgesia and cycloplegia (e.g. preservative free cyclopentolate 1% 3×/d).

Systemic treatment

Consider the addition of systemic antifungal treatment (e.g. oral fluconazole or voriconazole) should be considered for:

- severe disease (e.g. deep stromal lesions, threatened perforation, endophthalmitis), and in
- all immunocompromised patients.

Box 7.4 Systemic treatment in fungal keratitis

- First line: consider oral fluconazole (50–100mg 1×/d for 7–14d), which is effective against *Candida* and *Aspergillus*.
- In resistant cases or where *Aspergillus* has been identified: consider voriconazole (PO 400mg 2×/d for 2 doses then 200mg 2×/d but can ↑ to 300mg 2×/d; IV 6mg/kg 2×/d for 2 doses then 4mg/kg 2×/d; intrastromal injection 50 mcg/0.1ml).
- An alternative for invasive yeast infections is intravenous flucytosine (50mg/kg × 4/d; adjust as per plasma level monitoring).

Topical treatment should be continued. Liaise with a microbiologist for advice re drug selection, dosing, and monitoring. Systemic antifungals are associated with significant side-effects, including renal dysfunction (voriconazole), hepatotoxicity (fluconazole, voriconazole), and blood disorders (flucytosine, voriconazole). Monitoring should include FBC, U+E, and LFT before starting treatment, and at least weekly during treatment. In addition, dosing may need to be reduced in the presence of renal dysfunction and plasma level monitoring is required for flucytosine.

Ongoing treatment
- Taper treatment according to clinical improvement. Relapse is common and may signify incomplete sterilization or reactivation. Treatment is prolonged (12wks). In the healing phase topical corticosteroids (e.g. PF dexamethasone 0.1% 1x/d) are sometimes used; this should be at the direction of a corneal specialist and carefully monitored.
- Consider penetrating keratoplasty for progressive disease (to remove fungus/prevent perforation) or in the quiet but visually compromised eye.

Table 7.9 Antifungal agents

Class	Mechanism	Examples
Polyene	Destabilize cell wall	Natamycin, amphotericin
Imidazole	Destabilize cell wall	Clotrimazole, econazole, ketoconazole, miconazole
Triazole	Destabilize cell wall	Itraconazole, voriconazole, fluconazole
Pyrimidine	Cytotoxic	Flucytosine

1. Prakash G et al. Evaluation of intrastromal injection of voriconazole as a therapeutic adjunctive for the management of sleep recalcitrant fungal keratitis *Am J Ophthalmol* 2008; **146**:56–9

Herpes simplex keratitis (1)

The herpes simplex virus is a double-stranded DNA virus with two sero-types:

- HSV1 shows airborne transmission and classically causes infection of the eyes, face, and trunk;
- HSV2 infection is sexually transmitted, and usually causes genital herpes with rare ophthalmic involvement.

Primary infection is usually with a blepharoconjunctivitis, occasionally with corneal involvement. Following this the virus ascends the sensory nerve axon to reside in latency in the trigeminal ganglion. Viral reactivation, replication, and retrograde migration to the cornea results in recurrent keratitis, which may be epithelial, stromal, endothelial (discoid), or neurotrophic.

Potential intraocular involvement includes anterior uveitis and retinitis. Additionally, the resultant neurotrophic cornea is vulnerable to bacterial and fungal keratitis

Blepharoconjunctivitis

HSV1 infection is common (90% of the population are seropositive). Primary infection occurs in childhood with generalized viral malaise and is usually ophthalmically silent.

The most common ocular manifestation is a self-limiting blepharoconjunctivitis characterized by periorbital vesicular rash, follicular conjunctivitis, and preauricular lymphadenopathy. HSV keratitis in primary infection is rare; however, prophylactic topical (oc) aciclovir 3% 5×/d or oral aciclovir prophylaxis may be considered. The skin is treated with topical aciclovir 5% cream 3×/d.

Epithelial keratitis

Clinical features

- FB sensation, pain, blurred vision, lacrimation.
- Superficial punctate keratitis → stellate erosion → dendritic ulcer (branching morphology with terminal bulbs cf. pseudodendrites) → geographic ulcer (large amoeboid ulcer with dendritic advancing edges; more common if immunosuppressed/topical steroids). Ulcer base stains with fluorescein (de-epithelized); ulcer margins stain with Rose Bengal (devitalized viral-infected epithelial cells); ↓ corneal sensation.
- *Systemic*: may have associated orofacial or genital ulceration.

Investigation

This is usually a clinical diagnosis but where diagnostic uncertainty, investigate both for viral and other microbial (*see* Microbial keratitis: assessment, 📖 p.194) causes.

- Conjunctival and corneal swabs for molecular diagnosis (PCR and ELISA).
- Corneal scrapings: Giemsa stain (multinuclear giant cells).

Treatment

- Topical antiviral: aciclovir 3% oc initially 5×/day gradually tailing down but continued for at least 3d after complete healing; if resistant

consider trifluorothymidine 1% initially 9×/d but beware epithelial toxicity.
- Consider cycloplegia (e.g. cyclopentolate 1% 2×/d) for comfort/AC inflammation.
- If patient is on topical steroids for coexistent ocular disease reduce steroid dose (potency and frequency) where possible but do not stop until epithelium has healed.
- Where HSV keratitis is occurring in a corneal graft, reduction of topical steroids may increase the risk of graft rejection.
- If recurrent attacks consider oral antivirals (e.g. aciclovir 400mg PO 2×/d) as prophylaxis.

Stromal keratitis

Stromal keratitis may occur with or without epithelial ulceration.

Clinical features

- Multiple or diffuse opacities → corneal vascularization, lipid exudation, and scarring; or may → thinning; AC activity.
- *Complications*: ↑IOP; rarely perforation.

Treatment

- *Topical steroids*: defer (where possible) until epithelium intact; aim for minimum effective dose (e.g. prednisolone 0.1-1% 1-4×/d titrating down in frequency and strength).
- *Antiviral*: systemic aciclovir (initially 400mg 5×/d, then reduce; prophylactic dose is 400mg 2×/d). There is clear evidence that systemic aciclovir is beneficial and is useful in the prevention of recurrence. Consider in all patients with atopic keratoconjunctivitis, ocular surface disease, or frequent recurrences. Use of topical (3% oc 5×/d) is controversial and may be of benefit if stromal keratitis is associated with epithelial breakdown. Valciclovir or famciclovir may be considered in cases intolerant to aciclovir.
- Cycloplegia (e.g. cyclopentolate 1% 2×/d) for comfort/AC activity.
- Monitor IOP and treat as necessary.
- *Surgery*: may be indicated acutely for perforation (tectonic graft) or in the long term for scarring (usually penetrating keratoplasty).

Herpes simplex keratitis (2)

Disciform keratitis (endotheliitis)

Disciform keratitis probably results from viral antigen hypersensitivity rather than reactivation.

Clinical features
- Painless ↓VA, haloes.
- Central/paracentral disc of corneal oedema, Descemet's folds, mild AC activity, fine KPs; Wessely ring (stromal halo of precipitated viral antigen/host antibody).
- *Complications*: ↑IOP, chronic anterior uveitis.

Investigation
- If presentation is atypical and there is no previous history of herpetic keratitis, anterior chamber paracentesis and PCR of aqueous is of diagnostic benefit.
- Beware false negatives as long-term aciclovir will reduce HSV DNA copy number.

Treatment
- *Topical steroid*: defer (where possible) until epithelium intact; aim for minimum effective dose (e.g. dexamethasone 0.1% or prednisolone 0.5% 1–4×/d titrating down in frequency and strength); some patients may require low dose (e.g. prednisolone 0.1% alternate days –1×/d) for months or even maintenance. Use PF treatment if coexistent ocular surface disease.
- *Antiviral*: aciclovir either systemic (as above), or topical (3% oc 5×/d until ≥3d after complete healing); continue as prophylaxis (can frequency) until on low frequency/low strength topical steroid. Cycloplegia (e.g. cyclopentolate 1% 2×/d) for comfort/AC activity. Monitor IOP and treat as necessary.

Herpes zoster ophthalmicus

The varicella zoster virus is a double-stranded DNA virus of the herpes group.

Primary infection of the varicella zoster virus results in chicken pox (varicella). Reactivation of virus dormant in the sensory ganglion results in shingles (herpes zoster) of the innervated dermatome. Involvement of the ophthalmic branch of the trigeminal nerve occurs in 15% of shingles cases and results in HZO.

Transmission is by direct contact or droplet spread. Those never previously infected with VZV may contract chicken pox from contact with shingles. VZV infection may be more severe in the immunosuppressed, the elderly, pregnant women, and neonates. Maternal infection may also cause fetal malformations (3% risk in first trimester).

Systemic and cutaneous disease

Clinical features

Viral prodrome, preherpetic neuralgia (mild intermittent tingling to severe constant electric pain), rash (papules → vesicles → pustules → scabs) predominantly within the one dermatome (Va); Hutchinson's sign (cutaneous involvement of the tip of the nose indicating nasociliary nerve involvement and likelihood of ocular complications); may be disseminated in the immunocompromised. Additionally, the resultant neurotrophic cornea is vulnerable to bacterial and fungal keratitis.

Treatment

- *Systemic antiviral*: start as soon as rash appears either aciclovir PO 800mg 5x/d for 5d, valciclovir PO 1g 3x/d for 7d, or famciclovir PO 750mg 1x/d for 7d; if immunosuppressed then aciclovir IV 10mg/kg.
- Postherpetic neuralgia may cause depression (even suicide); treatments include amitriptyline, gabapentin, and topical capsaicin cream.

Keratitis

Clinical features

- *Epithelial*: superficial punctate keratitis + pseudodendrites often with anterior stromal infiltrates; acute (onset 2–3d after rash; resolve in few weeks); common.
- *Stromal*: nummular keratitis with anterior stromal granular deposits is uncommon and occurs early (10d); necrotizing interstitial keratitis with stromal infiltrates, thinning, and even perforation (cf. HSV) is rare and occurs late (3mths–yrs).
- *Disciform*: endotheliitis with disc of corneal oedema, Descemet's folds, mild AC activity, fine KPs (cf. HSV); late onset (3mths–yrs); chronic; uncommon.
- *Neurotrophic*: corneal nerve damage causes persistent epithelial defect, thinning, and even perforation; late onset; chronic; uncommon.
- *Mucus plaques*: linear grey elevations loosely adherent to underlying diseased epithelium/stroma; late onset (3mths–yrs); chronic.

Treatment
Ensure adequate systemic antiviral treatment.
- *Epithelial*: topical lubricants, usually preservative free (e.g. Celluvisc® 0.5–1% 8×/d).
- *Stromal and disciform*: topical steroid treatment (e.g. prednisolone 0.1–1% 1–4×/d titrating down in frequency and strength); some patients may require low dose (e.g. prednisolone 0.1% alternate days –1×/d) for months or even maintenance; threatened perforation may require gluing, bandage CL, or tectonic grafting.
- *Neurotrophic*: preservative free topical lubricants (e.g. Celluvisc® 0.5–1% 8×/d + Lacri-Lube® nocte) and consider tarsorrhaphy (surgical or medical with botulinum toxin-induced ptosis), amniotic membrane graft, or conjunctival flap.
- *Mucous plaques*: require mucolytics (e.g. acetylcysteine 5–10% non-preserved 3×/d).
- *Anterior uveitis*: topical steroid treatment and cycloplegia (e.g. cyclopentolate 1% 2×/d) for comfort/AC activity.
- *Monitor IOP*: assess whether due to inflammation or steroids and treat accordingly.
- *Corneal scarring*: axial scarring may require penetrating keratoplasty.

Other complications associated with HZO
- *Ocular*: conjunctivitis, secondary microbial keratitis, glaucoma, anterior uveitis, necrotizing retinitis (ARN, PORN), episcleritis, scleritis, optic neuritis, cranial nerve palsies.
- *Systemic*: strokes (cerebral vasculitis), neuralgia.

Thygeson's superficial punctate keratopathy

A rare condition, most commonly arising in young adulthood that may last anywhere from 1mth to 24yrs. The aetiology is idiopathic but a viral cause is suspected. It is bilateral but often asymmetric.

Clinical features

- Bilateral recurrent FB sensation, photophobia, and tearing.
- Coarse stellate grey–white epithelial opacities in a white quiet eye; the opacities appear slightly elevated but are classically non-staining with fluorescein or Rose Bengal. There may be a slight epithelial haze.

Treatment

- *Topical corticosteroids* (e.g. fluorometholone contact lens 0.1%), which can be rapidly tapered; sometimes a mild maintenance dose (even 1×/wk) is required to prevent further episodes.
- *Consider therapeutic contact lens*: for vision and comfort.

Recurrent corneal erosion syndrome

As clinical features may have resolved by the time the patient sees an ophthalmologist, a provisional diagnosis of RCES may be made on history alone. RCES is indicative of failure of epithelial to basement membrane re-adhesion and is defined as recurrent episodes of spontaneous breakdown of the corneal epithelium.

Risk factors
- Sharp trauma.
- Corneal dystrophies: anterior (especially epithelial basement membrane dystrophy and Reis–Buckler dystrophy) or stromal dystrophies.
- Post-keratoplasty.
- Diabetes, dry eye, ocular rosacea.

Clinical features
- Recurrent episodes of severe pain and photophobia usually starting on opening eyes after sleep; aggravated by blinking; resolves within hours; history of corneal trauma (often forgotten).
- Variable degree of epithelial irregularities (including loose epithelium without staining) or frank epithelial defects; may also have signs of underlying disease, e.g. microcysts, maps, dots, fingerprints, or stromal changes. When severe, may last for several days with pain accompanied by lid oedema, ciliary injection, extreme photophobia, and reduced vision.

NB May predispose to infection.

Pathology
Abnormalities of epithelial adhesion, defects in hemidesmosomes, basement membrane, which may exhibit thinning and reduplication. Excessive mucous membrane pemphigoid result in enzymatic degradation of adhesion complexes.

Treatment
Conservative
- *Topical*: lubricants (e.g. Celluvisc® 0.5–1% hourly during the day, oc Lacri-Lube® nocte ± cycloplegia (e.g. cyclopentolate 1% 2×/d), NSAID (e.g. ketorolac 3×/d) for comfort.
- *Therapeutic CLs*: extended wear silicone hydrogel.
- Tetracyclines (e.g. doxycycline 100mg 1×/d for 3mths or oxytetracycline 250mg 2×/d for 3 mths) may be beneficial as they inhibit matrix metalloproteinase activity and promote epithelial stability (contraindicated in children under 12, in pregnant/breast-feeding women, or in hepatic or renal impairment).

Surgical
- *Mechanical debridement*: consider mechanical debridement if heaped up, devitalized epithelium. Anaesthetize cornea, gently break away non-adherent grey epithelium with moistened cotton bud, or sponge; use post-procedure therapeutic CLs with preservative free chloramphenicol eye drops (0.5% 4×/d for 1wk to prevent secondary infection).

- *Alcohol delamination of the epithelium*: this promotes 'smoothing' of the stromal bed to improve epithelial adhesion. Technique involves 4-5 drops of 18% alcohol applied to a corneal well placed on top of a corneal for 30–40s followed by epithelial debridement of entire corneal epithelium with a cotton-tipped applicator.
- *Excimer laser phototherapeutic keratectomy*: consider this procedure for refractory or severe cases of RCES. Where therapeutic laser is not available, anterior stromal micropuncture may be considered for RCES outside the visual axis. Anterior stromal micropuncture is performed at the slit-lamp (if cooperative patient) or in theatre with topical anaesthesia, and using a bent 25-gauge needle to cover the defective area with closely packed micropunctures through epithelium and Bowman's layer.

Persistent epithelial defects

An epithelial defect is defined as persistent when it has failed to heal within a 2wk period.

Persistent corneal epithelial defects arise when there is a failure of the mechanisms promoting corneal epithelialization resulting in disassembly of hemidesmosomes. This is accompanied by degradation of Bowman's layer and stroma as a consequence of the disruption of the normally protective corneal microenvironment during a disease process.

Risk factors

Neurotrophic corneas, limbal stem cell deficiency, such as chemical injury or hereditary conditions (aniridia); and immune-mediated ocular surface disorders, including atopic keratoconjunctivitis, ocular mucus membrane pemphigoid, Stevens–Johnson syndrome and peripheral ulcerative sclerokeratitis.

Treatment

The treatment strategy must consider both the healing phase and then the maintenance phase (i.e. prevention of future epithelial defects). Treatment may include some of the following:

- Topical treatment:
  - oc chloramphenicol 1% with double-pad,
  - lubricants (e.g. Celluvisc® 0.5–1% hourly during the day, oc Lacri-Lube® nocte ± sodium hyaluronate preparations 4×/d).
  - If there is contributing ocular surface inflammation (e.g. OMMP, Wegener's) then consider topical steroids (± systemic steroids/immunosuppression).
  - For severe cases consider autologous serum drops.
- CL: extended wear silicone hydrogel or scleral CLs.
- Lid procedures: botulinum toxin induced tarsorrhaphy or surgical tarsorrhaphy; punctal plugs; punctal occlusion.
- Grafting procedures: amniotic membrane transplant, limbal stem cell transplantation, Gunderson flap, buccal mucous membrane graft.

Box 7.5 The role of amniotic membrane transplantation (📖 p.250) in persistent epithelial defects

- The use of amniotic membrane graft is usually reserved for cases where primary conservative measures (ocular lubricants, therapeutic CLs, and autologous serum (if available)) have failed, and/or when there has been loss of Bowman's layer, when amniotic membrane is used as a basement membrane substrate enabling corneal epithelial cell migration and closure of the epithelial defect.
- Beneficial effects of amniotic membrane graft appear to be independent of surgical technique employed (patch, bandage, or overlay).

Box 7.6 Developments in ocular lubricants

Most commercially available artificial tears do little more than lubricate, and fail to recapitulate other properties of natural tears, such as nutrition, promoting ocular surface renewal and immunological defence. However, there is evidence that newer agents, such as those containing carboxymethylcellulose or sodium hyaluronate preparations, do appear to have advantages beyond simple lubrication.

- *Carboxymethylcellulose (syn carmellose)*: these preparations have improved ocular surface retention and appear to be cytoprotective.
- *Sodium hyaluronate (hyaluronic acid)*: there is evidence that these preparations may be cytoprotective, promote basement membrane hemidesmosome formation, and have improved surface retention in inflamed eyes due to specific ligand binding to exaggerated CD44 (a transmembrane cell surface adhesion molecule) expression on the ocular surface during inflammation.[1,2] Hyaluronic acid itself is a ubiquitous naturally occurring extracellular matrix glycosaminoglycan, which plays an important part in wound healing, inflammation, and lubrication.

1. Haider AS et al. In vitro model of 'wound healing' analyzed by laser scanning cytometry: accelerated healing of epithelial cell monolayers in the presence of hyaluronate. *Cytometry A* 2003; **53**:1–18.

2. Gomes JA et al. Sodium hyaluronate (hyaluronic acid) promotes migration of human corneal epithelial cells in vitro *BJ Ophthalmol* 2004; **88**:821.

Limbal stem cell deficiency

The corneal limbus is thought to contain small numbers of limbal epithelial stem cells resident within a specialized stem-cell niche. The stem cells generate a continuous supply of daughter cells that, outside the stem cell niche, follow the normal paths of differentiation to replenish the ocular surface. This is vital to the maintenance of a healthy ocular surface not only in terms of recovery from trauma, but also in the face of daily wear and tear.

Deficiency of limbal epithelial stem cells leads to poor epithelialization, inflammation, vascularization, and scarring.

The presence of stem cells residing in a limbal niche at the palisades of Vogt explains a number of interesting clinical observations, notably the centripetal migration of healing epithelium, the circumferential migration of limbal epithelium, and that the columns of migration correspond to palisades of Vogt.

Although there is no specific marker for limbal epithelial stem cells, identification may be assisted by the absence of markers typical of corneal epithelium (such as cytokeratins K3 or K12) and the presence of progenitor markers such as ABCG2 (an ATP-binding-cassette-transporter protein) and P63 (a transcription factor).

Causes

Table 7.10 Causes of stem cell deficiency

Aniridia
Chemical injury
Thermal injury
UV/ionizing irradiation
CL wear
Preservative toxicity
Ocular surface malignancy
Neurotrophic cornea
Peripheral ulcerative keratitis
Inflammation
• Ocular mucous membrane pemphigoid,
• Atopic keratoconjunctivitis,
• Stevens–Johnson syndrome/TEN

Clinical features

• Conjunctivalization (invasion of conjunctival epithelium on to the corneal surface); 'corneal' epithelium that is opaque, irregular, thickened, and unstable after even minor trauma; persistent epithelial defects + corneal vascularization, inflammation, calcification.

• *Complications:* secondary corneal infection, perforation, and intraocular infection may render the eye permanently blind.

Investigations

Diagnosis can be confirmed on immunohistological studies (e.g. from impression cytology) demonstrating the presence of mucin-containing goblet cells on the cornea, and the absence of normal differentiation markers of corneal epithelium (such as cytokeratins K3 and K12).

Treatment

Table 7.11 An approach to the treatment of limbal stem cell deficiency

Deficiency	Additional features	Treatment options
Partial	Conjunctivalized metaplastic epithelium on cornea	*If visual axis not involved:* Observation
		If visual axis involved: Sequential sector conjunctival epitheliectomy + AMG
	With fibrovascular pannus	Sector limbal transplant + AMG
Total	Unilateral	Conjunctival limbal autograft from contralateral better eye
		Cultivated limbal corneal epithelial cells from contralateral better eye using carrier, e.g. AMG
	Bilateral	Living-related keratolimbal allograft (KLAL)
		Cadaveric KLAL
		Cultivated limbal corneal epithelial cells from cadaveric limbus using carrier, e.g. AMG

Allografts
Potential allograft donors are screened for hepatitis serology (hepatitis B surface antigen, antibodies to hepatitis C virus, hepatitis C virus nucleic acid testing), HIV I/II, human T-cell lymphoma virus and syphilis. Patients receiving allografts will require systemic immunosuppression (e.g. mycophenolate ± ciclosporin/rapamycin).

Cultivated limbal corneal epithelial cells
Cultivation of limbal corneal epithelial cells for transplantation into humans is an exciting development that requires meticulous care and is stringently regulated.

In the UK, for example, the following requirements have to be met: Class 100 clean room facilities, compliance with the Human Tissue Act 2004 and the European Union Tissues and Cells Directive, compliance with Good Manufacturing Practice and approval of the Medicines and Healthcare products Regulatory Agency (MHRA).

Corneal degenerative disease (1)

Arcus

A common, bilateral, degeneration secondary to progressive deposition of lipid in the peripheral stroma. It is usually age-related but may be associated with hyperlipidaemia.

Causes

Most bilateral cases have no systemic association but hyperlipidaemia (notably type II) should be ruled out in those presenting at a young age (arcus juvenilis). Unilateral arcus is rare and may signify ipsilateral carotid compromise or previous ocular hypotony.

Clinical features

Progressive peripheral opacity, starts (and remains thickest) at 3 o'clock and 9 o'clock but spreads circumferentially to form a complete ring of about 1mm thickness; typically, the central margin is blurred but the peripheral margin is sharp, leaving a zone of clear perilimbal cornea (which may show thinning).

Cornea farinata

A bilateral symmetrical degeneration of deep stromal, faint flour-like opacities that are prominent centrally but remain visually insignificant.

Crocodile shagreen

A faint reticular polygonal network of stromal opacities resembling crocodile skin. Anterior stromal shagreen is more common than posterior but both forms are innocuous and asymptomatic.

Vogt's limbal girdle

A common bilateral degeneration. There is chalky white peripheral corneal deposition at 3 o'clock and 9 o'clock. It may be separated from the limbus by a clear perilimbal zone (type I) or it may extend to the limbus (type II). Both types are innocuous and asymptomatic.

Primary lipid keratopathy

A rare idiopathic corneal deposition of cholesterol, fat, and phospholipids appearing as yellow–white stromal deposits with no associated vascularization. It is usually innocuous and non-progressive, and requires no treatment.

Secondary lipid keratopathy

Causes

This may accompany corneal vascularization following ocular injury or inflammation. Common causes include previous herpetic (simplex or zoster disciform) keratitis, trauma, and interstitial keratitis.

Clinical features

Corneal vascularization with associated yellow–white stromal deposition.

Treatment
Treat underlying cause of ocular inflammation. Long-term mild corticosteroid (e.g. fluorometholone) is occasionally useful. Consider feeder vessel occlusion or penetrating keratoplasty.

- *Occlusion of the feeder vessel*: may be by argon laser photocoagulation or direct needle point cautery under the operating microscope. Anterior segment fluorescein angiography may help identify the feeder vessel.
- *Penetrating keratoplasty*: it is performed if the disease is severe, persistent and once the eye is quiet. However, prognosis is guarded due to the poor condition of host tissue and preoperative vascularization.
- There is some evidence that topical or subconjunctival anti-VEGF therapy may be of benefit.

Corneal degenerative disease (2)

Band keratopathy

A common progressive subepithelial deposition of calcium phosphate salts that may be due to ocular or systemic causes.

Causes

Table 7.12 Causes of band keratopathy

Ocular	Anterior segment inflammation	Chronic anterior uveitis
		Chronic keratitis
		Chronic corneal oedema
		Silicone oil in AC
	Phthisis bulbi	
Systemic		Primary (familial)
		Senile
		Ichthyosis
		Hypercalcaemia
		Hyperphosphataemia
		Hyperuricaemia
		Chronic renal failure

Clinical features
- Often asymptomatic; FB sensation, pain, ↓VA.
- White opacities starting at 3 and 9 o'clock progressing centrally to coalesce to form a band.

Treatment
- Identify and treat underlying cause as appropriate.
- Consider therapeutic CL for comfort (often as a temporary measure).
- Remove calcium salts by: *chemical chelation* (disodium ethylenediamine tetra-acetic acid) followed by mechanical debridement (e.g. gentle scraping with no. 15 blade); or *excimer laser keratectomy*.

Salzmann nodular degeneration

An uncommon slowly progressive degeneration usually seen as a complication of chronic keratitis. It arises from replacement of Bowman's layer by eosinophilic material.

Causes

Chronic keratitis, including trachoma, phlyctenular keratitis, vernal keratitis, interstitial keratitis; post-corneal surgery; idiopathic.

Clinical features
- Glare, ↓VA, pain (if loss of overlying epithelium).
- Well-defined grey–white elevated nodules ± iron lines (indicate chronicity). There may be associated epithelial breakthrough and discomfort.

Treatment
- Identify and treat underlying keratitis.
- *Consider*: lubrication, therapeutic CL, or excimer laser keratectomy.

Corneal dystrophies: anterior

Epithelial basement membrane dystrophy
(syn Map-dot-fingerprint dystrophy, Cogan's microcystic dystrophy)

The most common corneal dystrophy with a prevalence of about 2.5%. Although there are pedigrees demonstrating autosomal dominant inheritance, most clinical presentations appear to be non-familial. There is a slight female predilection. It usually presents in early adulthood.

Pathophysiology

The basic defect appears to lie in epithelium-basement membrane interaction. In the absence of normal hemidesmosomes and anchoring fibrils there is continued secretion and intra-epithelial extension of basement membrane (maps), breakdown of desmosomes, degeneration of sequestered epithelial cells (dots or microcysts), and deposition of fibrillar material (fingerprints).

Clinical features

- Bilateral, asymmetrical; may be asymptomatic; but recurrent erosions in 10–33% (pain, lacrimation, photophobia).
- Epithelial maps (faint opacities), dots/microcysts, fingerprints (curvilinear ridges).

Treatment

See Recurrent corneal erosion syndrome ☐ p.212.

Reis–Buckler dystrophy

A relatively common autosomal dominant progressive dystrophy. It usually presents with recurrent erosions in early childhood. With age these become less painful (due to ↓corneal sensation) but central opacity may lead to ↓VA.

Pathophysiology

This is caused by a mutation in the keratoepithilin gene BIGH3 (Ch5q). There is progressive degeneration of Bowman's layer with subepithelial collagen deposition (stains blue with Masson trichrome). Thiel–Behnke (honeycomb dystrophy) is a similar but milder condition arising from a different mutation in BIGH3.

Clinical features

- Bilateral recurrent corneal erosions (pain, lacrimation, photophobia); later ↓VA.
- Multiple subepithelial grey reticular opacities usually starting centrally.

Treatment

See Recurrent corneal erosion syndrome ☐ p.212.
- *Consider* excimer laser superficial keratectomy, or lamellar/penetrating keratoplasty if ↓VA.

Meesman's dystrophy

A rare autosomal dominant dystrophy. It usually presents in adulthood.

Pathophysiology

This is caused by mutations in the genes for cytokeratins K3 (Ch12) and K12 (Ch17) that normally form the cytoskeleton of the epithelial cell.

Clinical features
- Initially asymptomatic; mild ocular irritation, photophobia, and mild ↓VA in adulthood.
- Discrete clear epithelial vesicles; initially central but spread peripherally (sparing the limbus).

Treatment
Treatment is not usually required; however, rarely lamellar keratoplasty may be considered in significant photophobia or visual impairment.

Corneal dystrophies: stromal (1)

Lattice dystrophy types I, II, III

Rare autosomal dominant dystrophies involving the progressive deposition of amyloid in the corneal stroma and sometimes elsewhere in the body.

- Type I is the commonest form and is isolated to the eye.
- Type II forms part of familial systemic amyloidosis (Meretoja syndrome).
- Type III is rare, isolated to the eye, and is seen in those of Japanese origin.

Pathophysiology

Type I lattice dystrophy is caused by a mutation in the keratoepithilin gene BIGH3 (Ch5q). Type II results from a mutation in the gene for the plasma protein gelsolin (Ch9q). In all types amyloid is deposited in the stroma, but in types I and II it may also disrupt the basement membrane and epithelium. Amyloid stains with Congo Red and demonstrates birefringence and dichroism at polarizing microscopy.

Clinical features

- ↓VA, recurrent erosions (pain, lacrimation, photophobia).
- Bilateral (often asymmetric) criss-cross refractile lines; later these may be obscured by a progressive central corneal haze (types I and II). In type III the lines are thicker and more prominent. The peripheral cornea is usually spared.

Systemic features

In type II lattice dystrophy with familial amyloidosis (Meretoja syndrome): mask-like facies, skin laxity, cranial nerve palsies (commonly VIIn with additional risk of corneal exposure), peripheral neuropathy, renal failure, and cardiac failure.

Treatment

See Recurrent corneal erosion syndrome 📖 p.212.

- *Consider* penetrating keratoplasty or excimer laser keratectomy if ↓VA. Recurrence after either procedure is common.
- If type II disease suspected refer to physician for assessment of systemic involvement.

Granular dystrophy

A rare autosomal dominant dystrophy involving deposition of hyaline material in the corneal stroma. It presents in adulthood.

Pathophysiology

Granular dystrophy is caused by a mutation in the keratoepithilin gene BIGH3 (Ch5q). Hyaline material (probably phospholipids) deposited in the stroma stains red with Masson trichrome.

Clinical features

- ↓VA; occasionally recurrent erosions.
- Bilateral (often asymmetric) white crumb-like opacities in otherwise clear stroma; initially central but progressively coalesce.

Treatment
See Recurrent corneal erosion syndrome 📖 p.212.
- If ↓VA consider penetrating keratoplasty, or lamellar keratoplasty if relatively superficial disease.
- Recurrence is common.

Avellino dystrophy

A very rare autosomal dominant dystrophy with some features of both granular and lattice dystrophies. It is usually seen in those originating out of Avellino, Italy.

Pathophysiology
Avellino dystrophy is caused by a mutation in the keratoepithilin gene BIGH3 (Ch5q). The stromal deposit stains both for hyaline (Masson tri-chrome) and amyloid (Congo Red; birefringence and dichroism at polarizing microscopy).

Clinical features
- ↓VA; recurrent erosions (pain, lacrimation, photophobia).
- Bilateral (often asymmetric) granular-type opacities in anterior stroma, and lattice-type lines in deeper stroma; may have a central subepithelial haze later.

Treatment
See Recurrent corneal erosion syndrome 📖 p.212.
- *Consider* penetrating keratoplasty if ↓VA.
- Recurrence is common.

Corneal dystrophies: stromal (2)

Macular dystrophy

A rare autosomal recessive dystrophy involving deposition of a glycosaminoglycan in the stroma. Abnormal stromal collagen packing causes loss of corneal translucency, usually from early adulthood.

Pathophysiology

This is effectively an ocular-specific mucopolysaccharidosis, arising from mutations in the gene for carbohydrate sulphotransferase (CHST6; Ch 16q). Abnormal glycosaminoglycans similar to keratan sulphate accumulate. These stain with alcian blue or colloidal iron. Macular dystrophy may be subclassified as type I (no keratan sulphate) and type II (low keratan sulphate).

Clinical features

- Gradual painless ↓VA; often incidental finding.
- Bilateral (often asymmetric) focal ill-defined grey–white stromal opacities superimposed on diffuse clouding; it may involve the whole cornea being superficial centrally, but potentially involving full stromal thickness peripherally. Cornea may be thinned.

Treatment

- If ↓VA consider penetrating keratoplasty, or lamellar keratoplasty if relatively superficial disease.
- Recurrence is rare.

Schnyder's crystalline dystrophy

This is a rare progressive dystrophy presenting in childhood with an autosomal inheritance pattern. Stromal crystals contain cholesterol and neutral fat (stains red with Oil red O). It may be associated with systemic hypercholesterolaemia.

Clinical features

- ↓VA, glare.
- Central anterior stromal yellow–white (often scintillating) crystals corneal haze and arcus.

Treatment

- *Consider* excimer laser keratectomy or penetrating keratoplasty if ↓VA.
- Recurrence may occur.
- Check fasting lipids.

Congenital hereditary stromal dystrophy (CHSD)

This is a very rare autosomal dystrophy that presents at birth with bilateral corneal clouding without oedema. It is non-progressive. It appears to arise due to abnormalities of stromal collagen but with normal anterior and posterior corneal layers. Corneal thickness is normal.

Treatment requires penetrating keratoplasty.

Other dystrophies of the corneal stroma

- *Central cloudy dystrophy*: autosomal dominant, similar changes to posterior crocodile Shagreen, visually insignificant.

- *Fleck dystrophy*: autosomal dominant, white flecks throughout stroma, visually insignificant.
- *Posterior amorphous corneal dystrophy*: autosomal dominant, grey sheets in deep stroma, non-progressive, rarely visually significant.

Corneal dystrophies: posterior

Fuchs' endothelial dystrophy (FED)

A common corneal dystrophy that may be autosomal dominant or sporadic. It is more commonly seen in females (F:M 4:1) and with increasing age. Presentation is usually gradual with ↓VA from middle-age but may be acute after endothelial injury (e.g. intraocular surgery). There appears to be an increased incidence of POAG.

Pathogenesis

Primary endothelial dysfunction associated with $Na^+K^+ATPase$ pump failure allows the accumulation of fluid. Mutation in the gene for the collagen VIII $\alpha2$ chain has been seen in patients with Fuch's endothelial dystrophy (FED) and with PPD. Microscopically there is irregular thickening of Descemet's membrane, protuberances (guttata), and flattening, irregularity in size, and loss of endothelial cells.

Clinical features

- Gradual ↓VA (often worse in morning); may arise after intraocular surgery.
- *Stage 1*: corneal guttata (appear centrally cf. the peripheral Hassall–Henle bodies which are normal with age); may extend to give 'beaten metal' appearance; pigment on endothelium.
- *Stage 2*: stromal oedema → Descemet's folds and epithelial bullae.
- *Stage 3*: recurrent corneal erosions → subepithelial vascular pannus and stromal haze.

Investigations

Specular microscopy: ↓cell count, ↑average cell diameter, ↓hexagons, ↑variation in cell size.

Treatment

Relieve corneal oedema and improve comfort

- Topical hypertonic agents: 5% NaCl.
- Treat ocular hypertension.
- Warm air blown on the eyes (e.g. hair dryer).
- Bandage CL for bullous change.

Visual rehabilitation

- Persistent corneal opacity may require PK.
- In the presence of coexisting cataract a triple procedure is performed (i.e. combined PK, lens extraction and PCIOL insertion).
- In the absence of any stromal scarring deep lamellar endothelial keratoplasty is an option.

Prevention

Corneal decompensation may be inadvertently accelerated by the ophthalmologist:

- *Cataract surgery*: consider (1) protecting the endothelium with additional heavy viscoelastic (soft shell technique) and (as always) minimizing phako-time, and (2) referring more severe cases to a corneal specialist for elective simultaneous penetrating keratoplasty/cataract extraction/IOL (triple procedure). **NB** Careful counselling re risk of decompensation is essential prior to surgery.

- *Ocular hypertension/glaucoma*: topical β-blocker preferred; topical carbonic anhydrase inhibitors may induce endothelial failure.

Congenital hereditary endothelial dystrophy (CHED)

CHED is an important cause of bilateral corneal oedema in otherwise healthy term neonates (see Common clinical presentations: cloudy cornea and leucocoria 📖 p.694). It is usually autosomal recessive. An autosomal dominant variant has been linked to the same region (Ch20q) as PPD. It appears to be a dysgenesis in which neural crest cells fail to complete differentiation into normal endothelium.

Clinical features
Autosomal recessive type
Bilateral marked corneal oedema from birth; stroma up to 3× normal thickness; severe ↓VA, amblyopia and nystagmus; not usually painful.

Autosomal dominant type
Bilateral mild corneal oedema from infancy with tearing and photophobia; milder ↓VA and no nystagmus; gradually progressive.

Treatment
Penetrating keratoplasty: visual outcome is often limited by amblyopia.

Posterior polymorphous dystrophy (PPD)

PPD is usually autosomal dominant but has a very variable expression. It is often asymptomatic and may in fact be much commoner than currently appreciated. It shares features with indocorneal endothelial (ICE) syndrome and the anterior segment dysgeneses, all of which may form part of a continuum of failed neural crest terminal differentiation.

Clinical features
Clusters or lines of vesicles, irregular broad bands or diffuse haze of the posterior cornea ± iridocorneal adhesion, corectopia, glaucoma (closed or open angle).

Treatment
- Treatment is not usually necessary.
- Consider penetrating keratoplasty if significant ↓VA.

Corneal ectasias

Keratoconus

A common corneal ectasia characterized by progressive *conical* distortion of the cornea with irregular astigmatism, axial stromal thinning, apical protrusion, and increasing myopia.

Prevalence estimates vary widely (0.05–5%) according to the population studied, the techniques used, and the definition adopted.

The aetiology is unclear but may be a combination of repeated trauma (e.g. eye-rubbing) and abnormalities of corneal stroma (e.g. in connective tissue disorders). Previously, only 10% of cases were thought to be familial. However, analysis by videokeratography suggests a high prevalence among asymptomatic family members consistent with autosomal dominant inheritance with variable penetrance.

Keratoconus usually presents in early adulthood; an earlier presentation is associated with a worse prognosis.

Risk factors

Table 7.13 Associations of keratoconus

Ocular		Leber's congenital amaurosis
		Vernal keratoconjunctivitis
		Floppy eyelid syndrome
		Retinitis pigmentosa
		Retinopathy of prematurity
Systemic	Atopy	Eczema
		Asthma
		Hay fever
	Connective tissue	Ehlers–Danlos syndrome
		Marfan syndrome
		Osteogenesis imperfecta
	Other	Down syndrome
		Crouzon syndrome
		Apert syndrome

Clinical features

- Usually bilateral (but asymmetric) progressive irregular astigmatism with ↓VA; progression continues into early adulthood but usually stabilizes by mid-30s.
- Corneal steepening/thinning (cone), Vogt's striae (vertical lines in the stroma, which may disappear on pressure), Fleischer ring (iron deposition at base of cone), conical distortion of lower lid on downward gaze (Munson's sign), abnormal focusing of a slit-lamp beam orientated obliquely across the cone from the temporal side (Rizutti's sign), scissoring reflex on retinoscopy, oil droplet reflex on ophthalmoscopy.
- *Complications*: acute hydrops (Descemet's membrane rupture → acute corneal oedema, may result in scarring); corneal scar.

Investigations
- *Videokeratography*: this has largely replaced manual keratometry. It is used for diagnosis and monitoring of disease. It may also classify keratoconic changes according to:
  - *severity*: mild (<48D), moderate (48–54D), and severe (>54D).
  - *morphology*: cone, nipple, oval, bow-tie, and globus.

Treatment
- *Counselling*: progressive nature of disease, frequent change in refractive error, potential impact on lifestyle (notably driving) and career. As disease usually stabilizes by mid-30s, a patient with good VA at age 35 is unlikely to need a keratoplasty. A promising new therapy to stabilize the progression of keratoconus is corneal collagen cross-linking using topical riboflavin and UVA light.
- *Mild astigmatism*: spectacle or contact lens correction.
- *Moderate astigmatism*: rigid gas permeable lens (8.7–14.5mm), scleral lens (PMMA). In CL-intolerant patients, insertion of intracorneal ring segments can flatten the cornea to improve vision and CL tolerance (Intacs): also collagen cross-linking.
- *Severe astigmatism*: deep lamellar keratoplasty (if normal Descemet's membrane) or penetrating keratoplasty. 90% of patients with primary keratoconus achieve clear transplants but postoperative astigmatism ± anisometropia often necessitate additional CL use. Coexistent atopy worsens prognosis.

Keratoglobus

A very rare bilateral ectasia characterized by global corneal thinning and significant risk of rupture at minor trauma. It may be acquired (probably as an end-stage keratoconus) or congenital (autosomal recessive associated with Ehlers–Danlos type VI and brittle cornea syndrome).

Treatment includes: protection from trauma, scleral CLs, and sometimes lamellar epikeratoplasty.

Pellucid marginal degeneration

A rare bilateral progressive corneal ectasia of the peripheral cornea. It results in crescentic thinning inferiorly and marked against the rule astigmatism. It presents in the 3rd–5th decade with non-inflammatory, painless visual distortion. Hydrops is rare.

Treatment is by hard CLs; it is usually uncorrectable with spectacles; surgical intervention is usually disappointing. Surgical techniques include eccentric penetrating keratoplasty, wedge resection, and lamellar keratoplasty.

Posterior keratoconus

A rare non-progressive congenital abnormality of the cornea in which there is abnormal steepening of the posterior cornea in the presence of normal anterior corneal surface. It is usually an isolated unilateral finding, but may be associated with ocular (e.g. anterior lenticonus, anterior polar cataract) or systemic abnormalities.

Treatment is not usually necessary, but requires penetrating keratoplasty if significant ↓VA.

Peripheral ulcerative keratitis

Peripheral ulcerative keratitis

PUK is an aggressive sight-threatening form of keratitis that is sometimes associated with underlying systemic disease. The aetiology is uncertain, although the rheumatoid model suggests that immune complex deposition at the limbus causes an obliterative vasculitis with subsequent corneal inflammation and stromal melt.

Causes

> **Box 7.7 Causes of peripheral ulcerative keratitis**
>
> Organ-specific autoimmune peripheral ulcerative keratitis (idiopathic)
> Rheumatoid arthritis (RA)
> Wegener's granulomatosis
> Systemic lupus erythematosus
> Relapsing polychondritis
> Polyarteritis nodosa
> Microscopic polyangiitis
> Churg–Strauss syndrome

Clinical features

- Variable pain and redness (may be none); ↓VA.
- Uni/bilateral peripheral corneal ulceration with epithelial defect and stromal thinning; associated inflammation at the limbus (elevated, injected) and either sectoral or diffuse scleritis.

NB Do not underestimate associated dry eye (may be severe and → filamentary keratitis).

- *Systemic features* (if associated disease): include degenerative joints (rheumatoid arthritis), saddle nose (Wegener's granulomatosis), skin changes (psoriasis, scleroderma, systemic lupus erythematosus), degenerative pinna cartilage (relapsing polychondritis).

Investigations

- As directed by systemic review. *Consider*: BP; FBC, ESR, U+E, LFT, Glu, CRP, vasculitis screen (including RF, ANA, ANCA, dsDNA), cryoglobulins, hepatitis C serology; urinalysis; CXR.

Treatment

- Emergency referral to corneal specialist and involve patient's physician/rheumatologist.
- Ensure adequate tear film: topical lubricants (e.g. carmellose or hyaluronate); if grossly reduced consider punctal plugs/cautery ± autologous serum.
- Systemic immunosuppression (liaise with physician/rheumatologist): may include corticosteroids (pulsed methylprednisolone or high-dose oral prednisolone), methotrexate, ciclosporin, mycophenolate, azathioprine, or cyclophosphamide.
- Doxycycline and oral vitamin C to promote a healing stromal environment (inhibit proteases, free radicals respectively).

- Topical immunosuppression: steroids (but use with caution in RA or if significant thinning as keratolysis may be accelerated.
- Ocular lubricants, topical antibiotics to prevent secondary infection (e.g. chloramphenicol PF 0.5% 4×/d), and cycloplegic (for pain and AC activity).
- Globe protection (e.g. glasses by day, shield at night).
- Consider therapeutic CL + cyanoacrylate glue for pending/actual perforation. Surgical options include conjunctival recession, amniotic membrane grafts, tectonic freehand lamellar keratoplasty, and occasionally conjunctival flaps.

Table 7.14 Corneal complications of rheumatoid arthritis

Marginal furrow	Peripheral thinning without inflammation or loss of epithelium; 'contact lens cornea'; does not perforate
Peripheral ulcerative keratitis	Peripheral inflammation, epithelial loss, infiltrate and stromal loss; may perforate
Acute stromal keratitis	Acute onset inflammation with stromal infiltrates but epithelium often preserved
Sclerosing keratitis	Gradual juxtalimbal opacification of corneal stroma bordering an area of scleritis
Keratolysis	Stromal thinning ('corneal melt') ± associated inflammation

Mooren's ulcer

This is a rare form of peripheral ulcerative keratitis that appears to be autoimmune. It is rarely associated with hepatitis C. It exists in two forms:
- the limited form is typically seen in middle-aged/elderly Caucasians and presents with unilateral disease that is fairly responsive to treatment;
- the more aggressive form is typically seen in young Africans with bilateral disease that may relentlessly progress despite treatment.

Clinical features
- Pain, photophobia, ↓VA.
- Uni/bilateral progressive peripheral ulceration; leading edge undermines epithelium; grey infiltrate at advancing margin; ulcer advances centrally and circumferentially; underlying stromal melt. **NB** No perilimbal clear zone and no associated scleritis (but conjunctival and episcleral inflammation).
- *Complications:* perforation; uveitis; cataract; at end-stage the cornea is thinned and conjunctivalized.

Investigations
Systemic work-up to rule out hepatitis C or any of the diseases associated with PUK.

Treatment
- Topical steroids (e.g. dexamethasone 0.1% PF hourly).
- Systemic immunosuppression: corticosteroids, cyclophosphamide, or ciclosporin (liaise with physician/rheumatologist); interferon if coexistent hepatitis C (as directed by a hepatologist).
- Also topical antibiotics, cycloplegia, globe protection, bandage CL ± glue, and surgical options as for peripheral ulcerative keratitis with systemic disease.

Other peripheral corneal diseases

Marginal keratitis

A common inflammatory reaction due to hypersensitivity to staphylococcal exotoxin. Often seen in patients with atopy, rosacea, or chronic blepharitis.

Clinical features
- Pain, FB sensation, redness (may be sectoral or adjacent to lid margins), photophobia, tearing, ↓VA.
- Sterile, white, subepithelial peripheral corneal infiltrate; most commonly at 2, 4, 8, and 10 o'clock but may spread circumferentially to coalesce; a perilimbal clear zone of cornea is preserved; epithelial ulceration (stain with fluorescein) and vascularization may occur.

Treatment
- Topical steroid/antibiotic (e.g. betamethasone 0.1% 4×/d for 1wk then 2×/d for 1wk, with chloramphenicol 0.5% 4×/d for 2wks) is commonly used to hasten resolution.
- Treat associated blepharitis or rosacea (see Blepharitis 🕮 p.130).

Rosacea associated keratitis

Acne rosacea is a chronic progressive disorder characterized by cutaneous telangiectasia and sebaceous hyperplasia. Affecting the face and eyes, rosacea presents in middle age, shows a female bias and is more common in the fair skinned.

Clinical features
- Telangiectasias at lids, meibomianitis, keratitis (ranges from inferior punctate epithelial erosions to marginal infiltrates to significant corneal thinning/perforation)
- Facial flushing is characteristically worse when consuming alcohol or spicy food.

Treatment
- Oral antibiotics, either a tetracycline (e.g. doxycycline 100mg 1×/d for 3mths or oxytetracycline 500mg 2×/d for 12wks; tetracyclines are contraindicated in children under 12, in pregnant/breast-feeding women, or in hepatic or renal impairment) or a macrolide (e.g. erythromycin 500mg 2×/d).
- Treat associated blepharitis: lid hygiene, ocular lubricants, topical antibiotics (for acute exacerbations).
- If moderately severe consider topical steroids ± antibiotics (e.g. dexamethasone 0.1% ± chloramphenicol 0.5%). Use with caution if significant stromal thinning as keratolysis may be accelerated.
- If very severe (threatened corneal perforation) systemic immunosuppression is usually necessary (e.g. azathioprine or mycophenolate).

Phlyctenulosis

These solitary limbal lesions are rare in the West but are relatively common in Africa. Children are more commonly affected than adults. Phlycten appear to be a hypersensitivity response, most commonly to staphylococcal or mycobacterial proteins, and rarely to adenovirus, fungi, *Neisseria*, lymphogranuloma venereum, and leishmaniasis. They may be located at the conjunctiva or the cornea. Conjunctival phlycten are inflamed nodules that may stain with fluorescein. They often resolve spontaneously. Corneal phlycten are grey nodules with associated superficial vascularization that may gradually move from limbus to central cornea.

Treatment: topical steroid (e.g. betamethasone 0.1% 4×/d).

Dellen

This is non-ulcerative corneal thinning seen adjacent to raised limbal lesions due to local drying and tear film instability. It is usually asymptomatic. Scarring and vascularization are rare.

Treatment: lubrication, and removal of precipitant (e.g. cessation of CL wear; removal of limbal mass).

Terrien's marginal degeneration

This is a rare cause of bilateral asymmetrical peripheral thinning, most commonly seen in young to middle-aged males (M:F 3:1). It is non-inflammatory and is, therefore, sometimes considered as an ectasia or degeneration.

Clinical features

- Initially asymptomatic; painless ↓VA (against the rule astigmatism).
- Initially there is yellow lipid deposition with fine vascularization at the superior marginal cornea; thinning occurs on the limbal side of the lipid line with a fairly steep leading edge; intact overlying epithelium; a perilimbal clear zone of cornea is preserved.
- *Complications*: opacification may spread circumferentially and rarely centrally. Rarely there may be associated inflammation (usually in younger men).

Treatment

- Spectacles/contact lenses for astigmatism.
- If severe thinning/risk of perforation consider surgical options, including crescentic or eccentric lamellar/penetrating keratoplasty.

Neurotrophic keratopathy

The ophthalmic branch of the trigeminal nerve is responsible for corneal sensation. Reduction of corneal sensation leads to:
- Loss of the normal feedback responsible for maintaining a healthy epithelium.
- Predisposition to inadvertent trauma and opportunistic infection.
- Impairment of epithelial repair.
- Delayed clinical presentation.

Causes

Table 7.15 Causes of corneal hyposthesia/anaesthesia

Congenital		Familial dysautonomia (Riley–Day syndrome)
		Anhydrotic ectodermal dysplasia
Acquired	Ocular	Herpes simplex keratitis
		Herpes zoster ophthalmicus
		Corneal scarring
		Corneal surgery (e.g. keratoplasty, refractive surgery)
		Contact lens wear
		Drugs (topical anaesthetics)
	Extraocular	Traumatic/surgical section of Vn
		Irradiation of Vn
		Compressive/infiltrative of Vn (e.g. acoustic neuroma)
	Systemic	Drugs (e.g. systemic β-blockers)
		Diabetes
		Age

Clinical features
- Painless red eye, ↓VA.
- ↓Corneal sensation; interpalpebral punctate epithelial erosions → larger defects with heaped grey edges, epithelial oedema; opportunistic microbial keratitis; perforation.

Investigation

If cause of corneal anaesthesia not yet established, patient will need full assessment (e.g. neurological referral, CT/MRI head scan, etc.).

Treatment
- Ensure adequate lubrication: consider ↑frequency or ↑viscosity; consider preservative free preparations.
- Treat any secondary microbial keratitis (see Microbial keratitis: treatment p.206).
- If significant ulcerative thinning consider admission, protective measures such as globe protection (e.g. glasses by day, shield at night), therapeutic CL, or tectonic grafting with amniotic membrane and measures to promote corneal healing such as tarsorrhaphy (surgical or botulinum toxin induced) and topical application of autologous serum (with caution).
- Some evidence that nerve growth factor is of benefit.

Prevention
- Assess corneal protective mechanisms: check corneal sensation, tear film, lid closure (VIIn), Bell's phenomenon; correct where possible.
- Warn patient of risk of corneal disease and that a red eye or ↓VA requires urgent ophthalmic assessment.

Exposure keratopathy

In exposure keratopathy there is failure of the lids' normal wetting mechanism with consequent drying and damage to the corneal epithelium. This most commonly arises due to incomplete closure of the eyelids at night (nocturnal lagophthalmos).

Causes

Table 7.16 Causes of exposure keratopathy

VIIn palsy	Idiopathic (Bell's palsy)
	Stroke
	Tumour (e.g. acoustic neuroma, meningioma, choleastoma, parotid, nasopharyngeal)
	Demyelination
	Sarcoidosis
	Trauma (temporal bone fracture)
	Surgical section
	Otitis
	Ramsay Hunt syndrome (herpes zoster)
	Guillan–Barré syndrome
	Lyme disease
Lid abnormality	Nocturnal lagophthalmos (commonest cause)
	Ectropion
	Traumatic defect in lid margin
	Surgical (e.g. overcorrection of ptosis)
	Floppy eyelid syndrome
Orbital disease	Proptosis
	Thyroid eye disease

Clinical features
- Irritable, red eye(s); may be worse in the mornings.
- Punctate epithelial erosions (usually inferior if underlying lagophthalmos; central if due to proptosis); → larger defects; opportunistic microbial keratitis; perforation.

Investigation
If cause of exposure keratopathy not yet established, patient will need further investigation as directed by full ophthalmic and systemic assessment.

Treatment
- Ensure adequate lubrication: consider ↑frequency or ↑viscosity; PF preparations preferred if >6×/d.
- Ensure adequate lid closure: temporary measures if early resolution anticipated (tape lids shut at night), intermediate (temporary lateral/central tarsorrhaphy; botulinum toxin-induced ptosis) vs permanent surgical procedures (e.g. lid weights or permanent tarsorrhaphy for lagophthalmos; orbital decompression if proptosis).
- Treat secondary microbial keratitis 📖 p.206.

- If significant ulcerative thinning consider admission, globe protection (e.g. glasses by day, shield at night), gluing, bandage CL, or lamellar grafting.

Prevention

- Assess corneal protective mechanisms: check corneal sensation, tear film, lid closure (VIIn), Bell's phenomenon; correct where possible.
- Warn patient of risk of corneal disease and that pain, photophobia, or ↓VA requires urgent ophthalmic assessment.

Deposition keratopathies

Wilson's disease (hepatolenticular degeneration)

This rare autosomal recessive condition arises due to deficiency in a copper-binding protein leading to low levels of caeruloplasmin and copper deposition throughout the tissues, including the cornea.

Clinical features

- Kayser–Fleischer ring (brownish peripheral ring at level of Descemet's membrane); starts superiorly and usually continuous with limbus; sunflower cataract (anterior and posterior subcapsular opacities).
- *Systemic*: liver failure, choreoathetosis (basal ganglia deposition), and psychiatric problems.

Vortex keratopathy

A number of drugs may result in deposits at the corneal epithelium. Similar appearances occur in Fabry's disease.

Causes

Amiodarone, chloroquine, suramin, indomethacin, tamoxifen, chlorpromazine, atovaquone, Fabry's disease.

Clinical features

- Asymptomatic; not an indication for withdrawing treatment.
- Swirling grey lines radiating from infracentral cornea.

Crystalline keratopathies

- *Infectious crystalline keratopathy* presents as feathery stromal opacities in the absence of significant inflammation. These are biofilms (i.e. slime) arising from the presence of *Streptococcus viridans*, or rarely *Staphylococcus epidermidis*, *Pseudomonas aeruginosa*, or *Candida* sp. Most commonly seen in graft tissue after a penetrating keratoplasty, they also occur in the presence of ocular surface disease (e.g. ocular mucous membrane pemphigoid, Stevens–Johnson syndrome).
- *Non-infectious crystalline keratopathy* includes deposition of gold (chrysiasis due to systemic treatment in rheumatoid arthritis), immunoglobulin (multiple myeloma, Waldenström's macroglobulinaemia, lymphoma), urate (gout), cysteine (cystinosis), and lipids (lipid keratopathy, Schnyder's crystalline dystrophy).

Mucopolysaccharidosis keratopathy

The mucopolysaccharidoses are a group of inherited enzyme deficiencies (usually autosomal recessive) in which there is an accumulation and deposition of glycosaminoglycans. This may be widespread causing skeletal abnormalities, organomegaly, and mental retardation (e.g. Hurler syndrome, MPS1) or limited (e.g. corneal deposition in macular dystrophy) (see Corneal dystrophies: stromal (2) 📖 p.226).

Table 7.17 Mucopolysaccharidoses associated with corneal clouding

Systemic		
	MPSI	Hurler, Scheie, Hurler–Scheie
	MPSIV	Morquio
	MPSVI	Maroteaux–Lamy
	MPSVII	Sly
Limited		Macular dystrophy

Keratoplasty: penetrating keratoplasty

Corneal grafting has been performed for over 100yrs and is the commonest of all transplantation procedures. It may be performed as an elective procedure to improve vision or as an emergency procedure for corneal perforation. It may involve full-thickness replacement of a button of corneal tissue (penetrating keratoplasty), partial-thickness replacement (lamellar keratoplasty), or of just the posterior layers (endothelial keratoplasty).

Although not necessary for low-risk procedures, systemic immunosuppression should be considered for high-risk grafts.

Penetrating keratoplasty

Indications

- *Visual*: keratoconus, pseudophakic/aphakic bullous keratopathy, Fuchs' endothelial dystrophy, other corneal dystrophies, scarring secondary to trauma, chemical injury, or keratitis.
- *Tectonic*: corneal thinning, threatened perforation, or actual perforation.

Cautions

Poor prognostic factors: corneal vascularization, reduced corneal sensation, active inflammation, peripheral corneal thinning, herpetic disease, ocular surface disease, uncontrolled glaucoma.

Methods

- *Consent*: explain what the operation does, the need for frequent postoperative visits, long-term follow-up, and the importance of immediate attendance if there are problems. Explain the nature of organ donation, that the donors are screened but that there is still a small risk of transmission of infectious agents. Explain the delay in visual rehabilitation and possible complications, including failure, graft rejection, infection, haemorrhage, worsened vision, and need for correction of astigmatism (contact lenses ± refractive surgery).
- *Preoperative*: miotic (e.g. pilocarpine 1%).
- *Preparation*: with 5% povidone iodine and drape.
- *Check donor material*: healthy looking corneoscleral ring in clear media.
- *Determine button sizes*: depends on corneal morphology and pathology, but commonly 7.5mm for the host, and 0.25–0.5mm larger for the donor.
- *Mark cornea*: measure height and width of cornea with calipers and mark centre with ink; consider marking periphery with radial keratotomy marker to assist with suture placement
- Perform paracentesis and fill AC with viscoelastic
- *Excise donor button*: cut from endothelial side using a trephine (types include hand-held, gravity, and vacuum-driven).
- *Excise host button*: cutting with the trephine (numerous designs) may be full-thickness or stopped at the first release of aqueous to perform a slower decompression with blade or corneal scissors.
- *Place cardinal sutures*: 4 × 10-0 nylon sutures to secure the donor button in position.

- *Complete suturing*: either additional interrupted sutures (often 16 in total) or a continuous running suture. Aim for 90% suture depth. Ensure suture tension even and attempt to minimize astigmatism.
- Refill AC with balanced salt solution.

Postoperative

Topical steroid and antibiotic; if low risk of rejection then a combined preparation (e.g. Tobradex® 4×/d) may be sufficient; if higher risk consider preservative free dexamethasone 0.1% q2h and chloramphenicol 4×/d.

Also consider oral acetazolamide in the immediate postoperative period (especially if coexistent glaucoma), and oral aciclovir (if HSV disease).

Follow-up

- As clinically indicated but commonly at 1d, 1wk, 1mth, and then 2–3monthly.
- Regular refraction/autorefraction and corneal topography permits adjustment/removal of sutures to minimize astigmatism. A continuous running suture should not usually be removed for at least a year.
- Use antibiotic/steroid cover to reduce risk of infection/rejection and check for wound leaks.

Keratoplasty: lamellar and endothelial keratoplasty

Deep lamellar keratoplasty

Indications
Visual: suitable for diseases in which host endothelium/Descemet's membrane is healthy, e.g. most keratoconus, stromal dystrophies, scarring; although longer surgical time than penetrating keratoplasty there is a reduced risk of rejection.

Method
Outline: a deep stromal pocket is formed from a superior scleral (or corneal) incision and filled with viscoelastic, so permitting a trephine to excise a deep but partial thickness button. Visualization of depth may be assisted by filling the AC with air.

Superficial lamellar keratoplasty

Indications
- *Tectonic*: reinforce thinned cornea in threatened perforation or post-pterygium excision.
- *Visual (uncommon)*: anterior stromal scarring.

Method
Outline: a trephine is used to cut to the desired depth before using a blade or microkeratome to separate the button at the base.

Endothelial keratoplasty

Indications
- Endothelial pathology such as Fuchs' endothelial dystrophy and pseudophakic bullous keratopathy.
- Advantages include shorter surgical time, corneal structural integrity, stable refraction, and faster visual recovery.
- Additional complications include pupillary block, donor endothelial damage, and donor graft detachment needing repositioning with air injection.

Method
Outline: the Descemet's membrane and endothelium are stripped off the recipient cornea, the donor endothelial graft is prepared and inserted through a small incision and apposed to the recipient stroma by air injection.

Triple procedure

Indications
Visual: visually significant cataract with disease that requires penetrating keratoplasty; most commonly Fuchs' endothelial dystrophy.

Method
Outline: a penetrating keratoplasty is performed with cataract extraction (usually by extracapsular 'open sky' rather than phakoemulsification) and IOL implantation.

Keratoplasty: complications

Early postoperative complications

Wound leak
- Seidel positive leak, shallow AC, soft eye.
- Consider lubricants, bandage CL, patching, or resuturing.
- ↑IOP—causes include retained viscoelastic, malignant glaucoma, choroidal effusion, choroidal haemorrhage.
- Identify and treat cause.

Persistent epithelial defect (i.e. defect >2wk duration)
See Persistent epithelial defects 📖 p.214
- Causes include ocular surface disease such as dry eye, blepharitis, rosacea, exposure, or systemic disease such as diabetes or rheumatoid arthritis.
- Identify and treat cause; ensure generous lubrication and that all drops are PF; consider taping lid shut/tarsorrhaphy.

Endophthalmitis
Rare, but sight-threatening ophthalmic emergency. Recognize and treat urgently, see Postoperative endophthalmitis 📖 p.292

Primary graft failure
Endothelial failure causes persistent graft oedema from day 1 in a quiet eye. Observe for 2–4wks; consider regraft if oedema persists.

Early graft rejection
See Graft rejection (📖 p. 247).

Urrets–Zavalia syndrome
A fixed dilated pupil may occur after either PK or deep lamellar kerotoplasty; it is presumed to be due to iris ischaemia.

Late postoperative complications

Astigmatism
Monitor with corneal topography; adjust running suture or remove interrupted sutures (at steepest axes), but ensure that wound is secure. Can be improved with hard CL ± arcuate keratotomies.

Microbial keratitis
Risk increased due to epithelial disturbance, sutures, and chronic steroid use. Recognize and treat urgently 📖 p.194.

Suture-related problems
Remove loose/broken sutures and check for wound leaks; use antibiotic/steroid cover to reduce risk of infection/rejection; if wound leak then may require resuturing; a continuous running suture should not usually be removed for at least a year.

Disease recurrence in graft
This is common with viral keratitis (e.g. HSV) and some corneal dystrophies (e.g. macular dystrophy). Identify and treat if possible (e.g. aciclovir for HSV); may require further graft.

Late graft rejection
See 📖 p.247.

Graft rejection

This is the commonest cause of graft failure. This is usually due to endothelial rejection that occurs in about 20% of grafts.

Rejection is dependent on the presence of appropriate antigen-presenting cells and CD4+ T cells. Owing to redundancy within the immune system, multiple independent mechanisms may result in rejection, e.g. rejection is not restricted to a pure Th1 or Th2 response.

Have a low threshold for admission—prompt and adequate treatment may save the graft. Anterior uveitis occurring in a patient with a corneal graft should be considered as graft rejection until proven otherwise.

Although for most cases topical steroid drops are sufficient, in severe rejection episodes or high-risk grafts consider oral prednisolone ± pulsed IV methylprednisolone.

Epithelial rejection

- Graft epithelium is replaced by host epithelium resulting in an epithelial demarcation line.
- ↑Topical steroids to at least double current regimen (e.g. dexamethasone PF 0.1%, up to hourly).

Stromal/subepithelial rejection

- This is indicated by subepithelial infiltrates.
- ↑Topical steroids to at least double current regimen (e.g. dexamethasone PF 0.1%, up to hourly).

Endothelial rejection

- This is indicated by corneal oedema, keratic precipitates, Khodadoust line (inflammatory cell/graft endothelium demarcation line), AC activity.
- Intensive topical steroids (e.g. dexamethasone PF 0.1% hourly day and night/steroid ointment at night); consider subconjunctival or systemic corticosteroids if fails to improve; cycloplegia (e.g. cyclopentolate 1% 3×/d).

Table 7.18 Summary of complications in keratoplasty

Early	Wound leak
	↑IOP
	Flat anterior chamber
	Iris prolapse
	Persistent epithelial defect
	Endophthalmitis
	Primary graft failure
	Early graft rejection
	Urrets–Zavalia syndrome
Late	Astigmatism
	Graft rejection
	Microbial keratitis
	Suture-related problems (loose, abscess, endophthalmitis)
	Disease recurrence in graft
	Glaucoma

Donor eye retrieval and eye banks

Corneal transplantation (see Keratoplasty 📖 pp.242–245) depends on the availability of screened cadaveric corneoscleral tissue preserved in optimal condition by a dedicated eye bank. In the UK the majority of corneas are stored by the Corneal Transplantation Service Eye Banks in Bristol and Manchester.

Retrieval

Eye retrieval should be carried out by somebody who is competent in enucleation (usually doctors or suitably trained ophthalmic nurses). Often there is a local Transplant Coordinator who will have already discussed consent and established the suitability of the donor. However, the person performing retrieval has a responsibility to check that both of these have been satisfactorily performed.

Consent

• This should be obtained from the most relevant life partner or closest family member. Consent should include confirmation: (1) that they agree to donation and that the deceased had no known objection to donation; (2) that they agree that the tissue may be used for research (if not suitable for transplantation); (3) that a blood test can be taken (if no pre-mortem blood test available) to check for infective risk; and (4) that further information about the deceased can be obtained from their medical records, or relevant medical professionals.

Screening

• This comprises gaining information on the likely suitability of the tissue for transplantation purposes, primarily with regard to avoiding transmission of infective agents or malignancy. Information may be gained from medical records, senior medical/nursing staff caring for the deceased, family of the deceased, primary healthcare practitioner, and post mortem. Serological tests for infective agents are also performed.

Enucleation

This procedure is carried out using aseptic technique and appropriate disinfection (e.g. povidone iodine 10%). Peritomy is performed to allow isolation and severing of the extraocular muscles (squint hook/strabismus scissors). A pair of enucleation scissors (closed) are then slid round the eye to sever the optic nerve, and allow the globe to be removed. After packing the sockets with cotton wool, the lids can be closed over plastic eye caps to restore the normal appearance of the lids.

Processing

Processing procedures must regard the potential infective risk of the donor material, and follow codes of Good Laboratory Practice and Good Manufacturing Practice. Donor eyes are cleaned (e.g. povidone iodine 10%) and the corneoscleral disc excised under sterile conditions (e.g. class II biological safety cabinet).

Storage

• *Corneoscleral discs*, options include:
  • Suspension in organ culture medium at 34°C; can be stored for 30d. *Advantages*: long storage time; infective risk can be screened for by routine sampling of culture medium at 7d.

- Hypothermic storage at 4°C: can be stored for 7–10d. *Advantages*: relatively simple. *Disadvantages*: shorter storage time; infective risk less easily identified.
- *Sclera:* storage in 70% ethanol; can be stored for up to 1yr.
- *Whole eyes:* for short-term storage (e.g. between removal and arrival at the eye bank)
  - *Moist-chamber storage:* whole eye placed on a stand with cornea uppermost, in a closed pot. Humidity is provided by moistened cotton wool. The pot is kept at 4°C (fridge or on ice during transit).

Issuing corneas

Three days before the scheduled date of transplantation, the corneal endothelium is examined. If endothelial cell count is at least 2200cells/ mm^2 the cornea is considered suitable for transplantation. It is placed back into medium and returned to 34°C. Two days before transplantation the medium may be sampled again to assess for infection. On the day before transplantation the corneas are sent in medium at ambient temperature to the operating hospital.

Table 7.19 Summary of contraindications to the use of ocular tissue in transplantation as outlined in the Royal College of Ophthalmologists' Guidance on the Retrieval of Ocular Tissue used in Transplantation and Research 2004[1]

Infection	*Known infection:* HIV, viral hepatitis (A, B, or C), viral encephalitis or encephalitis of unknown origin, viral meningitis, rabies, congenital rubella, tuberculosis, Reyes syndrome, progressive multifocal leucoencephalopathy, septicaemia, active malaria
	Seropositivity: HIV (1 or 2), HBsAg (hepatitis B surface antigen), hepatitis C virus, syphilis
	Behaviour leading to risk of contracting HIV, hepatitis B or C
Previous surgery	Receipt of an organ transplant (incl. dura, corneal, scleral, or limbal graft) or human pituitary derived hormones
	Brain/spinal surgery pre August 1992
CNS disorders and disorders of unknown aetiology	Motor neurone disease, chronic fatigue syndrome, CNS diseases of unknown aetiology (e.g. most dementias, multiple sclerosis, Parkinson's disease); death from unknown cause
Malignant/ premalignant disease	Leukaemia, lymphoma, myeloma, sideroblastic anaemia, polycythaemia
Ocular	Ocular inflammation, including known ocular involvement by systemic disease, e.g. sarcoidosis, rheumatoid arthritis
	Any ocular disorders that would preclude successful graft outcome (including previous refractive surgery)
	Malignant tumours

1. Royal College of Ophthalmologists. Guidance on the Retrieval of Ocular Tissue used in Transplantation and Research 2004 www.rcophth.ac.uk/docs/publications/published-guidelines/OcularTissueAndTransplantation_.pdf

Amniotic membrane transplantation

The amniotic membrane is part of the mammalian placenta, which has found numerous applications in ocular surface rehabilitation. It is widely available and, unlike most allografts (i.e. grafts from another individual), does not result in immunological rejection.

Histology

The placenta comprises a fetal component (the amniochorion) and a maternal component (the decidua). The amniotic membrane is an epithelial monolayer that secretes a thick basement membrane that is adjacent to an avascular stroma. This stroma comprises three collagenous layers: (1) a compact layer; (2) a fibroblast layer (also contains resident macrophages and serves to secrete components of the compact layer); and (3) an intermediate spongy layer (abundant in hydrated proteoglycans and glycoproteins).

In preparing the amniotic membrane for surgical use it is separated from the chorion along the natural cleavage plane of the intermediate spongy layer.

Function

The biological properties of amnion in ocular surface rehabilitation are thought to be primarily related to the amnion matrix and basement membrane substrate.

Amniotic membrane has anti-inflammatory, anti-angiogenic, and anti-scarring properties that promote inflammatory cell apoptosis, suppression of myofibroblast differentiation, inhibition of proteases and transforming growth factor signalling pathways. Other studies have indicated that amniotic membrane may also possess bactericidal properties.

Applications

Table 7.20 Applications of amniotic membrane transplantation

Common	Persistent corneal defects
	Reconstruction of conjunctival defects
	Chemical and thermal burns
	Limbal stem cell deficiency
	Bullous keratopathy
	Glaucoma surgery
Uncommon	Band keratopathy
	Post-refractive surgery haze
	Corneal hydrops
	Encasement of orbital prostheses
	Extraocular muscle surgery

Chapter 8

Sclera

Anatomy and physiology

The sclera is the tough outer coat of the globe covered by a loose connective tissue layer, the episclera.

The sclera develops from a condensation of mesenchymal tissue situated at the anterior rim of the optic cup. This forms first at the limbus at about week 7 and proceeds posteriorly to surround the optic nerve and form a rudimentary lamina cribrosa at week 12.

Sclera

Anatomy

The sclera is almost a complete sphere of 22mm diameter. Anteriorly it is continuous with the cornea, and posteriorly with the optic nerve. It is thickest around the optic nerve (1.0mm) and thinnest just posterior to the recti insertions (0.3mm).

Sclera consists of collagen (mainly types I, III, and V, but also IV, VI, VIII), elastin, proteoglycans, and glycoproteins. The stroma consists of a roughly criss-cross arrangement of collagen bundles of varying sizes (10–15µm thick, 100–150µm long). This renders it opaque but strong. The inner layer (lamina fusca) blends with the uveal tract, separated by the potential suprachoroidal space. The sclera itself is effectively avascular but is pierced by a number of vessels. It is innervated by the long and short ciliary nerves.

Physiology

The sclera provides a tough protective coat that is rigid enough to prevent loss of shape (with its refractive implications) but can tolerate some fluctuation in IOP. Scleral opacity is due to the irregularity of collagen and its relative hydration. The limited metabolic demands are supported by episcleral and choroidal vasculature. Inflammation of the sclera leads to engorgement of, mainly, the deep vascular plexus. This is relatively unaffected by the administration of topical vasoconstrictors (e.g. phenylephrine).

Episclera

Anatomy

This layer of connective tissue comprises an inner layer apposed to the sclera, intermediate loose connective tissue, and an outer layer that fuses with the muscle sheaths and the conjunctiva juxtalimbally. It is heavily vascularized with a superficial and deep anterior plexus (which underlie and anastamose with the conjunctival plexus) and a posterior episcleral plexus supplied by the short posterior ciliary vessels.

Physiology

The episclera gives nutrition to the sclera and provides a low friction surface assisting the free movement of the globe within the orbit. Inflammation of the episclera leads to engorgement of the conjunctival and superficial vascular plexus. These blanch with administration of topical vasoconstrictors (e.g. phenylephrine) leading to visible whitening.

Table 8.1 Scleral perforations

Location	Transmits
Anterior	Anterior ciliary arteries
Middle	Vortex veins
Posterior	Long + short ciliary nerves
	Long + short posterior ciliary arteries
Lamina cribrosa	Optic nerve

Episcleritis

This common condition is a benign, recurrent inflammation of the episclera. It is commonest in young women. It is usually self-limiting and may require little or no treatment. It is not usually associated with any systemic disease, although about 10% may have a connective tissue disease.

Simple episcleritis

Clinical features

- Sudden onset of mild discomfort, tearing ± photophobia; may be recurrent.
- Sectoral (occasionally diffuse) redness that blanches with topical vasoconstrictor (e.g. phenylephrine 10%); globe non-tender; spontaneous resolution 1–2wks.

Investigations

Investigations are not usually required unless there is a history suggestive of systemic disease.

Treatment

- *Supportive*: reassurance ± cold compresses.
- *Topical*: consider lubricants ± NSAID (e.g. ketorolac 0.3% 3×/d; uncertain benefit); although disease improves with topical steroids there may be rebound inflammation on withdrawal.
- *Systemic*: if severe/recurrent consider oral NSAID (e.g. flurbiprofen 100mg 3×/d for acute disease).

Nodular episcleritis

Clinical features

- Sudden onset of FB sensation, discomfort, tearing ± photophobia; may be recurrent.
- Red nodule arising from the episclera; can be moved separately from the sclera (cf. nodular scleritis) and conjunctiva (cf. conjunctival phlycten); blanches with topical vasoconstrictor (e.g. phenylephrine 10%); does not stain with fluorescein; globe non-tender (cf. scleritis); spontaneous resolution 5–6wks.

Investigations

Investigations are not usually required unless there is a history suggestive of systemic disease.

Treatment

As for simple episcleritis but there is a greater role for ocular lubricants.

Anterior scleritis (1)

This uncommon condition is a potentially blinding inflammation of the sclera. It is associated with systemic disease in about 50%, of which most cases are of a connective tissue disease. It is commonest in middle-aged women. Scleritis is bilateral in 50% cases, but both eyes may not be affected at the same time.

Classification

Table 8.2 Classification of scleritis and approximate frequency

Anterior	Non-necrotizing	Diffuse	50%
		Nodular	25%
	Necrotizing	With inflammation	10%
		Without inflammation	5%
Posterior			10%

Risk factors

- *Associated disease:* rheumatoid arthritis, Wegener's granulomatosis, relapsing polychondritis, systemic lupus erythematosus, sarcoidosis, polyarteritis nodosa, inflammatory bowel disease, psoriatic arthritis, ankylosing spondylitis, Cogan syndrome, rosacea, atopy, gout.
- *Infection:* e.g. syphilis, tuberculosis, VZV.
- *Local:* trauma, surgery (including surgically induced necrotizing scleritis).

Diffuse non-necrotizing anterior scleritis

Clinical features

- Subacute onset (over 1wk) of moderate/severe pain, redness, tearing photophobia.
- Diffuse injection of deep vascular plexus that does not blanch with vasoconstrictors (e.g. phenylephrine 2.5–10%), oedema; globe tender; usually non-progressive but may last for several months if untreated.

Investigations

- FBC, ESR, RF, ANA, ANCA, CRP, ACE, uric acid, syphilis serology, CXR, urinalysis.
- Anterior segment fluorescein angiograph: rapid arteriovenous transit time, rapid intense leakage from capillaries and venules.

Treatment

- *Oral:* NSAID (e.g. flurbiprofen 100mg 3×/d, can be tapered down once disease is controlled).
- If not controlled consider systemic immunosuppression: commonly corticosteroids (e.g. prednisolone 1mg/kg/d) ± other immunosuppressants (co-ordinate with a physician/rheumatologist).
- Topical corticosteroids are usually an adjunct to systemic therapy.

Nodular non-necrotizing anterior scleritis

Clinical features

- Subacute onset (over 1wk) moderate/severe pain, FB sensation, redness, tearing ± photophobia.
- Red nodule arising from the sclera; cannot be moved separately from underlying tissue (cf. nodular episcleritis); does not blanch with topical vasoconstrictor (e.g. phenylephrine 10%); globe tender.

Investigations

- As for diffuse anterior scleritis.

Treatment

- As for diffuse anterior scleritis, but add topical lubricants.

Box 8.1 Anterior scleritis: key points

- Pain (constant/deep/boring) can be so severe that it wakes the patient at night
- The globe may be very tender to touch
- Examine the eye under room light or in daylight prior to using the slit-lamp
- A bluish hue implies scleral thinning from previous active scleritis
- Topical phenylephrine 2.5–10% causes blanching of the more superficial episcleral vessels but does not change the engorgement of deeper sclera vessels and can help differentiate between scleritis and episcleritis.
- Scleral thinning may result in high degrees of astigmatism
- When seen in conjunction with peripheral corneal infiltrates, consider a diagnosis of Wegener's granulomatosis

Anterior scleritis (2)

Necrotizing anterior scleritis with inflammation

Clinical features
- Subacute onset (3–4d) severe pain, redness, tearing ± photophobia.
- White avascular areas surrounded by injected oedematous sclera; scleral necrosis → translucency revealing blue-black uveal tissue; anterior uveitis suggests very advanced disease.

NB scleral thinning and degree of scleral injection may be best appreciated under natural/room light.
- *Complications:* peripheral ulcerative keratitis, acute stromal keratitis, sclerosing keratitis, uveitis, cataract, astigmatism, glaucoma, globe perforation.

Investigations
- FBC, ESR, RF, ANA, ANCA, CRP, ACE, uric acid, syphilis serology, CXR, urinalysis.
- Anterior segment fluorescein angiograph: arteriovenous shunts with perfusion of veins before capillaries, and islands of no blood flow.

Treatment
- Systemic immunosuppression: commonly involves corticosteroids (e.g. prednisolone 1mg/kg/d tapering down, or 3 pulses IV methylyprednisolone 500–1000mg then oral corticosteroid) ± immunosuppressants such as cyclophosphamide, methotrexate, ciclosporin, azathioprine or mycophenolate mofetil; biologics, such as infliximab, adalimumab, rituximab; co-ordinate with a physician/rheumatologist.
- If risk of perforation protect globe (e.g. glasses by day, shield at night) and consider scleral patch graft.

Necrotizing anterior scleritis without inflammation (scleromalacia perforans)

Scleromalacia perforans is usually seen in severe chronic seropositive rheumatoid arthiritis.

Clinical features
- Asymptomatic.
- Small yellow areas of necrotic sclera coalesce to reveal large areas of underlying uvea in a quiet eye.
- Complications: although this does not usually result in perforation it may do so after minor trauma.

Investigations
- As for necrotizing anterior scleritis with inflammation.

Treatment
- Systemic immunosuppression: commonly involves corticosteroids ± other immunosuppressants (as discussed above); co-ordinate with a physician/rheumatologist.
- Topical: generous lubrication.
- If risk of perforation protect globe (e.g. glasses by day, shield at night) and consider scleral patch graft.

Relapsing polychondritis

Rare condition of recurrent inflammation of cartilage affecting the ear, nose, and most seriously trachea and larynx (risk of respiratory obstruction). The ophthalmic features include anterior uveitis, episcleritis scleritis, and rarely corneal involvement (keratoconjunctivitis sicca or peripheral ulcerative keratitis).

Posterior scleritis

Posterior scleritis is uncommon but is probably underdiagnosed. It is a potentially sight-threatening condition. It may be overlooked on account of more obvious anterior scleral inflammation or because there is isolated posterior disease and thus the eye appears white and quiet (often despite severe symptoms).

It is associated with systemic disease (usually RA or vasculitis) in up to one-third of cases.

Clinical features

- Mild–severe deep pain (may be referred to brow or jaw), ↓VA, diplopia, photopsia, hypermetropic shift.
- White eye (unless anterior involvement), lid oedema, proptosis, lid retraction, restricted motility; shallow anterior chamber, choroidal folds, annular choroidal detachment, exudative retinal detachments, macular oedema, disc oedema.

Investigation

- B-scan US: scleral thickening (see Opthalmic altrasonography images (2) 🕮 p.66) with fluid in Tenon's space (T-sign).
- Scleral thickening will also be seen on CT and MRI.

Treatment

- Oral: NSAID (e.g. flurbiprofen 100mg 3×/d, can be tapered down once disease controlled).
- If not controlled consider systemic immunosuppression: commonly involves corticosteroids (e.g. prednisolone 1mg/kg/d tapering down or 3 pulses IV methylprednisolone 500–1000mg then oral corticosteroid) ± immunosuppressants such as cyclophosphamide, methotrexate, ciclosporin, azathioprine, or mycophenolate mofetil; co-ordinate with a physician/rheumatologist.
- The response to therapy may be monitored by measuring the posterior scleral thickness on serial B-scan US.

Lens

Anatomy and physiology

The lens is a transparent, biconvex structure with an outer acellular capsule. It provides one-third of the refractive power of the eye. In the unaccommodated state it is about 4mm thick, with a 10mm anterior radius of curvature, a −6mm posterior radius of curvature, a refractive index of 1.386 (1.406 centrally), and an overall dioptric power of 18D.

Anatomy

Capsule

Unusually thick basement membrane, rich in type IV collagen; the anterior capsule arises from the epithelium and the posterior from the elongating fibre cells; the capsule is thicker at the equator than centrally, and thicker anteriorly (8–14μm, increasing with age) than posteriorly (2–3μm).

Epithelium

The lens epithelium lies just deep to the anterior capsule; centrally the epithelium is cuboidal and non-mitotic; peripherally, the epithelium is columnar and mitotic, producing almost 2 million transparent lens fibres over an adult's life.

Fibres

As the cells elongate (up to 10mm long) transparency is attained by loss of organelles, a tight regular arrangement, and a 90% crystallin composition. The nucleus (comprising embryonic and foetal parts) consists of the fibres laid down before birth; however, the clinical 'nucleus' observed at the slit-lamp also includes deep cortex. Lens sutures are formed by interdigitation of the ends of the fibres. The most visible example are the two Y-shaped sutures of the foetal nucleus—anterior Y, posterior λ. The cortex contains the more recently formed fibres and the nucleus contains the older non-dividing cells.

Zonules

These comprise sheets of suspensory fibres composed of fibrillin (Ch15q) that arise at the ciliary body and attach to the lens pre-equatorially, equatorially, and post-equatorially.

Physiology

The lens has a low water (65%) and high protein (35%) content. It has a resting pH of 6.9, a relatively low temperature, and is relatively hypoxic. Most energy production and active transport occurs at the epithelium, but peripheral lens fibres demonstrate significant protein synthesis (mainly of crystallins) and even central lens fibres show limited carbohydrate metabolism. Although oxidative phosphorylation occurs at the epithelium, most energy production is anaerobic (via glycolysis, pentose-phosphate pathway, and the α-glycerophosphate shuttle). Most glucose is thus converted to glucose-6-phosphate, and to a lesser degree sorbitol.

The high refractive index of the lens results from the crystallin content of its fibres. These proteins, of which α-crystallin is the commonest, are extremely stable and provide good short-range order (predominantly β-sheet secondary structure).

Clarity of the lens is attained by minimizing lens fibre scatter with: (1) narrow lens fibre membranes; (2) small interfibre spaces; (3) tightly packed regular contents (crystallin); (4) absence of blood vessels; and (5) loss of organelles.

Detoxification of free radicals is achieved by glutathione, supported by ascorbic acid (cf. hydrogen-peroxide catalase elsewhere in the body). In the process glutathione is oxidized to glutathione disulfide (GSSG), which would potentially form disulphide bonds with lens proteins were it not returned to its reduced state by glutathione reductase.

Cataract: introduction

Cataracts account for about 40% of global blindness representing about 16 million people. While cataract is ubiquitous, occurring in almost every aging population, the inequity of eye care means that 99% of these blinding cases are seen in developing countries.

Risk factors

The prevalence of cataract increases markedly with age. In the UK a visually significant cataract (VA <6/12) was present in 16% of those aged 65–69yrs, in 42% of those aged 75–79yrs, and in 71% of those aged >85yrs.

Other risk factors include: age, sunlight, smoking, alcohol, dehydration, radiation, corticosteroid use, diabetes mellitus.

Pathogenesis

How these factors cause cataracts is unclear, although a common pathway appears to be protein denaturation, e.g. by oxidation.

Metabolic disturbance (hyperglycaemia in diabetes mellitus or hyperuraemia in dehydration or renal failure), toxins (e.g. smoking, alcohol), loss of antioxidant enzymes, membrane disruption, reduced metabolism, failure of active transport, and loss of ionic/osmotic balance may all contribute to this process.

Clinical presentations

Common

- *Change in vision*: reducing acuity, contrast sensitivity, or colour appreciation, glare, monocular diplopia, polyplopia, or ghosting.
- *Change in refraction*: typically myopic shift in nuclear sclerosis or increased or changing astigmatism.
- *Change in fundal view*: optometrists and ophthalmologists may have difficulty 'looking in' long before the patient feels they have difficulties 'looking out'. This may be a problem when trying to monitor/treat posterior segment disease such as diabetic retinopathy.

Uncommon

Phakomorphic glaucoma

The large cataractous lens may cause anterior bowing of the iris with secondary angle closure. Presentation is as acute or chronic angle closure with high IOP, shallow AC, and fixed semi-dilated pupil. Distinguish it from PACG by the presence of an ipsilateral swollen cataractous lens and contralateral open angle with deep AC.

Phakolytic glaucoma

The hypermature cataract loses soluble lens proteins through the intact anterior capsule causing trabecular obstruction and subsequent secondary open angle glaucoma. Note raised IOP, lens protein in a deep AC (may form a pseudohypopyon), open angles, and hypermature cataract.

Phakoanaphylactic uveitis

This is an inflammatory response to lens protein, usually following traumatic capsular rupture or postoperative retention of lens material (when it must be distinguished from endophthalmitis). The IOP may be high, normal, or low.

Cataract: types

Cataracts may be classified according to age of onset, morphology, grade of opacification, and maturity.

Age of onset

Cataracts may be congenital (see Congenital cataract, 📖 p.704), juvenile/presenile (see Table 18.26, p.705), or age-related (senile).

Morphology

Cataract morphology (Table 9.1) may be divided into fibre-based (pattern relates to anatomical structure of the lens) or non-fibre based (a more random distribution). Fibre-based cataracts may be divided into sutural (pattern relates to lens sutures) and non-sutural types.

Table 9.1 Classification of cataract morphology

Fibre-based	Sutural	Congenital sutural
		Concussion
		Storage disorder
		Deposition
	Non-sutural	Lamellar
		Nuclear
		Cortical
Non-fibre based	Subcapsular	Lamellar
		Coronary
		Blue dot
		Christmas tree

Grade

Grading systems have been designed that aim to quantify the degree of opacification. These vary from simple assessment by direct ophthalmoscopy to more sophisticated methods such as the Lens Opacities Classification System II where silt-lamp examination is compared with a standard set of photographs (separate set for nuclear, cortical, and posterior subcapsular).

Maturity of cataract

- *Immature:* opacification is incomplete.
- *Mature:* opacification is total.
- *Hypermature:* lysis of cortex results in shrinkage, seen clinically as wrinkling of the capsule.
- *Morgagnian:* liquefaction of cortex allows the harder nucleus to drop inferiorly (but still within the capsule).

Table 9.2 Cataract types

Type		Properties	Cause
Sutural	(Y)	Congenital	Non-progressive
		Concussion	Often flower-shaped (lens fibre separation and fluid entry); anterior and posterior
		Storage disorder	Usually start posteriorly; • Fabry's disease, mannosidosis
		Deposition	Usually start anteriorly; • Copper, gold, silver, iron, chlorpromazine
Nuclear	(●)	Congenital	Non-progressive; limited to embryonic nucleus (cataracta centralis pulverulenta) or more extensive
		Age-related	Increased white scatter (light scattering) and brunescence (brown chromophores)
Lamellar	(0)	Congenital/infantile	Localized to a particular lamella (layer) ± extensions (riders) • Inherited, rubella, diabetes, galactosaemia, hypocalcaemia
Coronary	(⋮)	Sporadic	Round opacities in the deep cortex forming a 'crown' Occasionally inherited
Cortical	(◖)	Age-related	Spoke-like opacities in the superficial cortex, spreading along fibres at an unpredictable rate;
Subcapsular	(◯)	Age-related	Granular material just beneath capsule, posterior (more common and visually significant) or anterior • Diabetes, corticosteroids, uveitis, radiation
Polar	(◯)	Congenital	*Anterior*: with abnormalities of capsule ± anterior segment (persistent pupillary membrane, anterior lenticonus, Peters anomaly) *Posterior*: with abnormalities of capsule ± posterior segment (persistent hyperplastic primary vitreous, Mittendorf dots, posterior lenticonus)
Diffuse	(▨)	Congenital	Focal blue dot opacities are common and visually insignificant Also present in Lowe syndrome carriers
		Age-related	Christmas tree cataracts are highly reflective crystalline opacities

Cataract surgery: assessment

Surgical removal of cataracts is effective and safe. Overall, 92% patients attain best-corrected visual acuity (BCVA) ≥6/12 within 3mths of surgery and >80% are within 1D of predicted refraction.

Sight-threatening complications are rare. However, this is in part due to careful pre-operative preparation and postoperative assessment.

Referral

Referral may be by the primary care physician or, increasingly, directly from the optometrist.

Appropriate referral

- The cataract is likely to be responsible for the patient's visual complaint.
- The cataract is compromising the patient's lifestyle.
- The risks and benefits have been discussed with the patient and appropriate written information provided.
- The patient wants to have the operation.

All this information and a copy of a recent sight test should be included in the referral.

Out-patient appointment

Table 9.3 Initial assessment for cataract surgery

Visual symptoms	Blur at distance/near, glare, distortion, colour perception, 'second sight' (myopic shift)
POH	Previous acuity; history of amblyopia, strabismus, previous surgery (especially refractive surgery), trauma; concurrent eye disease; refraction from optometrist
PMH	Diabetes, hypertension, COPD; ability to lie flat and still for 30min; anaesthetic history (if GA considered)
SH	Occupation, driving, hobbies, daily tasks
Dx	Warfarin, antiplatelet agents, α_1-adrenoreceptor blockers, e.g.. tamsulosin; topical medication
Visual acuity	Distance/near, unaided/best-corrected/pin-hole
Pupils	Check for RAPD, adequate dilatation
Cataract	Morphology, density, maturity
Other factors	Globe (deep-set, small/large), lids (blepharitis, entropion, ectropion), nasolacrimal (mucocele), cornea (scarring, guttata), anterior chamber depth, IOP, iris (PXF, iridodonesis, posterior synechiae, inducible mydriasis), lens (PXF, phakodonesis, lens–vitreous interface) optic disc (e.g. glaucoma, neuropathy), macula (e.g. AMD), fundus

Appropriate listing for cataract surgery
- There is visually significant cataract responsible for the patient's complaint and compromising their lifestyle.
- There is no coexisting ocular disease precluding surgery; any disease that may affect surgery (e.g. PXF) or outcome (e.g. AMD) has been discussed with the patient and an appropriately guarded prognosis given.
- The patient wants to proceed and understands the risks.
- Informed consent is taken and a surgical plan is formulated (*see* Cataract surgery: consent and planning 📖 p.270).

The younger patient
In the younger patient also consider why they might have developed presenile cataracts (trauma, steroids, etc. *see Table 18.26* 📖 p.705).

Pre-operative assessment
For patient convenience this should be on the same day as the initial assessment. Aspects may be performed by suitably trained nursing staff according to local protocol.

History
- *General health*: PMH, Dx, Ax.
- *Social history*: support, telephone, transport, ability to manage topical medication.
- *Education*: surgery, postoperative care, information leaflet.

Investigation
- Biometry/IOL power calculations.
- Focimetry (unless recent copy of refraction).

Treatment
- Prescription of pre-operative treatments, e.g. for blepharitis.
- Prescription of mydriatic drops, e.g. cyclopentolate 1% + phenylephrine 2.5% + diclofenac 0.1%. to potentiate mydriasis.
- Prescription of postoperative treatment: steroid/antibiotic drops (e.g. Betnesol-N® 4×/d for 4wks); IOP-lowering agents (e.g. timolol 0.5% or acetazolamide 250mg stat dose post-operation).

Cataract surgery: consent and planning

Nature of the operation

Explain what a cataract is, 'The clear lens in your eye has become cloudy', and what the operation does, 'It replaces the cataract with a new plastic lens'.

General risk

For all patients warn of sight-threatening risks, notably endophthalmitis (0.1%), retinal detachment/tear (0.1%), and choroidal haemorrhage (0.1%). Also advise of the possibility of requiring a second operation GA (dropped nucleus/IOL (0.5%)). The commonest intra-operative complication is posterior capsule rupture with vitreous loss (4%), which may have a significant effect on outcome. The commonest postoperative complication is PCO (10% in 2yrs).

Anaesthetic options include topical, local (peribulbar or subtenons) or GA (see Ocular anasthesia 📖 p.828-831).

The risk of a GA will depend on the general health of the patient, and if necessary should be discussed with the anaesthetist ± physician before the day of surgery. Risks of local anaesthesia include globe rupture (0.006–0.1%) and life-threatening events such as brain stem anaesthesia or the oculocardiac reflex (0.03%).

Specific risk

Assess and warn of any additional risk, such as technical difficulties, guarded visual prognosis, and any increased risk of sight-threatening complications. Consider whether subspecialist review is indicated, e.g. for posterior polar cataracts or in the presence of endothelial dystrophies.

Common technical issues

Table 9.4 Common technical issues

Feature	Risk	Strategy
Positional		
Cervical spondylosis	Head-up posture	Tilt feet up
Deep-set eye	Poor access	Temporal approach
View		
Oily tear film	Aberrant reflexes	External methylcellulose
Poor red reflex	Difficult capsulorhexis	Vision blue
Access		
Short axial length	Crowded AC	High viscosity viscoelastic
Poor dilation	Inadequate access	Iris hooks/stretch techniques
Zonular integrity		
Age >90yrs	Zonular dehiscence	Minimize lens movement
Pseudoexfoliation	Zonular dehiscence	Minimize lens movement
Pre-operative phakodonesis	Zonular dehiscence	Vitreoretinal approach
White cataract	Zonular dehiscence	Consider ECCE/chopping
PC integrity		
Shallow AC depth	Iris/PC trauma	High viscosity viscoelastic
Posterior polar	PC rupture	Vitreoretinal approach

Guarded visual prognosis
Note history of amblyopia, or evidence of pre-existing corneal opacity, vitreous opacities, macular or optic nerve disease.

Increased risk of sight-threatening complications
- *Endophthalmitis*: note lid disease (blepharitis, trichiasis, entropion, ectropion), conjunctivitis, nasolacrimal disease (obstruction, mucocele, etc.), diabetes; pre-treat where possible, e.g. lid hygiene/antibiotics for blepharitis/conjunctivitis, surgery for lid malposition/nasolacrimal obstruction.
- *Retinal detachment*: note high myopia, lattice degeneration.
- *Choroidal haemorrhage*: possibly uncontrolled hypertension, age, arteriosclerosis.
- *Corneal decompensation*: note endothelial dystrophy (e.g. Fuchs').

Desired outcome
Consider the refractive needs of the patient.

When aiming for emmetropia (most patients) explain that while they may need no/weak glasses for distance they will need reading glasses. Patients with significant ametropia or astigmatism are more complex.

High ametropia
- *Complications*: anisometropia may lead to aniseikonia.
- *Pre-operatively*: with bilateral cataracts, discuss options re (1) aim for emmetropia and do the second eye within 6wks, or (2) aim to leave ametropic (but up to 2D nearer emmetropia than the other eye) with less immediate need for a second operation. If unilateral cataract, particularly where the second eye has good acuity and accommodative function consider aiming for emmetropia and using a contact lens on the second eye until surgery is indicated.

Astigmatism
Pre-existing astigmatism can usually be reduced by choosing to operate 'on-meridian'. For higher degrees of astigmatism additional refractive incisions can be placed at the time of cataract surgery (see Cataract surgery: perioperative 📖 p.272).

Cataract surgery: perioperative

Pre-operative check (on the day of surgery)

Patient preparation

- *Ensure mydriasis*: e.g. cyclopentolate 1% + phenylephrine 2.5% + diclofenac 0.1%.
- Check consent form complete.
- Check any new ophthalmic problems, especially evidence of active infection.
- Mark side of operation.
- Operating surgeon to confirm IOL type/power and axis/operating position.

Intraocular lens selection

- Check that the biometry does indeed belong to your patient.
- Check for *intraocular* consistency in axial length and K values (i.e. that they are similar and the standard deviation is low).
- Check for *interocular* consistency in axial length and K values. If axial length difference >0.3mm confirm by B-scan and if the difference in K readings >1D then consider corneal topography.
- Check appropriate formula used:

Table 9.5 Royal College of Ophthalmologists recommendations 2004

<22mm	Hoffer Q or SRK/T
22–24.5mm	SRK/T, Holladay, Haigis
>24.6	SRK/T

- Select appropriate lens power (usually but not always aiming for emmetropia); if previous refractive surgery enter corrected K values into SRK-T, Haigis, Hoffer Q, and Holladay 2 and select the highest IOL power suggested.

Astigmatic targeting

Some surgeons always operate 'from the top', but there are refractive advantages to a temporal clear corneal incision or scleral tunnel (relative astigmatic neutrality), or by operating 'on-meridian' (astigmatic targeting). If operating 'on-meridian' a clear corneal incision is placed on the steep corneal meridian. This should be based on keratometry as the refractive astigmatism may include a lenticular component that will be dealt with by lens removal. The astigmatic effect of the incision increases with depth and length of wound. It can be enhanced by an opposite refractive incision (on-meridian surgery) or by single or paired incisions at another meridian (off-meridian surgery).

Box 9.1 IOL selection after refractive surgery

Keratometric measurements performed after refractive surgery are unreliable in traditional biometric formulae. Methods to 'correct' the keratometry readings include:

Clinical history method

Corrected K = pre-laser K − change in refractive error at 6mths.

Contact lens method

- Measure refraction with and without a 40D hard contact lens.
- Corrected K = 40 + (refraction with CL—refraction without CL).
- These corrected Ks are entered into SRK-T, Haigis, Hoffer Q, and Holladay 2 formulae and the highest IOL power selected.

Cataract surgery: postoperative

Postoperative check (on the next day)

For most patients this has largely been replaced by a telephone assessment by a trained nurse. The first-day review is now generally reserved for higher-risk patients (complicated surgery, coexistent ocular disease).

Examination
- *Cornea*: wounds sealed (Seidel test negative), clarity
- *AC*: formed, activity
- *Pupil*: round
- *PCIOL*: centred and in the bag
- *Consider*: IOP check.

Give clear instructions re postoperative drops, use of a clear shield, what to expect (1–2d discomfort, watering), what to worry about (increasing pain/redness, worsening vision), and where to get help (including telephone number).

Final review (usually 2–4wks later)

Examination
- *VA*: unaided/pinhole
- *Cornea*: wounds sealed (Seidel test negative), clarity
- *AC*: depth and activity
- *Pupil*: round
- *PCIOL*: centred and in the bag
- *IOP*.
- *Fundus*: no CMO, flat retina.

If good result then either list for second eye or discharge to optometrist for refraction as appropriate.

If disappointing VA (unaided) perform refraction/autorefraction to look for 'refractive surprise' (see Refractive surprise 📖 p.296) and dilated fundoscopy to check for subtle CMO (especially if VA (pin hole) < VA (unaided)) and if in doubt, consider OCT.

Phakoemulsification (1)

Preparation

Povidone iodine (5% aqueous solution) cleansing of the skin and instillation into the conjunctival sac reduces bacterial load and risk of endophthalmitis. Careful draping maximizes surgical view, keeps lashes out of the surgical field, and prevents pooling of fluid.

Incision

Wound construction is critical. The wound needs to be large enough to allow easy access of instruments, but small enough to permit a stable AC and reduce risk of iris prolapse (e.g. 2.8mm). At the end of the operation it must seal to become water-tight.

Options for conventional phakoemulsification wounds include clear corneal incisions (which may be tri-, bi-, or uniplanar) and scleral tunnels. Scleral tunnels are fairly astigmatically neutral, whereas corneal incisions tend to cause flattening. This can be made use of by operating 'on-meridian' to reduce any pre-existing corneal astigmatism. With the advent of bimanual microincision cataract surgery (Box 9.3), wounds may be as small as 1.4mm.

Subsequent instrumentation should respect the shape of the wound to reduce the risk of stripping off Descemet's membrane.

Ophthalmic viscosurgical devices (viscoelastics)

OVDs are solutions of long-chain polymers with a range of viscosity and cohesive properties. Higher-viscosity cohesive OVDs are used for stabilizing the AC and opening the bag prior to IOL insertion. Lower-viscosity dispersive OVDs are used to isolate part of the surgical field e.g. protecting a vulnerable cornea in the 'soft-shell' technique (Box 9.2), or keeping iris or vitreous out of the way). Viscoadaptives are more advanced OVDs that can behave like a higher-viscosity cohesive OVD or like a dispersive according to AC fluid dynamics.

Table 9.6 Ophthalmic viscosurgical devices

Group	Subgroup	Content	Example	Molecular weight
Viscoadaptive		Hyaluronic acid	Healon 5	4000–8000kDa
Higher viscosity	Supervoscous	Hyaluronic acid	Healon GV	4000–8000kDa
	Viscous	Hyaluronic acid	Healon Provisc	1000–2000kDa
Lower viscosity	Medium viscosity	Hyaluronic acid	Viscoat	100–500kDa
	Very-low viscosity	HPMC	Occucoat	80–90kDa

Box 9.2 Options for the soft-shell technique

Traditional soft-shell technique

High-viscosity cohesive OVD to maintain AC
Low-viscosity dispersive OVD to coat cornea

Viscoadaptive soft-shell technique

Viscoadaptive OVD to achieve both maintenance of AC and protection of cornea. It is either used in combination with BSS (known as the 'ultimate soft-shell technique') or with a visco-dispersive OVD.

Phakoemulsification (2)

Continuous curvilinear capsulorhexis

The aim is to achieve a 5–6mm continuous central anterior capsulectomy via cystotome and/or forceps under viscoelastic. This is large enough to assist lens removal (and reduce risk of postoperative capsular phimosis) and small enough to stabilize the lens (and reduce risk of postoperative capsular opacification).

In the presence of poor red reflex or significant cortical opacities, visibility may be assisted by the use of trypan blue (often injected under air and irrigated after <60s). Decompress intumescent cataracts by puncturing the AC and aspirating lens matter.

A capsulorhexis that is running out to the periphery may be rescuable by deepening the AC/pushing the iris back with more or higher viscosity viscolelastic, e.g. Healon 5. If unable to bring the capsulorhexis back in, consider: tearing in the opposite direction from the start position; capsulorhexis scissors or a can-opener capsulotomy. Review whether to continue with cautious phakoemulsification or convert to ECCE.

A small capsulorhexis can be extended after insertion of the PCIOL by making a nick (e.g. with a cystotome) and then tearing with forceps as usual.

Hydrodissection

Injection of balanced salt solution under the anterior capsular rim separates the nucleus from the cortex and is seen as a wave passing posteriorly. If successful it permits rotation of the nucleus. If overly aggressive it may cause posterior capsule rupture, as may the use of a fine bore cannula (smaller than 27 gauge).

Managing the small pupil

Inadequate dilatation of pupil makes surgery technically more difficult and increases the risk of complications.

Causes

Common causes include diabetes, pseudoexfoliation, uveitis, the intraoperative floppy iris syndrome, and long-term pilocarpine usage.

Intra-operative strategies:
- Pupil stretch.
- Iris hooks.
- Intracameral mydriatics, e.g. intracameral lidocaine+ phenylephrine ± cyclopentolate.

Phakoemulsification (3)

Phakoemulsification

Rotate the probe to enter wound with minimal trauma.

Technique

- *Divide and conquer*: the groove should be about 1.5 phako-tips wide and as deep as safely possible (this is usually about 3mm deep centrally). An improving red reflex may assist in judging depth. Use a second instrument to rotate nucleus 90° to form the next groove, and continue until a cruciate configuration is formed. Insert both instruments deep into each groove, gently pulling apart to crack the nucleus into four segments. Use a higher vacuum setting to bring each segment centrally to be emulsified.
- *Phako chop*: use high vacuum and sufficient phako power to bury the phako tip into the nucleus just proximal to the centre and aiming steeply posterior. The second instrument is inserted under the anterior capsule and chopped through the stabilized nucleus against the phako probe. This is repeated to generate wedges that can then be emulsified as above.
- *Chip and flip*: sculpt to form a bowl and then flip it anteriorly to complete emulsification safely.

Pumps and fluidics

The traditional distinction between a vacuum pump (e.g. Venturi system) and a peristaltic pump has become blurred by hybrids such as the scroll pump.

- *Vacuum systems*: use a Venturi or a diaphragm pump to generate a low pressure relative to the anterior chamber. Flow is dependent on this pressure difference, and thus cannot be altered independently of vacuum.
- *Peristaltic systems*: the pressure gradient is generated by milking fluid along compressible tubing by a series of rollers. Flow and vacuum can be set separately. A low flow setting results in a more gradual, gentler response, so aiding cautious manipulation. This may be helpful in training. Higher flow results in a faster (but more aggressive) response from the phako-probe. Adjusting the vacuum level limits the maximum vacuum that will be generated once the tip is occluded.

Phako power modulation

Phako power can be delivered as continuous or intermittent. Intermittent modes are all directed at using phako power more efficiently, so reducing the effective phako time (EPT = phako time × percentage phako power used). These modes include pulse (usually linear control of energy with fixed/varying pulse rate), burst mode (fixed phako power with variable duration/interval), and assorted modifications such as sonolase (Whitestar), 'no burn' and 'cool' phako.

Dual linear

This permits simultaneous foot control of both phako power (pitch, i.e. up/down) and aspiration (yaw, i.e. left/right). This is particularly useful for the phako chop technique.

Irrigation and aspiration

This is usually automated (straight/curved/45°/90° tips) and can be combined or split (bimanual). Manual irrigation and aspiration is an alternative (Simcoe). Cortex is engaged peripherally and dragged centrally where the vacuum can be increased under direct view.

Intraocular lens

Enlarge the wound sufficient to allow the introduction of the lens (e.g. 3.5mm for a foldable IOL) before introducing it with either a special forceps or an injector. Pre-fill the bag with viscoelastic before implanting the lens, placing the lead haptic directly into the bag before dropping/dialling in the second haptic. The choice of lens is in part due to capsular integrity (and therefore type of operation). (*See* Intraocular lenses (1), 📖 p. 284.)

Wound closure

Well-constructed wounds sized for foldable lenses are usually self-sealing, but may be assisted by stromal hydration. If in any doubt suture the wound closed.

Peri-operative antibiotics

At the end of the procedure, antibiotics (± corticosteroids) are routinely given. Traditionally this has been topical, subconjunctival, or sub-tenons, intracameral cefuroxime has been increasingly popular since the ESCRS study found a 5-fold reduction in the rate of endophthalmitis.[1]

Common regimens include: subconjunctival – cefuroxime or gentamicin ± dexamethasone; intracameral – cefuroxime (1mg).

Box 9.3 Bimanual microincision cataract surgery

In essence bimanual microincision cataract surgery uses separate handpieces for irrigation and phakoemulsification/aspiration. The technique requires two limbal incisions of 1.2 × 1.4 mm made with a trapezoidal blade. *Advantages include:*

- Smaller incision (e.g. 1.45mm) due to narrower handpieces leads to fewer wound complications.
- More stable anterior chamber.
- Improved fluid dynamics: the irrigation does not propel the pieces of nucleus away from the tip of the phako probe.
- Improved accessibility (e.g. easier removal of soft lens matter (SLM) as the probes can be interchanged between the two wounds).
- Reduced 'phako time/power'.

---

1. Barry P et al. ESCRS study of prophylaxis of postoperative endophthalmitis after cataract surgery. *J Cataract Refract Surg* 2006;**32**:407–10.

Extracapsular and intracapsular cataract extraction

Extracapsular cataract extraction

This is removal of the lens while retaining the posterior capsule and integrity of the anterior vitreous face. The operation requires a superior 10mm biplanar corneal (or limbal) incision, injection of viscoelastic to form the AC, anterior capsulotomy (usually can-opener technique), hydrodissection, nucleus expression (gentle digital pressure or irrigating vectis), aspiration of cortex and lens implantation (usually rigid PMMA lens into the bag).

Table 9.7 Types of cataract extraction

Technique	Advantages	Disadvantages
Intracapsular	No PCO Can deal with zonular dialysis	Higher rates of CMO and retinal detachment Higher rate of rubeosis in diabetic eyes ACIOL, sutured lens or aphakia Sutures required
Extracapsular	PCIOL Lower rate of CMO and retinal detachment	PCO Sutures required
Phakoemulsification	More stable AC/IOP PCIOL Lower rate of CMO, retinal detachment, and expulsive haemorrhage Sutureless wound Reduced astigmatism Faster visual rehabilitation Reduced postoperative inflammation Topical anaesthesia possible	PCO Expensive equipment Dropped lens fragments

Intracapsular cataract extraction

This is removal of the whole lens including capsule and was widely practised during the 1960s and 1970s. The operation requires a 150° corneal (or limbal) incision, a peripheral iridectomy, zonular digestion (α-chymotrypsin), forceps or cryoprobe removal of the lens and insertion of an ACIOL (angle or iris-supported), a sutured lens or aphakic correction (spectacles or contact lenses).

Intraocular lenses (1)

Choice of lens

Phakoemulsification with intact posterior capsule and anterior capsulorhexis permits use of a foldable PCIOL (smaller wound, usually sutureless), which can be placed in the bag (preferable optically and physiologically).

In the presence of a small tear in the anterior or posterior capsule it may still be possible to implant the lens in the bag. If there is a significant PC tear but intact anterior capsule, consider sulcus fixation. If anterior and posterior capsular damage, consider ACIOL. For extracapsular cataract extraction the larger incision is sufficient for implantation of a rigid PMMA lens into the bag or sulcus.

Posterior chamber intraocular lens

IOLs may be classified according to their material (silicone or acrylic), interaction with water (hydrophilic or hydrophobic), and design (one-piece or three-piece; spherical or toric; rounded or square-edged). Lens behaviour therefore arises from a number of contributing factors. For example, hydrophilic acrylic lenses appear to be the most biocompatible with little attachment of inflammatory cells. However, the hydrophobic acrylic IOLs appear to have the lowest PCO rates, but this may be due to their square-edge design rather than the material.

Material

Table 9.8 Types of PCIOL

Material	Advantages	Disadvantages
Rigid		
PMMA	Follow-up>50yrs Stable	Large incision needed Higher rate of PCO
Foldable		
Silicone	Follow-up >15yrs Folds easily	Rapid unfolding Poor handling when wet Adherence to silicone oil
Hydrophobic acrylic	Higher *n* allows thinner lenses Slow unfolding Low PCO rate (some designs)	Glistenings in optic (some lenses)
Hydrophilic acrylic	Slow unfolding Low inflammatory cell attachment Resistant to YAG laser damage	Calcium deposition on/in optic (some lenses)
n = refractive index		

Table 9.9 PCIOL materials

Lens type	Material	Refractive index (n)
Rigid		
PMMA	Polymethyl methacrylate	1.49
Flexible		
Silicone	Silicone polymers	1.41–1.46
Hydrophobic acrylic	Acrylate + methacrylate	1.54
Hydrophilic acrylic	Poly-hydroxyethyl-methylacrylate + hydrophilic acrylic monomer	1.47

Design

Square-edged vs rounded
IOL optics with square posterior edges appear to reduce posterior capsular opacification by reducing migration of lens epithelial cells, although dysphotopsia (crescentic glare in certain ambient light conditions) from edge reflections can be bothersome with 'very' square edged lenses.

Toric vs spherical
Toric IOLs can correct for pre-operative astigmatism but may cause problems if not perfectly positioned.

Short wavelength filtration
Some recent IOLs filter out short wavelength blue light as this may be linked to accelerated age-related macular changes in pseudophakic patients. They are also reported to increase contrast and reduce glare.

Thin vs standard
Thin IOLs are designed for use with the smaller incisions of microincision cataract surgery. They are reported as also causing less aberration, glare, and haloes than standard lenses.

Pseudo-accommodative and accommodative lenses
- *Pseudo-accommodative lenses* are multifocals that may be diffractive or refractive in nature. They are attended by a loss of contrast sensitivity, and are not always tolerated.
- *Accommodative IOLs* alter their focal length by anteroposterior movement within the capsular bag.

Intraocular lenses (2)

Anterior chamber intraocular lens

ACIOL use is mainly associated with intracapsular cataract extraction but may still be of use where there has been unintentional disruption of capsular support. These may be angle-supported or iris-supported. Angle-supported lenses are sized to the anterior chamber (measure 'white-to-white'). In earlier designs sizing was critical: too large and they would cause inflammation and local destruction; too small and they would be unstable and again cause irritation. Modern one-piece lenses with three-/four-point fixation are much better tolerated and sizing is less critical. ACIOLs may be introduced by means of a glide. A peripheral iridectomy should be performed at the time of surgery.

Some surgeons feel that allowing the eye to settle and then 4–6wks later performing a secondary insertion of ACIOL and PI provides for a more stable and safer surgical environment.

Accommodative/pseudo-accommodative intraocular lens

Pseudo-accommodative (multifocal)

Types
- *Refractive type*: concentric zones of different optical power; may be near dominant or far dominant; e.g. AMO Rezoom.
- *Diffractive type*: annular grooves cut in surface of IOL cause diffraction and multiple foci, e.g. Acrysof Restor—good distance and near vision.

Disadvantages

Loss of contrast sensitivity, glare, night vision problems, visual adaptation, and good outcome relies on very accurate spherical targeting (just +0.125 side of emmetropia) and less than 0.50DC or residual astigmatism for the lenses to work. As these postoperative refractive errors increase, so the lens efficacy reduces, yet the side-effects remain. Therefore, careful consideration should be exercised when using these lenses.

Accommodative

Accommodative IOLs alter their focal length by anteroposterior movement within the capsular bag due to their thin, flexible hinge at the haptic–optic junction that permits forward movement of the optic with haptic compression, e.g. 1 CU IOL, Crystalens.

Disadvantages

Longer-term results (1–2yrs) have so far been disappointing due to high levels of capsular fibrosis restricting optic movement.

Phakic intraocular lenses

Phakic IOLs may be used to correct refractive error or as a treatment for presbyopia.

Angle-supported

- *Examples*: Thinoptix, I-Care IOL, Multifocal ACIOL for Presbyopia.
- *Disadvantages*: endothelial cell loss, pupil ovalization, decentration.

Iris supported
These IOLs clip to midperipheral iris.
- *Examples:* Verisyse, Artisan, Toric Artisan , Artiflex.
- *Disadvantages:* endothelial cell loss, night vision problems.

Lens supported
- *Examples:* ICL, ICL toric, PRL.
- *Disadvantages:* Lens changes, pigment dispersion, meridional alignment for toric versions.

Box 9.4 Intraocular refractive surgery

This is any intraocular surgical procedure done with the intention of inducing refractive or optical change to the dioptric value of the eye.

Phakic intraocular lens insertion
For correction of myopia, hypermetropia, astigmatism, presbyopia.

Refractive lens surgery
Either cataract surgery or refractive lens exchange (no significant cataract).

For spherical correction
- Choice of lens power.

Astigmatic correction
- Operate on-meridian.
  - Place main incision on steep axis.
- Limbal relaxing incisions (LRI):
  - For astigmatism ≤3D; single or paired incisions on the steep axis anterior to the palisade of Vogt; use nomogram to determine number and length of LRI.
  - *Advantage:* easier to do, less risk of overcorrection (vs corneal relaxing incisions).
  - *Disadvantage:* regression (loss of effect with time).
  - *Complications:* infection, perforation, misalignment of axis.
- Corneal relaxing incisions:
  - For astigmatism >3D.
  - *Disadvantage:* less predictable (vs LRI), overcorrection, induction of higher-order aberrations (irregular astigmatism).
- Toric IOLs:
  - *Advantage:* no regression
  - *Disadvantage:* precise axis placement necessary (10° rotation can reduce effect by 30%; 30° rotation keeps same astigmatic magnitude but 'flips' it to a new meridian.

Cataract surgery and concurrent eye disease

Diabetes

- *Complications*: fibrinous anterior uveitis, PCO, progression of retinopathy, and macular oedema. Risk of complications increases with degree of retinopathy.
- *Pre-operative*: if severe PPDR/PDR then treat (PRP) prior to surgery where possible. Treat clinically significant macular oedema (focal/grid laser) 12wks before surgery.
- *Postoperative*: consider topical NSAID (e.g. ketorolac 0.3% 3×/d 6/52). An extended course of topical steroids may be required. See at 1d, 1wk, and then 6wks.

Glaucoma

- *Complications*: postoperative pressure spike, progression of field loss.
- *Pre-operative*: stabilize IOP control.
- *Postoperative*: consider extended use of postoperative acetazolamide to minimize postoperative pressure spike (and risk of 'wipe out' to a vulnerable optic nerve). Although there have been concerns re CMO, the continuation of prostaglandin analogues postoperatively is probably safe. In the short eye beware aqueous misdirection syndrome. See at 1d, 1wk, and then 6wks.
- A potential advantage with uncomplicated surgery is a small lowering of intraocular pressure.

Uveitis

- *Complications*: exacerbation of inflammation, fibrinous anterior uveitis, synechiae, raised IOP, macular oedema, PCO.
- *Pre-operative*: control inflammation and IOP as far as possible. In well-controlled anterior uveitis consider intensive topical steroids for 2wks prior to surgery (e.g. dexamethasone 0.1% 2-hourly). In patients with chronic uveitis consider 500mg IV methylprednisolone 1h prior to surgery, or prednisolone 40mg 1×/d for 2wks prior to surgery.
- *Intra-operative*: ensure adequate pupillary access (synechiolysis, iris hooks, iris stretching) but avoid unnecessary iris manipulation. Ensure meticulous cortical clearance. Perform a well-centred 5–6mm capsulorhexis (vs postoperative phimosis, iris-capsule synechiae). Foldable lenses (e.g. acrylic or silicone) may be used. Give subconjunctival steroid (e.g. betamethasone 4mg).
- *Postoperative*: frequent potent topical steroid (e.g. dexamethasone 0.1% 2-hourly) and taper slowly; if oral steroids were started/increased pre-operatively these should be tapered slowly to zero/maintenance dose. Consider mydriatic (e.g. cyclopentolate 1% nocte). In persistent fibrinous uveitis consider intracameral recombinant tissue plasminogen activator. See at 1d, 1wk, and then 6wks.

Post-vitrectomy

- *Complications*: PCO, retinal (re)detachment, vitreous haemorrhage.
- *Pre-operative*: silicone oil slows sound transmission (estimated at 987m/s), and this must be incorporated when calculating axial length from an A-scan. Additionally, the axial length may not be stable within a year of encirclement procedures and may be unpredictable post-macular surgery.
- *Intra-operative*: use clear corneal incision (rather than scleral tunnel). Poor mydriasis may require iris hooks/stretching. Fluctuation of AC depth and the risk to the flaccid PC may be minimized by well-constructed wounds, lower bottle height, reduced vacuum, and lifting the iris with second instrument. Minimize nucleus manipulation to protect damaged zonules. Use acrylic or PMMA lenses (*not* silicone), placing in the bag or sulcus.
- *Postoperative*: give retinal detachment warning, dilate at follow-up review.

Prostatism, α-blockers, and the intra-operative floppy iris syndrome

Intra-operative floppy iris syndrome occurs in patients using α_1-adrenergic blocking agents, e.g. tamsulosin, alfuzosin used in the treatment of benign prostatic hypertrophy.

It is characterized by iris prolapse and progressive narrowing of the pupil during surgery thus increasing the risk of complications. Intra-operative strategies include use of iris hooks and intracameral phenylephrine. It can also be useful to keep the side port incision as small as possible and consider moving both incisions anteriorly into the cornea by 1mm to help with flow dynamics and reduce prolapse. This is also useful in the hypermetropic eye.

Cataract surgery: complications

Intraoperative

Posterior capsule rupture without vitreous loss (about 2%)

The main aims when confronted with a PC tear (± vitreous loss) are to maintain as much capsule as possible and to clear any vitreous. If PC tear is small and well-defined the PCIOL may still be placed in the bag either at the time of surgery or as a secondary procedure. However, with larger, poorly defined PC tears it is safer to place the lens in the sulcus providing sufficient anterior capsule remains to stabilize it.

NB Assuming equal A-constants, a sulcus fixated lens should be 0.5D lower power than that calculated for fixing in the bag.

Posterior capsule rupture with vitreous loss (1%)

Clear the wound and AC of vitreous with manual (sponge/scissors) and/or automated vitrectomy while maintaining as much posterior capsule as possible. If sufficient anterior capsule remains place the lens in the sulcus else consider an ACIOL (+ PI). The crucial role of the cataract surgeon under these circumstances is to:

- maintain all the capsule possible (this may facilitate PCIOL insertion 4wks later), and
- clear vitreous from the AC and wounds; intracameral triamcinolone can be very useful as it will highlight any remaining vitreous.

Anterior capsule problems

The capsulorhexis has a tendency to 'run out' in a number of situations: shallow AC, positive posterior pressure, young patients, intumescent cataracts. Stabilize the AC with a more viscous viscoelastic, e.g. Healon 5. Decompress intumescent cataracts by puncturing the AC and aspirating lens matter. If unable to bring the capsulorhexis back in, options include returning to the start and attempting a second tear in the opposite direction, the use of capsulorhexis scissors and switching to a can-opener technique. Depending on the security of the resulting capsulorhexis either continue with cautious phakoemulsification or convert to ECCE.

Zonular dehiscence

Consider stabilizing with iris hooks (secure the capsule in the area of dialysis) or a capsular tension ring (stabilizes the bag and redistributes forces away from individual zonules). If associated with vitreous loss an anterior vitrectomy will be required.

Loss of nuclear fragment posteriorly (0.3%)

Nuclear material is inflammatory. Very small fragments can be observed but may require prolonged topical steroids. Larger fragments require removal via a pars plana vitrectomy, ideally within 1–2wks. Refer immediately to a VR surgeon. Start on their preferred regimen to control inflammation, reduce risk of infection, and prevent ↑IOP (partly to preserve corneal clarity). One example is dexamethasone 0.1% 2-hourly, chloramphenicol 0.5% 4×/d, acetazolamide SR 250mg bd.

Choroidal haemorrhage (0.1%)

- Suspect this if there is sudden increase in IOP with AC shallowing, iris prolapse, loss of vitreous, and loss/darkening of the red reflex. This is often associated with patient complaining of severe pain.

- Immediately suture all wounds closed, give IV pressure lowering treatment (e.g. acetazolamide or mannitol), and start on intensive topical steroids.
- Prognosis is poor with only 45% achieving VA ≥6/60 in that eye.

Postoperative: early

Corneal oedema (10%)
Control IOP and inflammation with topical treatment ± acetazolamide.

Elevated IOP (2–8%)
- Control with topical treatment ± acetazolamide.
- In extreme cases consider releasing fluid from the paracentesis wound under aseptic conditions.

Increased anterior inflammation (2–6%)
If greater than expected increase topical steroids, maintaining normal antibiotic cover (e.g. chloramphenicol 0.5% 4×/d), but always have a low threshold of suspicion for endophthalmitis.

Wound leak (1%)
Return to theatre and suture wound closed if persistent or severe (AC shallow with iris prolapse or iridocorneal touch).

Iris prolapse (0.7%)
Return to theatre, assess vitality of extruded iris (may need abscising) reform AC and suture wound closed.

Endophthalmitis (0.1%) (see Postoperative endophthalmitis 📖 p.292)

Postoperative: late

Posterior capsule opacification (10% by 2yrs)
- Consider YAG posterior capsulotomy if opacification is causing reduced vision, monocular diplopia, or is preventing assessment/treatment of fundal pathology.
- In uveitic patients defer until opacification causing VA ≤6/12 or preventing fundal view *and* 6mths post-surgery *and* 2mths since last exacerbation.
- Do not perform a posterior capsulotomy if there is any question of lens replacement being required.

Cystoid macular oedema (1–12%) (see Postoperative cystoid Macular oedema 📖 p.294)

Retinal detachment (0.7%)
Risk is increased in myopes, with lattice degeneration and particularly if there has been vitreous loss. Refer immediately to VR surgeon.

Corneal decompensation
Risk is increased if pre-existing endothelial dystrophy, diabetes, intraoperative endothelial trauma/phakoburn, long phako time/power or long irrigation time, or ACIOL. Control IOP and inflammation. Consider hypertonic drops (e.g. sodium chloride 5%), bandage CL (for comfort in bullous keratopathy), or penetrating/endothelial keratoplasty.

Chronic endophthalmitis (see Postoperative endophthalmitis 📖 p.242.)

Postoperative endophthalmitis

Acute postoperative endophthalmitis

A sight-threatening emergency requiring rapid assessment and treatment. Onset is usually 1–7d after surgery. The most common organisms are *Staphylococcus epidermidis*, *Staphylococcus aureus*, and *Streptococcus* species.

Suspect if:

Pain, worsening vision, disproportionate/increasing postoperative inflammation (including hypopyon), posterior segment inflammation, lid swelling. RAPD and inaccurate light projection suggest a poor prognosis. Risk factors include patient flora (blepharitis, conjunctivitis, nasolacrimal disease), comorbidity (diabetes) and complicated surgery (PC rupture with vitreous loss, ACIOL, prolonged surgery).

Diagnosis

AC tap and vitreous biopsy (with simultaneous intravitreal antibiotics); use automated vitrector to perform the vitreous biopsy. Consider B-scan ultrasound to indicate degree of vitritis and integrity of retina.

Treatment
- *Admit:*
  - *Intravitreal antibiotics*: consider vancomycin 1mg in 0.1ml (Gram-positive cover) combined with either amikacin 0.4mg in 0.1ml or ceftazidime 2mg in 0.1ml (Gram-negative cover). Ceftazidime can precipitate with vancomycin and so needs a different syringe.
  - *Vitrectomy*: if VA ≤ PL (the Early Vitrectomy Study found a significant 3-fold improvement in attaining 6/12 for this group; in diabetics there was a trend towards benefit whatever the baseline VA).
- *Consider:*
  - *Topical antibiotics*: possibilities include hourly fortified vancomycin (50mg/ml), amikacin (20mg/ml), or ceftazidime (100mg/ml) with a view to increasing anterior segment concentration of the intravitreal drugs. No evidence of clinical benefit.
  - *Corticosteroids*: may be topical (e.g. dexamethasone 0.1% hourly), intravitreal (dexamethasone 0.4mg in 0.1ml), or systemic (prednisolone PO 1wk). While steroids reduce inflammation and some sequelae of endophthalmitis there is no evidence that it improves VA.
- *If failure to respond at 24h*: consider repeating AC tap, vitreous biopsy, and intravitreal antibiotics.

Chronic postoperative endophthalmitis

Onset is usually 1wk to several months after surgery. The most common organisms are *Propionobacterium acnes*, partially treated *S. epidermidis,* and fungi.

Suspect if

Chronic postoperative inflammation, which flares up whenever steroid treatment is reduced. A white plaque on the posterior capsule suggests *P. acnes* infection.

Diagnosis

Perform an AC tap, vitreous biopsy, and consider removal of posterior capsule. Send sample for smears (Gram's, Giemsa, and methenamine-silver stain) and culture (blood, chocolate, Sabouraud's, thioglycolate broth, and solid anaerobic medium; the last is especially important for *P. acnes*). PCR may also be helpful.

Treat

For *P. acnes* or low-grade *S. epidermidis* consider vitrectomy, intravitreal vancomycin, and if necessary IOL removal. For suspected fungal infection consider vitrectomy, intravitreal amphotericin B (5–10µg), and subsequent topical ± systemic antifungals according to sensitivity.

Box 9.5 Summary of Royal College of Ophthalmologists Focus on Endophthalmitis 1996 and 2004

Prophylaxis

- Skin and conjunctival sac preparation with 5% aqueous povidone iodine at least 5min before surgery. It is safe and effective in significantly reducing ocular surface flora. Additional benefit may be gained by postoperative instillation into the sac.
- Identifying and treating risk factors such as blepharitis, conjunctivitis, or mucocoele is probably more useful than universal antibiotic prophylaxis. The use of antibiotics in irrigating solutions is controversial.

Treatment

- *VA > PL*: single-port vitreous biopsy via the pars plana should be performed using a vitreous cutting-suction device. The specimens are directly smeared, for Gram stain, etc., and plated for culture. Directly inject amikacin and vancomycin (or gentamicin and cefuroxime).
- *VA ≤ PL*: three port pars plan vitrectomy and intravitreal antibiotics. High-dose systemic prednisolone may be given, e.g. 60–80mg daily, rapidly reducing to zero over a week to 10d. Steroids are contraindicated if there is a fungal infection.
- If the clinical course warrants it, the biopsy and intravitreal antibiotic injection may be repeated after 48–72hr.

Postoperative cystoid macular oedema

Irvine–Gass syndrome

Suspect if

Worsening vision (may decrease with pin-hole), perifoveal retinal thickening ± cystoid spaces. Increased risk in patients with diabetes, complicated surgery, postoperative uveitis, or previous CMO (in the other eye post-routine surgery). The classical presentation is excellent vision immediately post-operation and for a few days, then declining.

Diagnosis

Clinical appearance (but may be subclinical) and/or OCT/FFA findings:

- *Clinical appearance*: Loss of foveal contour, retinal thickening, cystoid spaces; central yellow spot, small intraretinal haemorrhages, and telangiectasia (occasional).
- *OCT*: in addition to detecting cystoid spaces, can measure degree of retinal thickening and specific pathology, e.g. vitreomacular traction.
- *FFA*: typically dye leakage from both the parafovea into the cystoid spaces—petalloid pattern—and from the optic disc.

Prophylaxis

Consider adding topical NSAID (e.g. ketorolac 0.3% 3×/d 6wks) to usual postoperative steroid regimen for high-risk groups (diabetes, uveitis, previous CMO, complicated surgery with vitreous loss).

Treatment

A step-wise approach is recommended. Review the diagnosis (e.g. OCT, FFA) if atypical or slow to respond. One approach is as follows:

1. Topical: steroid (e.g. dexamethasone 0.1% 4×/d) + NSAID (e.g. ketorolac 0.3% 3×/d);
   Review in 4–6wks; if persisting then:
2. Periocular steroid (e.g. subtenons triamcinolone) and continue topical treatment;
   Review in 4–6wks; if persisting then:
3. Consider: repeating periocular or giving intravitreal steroid; vitrectomy; systemic steroids (e.g. prednisolone 40 mg 1×/d, titrating over 3wks; or IV methylprednisolone 500mg single dose); oral acetazolamide (500mg/d; limited evidence).

Refractive surprise

Failure to achieve the estimated/target refraction is disappointing for the patient and the surgeon. A careful systematic approach will help identify the source of the problem.

In patients where the refractive outcome is harder to predict (high ametropia, previous corneal refractive surgery), review patients early (1wk) with refraction to permit the option of an early IOL exchange if a large discrepancy noticed. It should be noted that retention of OVD (e.g. healon) in the capsular 'bag' in the early postoperative period may distort the true post operative refraction.

> **Box 9.6 An approach to the assessment of the patient with refractive surprise**
>
> *Verify the problem:*
> - What is the postoperative refraction?
>   - Have it checked by a clinician experienced at refraction.
>
> *Case notes review:*
> - Was the correct IOL selected intra-operatively?
> - Was the preoperative biometry/lens selection valid?
>   - Check biometry used does indeed belong to your patient.
>   - Look for *intraocular* consistency in axial length and K values (i.e. that they are similar and the standard deviation is low).
>   - Look for *inter-ocular* consistency in axial length and K values.
>   - Check appropriate formula used.
>   - Had they had previous refractive surgery?
>
> *Clinical examination:*
> - Has there been a change in the corneal curvature (K readings) since the operation?
>   - Wounds: poorly constructed wounds or use of limbal relaxing incisions; LRI will rarely change the spherical equivalent when treating ≤3DC but have a hypermetropic effect when treating higher levels of astigmatism.
>   - Corneal oedema.
>   - Other corneal pathology (previously unrecognized), e.g. keratoconus, previous refractive surgery; CL use.
> - Is the IOL correctly positioned?
>   - Check IOL centred and completely in the bag.
>   - Is there retention of healon within the bag?
>   - Is early capsule healing/phimosis affecting IOL position.
>
> *Investigations:*
> - Repeat biometry ± B-scan to confirm axial length (on psuedophakic mode).
> - Repeat keratometry ± corneal topography.

Treatment
Small errors
Depending on the cause of the refractive surprise the following options may be considered:
- *Observation*: postoperative change in corneal curvature may improve as oedema settles and wounds heal.
- *Trial of spectacles*.
- *Intervention for specific problem*: surgical repositioning of poorly placed IOL, YAG laser for capsular phimosis.

Large errors
For large errors the following may be considered:
- *Contact lens*.
- *IOL exchange*: preferred option if recognized early, but becomes increasingly difficult surgically if delayed.
- *Secondary piggyback IOL*: eliminates guesswork of IOL power as power now based on postoperative refraction.
- *Laser refractive surgery for residual errors*.

NB It is important to recognize refractive surprise and accept—particularly with hypermetropic surprise—that the patient is unhappy for that reason. Do not be tempted to try to improve their vision by performing a YAG posterior capsulotomy, thereby reducing the surgeon's options and the patient's chance of a satisfactory outcome.

Abnormalities of lens size, shape, and position

Abnormalities of size, shape, and position may affect both the refractive power of the lens and increase optical aberration. In addition, most of these abnormalities are associated with lens opacity. Commonest among this group are disorders of lens position, i.e. ectopia lentis.

Ectopia lentis

This may be complete (dislocation or luxation) or partial (displacement or subluxation). Do not neglect possible acquired causes of ectopia lentis.

Complications
- Refractive (edge effect, lenticular astigmatism, lenticular myopia, aphakic hypermetropia, diplopia).
- Anterior dislocation → glaucoma, corneal decompensation, uveitis.

Treatment
- *Refractive*: CLs, spectacles.
- *Dislocation*: into the posterior segment (followed by aphakic correction) either by (1) YAG zonulolysis, or (2) mydriatics + lie the patient on their back if lens already dislocated anteriorly.
- *Lensectomy* (followed by aphakic correction).

Causes
Congenital
- *Familial ectopa lentis (AD)*: uni/bilateral superotemporal lens subluxation; no systemic abnormality.
- *Ectopia lentis et pupillae (AR)*: superotemporal dissociation with pupil displacement in the opposite direction; no systemic abnormality.
- *Marfan syndrome (AD, Ch15, fibrillin)*: bilateral superotemporal lens subluxation with some preservation of accommodation, lattice degeneration, retinal detachment, anomalous angles, glaucoma, keratoconus, blue sclera, axial myopia; musculoskeletal (arachnodactyly, disproportionately long-limbed, joint laxity, pectus excavatum, kyphoscoliosis, high arched palate, herniae); cardiovascular (aortic dilatation, aortic regurigation, aortic dissection, mitral valve prolapse).
- *Weill–Marchesani syndrome (AR)*: bilateral anteroinferior lens subluxation, microspherophakia, retinal detachment, anomalous angles; musculoskeletal (short stature, brachydactyly); neurological (reduced IQ).
- *Homocystinuria*: (AR, cystathionine synthetase abnormality → homocysteine and methionine accumulation)—bilateral inferonasal lens subluxation, myopia, glaucoma; skeletal ('knock-kneed', Marfanoid habitus, osteoporosis); haematological (thromboses, especially associated with general anaesthesia); facies (fine, fair hair); neurological (low IQ).
- *Hyperlysinaemia*: (AR, lysine α-ketogluatarate reductase)—lens subluxation, microspherophakia; musculoskeletal (joint laxity, hypotonia); neurological (epilepsy, low IQ).
- *Sulphite oxidase deficiency (AR)*: lens subluxation; neurological (hypertonia, low IQ); life expectancy less than 5yrs.

Acquired
- These include trauma, high myopia, (hyper)mature cataract, pseudoexfoliation, buphthalmos, and ciliary body tumour.

Table 9.10 Abnormalities of lens size, shape, and position

Abnormality	Condition	Associations
Size	Microphakia (small lens)	Lowe syndrome
	Microspherophakia (small spherical lens)	Familial microspherophakia (AD)
		Peters anomaly
		Marfan syndrome (AD)
		Weill–Marchesani syndrome (AR)
		Hyperlysinaemia (AR)
		Alport syndrome (XD)
		Congenital rubella
Shape	Coloboma (inferior notch)	Iris/choroid colobomata Giant retinal tears
	Anterior lenticonus (bulge in anterior lens)	Alport syndrome
	Posterior lenticonus (bulge in posterior lens)	Unilateral: usually sporadic
		Bilateral: familial (AD/AR/X)
		Lowe syndrome (X)
	Lentiglobus (extreme lenticonus)	Posterior polar cataract
Position	Ectopia lentis (congenital)	Familial ectopia lentis (AD)
		Marfan syndrome (AD)
		Weill–Marchesani syndrome (AR)
		Homocystinuria (AR)
		Familial microspherophakia (AD)
		Hyperlysinaemia (AR)
		Sulphite oxidase deficiency (AR)
		Stickler syndrome (AD)
		Sturge–Weber syndrome (sproradic)
		Crouzon syndrome (sporadic)
		Ehlers–Danlos syndrome (AD/AR)
		Aniridia
	Ectopia lentis (acquired)	Trauma
		High myopia
		Buphthalmos
		Ciliary body tumour
		Hypermature cataract
		Pseudoexfoliation

Glaucoma

Anatomy and physiology

Glaucoma is a progressive optic neuropathy with characteristic changes in the optic nerve head and corresponding loss of visual field. It represents a final common pathway for a number of conditions, for most of which raised IOP is the most important risk factor. In Western countries glaucoma is present in 1% of those over 40 and 3% in those over 70yrs old. It is the second leading cause of blindness worldwide.

Anatomy

- *AC angle*: extends from Schwalbe's line (the termination of Descemet's membrane on the peripheral cornea) posteriorly to the trabecular meshwork, scleral spur, and in some cases ciliary body where an acute angle is formed with the peripheral iris.
- *Trabecular meshwork*: this is a reticulated band of fibrocellular sheets, with a triangular cross-section, base towards the scleral spur.
- *Scleral spur*: firm fibrous projection from the sclera, with Schlemm's canal at its base and the longitudinal portion of the ciliary muscle inserting into its posterior surface.
- *Schlemm's canal*: circumferential septate drain with an inner wall of endothelium containing giant vacuoles and an outer wall obliquely punctuated by collector channels that drain into the episcleral veins.
- *Ciliary body*: comprises the ciliary muscle and ciliary epithelium, arranged anatomically as the pars plana and pars plicata (containing the ciliary processes). Contraction of the ciliary muscle permits accommodation and increases trabecular outflow. The ciliary epithelium is a cuboidal bilayer arranged apex to apex with numerous gap junctions. The inner layer is non-pigmented, with high metabolic activity and posteriorly is continuous with the neural retina. The outer layer is pigmented and posteriorly is continuous with the RPE.

Physiology

Aqueous production

Aqueous humour is a clear, colourless, plasma-like balanced salt solution produced by the ciliary body. It is a structurally supportive medium providing nutrients to the lens and cornea. It differs from plasma in having lower glucose (80% of plasma levels), low protein (assuming an intact blood aqueous barrier), and high ascorbate, It is formed at about 2.5μl/min by a combination of active secretion (70%), ultrafiltration (20%), and osmosis (10%). Active secretion is complex, involving the maintenance of a transepithelial potential by the Na^+K^+ pump, ion transport by symports and antiports (including the important $Na^+/K^+/2Cl^-$ symport), calcium- and voltage-gated ion channels, and carbonic anhydrase.

Aqueous outflow

While the trabecular route is the major outflow, the uveoscleral contribution may be as much as 30%.

Trabecular (conventional) route

Most aqueous humour leaves the eye by this passive pressure-sensitive route. About 75% of outflow resistance is due to the trabecular meshwork itself, with the major component being the outermost (juxtacanalicular) portion of the trabecular meshwork. This comprises several layers of endothelial cells embedded in ground substance which appears to act as a filter, which is continually cleaned by endothelial cell phagocytosis. Onward transport into Schlemm's canal is achieved by pressure-dependent trans-cellular channels (seen as giant vacuoles of fluid crossing the endothelium) and paracellular pores. Aqueous is then transported via collector channels to the episcleral veins and on to the general venous circulation.

Uveoscleral (unconventional) route

The aqueous passes across the iris root and ciliary body into the supra-ciliary and suprachoroidal spaces from where it escapes via the choroidal circulation.

Intraocular pressure

$$\text{Flow in} = \text{Flow out} = C(IOP - Pv) + U$$

where C is the pressure-sensitive outflow facility (via trabecular mesh-work), U is the pressure-independent outflow (via uveoscleral route), and Pv is the episcleral venous pressure. Typical values are:

2.5μl/min = **0.3**μl/min/mmHg (**16–9**mmHg) + **0.4**μl/min

Variation in intraocular pressure

Within the population

Normal IOP within the population is generally taken to be: Mean IOP ± 2 SD = 16 ± 2 (2.5), i.e. a range of 11–21mmHg. However, there is a positive skew to this distribution.

Within the individual

Mean diurnal variation is up to 5mmHg in normals, but 10–15mmHg in primary open angle glaucoma (POAG). IOP tends to peak in the morning in most individuals. Posture, pulse pressure, respiration, extremes of BP, and season also have an effect. The effect of posture on IOP may have sig-nificant clinical impact, with some studies showing a glaucoma progression to be more strongly associated with supine (vs sitting) IOP, and to corre-late with the magnitude of the increase in IOP caused by posture.

Glaucoma: assessment

Over 1 million sight tests are performed each year in the UK. Of these, about 60 000 people are referred to ophthalmologists for assessment of possible glaucoma. Of these, about one-third will be diagnosed with glaucoma, one-third with ocular hypertension, and one-third will be discharged. At initial consultation consider: (1) evidence for glaucoma vs normal variant or alternative pathology (Table 10.3); (2) evidence for underlying cause (i.e. type of glaucoma); (3) factors that may influence treatment. Be cautious of interpreting any one abnormality in isolation: e.g. apparent field defects may be artefactual and disappear with repeated testing due to the ' learning effect'.

Table 10.1 An approach to assessing possible glaucoma

Visual symptoms	Asymptomatic; haloes 9 ache, precipitants (dim light, reading, exercise); subjective loss of vision/field
POH	Previous surgery (incl. refractive) or trauma; concurrent eye disease; refractive error
PMH	Diabetes, hypertension, smoking; migraine, Raynaud's phenomenon; vascular disease; asthma/COPD, renal disease
FH	Family members with glaucoma and their outcome (e.g. any glaucoma-related blindness)
Dx	Current/previous topical medications, current drugs (interactions), systemic β-blockers, current/previous use of steroids (any route)
Ax	Allergies or relevant drug contraindications
Visual acuity	Best-corrected
Visual function	Check for RAPD, colour vision
Cornea	Pigment deposition, guttata, pachymetry
AC	Peripheral/central depth, cells, pigment
Gonioscopy	Angle configuration, iris approach, abnormal pigmentation, PAS, rubeosis
Tonometry	IOP
Iris	Transillumination defects, PXF, heterochromia, rubeosis, configuration
Lens	Cataract (swollen, hypermature), ACIOL
Optic disc	Size, vertical cup:disc ratio, colour, flat/elevated/tilted, neuroretinal rim (incl. contour, notches, haemorrhages), pits/colobomata/drusen
Disc vessels	Baring, bayonetting
Peripapillary area	Haemorrhages, atrophy, pigmentation, retinal nerve fibre layer defects
Fundus	Chorioretinal scarring, retinoschisis, retinal detachment (can cause field loss)

Table 10.2 The 'glaucoma triad'

Evidence for glaucoma	Features
Raised IOP	>21mmHg
Abnormal disc	Cup:disc ratio asymmetry
	Large cup:disc ratio for disc size
	Neuroretinal rim notch/thinning (ISNT rule)
	Disc haemorrhage
	Vessel bayoneting/nasally displaced
	Peripapillary atrophy (β-zone)
Visual field defect	Nasal step
	Paracentral scotoma
	Arcuate scotoma
	Altitudinal scotoma
	Residual temporal or central island of vision

'ISNT rule' describes the normal contour of the disc rim, being thickest inferiorly, thinner superiorly, then nasally and thinnest temporally.

Table 10.3 A short differential diagnosis of the 'glaucoma triad'

IOP	Discs	Visual field	Consider
Raised IOP	Normal	Normal	Ocular hypertension
	Borderline	Normal	Glaucoma suspect/pre-perimetric glaucoma
	Borderline	Consistent defect	Highly suspicious: treat as glaucoma
	Abnormal	Consistent defect	Glaucoma
Normal IOP	Normal	Normal	Normal
	Borderline	Normal	Physiological cupping
	Stable abnormality	Stable defect	Congenital disc anomaly Previous optic disc insult
	Evolving abnormality	Evolving defect	Normal tension glaucoma Other optic neuropathy

Box 10.1 Significant glaucomatous field loss

The European Glaucoma Society recommend that the following abnormalities be regarded as significant:

- Abnormal Glaucoma Hemifield test.
- 3 abnormal points at $p<5\%$ level, one of which should be at $p<1\%$ level and none of which should be contiguous with the blind spot.
- Corrected pattern standard deviation <5% if the visual field is otherwise normal *provided that* they are confirmed on two consecutive tests *and* there is no other retinal or neurological disease affecting the visual field.

Ocular hypertension

Ocular hypertension describes an IOP >21mmHg (representing 2SD above the population mean) in the presence of a healthy optic disc and normal visual field. This population is positively skewed, with 5–7% of those aged >40 having an IOP >21mmHg. In the absence of glaucomatous damage, it is difficult to differentiate those in whom such an IOP is physiological from those in whom it is pathological (i.e. will 'convert' to POAG).

Risk of 'conversion' to primary open angle glaucoma

In the Ocular Hypertension Treatment Study the 'conversion rate' was found to be 9.5% over 5yrs (untreated). If treated with topical medication (to reduce IOP by >20% and to achieve ≤24mmHg) this 'conversion rate' was reduced to 4.4%.

Risk factors (and their hazard ratios, HR) demonstrated in the OHTS trial include:
- *Older age*: HR 1.2 per decade.
- *Higher IOP*: HR 1.1 per mmHg.
- *Larger C/D ratio*: HR 1.2 per 0.1.
- *Greater pattern standard deviation*: HR 1.3 per 0.2dB.
- *Thinner CCT*: HR 1.7 per 40μm.

Thinner CCT may lead to underestimation of IOP; thus the true risk factor here may be higher than recognized IOP. Other possible risk factors include African-Caribbean race, FH, myopia, and other suspicious disc/peripapillary changes.

Who to treat?

There is considerable variation in practice. Some practitioners treat all >21mmHg. Consider treating:
- *Isolated OHT*: if IOP >30mmHg.
- *OHT and suspicious disc*: if IOP >21mmHg.
- *OHT and thin cornea*: if IOP >21mmHg.

Relatively thin corneas (CCT < 555μm) were associated with a 3-fold risk of 'conversion' to POAG vs thick corneas (>588μm). Some practitioners therefore use pachymeter routinely and 'correct' the IOP for corneal thickness. One estimate is that for every 20μm that the CCT is less than 550μm (mean population CCT) the IOP is under-read by 1mmHg; interestingly, this calculation reclassifies many normal tension glaucoma patients as high-tension POAG, and OHT patients as normals.

Other factors that may suggest a lower threshold for treatment include:
- OHT and only eye.
- OHT and CRVO or AION in either eye.
- OHT and FH glaucoma (especially of blinding disease).

Monitoring

For those not requiring treatment, follow up 6–12/12 (IOP, disc appearance) and perform perimetry every 6–12/12. If stable consider shared care with technician/optometrist.

For those requiring treatment, follow-up as per POAG (see Primary open angle glaucoma 📖 p.308).

Box 10.2 Devices used to measure IOP

Measurement of IOP may be affected by central corneal thickness (CCT), corneal hysteresis (a measure of structural rigidity), corneal curvature and axial length. Different methods of measuring IOP are variably affected by these factors. As the accurate estimation of IOP is fundamental to the management of glaucoma, it is important to appreciate the limitations of the devices in common usage.

- Goldmann applanation tonomtery (GAT; Haag-Streit, Bern, Switzerland): the ubiquitous slit-lamp mounted contact applanation device; it is calibrated for measuring IOP in subjects with an average CCT, and is significantly affected by deviations in CCT.
- Reichert Ocular Response Analyser (ORA; Reichert Ophthalmic Instruments, Buffalo, USA): automated non-contact device that scans the central cornea during deformation by an air-pulse, and estimates the IOP both from the applanation point achieved during deformation and during recovery. The average of these two points—known as the Goldmann-correlated IOP value—is indicated as IOPg. A more sophisticated estimate—the corneal compensated IOP (IOPcc)—takes into account the difference between the two applanation values, which indicates the corneal hysteresis and reflects the structural rigidity of the cornea.
- Pascal dynamic contour tonometer (Swiss Microtechnology AG, Bern, Switzerland): a slit-lamp mounted digital device that provides a direct trans-corneal measurement of diastolic IOP; it also measures ocular pulse amplitude, enabling an estimate of systolic IOP. It is less affected by CCT than Goldmann applanation tonometry.
- TonoPen XL (Reichert Ophthalmic Instruments, Buffalo, USA): a portable contact instrument that estimates the IOP based on the Mackay–Marg principle. It displays the average of four independent readings. Like GAT it is affected by CCT, but is less affected by corneal curvature and can be useful in irregular corneas.
- ICare tonometer (Icare Finland, Espoo, Finland): a portable contact instrument that is the only contact device not to require topical anaesthesia. Like GAT and the TonoPen it is affected by CCT, but is less affected by corneal curvature and can be useful in irregular corneas and those who do not tolerate other contact methods.

Primary open-angle glaucoma

This is an adult-onset optic neuropathy with glaucomatous disc and/or field changes, open angles, and no other underlying disease (cf. secondary open-angle glaucomas). The term is usually reserved for those with 'high tension' glaucoma, i.e. IOP>21mmHg (cf. normal tension glaucoma). It is present in 1% of the population.

Risk factors

- *Age*: increasing age (uncommon <40yrs).
- *Race*: African-Caribbean: more frequent, younger onset, more severe.
- *FH*: first degree relative confers 1 in 8 risk; higher in siblings.
- *Steroid-induced IOP elevation*: more common in POAG and those with FH of POAG.
- *Other possible risk factors* include vascular disease (e.g. diabetes and hypertension) and myopia (the disc is said to be more vulnerable due to the scleral canal morphology).

Clinical features

- Usually asymptomatic (rarely eye ache and haloes—transient corneal oedema if ↑↑IOP).
- IOP>21mmHg, often with high diurnal variability.
- Disc changes: C/D asymmetry, high C/D for disc size, vertical elongation of the cup, NRR notch/thinning (does not follow 'ISNT' rule 📖 p.305), disc haemorrhage, vessel bayoneting/nasally displaced, peripapillary atrophy (β-zone). β-zone peripapillary atrophy describes choroidal atrophy immediately adjacent to the disc; it may correspond to areas of ganglion cell loss and field defects. α-zone is more peripheral, irregularly pigmented, and less specific for glaucoma.
- Visual field defects: (1) focal defects respecting the horizontal meridian, including nasal step, baring of the blind spot, paracentral scotomas, arcuate defects, and altitudinal defects; (2) generalized depression.

Treatment

- *Counselling* (see 📖 Box 10.3).
- *Medical*: topical—prostaglandin analogue, β-blocker, α2-agonist, carbonic anhydrase inhibitor. All have contraindications and side-effects.
- *ALT*: may be appropriate first-line for those who are frail or in whom compliance is likely to be an issue; it is most effective in those with moderate trabecular pigmentation (e.g. in PXF, PDS). IOP control fails with time, with 50% failure rate at 5yrs.
- *Trabeculectomy* (± augmented): may be appropriate first-line for those who hope to be 'drop free' or with high risk of progression; otherwise use if failure of maximal medical therapy (see Filtration surgery: trabeculectomy 📖 p.342). In resistant cases consider:
  - Shunt procedures (e.g. Molteno or other tubes); destructive procedures to the ciliary body (cyclodiode, cyclocryotherapy) (see Laser procedures for glaucoma 📖 p.338).

Box 10.3 An approach to the medical treatment of primary open angle glaucoma

(1) Counsel patient
Nature and natural history of condition; implications for driving; effect of drops; important side-effects; importance of compliance; probability of lifetime treatment; that they will not notice any day-to-day benefit.

(2) Define target IOP
Usually ≥20% reduction initially; target IOP should be lower if there is already advanced damage, disease continues to progress or other risk factors are present.

(3) Select drug
First line consider: prostaglandin agonist or β-blocker. Note contra-indications.

(4) Teach how to administer drops (incl. nasolacrimal occlusion)

(5) Review treatment (e.g. 6 wks later)
- *Effects*: is there significant IOP reduction and has the target IOP been reached. Some advocate a treatment trial of one eye so that therapeutic efficacy can be gauged against the other eye (which controls for diurnal variation).
- *Side-effects*: local (e.g. allergic) and systemic (e.g. lethargy, dizziness, wheeze, etc.).

(6) Decide re further treatment
- If no significant reduction in IOP → stop drop and try another first line agent; check compliance.
- If significant reduction but target IOP not met → augment with another agent (another first line drug or second line such as topical carbonic anhydrase inhibitor).
- If target IOP achieved → continue; review (e.g. 3mths).
- If target IOP achieved BUT disc or field continues to progress then target may need to be lowered. Consider other risk factors such as pressure spikes (may need IOP phasing), systemic hypotension, or poor compliance.

Normal tension glaucoma

Normal tension glaucoma is generally regarded as a subcategory of POAG, although some have suggested a distinct pathogenesis, such as vascular anomalies, systemic hypotension, and inherited abnormalities of the optic nerve. It is present in 0.1% of the population.

Risk factors

- *Age*: more common in the elderly, but up to one-third may be <50yrs.
- *Race*: more common in Japan.
- *Sex*: possible female preponderance.

Clinical features

- Usually asymptomatic.
- IOP <21mmHg.
- *Disc changes*: as for POAG, although disc haemorrhages and acquired pits may be more common and the cup may be larger and shallower.
- *Visual field defects*: as for POAG, although (1) focal defects are more often in the superior hemifield (especially superonasal) and are said to be deeper, steeper, and closer to fixation; (2) generalized depression is less marked than in high-tension POAG.

Differential diagnosis and investigations

- *POAG*: perform pachymetry (permits estimation for potential 'under-reading' of IOP (see Ocular hypotension 📖 p.306) and phasing to assess IOP range. Phasing constitutes regular IOP checks (e.g. 2-hourly) over an extended period of the day (e.g. 0800–1800h or later; less commonly for a full 24h).
- *Secondary glaucoma*: clinical assessment.
- *Compressive optic neuropathy*: consider MRI optic nerves/chiasm if disc and field defects do not correlate, if atypical field defect, or if VA/colour vision affected.
- *Other optic neuropathies*: consider sending blood for FBC, B12, folate, ESR, VDRL, TPHA, ACE, ANA, ANCA, CRP, Lebers; CXR (see Table 16.3 📖 p.586).
- *Nocturnal hypotension*: consider 24h ambulatory BP monitoring especially if on topical or systemic β-blockers (see below).

Who to treat?

The Collaborative Normal Tension Glaucoma study demonstrated that considering the group as a whole, an IOP reduction by >30% slows the rate of field loss, but that even without treatment 50% of normal tension glaucoma patients actually show no progression of field defects at 5yrs. Risk factors for progression were:

- Female sex.
- Migraine.
- Disc haemorrhage at diagnosis.

Treatment

Generally as for POAG, although some clinicians emphasize the role of optic nerve head perfusion and the possible role of nocturnal dips in BP. This may be confirmed on 24h ambulatory BP monitoring. On this basis consider using prostaglandin analogues (better IOP control at night) rather than non-selective β-blockers (may reduce blood flow at night), and for treatment of systemic hypertension, β-blockers may be avoided in favour of calcium-channel blockers.

Primary angle closure glaucoma

Primary angle closure glaucoma is a significant cause of blindness world-wide. It is present in about 0.1% of the general population over 40yrs old, but up to 1.5% of the Chinese population over 50. Acute primary angle closure is an ophthalmic emergency. The terminology surrounding this condition has been reassessed by a consensus panel of glaucoma experts in the light of epidemiological studies,[1] and is outlined below.

Risk factors

Epidemiological

- *Age*: >40yrs old; mean age of diagnosis ± 60yrs.
- *Female sex*.
- *Race*: Chinese, SE Asians, Inuit.

Anatomical

Pupil block mechanism

- Narrow angle shallow AC, relatively anterior iris–lens diaphragm, large lens (older, cataractous), small corneal diameter, short axial length (usually hypermetropic); risk increases with increasing lens thickness to axial length ratio.
- In pupillary block apposition of the iris to the lens impedes aqueous flow from PC to AC, causing relative build up of pressure behind the iris, anterior bowing of the peripheral iris, and subsequent angle closure.

Plateau iris mechanism

- Plateau iris configuration (relatively anterior ciliary body that apposes the peripheral iris to the trabeculum; AC depth normal centrally, shallow peripherally with flat iris plane).
- Mild forms of plateau iris configuration are vulnerable to pupil block, but 'higher' plateau configurations may result in plateau iris syndrome where the peripheral iris bunches up and blocks the trabeculum directly. This means that angle closure can occur despite a patent PI.

Terminology

The following hierarchy has been suggested:

(1) *Anatomically narrow drainage angle* (ANDA): defined on gonioscopy.
(2) *Iridotrabecular contact* (ITC): defined on gonioscopy.
(3) *Primary angle closure* (PAC): iridotrabecular contact with ↑IOP or PAS or symptoms suggestive of episodes of acute primary angle closure.
(4) *Acute primary angle closure*(APAC): iridotrabecular contact with acute symptomatic ↑↑IOP.
(5) *Primary angle closure glaucoma* (PACG): primary angle closure with glaucomatous damage (changes in the optic disc and visual field).

Acute primary angle closure

Clinical features

- Pain (periocular, headache, abdominal), blurred vision, haloes, nausea, vomiting.
- *Ipsilateral*: red eye, raised IOP (usually 50–80mmHg), corneal oedema, angle closed, fixed semi-dilated pupil; glaucomflecken; contralateral angle narrow; bilateral shallow AC.

Differential diagnosis
Consider: secondary angle closure (e.g. phacomorphic, inflammatory, neo-vascular) or acute glaucoma syndromes such as Posner–Schlossman syndrome or PDS (Table 10.2).

Treatment
As per Box 10.4.

Primary angle closure
Clinical features
- Narrow angles with iridotrabecular contact and one or more of:
  ↑IOP, PAS or symptoms suggestive of episodes of acute primary angle closure.

Treatment
- Treat with 'prophylactic' Nd-YAG PIs.

Primary angle closure glaucoma
This may occur due to (1) synechial closure, which is either asymptomatic ('creeping') or follows episodes of acute/subacute angle closure, or (2) a POAG-like mechanism, but in the context of narrow angles.
Clinical features
- As for primary angle closure with evidence of glaucomatous optic neuropathy (characteristic optic disc and visual field changes (see Glaucoma assessment 📖 p.304).

Treatment
- Treat with Nd-YAG PIs (although beware IOP spike if extensive PAS); medical treatment (as for POAG) and surgical therapy (consider lens extraction and/or trabeculectomy, but note ↑risk of aqueous misdirection syndrome) as required.

1. Foster PJ, Buhrmann R, Quigley HA, Johnson GJ. The definition and classification of glaucoma in prevalence surveys. *Br J Ophthalmol* 2002;**86**:238–42.

Acute primary angle closure

Acute primary angle closure is an ophthalmic emergency requiring urgent treatment to prevent irreversible optic nerve damage. The clinical features and differential diagnosis are outlined earlier (see Primary angle closure glaucoma 📖 p.312). An approach to treatment is given below.

> **Box 10.4 An approach to the treatment of acute primary angle closure**
>
> *Immediate*
> - Systemic: acetazolamide 500mg IV stat (then 250mg PO 4×/d)
> - Ipsilateral eye:
>
> | | |
> |---|---|
> | β-blocker | (e.g. timolol 0.5% stat then 2×/d) |
> | Sympathomimetic | (e.g. apraclonidine 1% stat) |
> | Steroid | (e.g. prednisolone 1% stat then q30–60min) |
> | Pilocarpine 2% | (once IOP<50mmHg; e.g. twice in first h then 4×/d) |
>
> - Admit patient
> - Consider: corneal indentation with a 4-mirror goniolens may help relieve pupil block; lying the patient supine may allow the lens to fall back away from the iris; analgesics and anti-emetics may be necessary.
>
> Pilocarpine 1% is often given to the contralateral eye while awaiting Nd-YAG PI (although some glaucoma specialists advise against this due to a risk of inducing reverse pupil block). In either case the priority is for prompt bilateral PIs.
>
> *Intermediate*
> - Check IOP hourly until adequate control.
> - If IOP not improving: consider systemic hyperosmotics (e.g. glycerol PO 1g/kg of 50% solution in lemon juice or mannitol 20% solution IV 1–1.5g/kg).
> - If IOP still not improving: consider acute Nd-YAG PI (can use topical glycerin to temporarily reduce the corneal oedema).
> - If IOP still not improving:
>   - review the diagnosis (e.g. could this be aqueous misdirection syndrome with a patent PI?)
>   - consider repeating Nd-YAG PI, or proceeding to surgical peripheral iridectomy, argon laser iridoplasty, paracentesis, cyclodiode photocoagulation or emergency cataract extraction/ trabeculectomy.
>
> *Definitive*
> - Bilateral Nd-YAG or surgical PI.
>
> **NB** Some eyes may develop chronic ↑IOP either from synechial closure or from a POAG-like mechanism, and will require long-term medical ± surgical treatment.

Table 10.4 Glaucoma syndromes that may present acutely with symptomatic ↑IOP (selected)

Glaucoma type	Critical features	Additional features
Closed angle		
Primary angle closure	Closed angle, shallow AC; fixed mid-dilated pupil; iris bombé	Corneal oedema; contralateral angle narrow; may have plateau iris
Angle pulled shut (anterior pathology)		
Neovascular	Rubeosis ± zipped shut	Signs of underlying pathology, e.g. diabetes, CRVO
Inflammatory closed angle	Angle zipped shut by PAS	Signs of uveitis
Angle pushed shut (posterior pathology)		
Phacomorphic	Ipsilateral intumescent lens	Appositional closure; contralateral open angle
Lens dislocation	Poor lenticular support permits anterior dislocation	Abnormalities of zonules or lens size
Aqueous misdirection	Shallow AC despite patent PI; no iris bombé	Usually post-surgery in hypermetropic eyes
Choroidal pathology	Choroidal detachment, haemorrhage, or effusion	Recent history of surgery/ extensive laser
Open angle		
Inflammatory open angle	Elevated IOP with significant flare/cells; open angle	Other signs of cause, e.g. uveitis, trauma, surgery
Steroid-induced	↑IOP associated with steroid use (but may be lag of days or weeks)	Signs of underlying pathology, e.g. uveitis
Posner–Schlossman syndrome	Recurrent unilateral IOP spikes in fairly quiet, white eye	Corneal oedema
Pigmentary	Mid-peripheral spoke-like trans-illumination (TI) defects; trabecular pigmentation	Pigment in AC, on cornea, lens, iris, male myopes; 20–45yrs; post-exercise
Red cell	Hyphaema	Corneal staining
Ghost cell	Vitreous haemorrhage; bleached erythrocytes in AC	
Phakolytic	Lens protein in AC with (hyper)mature cataract	AC cells + flare, open angle ± clumps of macrophages
Lens particle	Retained lens fragment in AC post-surgery/trauma	AC inflammation
Intraocular tumour	Posterior segment tumour	± Cataract; mass seen on US

Pseudoexfoliation syndrome

PXF is a common but easily missed cause of secondary glaucoma. The term was originally chosen to distinguish it from 'true' exfoliation syndrome, in which heat or infrared radiation caused damage to the lens capsule (e.g. in glass blowers). Confusingly, this distinction has become blurred with PXF increasingly being referred to as exfoliation syndrome.

PXF is a systemic condition in which a whitish dandruff-like material is deposited over the anterior segment of the eye and other organs such as skin, heart, lungs, kidneys, and meninges. Although its exact nature is unclear, it appears to include abnormal elastic microfibrils, basement membrane material, and glycosaminoglycans. A number of small studies have suggested an association with cardiovascular and cerebrovascular disease, possibly via elevation of plasma homocysteine levels. In some parts of Scandinavia PXF is present in up to 20% of the general population, and up to 90% of the glaucoma population.

Risk factors
- *Age*: >40yrs old; increases with age.
- *Female sex.*
- *Race*: North European (Finnish, Icelandic); Mediterranean (Cretan); possibly any population in which it is carefully looked for.

Clinical features
- Dandruff-like material on pupillary border and anterior lens capsule (centrally and peripherally with a clear intermediate zone), peripupillary transillumination defects, poor mydriasis, iridodonesis/phacodonesis (**NB** risk of zonulodialysis during cataract surgery), pigment in the AC, pigment and pseudo-exfoliative material on the endothelium.
- *Gonioscopy*: irregular pigment deposition in the trabeculum and anterior to Schwalbe's line (Sampaolesi's line), PXF material in the angle; angle is usually open but may be narrow.

Pseudoexfoliation syndrome glaucoma (glaucoma capsulare)

Glaucoma occurs in up to 25% of patients with PXF (i.e. up to 10-fold increased risk). Although the disease presents similarly to POAG, the disease course is more severe with poorer response to medication, and more frequent need for surgery.

Mechanism of glaucoma
- *Open angle*: deposition of PXF material and pigment in the trabecular meshwork.
- *Narrow angle (rare)*: weak zonules with anterior movement of the lens–iris diaphragm; posterior synechiae.

Clinical features
- Features of PXF (see above), ↑IOP, disc changes, and field defects as for POAG (see Primary open angle glaucoma 🕮 p.308).

Treatment of PXF glaucoma (open angle type)
- *Medical*: as for POAG, but generally less effective; greater role for miotics (e.g. pilocarpine).
- *ALT*: particularly effective early on; >50% failure rate by 5yrs.
- *Trabeculectomy*: higher complication rate but similar overall success to trabeculectomy in POAG.

Pigment dispersion syndrome

This describes the release of pigment from the mid-peripheral posterior surface of the iris, from where it is distributed around the anterior segment. Pigment release is thought to occur as a result of posterior-bowing of the mid-peripheral iris rubbing against the zonules. This unusual iris configuration may be due to 'reverse pupil block' in which there is a transient ↑IOP in the AC relative to the PC; this is supported by an observed improvement when treated with miotics or Nd-YAG PIs. PDS is inherited as an autosomal dominant trait (Ch7q36), with a possible second locus on Ch18q; the exact gene(s) have not yet been identified.

Risk factors
- *Myopia.*
- *Age*: 20–40.
- *Male sex.*
- *Race*: caucasian.

Clinical features
- Pigment on the corneal endothelium (sometimes in a vertical line—Krukenberg spindle), pigment elsewhere (e.g. in the AC, posterior lens capsule), mid-peripheral spoke-like transillumination defects; increased rate of lattice degeneration (so check peripheral retina).
- *Gonioscopy*: open angle, concave peripheral iris, 360° homogeneous pigmentation of the trabeculum, and may be anterior to Schwalbe's line inferiorly.

Pigmentary glaucoma

Glaucoma may develop in 33–50% of patients with PDS.

Clinical features
- Usually asymptomatic, but blurred vision, haloes, and red eye(s) may occur after acute pigment shedding following mydriasis or exercise.
- ↑IOP ± corneal oedema (if acute); features of PDS (see above); disc changes and visual field defects as for POAG (see Primary open angle glaucoma 📖 p.308).

Treatment
- *Topical*: as for POAG; miotics have theoretical benefits (minimize irido-zonular contact), but tend to be poorly tolerated in this age group and carry a small risk of inducing retinal detachment (myopia, lattice degeneration).
- *ALT*: particularly effective early on; >50% failure rate by 5yrs.
- *Trabeculectomy*: similar success rate to surgery in POAG, but increased risk of hypotensive maculopathy (especially if augmented).
- *PI*: controversial; despite theoretical benefits no trial data to support its use.

Table 10.5 Chronic glaucoma syndromes (selected)

Glaucoma type	Critical features	Additional features
Open angle		
Primary open angle	↑IOP; disc cupping; visual field defect; normal open angle	Other glaucomatous disc changes
Normal tension	Normal IOP; disc cupping; visual field defect; normal open angle	Other glaucomatous disc changes
Pseudoexfoliation	Dandruff-like material on pupil margin and lens surface;	Unevenly pigmented trabeculum; peripupillary TI defects
Pigmentary	Mid-peripheral spoke-like TI defects; trabecular pigmentation	Pigment in AC, on cornea, lens, iris, male myopes aged 20–45yrs
Steroid-induced	↑IOP associated with steroid use (but may be lag of days or weeks)	Signs of underlying pathology, e.g. uveitis, eczema
Angle-recession	Recessed iris	Other signs of trauma
↑episcleral venous pressure	Engorged episcleral vein(s)	Vascular abnormalities according to underlying pathology
Intraocular tumour	Posterior segment tumour	Cataract; mass seen on US
Schwartz syndrome	RRD	Mild AC inflammation
Closed angle		
Chronic angle closure	PAS	May have had subacute attacks of angle closure
Angle pulled shut (anterior pathology)		
Neovascular	Rubeosis ± zipped shut	Signs of underlying pathology e.g. diabetes, CRVO
Inflammatory closed angle	Angle zipped shut by PAS	Signs of uveitis
ICE syndrome	Abnormal endothelial growth over angle	Iris distortion/atrophy; corneal hammered-metal appearance
Epithelial downgrowth	Epithelial downgrowth through wound to spread over angle	Surgical/traumatic wound
Angle pushed shut (posterior pathology)		
Phakomorphic	Ipsilateral intumescent lens	Appositional closure; contralateral open angle
Aqueous misdirection	Shallow AC despite patent PI; no iris bombe	Usually post-surgery in hypermetropic eyes

Other glaucoma syndromes, which may also present in an insidious manner, include inflammatory open angle, red cell, ghost cell, phacolytic, Posner–Schlossman syndrome (all open angle) and surgically induced angle closure (tight scleral buckle, penetrating keratoplasty). See ▢ Table 10.4 for syndromes that typically present in an acute/subacute manner.

Neovascular glaucoma

Posterior segment ischaemia drives neovascularization of the angle leading to a fibrovascular membrane. Initially, this overlies the trabecular meshwork so that the angle appears open, but with time PAS form and the membrane contracts to zip the angle shut. Ischaemic CRVO and diabetes each account for about a third of the cases of neovascular glaucoma (NVG). The advent of anti-VEGF therapies is an exciting new development in the management of NVG.

Causes include
- Ischaemic CRVO (common); risk of progression to NVG is 50%.
- Diabetic retinopathy (common); risk of NVG highest in PDR.
- Other vascular disorders: ocular ischaemic syndrome, CRAO, BRVO.
- Other retinal disease: chronic retinal detachment, sickle cell retinopathy.
- Retinal or choroidal tumours.

Clinical features:
- Pain is often a feature and may be severe; predisposing condition may be known, or may be suggested by the history (e.g. sudden loss of vision a couple of months previously in cases of CRVO).
- *Iris rubeosis*: abnormal/non-radial vessels at pupil; ↑IOP; AC flare/cells, hyphaema; ectropion uvea; conjunctival injection and corneal oedema if acute ↑IOP or decompensating; disc changes and field loss as for POAG (see Primary open angle glaucoma, 📖 p.308).
- *Gonioscopy*: abnormal vessels in the angle; fibrovascular membrane overlying the trabeculum (open angle type) or membrane + PAS zipping angle shut (angle closure type).

Investigation (to determine cause)
- Dilated fundoscopy in all cases ± FFA.
- Carotid dopplers: if no retinal pathology or asymmetric diabetic retinopathy.
- B-scan ultrasound: if poor fundal view (cataract may be associated with chronic retinal pathology such as tumours, detachment, inflammation).

Treatment
- Treatment of NVG has often been challenging and unsatisfactory, but is undergoing a positive transformation with the advent of anti-VEGF therapies.

Of underlying cause:
For example:
- PRP for retinal ischaemia;
- retinal reattachment for RD;
- carotid endarterectomy for suitable carotid artery stenosis.

Of neovascularization
- Anti-VEGF therapies have been shown to have a significant impact on neovascularization. Small retrospective studies using intravitreal bevacizumab have shown regression of neovascularization and ↓IOP both when used alone[1] or in combination with PRP.[2]

Of ↑IOP:
- mydriatic (e.g. atropine 1% 2×/d) + topical steroid (e.g. prednisolone 1% 1–4-hourly) + ocular hypotensive agents as for POAG;
- if medical treatment fails consider trabeculectomy, tube-shunt procedures or cyclodestruction (e.g. cyclodiode/cyclocryotherapy) depending on *visual prognosis*.

Of pain:
- if the eye is blind and painful consider retrobulbar alcohol or evisceration/enucleaton.

1. Wakabayashi T *et al.* Intravitreal bevacizumab to treat iris neovascularization and neovascular glaucoma secondary to ischemic retinal diseases in 41 consecutive cases. *Ophthalmology* 2008;**115**:1571–80.

2. Ehlers JP *et al.* Combination intravitreal bevacizumab/panretinal photocoagulation versus panretinal photocoagulation alone in the treatment of neovascular glaucoma. *Retina* 2008;**28**:696–702.

Inflammatory glaucoma: general

Raised IOP in the context of intraocular inflammation is a common clinical problem. The challenge is to elucidate the time-course (acute vs chronic ↑IOP), the state of the angle (open vs appositional closure vs synechial closure), and the underlying mechanism.

Therapy may be made difficult due to marked fluctuations in IOP (ciliary body shutdown → IOP↓, trabeculitis → IOP↑) and concerns over whether the treatment could be making things worse (steroid-induced glaucoma).

Open angle type

Acute

Mechanism: acute trabeculitis (particularly with HSV, VZV), trabecular meshwork blockage.

Clinical features

- ↑IOP; open angle; signs of uveitis ± keratitis; IOP returns to normal after acute episode of inflammation.

Treatment

- *Of inflammatory process*: treatment of underlying cause may be sufficient (e.g. topical steroids and mydriatic for AAU, *see* Acute anterior uveitis 📖 p.368).
- *Of ↑IOP*: if features of concern (e.g. IOP >30mmHg; sustained ↑IOP; vulnerable optic disc) consider topical (e.g. β-blocker, carbonic anhydrase inhibitor) or systemic (e.g. acetazolamide) medication for as long as required.

Chronic

Mechanism: trabecular scarring; chronic trabeculitis.

Clinical features

- ↑IOP; open angle; no active inflammation but may have signs of previous episodes; ± disc changes or field defects, *see* Glaucoma assessment (📖 p.304).

Treatment

- *Medical*: as for POAG; some practitioners may avoid PG agonists.
- If medical treatment fails consider trabeculectomy (poorer results than for POAG, but improves if augmented or tube procedure). However, to improve outcome of the operation, tight control of inflammation should first be achieved.
- If surgical treatment fails consider cyclodestruction (e.g. cyclodiode), but significant risk of phthisis.

Steroid-induced glaucoma

Although related to the treatment rather than the underlying disease process, this is an important differential diagnosis of inflammatory glaucoma. Raised IOP due to steroids requires a reduction in the potency and frequency of topical corticosteroids (± use of steroid-sparing agents), whereas if it is due to uncontrolled inflammation the steroid dose may need to be increased.

Angle closure type

With seclusio pupillae

Mechanism: 360° posterior synechiae (seclusio pupillae) blocks anterior flow of aqueous humour causing iris bombé and appositional angle closure.

Clinical features

- ↑IOP; seclusio pupillae; iris bombé; shallow AC; angle closure (appositional); signs of previous inflammatory episodes

Treatment

- *Of inflammatory process*: minimize posterior synechiae formation by rapid and effective treatment of anterior uveitis (consider subconjunctival betnesol and mydricaine if required).
- *Of ↑IOP*: Nd-YAG PI—PI should be larger (or multiple) than is necessary for acute angle closure glaucoma (**NB** AC will be shallow so watch out for the corneal endothelium) and surgical PI may be necessary if Nd-YAG PI closes. Consider topical (e.g. β-blocker, carbonic anhydrase inhibitor) or systemic (e.g. acetazolamide) medication as a temporary measure or for as long as required.

With synechial closure

Mechanism: PAS may zip the angle closed; risk of synechial closure is increased in presence of granulomatous inflammation and possibly pre-existing narrow angles.

Clinical features

- ↑IOP, shallow AC, PAS with angle closure, signs of previous inflammatory episodes

Treatment

- *Medical*: as for POAG, but some practitioners would advise caution with prostaglandin agonists.
- If medical treatment fails consider trabeculectomy (augmented).
- If surgical treatment fails consider cyclodestruction (e.g. cyclodiode), but significant risk of phthisis.
- If >25% of angle remains open consider Nd-YAG PI to deal with any pupil block component.

Inflammatory glaucoma: syndromes

Posner–Schlossman syndrome

This is a syndrome of recurrent unilateral episodes of painless high IOP occurring in a 'white' eye. It typically affects young males. The cause is not known; acute trabeculitis has been postulated, possibly secondary to HSV.

Clinical features
- Blurring of vision, haloes, painless.
- ↑IOP (40–80mmHg), white eye, minimal flare, occasional cells/keratic precipitates, no synechiae (PS or PAS), open angle.

Treatment
- *Of inflammatory process*: topical steroid (e.g. dexamethasone 0.1% 4×/d).
- *Of ↑IOP*: consider topical (e.g. β-blocker, α2-agonist, carbonic anhydrase inhibitor) or systemic (e.g. acetazolamide) according to IOP level.

NB Chronic recurrent inflammatory episodes may lead to sever angle damage.

Fuchs' heterochromic uveitis (syn Fuchs' heterochromic cyclitis)

Fuchs' heterochromic uveitis (see Anterior uveitis syndromes (1) 📖 p.372; syn Fuchs' heterochromic cyclitis)is a syndrome of mild chronic anterior uveitis, iris heterochromia, and cataract may be complicated by glaucoma in 10–30% cases.

It typically affects young adults and there is no sex bias. It is unilateral in >90% cases.

Clinical features
- ↓VA due to cataract; floaters; often asymptomatic.
- White eye, white stellate Keratic precipitates (KPs) over whole corneal endothelium, mild flare, few cells, iris atrophy (washed out, moth-eaten), transillumination defects, abnormal iris vessels, iris heterochromia ('becomes bluer'; more obvious if observed in natural light), iris nodules, cataract (posterior cortical/subcapsular), vitritis, ↑IOP.
- *Gonioscopy*: open angle; ± twig-like neovascularization of the angle.

Treatment
- *Of inflammatory process*: not usually necessary.
- *Of ↑IOP*: treat as for POAG 📖 p.308.

Lens-related glaucoma

Lens-related glaucoma

Lens-related glaucoma may result from abnormalities of lens size, lens position, release of lens protein (mature cataract/trauma/surgery), and/or the consequent inflammatory response.

Phacomorphic glaucoma

Mechanism: the enlarging lens causes pupil block and anterior bowing of the iris with secondary angle closure. In an eye of normal axial length this occurs secondary to an intumescent cataractous lens; in a short eye this may result simply from the normal increase in lens size with age.

Clinical features
- ↑IOP, shallow AC, fixed semi-dilated pupil, swollen cataractous lens.
- Ipsilateral closed angle (appositional; sigma sign may be seen on indentation gonioscopy).
- Contralateral angle may be open with deep AC (in contrast to primary angle closure glaucoma); however, this helpful sign may not be present if contralateral eye also has significant cataract.

Treatment
- Medical (topical and systemic): as for primary angle closure glaucoma.
- Nd-YAG PI to reverse pupil block component.
- Early cataract extraction is the definitive treatment.

Phacolytic glaucoma

Mechanism: the hypermature cataract loses soluble lens proteins through the anterior capsule causing trabecular obstruction and subsequent secondary open angle glaucoma.

Clinical features
- ↑IOP, lens protein in a deep AC (may form a pseudohypopyon), hypermature/mature cataract, open angle (with lens protein); AC tap reveals lens protein and foamy macrophages.

Treatment
- *Medical*: topical (e.g. β-blocker, α2-agonist, carbonic anhydrase inhibitor) or systemic (e.g. acetazolamide) agents as required; consider topical steroids vs associated inflammation.
- Early cataract extraction—usually ECCE.

Phacoanaphylactic uveitis

Mechanism: this is an inflammatory reaction to lens protein, usually following traumatic capsular rupture or postoperative retention of lens material (when it must be distinguished from endophthalmitis). This insult may also cause sensitization such that lens protein exposure in the contralateral eye (surgery, hyper/mature cataract) may be associated with an aggressive response.

Clinical features
- Recent trauma/surgery, exposed lens protein, AC flare + cells ± hypopyon, KPs, synechiae (PS + PAS), angle usually open (but ± PAS); IOP may be high, normal or low.

Treatment
- *Of inflammatory process*: topical steroid (e.g. dexamethasone 0.1% hourly) and surgical removal of any retained lens fragments.
- *Of ↑IOP*: Medical: topical (e.g. β-blocker, α2-agonist, carbonic anhydrase inhibitor) or systemic (e.g. acetazolamide) agents as required.
- *For contralateral cataract*: consider removal by ICCE to reduce lens protein exposure.

Glaucoma secondary to lens subluxation/dislocation

Mechanism: pupil block by anterior lens subluxation or complete dislocation into the AC; there may also be a coincident angle abnormality (e.g. Marfan syndrome).

Clinical features
- ↑IOP, subluxed/dislocated lens, ± corneal oedema (if acute or lenticulo-corneal touch); lenticular astigmatism and variable refraction

Treatment
- *Positional*: dilate and lie patient supine (to encourage posterior movement of lens), and constrict (to keep lens safely behind pupil); long-term miotic therapy may be needed unless the lens dislocates safely into the vitreous.
- *Early lens extraction*: if positional measures fail, if complete dislocation into the AC, if cataract or if recurrent problem.

Other secondary open angle glaucoma

Steroid-induced

Exogenous and occasionally endogenous steroids may decrease outflow facility leading to ↑IOP after a few days or weeks. In the normal population 5% will have an IOP increase of >15mmHg and 30% will have an increase of 6–15mmHg if given topical steroids for up to 6wks. POAG patients are often particularly sensitive to this steroid-effect.

Possible mechanisms include prostaglandin inhibition (e.g. PGF2α) and structural changes in the extracellular matrix (glycosaminoglycans) and trabecular meshwork (cross-linking of actins). A history of steroid administration should be specifically asked for as patients may not volunteer use of steroid-containing anabolics, skin creams or episodic courses of steroids (e.g. for exacerbations of asthma/COPD).

Treatment: ideally decrease frequency/potency or stop steroid (± steroid-sparing agent) to normalize IOP—liaise with prescribing physician. If corticosteroids essential/IOP still elevated then treat as POAG (see Primary open angle glaucoma 📖 p.308).

Red cell glaucoma

Hyphaema (usually traumatic) leads to blockage of the trabecular meshwork by red blood cells. In 10% cases a rebleed may occur, usually at about 5d. Patients with sickle cell disease/trait do worse and are harder to treat (e.g. sickling may be worsened by the acidosis from carbonic anhydrase inhibitors).

Treatment

- *Of hyphaema*: strict bed-rest, topical steroid (e.g. dexamethasone 0.1% 4×/d), mydriatic (e.g. atropine 1% 2×/d) (see Hyphaema 📖 p.120).
- *Of IOP*: topical (e.g. β-blocker, α2-agonist, carbonic anhydrase inhibitor) or systemic (e.g. acetazolamide) agents as required
  - *Surgical*: AC paracentesis ± AC wash-out.

Ghost cell glaucoma

Vitreous haemorrhage leads to blockage of the trabecular meshwork by degenerate red blood cells, usually 2–4wks after the haemorrhage. These cells, which may be seen in the AC and the angle, are tan-coloured, having lost haemoglobin.

Treatment: Medical treatment (as for POAG, see 📖 p.308) is usually sufficient. If this fails consider AC wash-out + vitrectomy to remove persistent vitreous haemorrhage.

Angle recession glaucoma

Blunt trauma may cause angle recession and associated trabecular damage. Traumatic angle recession carries a 10% risk of glaucoma at 10yrs, the risk increasing with extent of recession. Look for asymmetry of AC depth, pupil, and angle.

- *Screening*: periodic IOP check (e.g. 3mths, 6mths, yearly) if known angle recession.
- *Treatment*: as for POAG (see 📖 p.308).

Raised episcleral venous pressure

Aqueous drainage is reduced as episcleral venous pressure increases (*see* Anatomy and physiology p.302). This may occur as a result of vascular abnormalities in the orbit (Sturge–Weber syndrome, orbital varices), cavernous sinus (arteriovenous fistulae) or SVC (SVC obstruction). Episcleral venous pressure manifests as unilateral/bilateral engorged episcleral veins, chemosis, proptosis, with blood in Schlemm's canal on gonioscopy.

Treatment: primarily directed at the underlying pathology, although medical and occasionally surgical lowering of IOP may be necessary.

Tumours

Tumours may cause ↑IOP via open angle mechanisms (clogging or infiltration of trabecular meshwork with tumour cells) or, for larger posterior segment tumours, rubeosis (secondary to ischaemia), or secondary angle closure (anterior displacement of lens–iris diaphragm).

Suspect in atypical unilateral glaucoma; if poor view of posterior segment (usually due to cataract) a B-scan ultrasound is essential. About 20% of malignant melanoma is associated with ↑IOP.

Treatment: directed by the underlying tumour, although ↑IOP itself suggests a poor prognosis.

Schwartz syndrome

This is the uncommon association of anterior segment inflammation (mild) and ↑IOP (with an open angle) arising from a rhegmatogenous retinal detachment. It is discussed further, *see* Anterior uveitis syndromes (1) (p.372). The ↑IOP and anterior uveitis may be treated medically in the interim but tend to resolve rapidly with surgical repair of the retinal detachment.

Other secondary closed angle glaucoma

Iridoschisis

Bilateral splitting and atrophy of anterior iris leaf is associated with ↑IOP usually secondary to angle closure (due to pupil block), but sometimes due to debris blocking the trabecular meshwork (open angle). It is uncommon, and usually occurs in the elderly.

Treatment

- Angle closure type with Nd-YAG PI.
- Open angle type as for POAG (see Primary open angle glaucoma 📖 p.308).

Iridocorneal endothelial syndrome (ICE)

A unilateral condition in which abnormal corneal endothelium migrates across the angle, the trabecular meshwork, and the anterior iris so causing significant anterior segment distortion. ICE syndrome is rare, usually occurs in 20–40yr old females and carries a 50% risk of glaucoma. HSV has been proposed as a causative agent.

  Three overlapping syndromes are described: Chandler syndrome (predominantly corneal), essential iris atrophy (predominantly iris changes), and iris naevus (Cogan–Reese) syndrome (appearance of a diffuse naevus or pigmented nodules, which probably represent protrusions of iris stroma).

Clinical features

- Unilateral pain, blurred vision.
- Unilateral fine corneal guttata ('beaten-metal'), corneal oedema. (± ↑IOP), iris atrophy corectopia (displaced pupil), pseudopolycoria (accessory pupil).
- *Gonioscopy*: broad-based PAS that may insert anterior to Schwalbe's line.

Investigation

Consider specular microscopy to demonstrate endothelial changes.

Treatment

- Medical (e.g. β-blocker, α2-agonist, carbonic anhydrase inhibitor, prostaglandin agonist), surgery (trabeculectomy ± augmented or tube procedures), or cyclodestruction as required.

Posterior polymorphous dystrophy (PPD)

A bilateral condition in which abnormal corneal endothelium may form extensive irido-corneal adhesions with angle closure. Clinically, it may appear similar to ICE syndrome but is dominantly inherited, bilateral, and usually detectable in childhood (although may only be symptomatic later). PPD carries a 15% risk of glaucoma. Treat glaucoma as for POAG (see Primary open angle glaucoma 📖 p.308).

Epithelial downgrowth

A deranged healing response in which trauma or surgery (poorly constructed wound, vitreous incarceration) allows epithelium to proliferate down through the wound and onto the endothelial surface. Once free of its normal environment it may proliferate unchecked across the corneal endothelium and angle so causing glaucoma in a similar manner to ICE syndrome.

Treatment is very difficult: lower IOP as for POAG; intracameral antifibrotic agents have been used. Prognosis for vision is poor.

Fuchs' endothelial dystrophy

In Fuchs' endothelial dystrophy (see Corneal dystrophies: posterior 📖 p.228) oedema of the peripheral cornea may cause secondary angle closure, especially in at-risk eyes with pre-existing shallow ACs.

Iatrogenic glaucoma

Malignant glaucoma (syn aqueous misdirection syndrome, ciliary block, ciliolenticular block)

Mechanism:

it is thought that posterior misdirection of aqueous into the vitreous causes anterior displacement of vitreous, ciliary processes, and lens/PCIOL with secondary angle closure.

Risk factors

- Short axial length, chronic angle closure, previous acute angle closure.
- Post-procedure: surgery (trabeculectomy, tube-procedures, cataract extraction, peripheral iridectomy); laser (Nd-YAG PI).
- Miotic therapy (rare).

Clinical features

- Often ↓VA due to acute ↑/very high IOP; may be asymptomatic.
- ↑IOP (may be normal initially), shallow/flat AC, no pupil block (so no iris bombé and occurs despite a patent PI), no choroidal/suprachoroidal cause (detachment/haemorrhage).

Treatment

- Ensure that a patent PI is present (repeat Nd-YAG PI if necessary).
- Dilate (atropine 1% 3×/d + phenylephrine 2.5% 4×/d).
- *Systemic ↓IOP*: acetazolamide 500mg IV stat (then 250mg PO 4×/d) ± mannitol/glycerol.
- *Topical ↓IOP*: β-blocker (e.g. timolol 0.5% stat then 2×/d) + sympathomimetic (e.g. apraclonidine 1% stat then 3×/d).

If medical treatment fails consider:

Laser

- YAG disruption of anterior vitreous face (if aphake/pseudophakia perform posterior capsulotomy/hyaloidotomy; if phakic a hyaloidotomy can be attempted through the patent PI).
- Argon laser to the ciliary processes (through the patent PI; relieves block by causing shrinkage of the processes).
- Trans-scleral cyclodiode photocoagulation of the ciliary body may also be successful in breaking the acute attack.[1]

Surgery

- The aim in surgery is to achieve adequate posterior–anterior communication to re-establish aqueous humour (AqH) flow, for which the key surgical step is peripheral zonulohyaloidectomy:
- *If phakic*: cataract extraction (phacoemulsification or ECCE), posterior capsulotomy, and anterior vitrectomy; cataract surgery in these situation can be facilitated by preliminary pars plana vitreous debulking as part of a vitrectomy–phacoemulsification–vitrectomy procedure[2].
- If aphakic/pseudophakic: pars plana vitrectomy and posterior capsulotomy.

Post-cataract surgery

Acute postoperative ↑IOP may be due to retained viscoelastic, lens fragments or inflammation. A single dose of acetazolamide SR 250mg may be used prophylactically against the risk of an early postoperative pressure spike. Less commonly glaucoma may arise due to suprachoroidal haemorrhage, phacolysis, phacoanaphylaxis (see Lens related glaucoma 📖 p.326), Amsler haemorrhage in Fuchs heterochronic uveitis (see Inflammatory glaucoma: syndromes 📖 p.324), epithelial downgrowth (see Other secondary closed angle glaucoma 📖 p.330) syndrome, aqueous misdirection or the UGH syndrome.

Post-vitreoretinal surgery

- *With intra-ocular gases*: acute postoperative ↑IOP is usually due to expansion/overfill of SF6 or C3F8. *Treatment*: decide according to IOP and half-life of gas, but usually short-term medical treatment sufficient (e.g. acetazolamide SR 250mg 2×/d for 5/7); or else remove some of the gas.
- *With scleral buckles*: secondary angle closure may occur due to ciliary body swelling and choroidal detachment (possibly due to pressure on the vortex veins). *Treatment*: usually resolves spontaneously; treat medically in the interim.
- *With silicone oil*: oil in the AC blocking the trabecular meshwork (and possibly other mechanisms) may cause an ↑IOP, presenting from days to months after surgery. *Treatment*: sometimes resolves spontaneously; treat medically in the interim; consider cyclodestruction if persists. **NB** Early removal of oil (<6mths) may ↓IOP. After this period removal of oil makes little difference due to incorporation of oil by macrophages.
- *Vitrectomy*: may facilitate ghost cell glaucoma (see Other secondary open angle glaucoma 📖 p.328) and increase the risk of rubeosis in proliferative diabetic retinopathy.

1. Stumpf TH *et al.* Transscleral cyclodiode laser photocoagulation in the treatment of aqueous misdirection syndrome. *Ophthalmology* 2008;**115**:2058–61.

2. Sharma A, Sii F, Shah P, Kirkby GR. Vitrectomy-phacoemulsification-vitrectomy for the management of aqueous misdirection syndromes in phakic eyes. *Ophthalmology* 2006;**113**:1968–73.

Pharmacology of intraocular pressure lowering agents

Prostaglandin analogues

These analogues of $PGF_{2\alpha}$ increase uveoscleral outflow.

- *Ocular side-effects*: *common*: hyperaemia, increased pigmentation of iris (and rarely lid skin), thickening and lengthening of lashes; *rare*: uveitis, CMO.
- *Contraindications*: may be associated with CMO after complicated cataract surgery (possibly active uveitis).

β-blockers

These reduce aqueous production probably by acting on β-receptors on the non-pigmented ciliary epithelium and vasoconstriction of the arterioles supplying ciliary processes.

- *Ocular side-effects*: uncommon; allergic blepharoconjunctivitis, punctate keratitis.
- *Contraindications*: asthma/COPD (bronchospasm may occur even with selective β1-agents), heart block, bradycardia or cardiac failure. Try to avoid in nursing mothers as it is secreted in breast milk.
- *Drug interactions*: concurrent use of cardiac-directed Ca^{2+} antagonists, such as verapamil, may compound bradycardia, heart block, and hypotension.

Carbonic anhydrase inhibitors

These reduce aqueous production by inhibiting carbonic anhydrase isoenzyme II (and hence bicarbonate production) in the non-pigmented ciliary epithelium.

- *Ocular side-effects*: common; burning, tearing, allergic blepharoconjunctivitis (up to 10%).
- *Contraindications*: sulphonamide sensitivity; renal failure, liver failure (systemic acetazolamide).
- *Drug interactions*: K^+ losing diuretics (e.g. thiazide) may cause profound hypokalaemia if used concurrently with acetazolamide. K^+ supplementation is not usually required for acetazolamide used alone.

Sympathomimetics

The highly α2-selective brimonidine is well tolerated and apraclonidine (α1 + α2) is useful for short-term use, e.g. after laser iridotomy. Non-selective sympathomimetics such as adrenaline (epinephrine), dipivefrine, and the adrenergic neurone blocker guanethidine are now seldom used due to their frequent side-effects.

- *Ocular side-effects*: *common*: allergic blepharoconjunctivitis (up to 15% for brimonidine, 30% for apraclonidine); *older agents*: scarring, mydriasis, adrenochrome; *uncommon*: CMO in aphakia (possibly pseudophakia).
- *Contraindications*: heart block, bradycardia.
- *Drug interactions*: monoamine oxidase inhibitors.

Miotics (parasympathomimetics)

Muscarinic receptor agonism leads to ciliary muscle contraction, which pulls on the scleral spur to open the trabecular meshwork. Pilocarpine is used first line in narrow angle glaucoma; sometimes still used in POAG.

- *Ocular side-effects*: fluctuating myopia, miosis (constricted visual field, worse night vision.
- *Contraindications*: inflammatory or malignant glaucoma.

Table 10.6 Pharmacological groups

Group	Mechanism	Advantages	Systemic side-effects	Examples
Topical				
Prostaglandin analogues	Increase uveoscleral outflow	↓IOP by 930% well-tolerated	Bronchospasm (rare)	Latanoprost 0.005% Travaprost 0.004% Bimatoprost 0.03%
β-blocker	Decrease aqueous production	20yr follow-up ↓IOP by ±25% Well-tolerated (in most cases)	Bronchospasm Bradycardia Heart block Hypotension Glucose intolerance Lethargy Impotence	*Non-selective* Timolol 0.25/0.5% Carteolol 1% Levobunolol 0.5% *β1-selective* Betaxolol 0.25/0.5%
Carbonic anhydrase inhibitors	Decrease aqueous production	↓IOP by ±20%	Metallic taste See list below (for systemic)	Brinzolamide 1% Dorzolamide 2%
α2-agonists	Decrease aqueous production Increase uveoscleral outflow	↓IOP by ±20%	Bradycardia Hypotension Insomnia Irritability GI disturbance	Brimonidine 0.2% Apraclonidine 0.5/1%
Miotics	Increase trabecular outflow		Sweating Sialorrhoea Nausea Headache Bradycardia	Pilocarpine 0.5–4%
Systemic				
Carbonic anhydrase inhibitor	Decrease aqueous production Acidosis may cause hypotension	↓IOP by ≤65%	Lethargy Depression Anorexia Hypokalaemia Renal calculi Blood dyscrasia	Acetazolamide
Hyperosmotic agents	Creates an osmotic gradient	Rapidly ↓IOP (onset 30min)	Hypertension Vomiting Cardiac failure MI Hyperglycaemia (mannitol) Urinary retention	Mannitol Glycerol

Laser procedures for glaucoma (1)

Nd-YAG peripheral iridotomy

Indication

- *Treatment*: angle closure with pupil block—may be acute/subacute/chronic, primary/secondary.
- *Prophylaxis*: occludable narrow angles (including fellow eye in angle closure).

Method

- *Consent*: explain what the procedure does, why you are treating both eyes and possible complications, including failure/need for retreatment, bleeding, inflammation, corneal burns, visual effects (e.g. monocular diplopia).
- *Instil* pilocarpine 2% (tightens the iris) + apraclonidine 1% (prevents IOP spike and may reduce bleeding) + topical anaesthetic (e.g. oxybuprocaine).
- *Set laser (varies according to model)*: commonly bursts of two or three pulses of 3–6mJ (greater energy required for irides, which are thick, velvety, and heavily pigmented); the beam should be angled (i.e. not perpendicular).
- *Position CL* (usually the Abraham lens; require coupling agent).
- *Identify suitable iridotomy sites*: superior (hidden by the normal lid position), peripheral and ideally in an iris crypt (less energy required).
- *Focus and fire laser*: success is indicated by a forward gush of pigment-loaded aqueous. This usually takes 2–6 shots.

Post-procedure

- Topical steroid (e.g. dexamethasone 0.1% stat, then 6×/d for 1wk).
- Consider early post-procedure IOP check (e.g. at 1–2h) or prophylactic IOP lowering treatment.
- Review within 10d to recheck IOP and inflammatory response.

Complications

Bleeding (stops with maintained pressure on lens), anterior inflammation (increase topical steroids), corneal burns (caution with a flatter AC), glare (avoid interpalpebral iris).

Argon laser trabeculoplasty

Indication

- Open angle glaucoma with pigmented trabeculum—commonly POAG/PXF glaucoma/PDS glaucoma.
- Medical and surgical options undesirable or ineffective.

Method

- *Consent*: explain what the procedure does and possible complications, including failure (short and long term), bleeding, and inflammation.
- Instil apraclonidine 1% (vs IOP spike; alternatively give 250mg acetazolamide 30min beforehand) + topical anaesthetic (e.g. oxybuprocaine).

- Set laser (varies according to model): argon—commonly 50μm spot size, 0.1s duration, 300–1000mW power (start low, increase as required); Diode—commonly 100μm spot size, 0.1–0.2s duration, 800–1200mW power.
- Position goniolens (antireflective laser lens).
- *Identify trabeculoplasty site*: aim for the anterior border of the pigmented trabecular meshwork.
- *Focus and fire laser*: the ideal reaction is a mild blanching or small bubble; the more pigmented the angle the less power is usually required. Place 50 equally spaced shots over 180°.

Post-procedure

- All usual glaucoma medication should be continued; topical steroid (e.g. betamethasone 4×/d for 1wk) may be prescribed.
- Consider early post-procedure IOP check (e.g. at 1–2h) or prophylactic IOP lowering treatment (e.g. oral acetazolamide).
- *Review in 2–6wks*: if inadequate IOP response consider ALT on the remaining 180°.
- Failure occurs at a rate of 6–10% per year and is often sudden[1]. Long-term follow-up is necessary.

Complications

Bleeding (stops with maintained pressure on lens), anterior inflammation (usually mild), PAS, pressure spike, may worsen outcome of subsequent trabeculectomy.

Selective laser trabeculoplasty

An alternative to the ALT, selective laser trabeculoplasty uses a Q-switched frequency-doubled Nd-YAG laser to selectively target the pigmented cells, and to minimize damage to angle structures (cf. ALT). The usual strategy is to place 50 non-overlapping spots (400μm spot size, 3ns duration, 0.8mJ initial energy) centred on the trabecular meshwork over the inferior 180°. The power is adjusted to be 0.1mJ below the level that causes bubble formation.[2] Pre- and post-procedure management is similar to ALT.

Laser iridoplasty

In laser iridoplasty a ring of Argon laser burns shrinks the peripheral iris stroma to widen the angular approach. It is the procedure of choice for plateau iris syndrome, and can also be used to break the acute attack of acute primary angle closure. A CL (e.g. Abraham or Goldmann (central part rather than mirrors)) is used to direct argon laser to the most peripheral iris. Typical applications are 20–50 burns over 360° (with ≥ 2 spot sizes between burns) of 200–500μm spot-size, 0.2–0.5s duration, and 200–400mW power.

1. Spaeth GL *et al.* Argon laser trabeculoplasty controls one third of progressive uncontrolled open angle glaucoma for 5 years. *Arch Ophthalmol* 1992;110:491–4.

2. Damji KF *et al.* Selective laser trabeculoplasty vs argon laser trabeculoplasty: a randomized controlled trial. *Br J Ophthalmol* 1999;**83**:718–22.

Laser procedures for glaucoma (2)

Trans-scleral diode laser cyclophotocoagulation (*syn* 'cyclodiode')

Selective destruction of the ciliary body was traditionally achieved by cyclocryotherapy, but is now usually achieved with either a diode or less commonly a Nd:YAG laser. The procedure for a trans-scleral diode laser cyclophotocoagulation is outlined here.

Indication

Most commonly used for intractable ↑IOP, e.g. in rubeotic or synechial angle closure where other treatment modalities have failed; also used as an alternative to incisional surgical procedures (e.g. where the patient is too systemically unwell to tolerate surgery), and has been used to break the acute attack of acute primary angle closure.

Methods

- *Consent*: explain what the procedure does and possible complications including failure/need for retreatment, hypotony, inflammation, bleeding and adverse effect on vision; sympathetic ophthalmia has now also been described after cyclophotocoagulation.
- *Set laser (varies according to model)*: commonly 1500mW power, 1.5s duration.
- *Identify ciliary body 0.5–2mm from limbus*: transillumination helps to identify the dark ciliary body. Place the contact probe (of the diode laser) in an anteroposterior manner against the globe, adjusting its position so that the probe is directed at the ciliary body.
- Fire laser: aim to treat up to three quadrants, using 5–10 shots per quadrant; if laser burn is audible ('pop') decrease power; avoid the 3 and 9 o'clock positions.

Post-procedure

Topical steroid (e.g. dexamethasone 0.1% 4×/d for 1wk) and all usual glaucoma medication. Review in 1–2wks.

Complications

Anterior inflammation (may get hypopyon with neovascular glaucoma), hypotony, haemorrhage, scleral thinning, cataract, and phthisis.

Surgery for glaucoma

Surgery for glaucoma

Glaucoma surgery includes iris procedures (surgical iridectomy), angle procedures (goniotomy, trabeculotomy), filtration procedures (trabeculectomy, deep sclerectomy), artificial drainage tubes, and cyclodestruction (cyclodialysis). In adult glaucoma the commonest operation is trabeculectomy with/without augmentation. This filtration procedure steers between the excessive drainage of the unguarded sclerostomy and the often inadequate drainage of a deep sclerectomy (non-penetrative). Augmentation with antifibrotics is indicated according to risk of fibrosis and previous failure. Artificial drainage tubes (or setons) require considerable experience and are reserved for resistant cases.

Surgical iridectomy and surgical cyclodialysis have become less common since the advent of laser PI and cyclodiode. Goniotomy and trabeculotomy are generally restricted to congenital glaucoma (see Glaucoma in children pp.712–714).

Table 10.7 Common surgical procedures in glaucoma

Procedure	Mechanism	Indication
Iris procedures		
Peripheral iridectomy	Relieves pupil block	Laser PI not possible (patient cooperation, thick iris, poor view, e.g. persistent oedema)
Angle procedures		
Goniotomy	Opens the abnormal angle (probably)	Primary congenital glaucoma (primary trabecular meshwork dysgenesis)
Trabeculotomy	Opens Schlemm's canal directly to anterior chamber	Congenital glaucoma, including primary congenital glaucoma and anterior segment dysgenesis
Filtration procedures (penetrating)		
Trabeculectomy	Forms new drainage channel from AC to sub-Tenon's space	Has a place in most chronic glaucomas (adult and paediatric)
Augmented trabeculectomy	Trabeculectomy with antifibrotic to reduce scarring	Standard trabeculectomy has failed/would be likely to fail
Artificial drainage tubes	Silicone tube flows from AC to episcleral explant	Augmented trabeculectomy has failed/would be likely to fail
Filtration procedures (non-penetrating)		
Deep sclerectomy	Exposes the trabecular meshwork and removes the internal wall of Schlemm's canal	Alternative to penetrative filtration procedures
Viscocanalostomy	As above + viscoelastic injected to open up Schlemm's canal	Alternative to penetrative filtration procedures

Filtration surgery: trabeculectomy

Indication

- *When to operate*: may be first line if high risk of progression or patient aims to be 'drop-free'; more commonly reserved when medical therapy is proving inadequate.
- *Which operation*: assess risks of operation failure (e.g. from scarring) against the increased risk of complications in augmented or tube procedures.

Method (standard trabeculectomy with fornix-based flap described)

- *Consent*: explain what the operation does and possible complications including scarring with return to high IOP, hypotony, infection, haemorrhage, and worsened vision.
- *Pre-operative*: consider preoperative steroid treatment.
- *Preparation*: with 5% povidone iodine and drape.
- *Place traction suture*: either corneal (avascular but care re cheese wiring or penetration) or superior rectus (risk of haematoma).
- *Form conjunctival flap*: incise at limbus with 6–10mm arc.
- *Form scleral flap (rectangular/square/triangular)*: incise the outline of the flap to a depth of 1/2 scleral thickness, before anterior lamellar dissection to free the posterior and lateral aspects of the flap.
- *Place a paracentesis*: oblique in the temporal cornea.
- *Form sclerostomy*: make a perpendicular incision at the sclerolimbal junction to form the anterior margin of the sclerostomy. Complete sclerostomy posteriorly by removing a block of sclerolimbal tissue with the punch (e.g. Khaw or Kelly punch) or blade/scissors (e.g. Vannas).
- *Perform peripheral iridectomy*: this should be broad-based but short and peripheral. This stage is primarily to prevent iris blockage of the trabeculectomy, although it will also relieve any coincident pupil block.
- *Suture scleral flap*: sutures can either be fixed, releasable (leave access via a corneal groove) or adjustable (can be loosened by massaging posterior aspect of scleral flap). This can be greatly assisted by having 'pre-placed' these scleral flap sutures. Assess opening pressure of flap by injecting balanced salt solution via the paracentesis.
- *Close conjunctiva and Tenon's layer securely* to prevent retraction and consequent leak. This can be achieved with two lateral interrupted sutures and a central mattress sutures.
- *Postoperative*: subconjunctival steroid (e.g. betamethasone) and antibiotic (e.g. cefuroxime).

Post-procedure

Topical antibiotic (e.g. chloramphenicol 0.5% 4×/d) and steroid (e.g. prednisolone acetate 1% 2 hourly initially tapering down over 2mths).
Review at 1d and 1wk, then according to result.

Fixed, releasable, and adjustable sutures

Optimal bleb drainage is not always achieved. Postoperatively bleb drainage may be increased by removing or loosening selected scleral sutures. The technique depends on the suture type used:

- *Fixed sutures*: if the suture can be visualized through Tenon's layer it may be released by Argon laser suture lysis.
- *Releasable sutures*: these are tied with a slip-knot and loop into a corneal groove to permit access; they can be released at the slit-lamp without disturbing the conjunctival flap.
- *Adjustable sutures*: these can be loosened by massaging the posterior aspect of the scleral flap at the slit-lamp.

Table 10.8 Choice of filtration procedure

Procedure	Indication
Trabeculectomy	
Standard	Low risk of scarring
	Low risk of failure from other causes
Augmented trabeculectomy	
5-FU (50mg/ml) or MMC (0.2mg/ml)	Moderate risk of scarring
	Planned combined trabeculectomy/cataract surgery
	Previous surgery involving the conjunctiva (not trabeculectomy)
MMC (0.4mg/ml)	High risk of scarring
	Previous failed trabeculectomy
	Chronic inflammation (conjunctival or intraocular)
	High-risk glaucoma (including aphakic, active neovascular)
Tube procedures	
Molteno and alternatives	Previous failed augmented trabeculectomy
	Multiple further operations likely to be necessary
	Inadequate healthy conjunctiva for trabeculectomy
	High-risk glaucoma (including aphakic, active neovascular, aniridia, cellular overgrowth, e.g. ICE, epithelial downgrowth syndrome)

Table 10.9 Comparison of fornix vs limbal-based flaps for trabeculectomy

	Fornix-based	Limbal-based
Operative	Easier	Access can be difficult
	Faster	Slower
	Good sclerostomy exposure	Adequate sclerostomy exposure
Use of antifibrotics	Take care to avoid wound margin	Relatively safe
Postoperative manipulation	Easier	More difficult
Postoperative	More conjunctival wound leaks Less posterior scarring	Fewer conjunctival wound leaks More posterior scarring → 'ring of steel'

Filtration surgery: antifibrotics

The control of wound healing is critical to the success of glaucoma filtration surgery. Antifibrotics such as 5-fluorouracil (5-FU) and mitomycin-C (MMC) permit the surgeon to inhibit the fibrosis and scarring that may 'close off' an otherwise satisfactory trabeculectomy.

As this fibrotic response will vary between patients the use of antifibrotics is titrated according to the predicted risk of scarring (Table 10.8). They should not be used indiscriminately as they may cause significant side-effects (Box 10.5).

Agents
- *5-FU*: inhibits DNA synthesis and RNA function; usual dose 50mg/ml.
- *MMC*: alkylates DNA, inhibits DNA and RNA synthesis; usual dose 0.2–0.4mg/ml

Indications
- *Moderate risk of scarring*: 5-FU (50mg/ml) or MMC (0.2mg/ml).
- *High risk of scarring*: MMC (0.4mg/ml)
- If very high risk or failed augmented trabeculectomy consider a tube procedure (Table 10.8).

Risk factors for scarring
- *Age*: <40.
- *Race*: African-Caribbean, Indian subcontinent.
- *Previous surgery involving conjunctiva*: includes trabeculectomy, cataract surgery with scleral tunnel, vitreoretinal surgery.
- *Glaucoma type*: neovascular, aphakic, inflammatory.
- *Chronic inflammation*: chronic conjunctivitis, uveitis.
- *Topical treatment*: β-blockers (low risk), pilocarpine, dipivefrine (moderate risk).

Intraoperative use (as part of trabeculectomy, see *Filtration surgery: trabaculectomy* 🕮 *p.342*)
- Select agent and concentration (50mg/ml 5-FU; 0.2–0.4mg/ml MMC) according to patient risk of fibrosis.
- *Prepare sponges*: sponges need to be cut to size and then soaked in the antifibrotic of choice; polyvinyl alcohol sponges may be preferred as they disintegrate less than those made of methyl cellulose.
- During trabeculectomy place sponge under the conjunctival/Tenon's flap (± scleral flap in resistant cases) for appropriate duration (5min for 5-FU; 2–5min for MMC); avoid contact with cornea and conjunctival wound edge; ensure no intraocular administration.
- Remove sponges; all cytotoxics/used sponges require safe disposal separate to clinical waste.
- Irrigate eye well.

Postoperative use
- Select agent (usually 5-FU).
- Using a small calibre needle (29–30G) on a 1ml syringe administer antifibrotic as posteriorly as possible adjacent *but not into* the bleb.
- The usual dose is 5mg of 5-FU (usually 0.1ml of 50mg/ml 5-FU); MMC is occasionally used (at a dose of 0.02mg) but there are concerns over its potential toxicity.

Box 10.5 Potential complications of antifibrotics

Epithelial erosions
Wound leak
Bleb leak
Hypotony
Blebitis
Endophthalmitis
Scleritis
Limbal stem cell failure

Filtration surgery: complications of penetrating procedures (1)

Intraoperative complications

- *Conjunctival flap damage:* may get persistent leak especially if exposed to antifibrotics, button-holes especially if previous surgery.
- *Scleral flap damage:* may not close in controlled manner.
- *Bleeding:* may be conjunctival, scleral, from the iris, or, most seriously, suprachoroidal.
- *Vitreous loss:* increased risk with posterior sclerostomy.
- *Wound leak:* from damaged conjunctiva or inadequate closure.

Early postoperative complications

Shallow anterior chamber

Grade according to corneal contact: with peripheral iris only (I), with whole iris (II), or with lens (III). Examination ± ultrasound should identify the reason for a shallow AC (Table 10.10). If the AC is very shallow it may not be possible to see if the PI is patent or not.

Table 10.10 Differential diagnosis of shallow AC after trabeculectomy

	IOP	Seidel	PI	Bleb
Wound leak	Low	+	Patent	Poor/flat
Ciliary body shutdown	Low	−	Patent	Poor/flat
Overfiltration	Low	−	Patent	Good
Pupil block	High	−	Non-patent	Flat
Malignant glaucoma	High	−	Patent	Flat
Suprachoroidal haemorrhage	Variable	−	Patent	Variable

Specific treatment will depend on the underlying cause, but in general when there is a risk of corneal decompensation from lenticulo-corneal touch, urgent measures are required to reform the AC (e.g. balanced salts, viscoelastic, or gas). Otherwise, there is a risk of early cataract formation.

Low intraocular pressure/hypotony

- IOP <6mmHg is associated with flat AC, choroidal detachment, suprachoroidal haemorrhage, hypotonous maculopathy and corneal oedema.
- *General treatment:* topical steroids + mydriatic; stop IOP lowering agents; consider surgery (reform AC ± drain choroidal effusions) if corneal decompensation from lens touch (absolute indication), 'kissing' choroidal detachments, or marked AC inflammation (relative indications).

Wound leak
In milder cases where antifibrotics have not been used resolution is likely within 48h; in the interim a bandage CL may be applied and topical steroids may be temporarily stopped. However, more severe wound leaks (particularly with antifibrotics) usually require surgical intervention (a suture).

Ciliary body shutdown
This rare complication is associated with postoperative inflammation, requiring treatment with systemic corticosteroids. The AC should be reformed with viscoelastic.

Overfiltration
In milder cases a scleral shell or autologous blood injection may be sufficient. However, more severe cases (e.g. where maculopathy) need surgical intervention (resuturing of scleral flap).

High intraocular pressure
- *Pupil block*: PI is either incomplete or blocked by inflammatory debris
  - perform a new Nd-YAG PI (or complete old iridectomy); then topical mydriatic + steroids.
- *Malignant glaucoma*: aqueous misdirection may occur especially in short eyes (see Iatrogenic glaucoma 🕮 p.332).
- *Filtration failure*: obstruction of the sclerostomy and scleral flap may be internal (incarceration of iris, ciliary processes, or vitreous), scleral (fibrin, blood) or external (overly tight scleral flap sutures).
- Consider bleb massage, removal of releasable suture(s), loosening of adjustable suture(s), argon laser lysis of fixed suture(s)

Infection
Blebitis
Presents as an painful red eye, possibly with mucus discharge and photophobia; the bleb is milky with loculations of pus, conjunctival injection (especially around the bleb), and increasing IOP; ± AC activity (cells/flare ± hypopyon).
- *Identify organism*: swab bleb ± AC tap.
- Treat with intensive topical antibiotics (e.g. ofloxacin and penicillin hourly) and systemic antibiotic (e.g. ciprofloxacin 750mg 2×/d); adjust according to response and organism identified (commonly *Staphylococci* if early and *Streptococci* and *Haemophilus* if late); consider addition of topical steroids after 24h and add mydriatic if AC activity.

Endophthalmitis
- Clinical features as for blebitis but more severe, ↓VA, and vitritis.
- Investigate and treat as for other postoperative endophthalmitis (see Postoperative endophthalmitis 🕮 p.292). However, endophthalmitis occurring after trabeculectomy tends to run a more aggressive course with a worse prognosis than after cataract surgery.

Visual loss
'Wipe-out' of the remaining field may occur in the presence of a vulnerable optic nerve (associated with ↑IOP or hypotony) or hypotonous changes may lead to reduced acuity (e.g. from maculopathy).

Filtration surgery: complications of penetrating procedures (2)

Late postoperative complications

- *Filtration failure*: subconjunctival fibrosis ('ring of steel') especially with limbal-based flaps may lead to a poorly filtering encapsulated bleb (tense localized dome). Treat with bleb needling revision + subconjunctival antifibrotic (usually 5-FU) and post-procedure topical steroids/antibiotics.
- *Leaky bleb*: sweaty or leaky blebs are more common in augmented or non-guarded filtration surgery. If small leak, low risk of infection, and not hypotonous then may be monitored initially. Otherwise consider bandage CL, autologous blood injection, compression sutures, or refashioning of bleb.
- *Infection*: (blebitis/endophthalmitis)—see Filtration surgery: complications of penetrating procedures (1) (🕮 p.346) and also Postoperative endophthalmitis (🕮 p.292).
- *Visual loss*: postoperative lens opacities probably account for most of the postoperative drop in acuity—unfortunately, cataract surgery carries a 10–30% risk of bleb failure; astigmatism.
- *Ptosis*: often resolves spontaneously; more common with superior rectus traction sutures (rather than corneal) and in revised trabeculectomies where conjunctiva has been mobilized from superior fornix.

Non-penetrating glaucoma surgery

Non-penetrating glaucoma surgery describes a group of techniques in which improved aqueous drainage is achieved surgically without penetrating into the intraocular space. In some parts of the world, they have overtaken penetrating filtration procedures (such as trabeculectomy) in part due to their better safety profile. Controversy continues regarding their long-term success rate, partly due to the long learning curve associated with this challenging technique. It is likely that in experienced hands non-penetrating glaucoma surgery with augmentation can achieve a similar long-term success to that seen with penetrating glaucoma surgery.

Deep sclerectomy

Mechanism

Deep sclerectomy is effectively a form of guarded filtration (such as trabeculectomy) but with the rate of drainage being controlled at the level of the trabecular meshwork/Descemet's membrane rather than at the scleral flap.

Outline

Deep sclerectomy involves the formation of conjunctival and superficial scleral flaps, followed by a deep (90% depth) scleral flap to expose Schlemm's canal. Schlemm's canal is then deroofed and its endothelium and juxtacanalicular trabecular meshwork peeled off to improve drainage. Part of the deep scleral flap is then excised to form the deep sclerectomy space. At this stage antifibrotics may be applied and an implant may be inserted. The conjunctival flap is then closed.

Variations

- *Antifibrotics*: in high-risk cases antifibrotic agents are sometimes applied to the deep scleral flap to reduce intrascleral scarring. Although no benefit was demonstrated with 5-FU, some small studies have shown improved IOP control with use of MMC.[1]
- *Implants*: implants may be inserted into the deep scleral space to maintain the space during healing and effectively form an 'intrascleral bleb'. Implants may either be absorbable (e.g. Aquaflow or SKGel) or non-absorbable (e.g. T Flux). Implant use is associated with better IOP control than deep sclerectomy alone: 69% vs 39% achieving IOP <21mmHg off medication at 4yrs.[2]
- *Goniopuncture*: Nd-YAG goniopuncture is usually used as a secondary procedure where sufficient IOP control has not been achieved by the surgical procedure alone; this effectively converts it to a penetrating procedure. In one longer study, goniopuncture was performed in about half of all cases, on average 21mths post-surgery.

Complications

Moderate hypotony (with a deep AC) is to be expected and may transiently affect vision. Causes of high IOP include: (1) inadequate dissection of the trabecular meshwork/Descemet's membrane (treated with Nd:YAG goniopuncture); (2) rupture of the trabecular meshwork/Descemet's membrane by mild ocular trauma (e.g. rubbing, Valsalva manoeuvre) causing iris prolapse and blockage of the drainage site (requires revision of the drainage site and conversion to a conventional trabeculectomy); (3) PAS formation blocking the drainage site (may be reversible with laser iridoplasty). Very rarely detachment of Descemet's membrane may occur. Other complications relating to filtration surgery (see Filtration surgery: complications of penetrating procedures 🕮 pp.346–348) are uncommon in non-penetrating glaucoma surgery.

Viscocanalostomy

Mechanism

Viscocanalostomy, is proposed to work by increasing flow into Schlemm's canal; there is, however, little evidence to support this.

Outline

The procedure is similar to deep sclerectomy with the creation of conjunctival, superficial scleral and deep scleral flaps, and deroofing of Schlemm's canal. However the key feature is that Schlemm's canal is then opened with a viscoelastic, which, it is argued, directly improves drainage by this route, without the need for further thinning of trabecular meshwork. The superficial scleral flap is tightly sutured to minimize filtration into the sub-Tenon's space and to rather encourage drainage into Schlemm's canal.

Variations

• *Antifibrotics and implants*: as with deep scleretomy, both antifibrotics and implants may be used in viscocanalostomy.

Complications

Complications are similar to that seen with deep sclerectomy. Detachment of Descemet's membrane (associated with overvigorous injection of viscoelastic) occurs more commonly than in deep sclerectomy, but is still uncommon.

1. Kozobolis VP *et al.* Primary deep sclerectomy versus primary deep sclerectomy with the use of mitomycin C in primary open angle glaucoma. *J Glaucoma* 2002;**11**:287–293.

2. Shaarawy T, Mermoud A. Deep sclerectomy in one eye vs deep sclerectomy with collagen implant in the contralateral eye of the same patient: long-term follow-up. *Eye* 2005;**19**:298–302.

3. Shaarawy T, *et al.* Long-term results of deep sclerectomy with collagen implant. *J Cataract Refract Surg* 2004;**30**:1225–31.

Uveitis

Anatomy and physiology

Uveitis describes intraocular inflammation both of the uveal tract itself and of neighbouring structures (e.g. retina, vitreous, optic nerve).

Uveitis is relatively common with an incidence of about 15 new cases per 100 000 population per year, and acute presentations (often recurrences) making a significant contribution to the emergency ophthalmic workload.

Anatomy

The uveal tract comprises the iris, ciliary body, and choroid.

Iris

This is the most anterior part of the uveal tract. It extends from its relatively thin root in the AC angle to the pupil. It is divided by the collarette into the central pupillary zone and the peripheral ciliary zone.

The anterior surface is of connective tissue with an incomplete 'border layer' overlying the stroma, which contains the vessels, nerves, and sphincter pupillae. The sphincter pupillae is a ring of true smooth muscle supplied by the short ciliary nerves (III) under parasympathetic control. The posterior surface comprises an epithelial bilayer. The anterior layer of this is lightly pigmented and contains the radial myoepithelial processes of the dilator pupillae, which extend from the iris root. These are supplied by two long ciliary nerves (Va) under sympathetic control.

The anterior layer is continuous with the pigmented outer layer of the ciliary body.

The posterior epithelial layer is cuboidal, densely pigmented, and is continuous with the non-pigmented inner layer of the ciliary body.

Ciliary body

This comprises the ciliary muscle and ciliary epithelium, arranged anatomically as the pars plana and pars plicata (containing the ciliary processes).

The ciliary epithelium is a cuboidal bilayer arranged apex to apex with numerous gap-junctions.

The inner layer is non-pigmented, with high metabolic activity and posteriorly is continuous with the neural retina. The outer layer is pigmented and posteriorly is continuous with the RPE.

Choroid

This is a vascular layer extending from the ora serrata (where it is 0.1mm thick) to the optic disc (0.3mm thick).

From the inside-out it comprises Bruch's membrane (RPE basement membrane, collagen, elastin, collagen, choriocapillaris basement membrane), the choriocapillaris (capillary layer), the stroma (medium-sized vessels in Sattler's layer, large vessels in Haller's layer), and the suprachoroid (a potential space).

Physiology

Iris

Pupillary functions include light regulation, depth of focus, and minimizing optical aberrations. The iris also maintains the blood–aqueous barrier (tight junctions between iris capillary endothelial cells) and contributes to aqueous circulation and outflow (uveoscleral route).

In inflammation there is breakdown of the blood–aqueous barrier leading to flare and cells in the AC.

Ciliary body

The non-pigmented layer contributes to the blood–aqueous barrier (tight junctions between non-pigmented epithelial cells). The non-pigmented and pigmented layers together are responsible for aqueous humour production.

Contraction of the ciliary muscle permits accommodation and increases trabecular outflow. The ciliary body also contributes to the uveoscleral outflow route.

Choroid

With 85% of the ocular blood flow (cf. <5% for the retina) the choroid provides effective supply of oxygen/nutrients, removal of waste products, and heat dissipation. It may also have a significant role in ocular immunity.

Classification of uveitis (1)

The classification of uveitis may be anatomical, clinical, pathological, or aetiological, and all of these may be useful in defining a uveitis entity. Anatomical classification has been formalized by the International Uveitis Study Group and amended by the Standardization of Uveitis Nomenclature Group (2005). Anterior uveitis accounts for the majority of uveitis in Western populations; a much smaller proportion is made up of posterior, intermediate, and panuveitis.

Anatomical classification

Table 11.1 Anatomical classification of uveitis[1]

Type	Primary site of inflammation	Includes
Anterior uveitis	Anterior chanber	Iritis Iridocyclitis Anterior cyclitis
Intermediate uveitis	Vitreous	Pars planitis Posterior cyclitis Hyalitis
Posterior uveitis	Retina or choroid	Focal, multifocal, or diffuse choroiditis Chorioretinitis Retinochoroiditis Retinitis Neuroretinitis
Panuveitis	Anterior chanber, vitreous, and retina or choroid	

1. Jabs DA et al; Standardization of uveitis Nomenclature (SUN) Working Group Am J Ophthalmol 2005; 14: 509–16

Clinical classification

The most recent clinical classification of uveitis is outlined in Table 11.2. Clinical behaviour may be further described in terms of onset, duration, and course of uveitis (Table 11.3).

Table 11.2 IUSG clinical classification of uveitis[1]

Group	Subgroup
Infectious	Bacterial Viral Fungal Parasitic Others
Non-infectious	Known systemic association No known systemic association
Masquerade	Neoplastic Non-neoplastic

1. Deschenes J, Murray PI, Rao NA, Nussenblatt RB; International Uveitis Study Group. International Uveitis Study Group (IUSG): clinical classification of uveitis. *Ocul Immunol Inflamm* 2008;**16**:1–2.

Table 11.3 Descriptors of uveitis[1]

Type	Descriptor	Definition
Onset	Sudden Insidious	
Duration	Limited Persistent	≤ 3mths >3mths
Course	Acute Recurrent Chronic	Sudden onset + limited duration Repeated episodes; inactive periods ≥3mths off treatment Persistent; relapse in <3mths off treatment

1. *Jabs DA et al; Standardization of uveitis Nomenclature (SUN) Working Group Am J Ophthalmol 2005; 14: 509–16.*

Pathological classification

Pathological classification separates granulomatous and non-granulomatous uveitis.

The term 'granulomatous' is sometimes used in the clinical context to describe uveitis with large, greasy 'mutton fat' keratic precipitates (macrophages), and iris nodules (which may include Koeppe and Busacca nodules). However, this is strictly a histological term and is not accurate as a clinical descriptor. Indeed this clinical picture may be seen in diseases with non-granulomatous histopathology, and true granulomatous diseases may present with 'non-granulomatous' uveitis.

Aetiological classification

An aetiological classification helps define the cause, context, and treatment options for the disease, but in many patients a 'true' aetiology is not found.

Classification of uveitis (2)

Differential diagnosis of uveitis by anatomical type

Table 11.4 Differential diagnosis of uveitis by anatomical location (selected)

Anatomical type			Diagnoses
Anterior			Idiopathic
			HLA-B27 group
			JIA
			FHU
			Sarcoidosis
			Syphilis
			Posner–Schlossman
Intermediate			Idiopathic (pars planitis)
			MS
			Sarcoidosis
			IBD
			Lyme disease
Posterior	**Retinitis**	**Focal**	Idiopathic
			Toxoplasma
			Onchocerciasis
			Cysticercosis
			Masquerade
		Multifocal	Idiopathic
			Syphilis
			HSV
			VZV
			CMV
			Sarcoidosis
			Masquerade
			Candidiasis
	Choroiditis	**Focal**	Idiopathic
			Toxocariasis
			TB
			Masquerade
		Multifocal	Idiopathic
			Histoplasmosis/POHS
			Sympathetic ophthalmia
			VKH
			Sarcoidosis
			Serpiginous
			Birdshot
			Masquerade
			MEWDS
Pan			Idiopathic
			Sarcoidosis
			Behçet's disease
			VKH
			Infective endophthalmitis
			Syphilis

Uveitis: assessment

All patients require a detailed history (ophthalmic and general) and a thorough ophthalmic examination, including dilated fundoscopy of both eyes (Table 11.5).

In some cases a systemic examination may also be necessary. For example, an apparently classic AAU may have posterior segment involvement (notably CMO), be part of a panuveitis and have systemic involvement (e.g. sarcoid).

Table 11.5 An approach to assessing uveitis

Symptoms	Anterior: photophobia, redness, watering, pain, ↓VA; may be asymptomatic Intermediate: floaters, photopsia, ↓VA Posterior: ↓VA, photopsia, floaters, scotomata
POH	Previous episodes and investigations; surgery/trauma
PMH	Arthropathies (e.g. ankylosing spondylitis), chronic infections (e.g. HSV, tuberculosis), systemic inflammation (e.g. sarcoid, Behçet's disease)
SR	Detailed review of all systems
FH	Family members with uveitis or related diseases
SH	Travel/residence abroad, pets, IV drugs, sexual Hx
Dx	Including any systemic immunosuppression
Ax	Allergies or relevant drug contraindications
Visual acuity	Best-corrected/pin-hole; near
Visual function	Check for RAPD, colour vision
Conjunctiva	Circumcorneal injection
Cornea	Band keratopathy, keratic precipitates (distribution, size, pigment)
AC	Flare/cells, fibrin, hypopyon
Gonioscopy	PAS (consider if ↑IOP)
Iris	Transillumination defects/sectoral atrophy, miosis, posterior synechiae, heterochromia, Koeppe or Busacca nodules
Lens	Cataract, aphakia/pseudophakia
Tonometry	
Dilated fundoscopy	(non-contact handheld lens ± indirect/indenting)
Vitreous	Haze, cells, snowballs, opacities, subhyaloid precipitates (KP-like but on posterior vitreous face)
Optic disc	Disc swelling, glaucomatous changes, atrophy
Vessels	Inflammation (sheathing, leakage), ischaemia (BRAO, B/CRVO, retinal oedema), occlusion
Retina	CMO, uni/multifocal retinitis (blurred white lesions may progress to necrosis, atrophy, or pigmentation)
Choroid	Uni/multifocal choroiditis (deeper yellow-white lesions), associated exudative retinal detachment

Grading of activity

Grading of AC cells and flare (Tables 11.6 and 11.7) is easy and a useful indicator of disease activity. Activity within the vitreous is harder to assess: quantification of vitreous cells is of limited use due to their persistence; degree of vitreous haze is a more useful indicator.

Table 11.6 Grading of AC flare[1]

Grade	Description
0	None
1+	Faint
2+	Moderate (iris + lens clear)
3+	Marked (iris + lens hazy)
4+	Intense (fibrin or plastic aqueous)

1. Jabs DA et al; Standardization of uveitis Nomenclature (SUN) Working Group Am J Ophthalmol 2005; 14: 509–16

Table 11.7 Grading of AC cells (counted with 1mm × 1mm slit)[1]

Activity	Cells
0	<1
0.5+	1–5
1+	6–15
2+	16–25
3+	26–50
4+	>50

1. Jabs DA et al; Standardization of uveitis Nomenclature (SUN) Working Group Am J Ophthalmol 2005; 14: 509–16

Uveitis: systemic review

Table 11.8 Systemic review (not exhaustive), which may provide clues to underlying disease

System	Symptom	Associated disease
CVS	Chest pain—pericarditis	TB, RA, SLE
	Chest pain—myocarditis	Syphilis
	Palpitations	Sarcoidosis, ankylosing spondylitis, syphilis, RA, SLE, HIV
	Oedema—cardiac failure	TB, sarcoidosis, syphilis, RA, SLE, HIV
	Oedema—IVC obstruction	Behçet's disease
RS	Cough	TB, sarcoidosis, Wegener's, HIV, toxocariasis
	Haemoptysis	TB, Wegener's, HIV, RA, SLE, sarcoidosis
	Stridor	Relapsing polychondritis
	Chest pain—pleuritic	Sarcoidosis, TB, Wegener's, SLE, RA, lymphoma, HIV
	Shortness of breath	Sarcoidosis, TB, Wegener's, SLE, RA, HIV
GI	Diarrhoea	IBD, Behçet's, HIV
	Blood/mucus in stools	IBD, Behçet's, HIV
	Jaundice	IBD (with cholangitis or hepatitis) toxoplasmosis, HIV
GU	Dysuria/discharge	Reiter's, syphilis, TB
	Haematuria	Wegener's, IgA nephropathy, TINU, SLE, TB
	Genital ulcers	Behçet's, syphilis, HLA-B27-related disease
	Testicular pain	Behçet's, HLA-B27-related disease
ENT	Deafness/tinnitus	VKH, sympathetic ophthalmia, Wegener's
	Earlobe pain/swelling	Relapsing polychondritis
	Oral ulcers	Behçet's, HSV, HLA-B27-related disease, SLE
	Sinus problems	Wegener's
	Recurrent epistaxis	Wegener's
Musculo-skeletal	Joint pain/swelling/stiffness	HLA-B27-related arthropathies, JIA, sarcoidosis, RA, SLE, Behçet's, relapsing polychondritis, Wegener's, Lyme
	Lower back pain	HLA-B27-related arthropathies, TB
Skin	Rash—erythema nodosum	Sarcoidosis, Behçet's, TB, IBD
	Rash—vesicular	HSV, VZV
	Rash—other	Psoriasis, syphilis, Lyme, SLE, Behçet's, Reiter's, JIA, TB
	Photosensitivity	SLE
	Vitiligo	SLE, VKH, sympathetics opthalmia, leprosy

Table 11.8 (Continued)

System	Symptom	Associated disease
	Alopecia	SLE, VKH
	Raynaud's phenomenon	SLE, RA
CNS	Headaches	Sarcoidosis, VKH, Behçet's, TB, SLE, lymphoma
	Collapse or fits	Sarcoidosis, VKH, Behçet's, SLE, HIV, toxoplasmosis, lymphoma
	Weakness	MS, sarcoidosis, Behçet's, HIV, leprosy, syphilis, toxoplasmosis, lymphoma
	Numbness/tingling	MS, sarcoidosis, Behçet's, HIV, leprosy, lymphoma
	Loss of balance	MS, sarcoidosis, Behçet's, VKH, HIV, syphilis, lymphoma
	Speech problems	MS, sarcoidosis, Behçet's, HIV, lymphoma
	Behaviour change	VKH, sarcoidosis, Behçet's, SLE, Wegener's, HIV, TB, syphilis, lymphoma
General	Fever/night sweats	JIA, lymphoma, VKH, SLE, RA, IBD, sarcoidosis, Kawasaki
	Swollen glands	Sarcoidosis, lymphoma, HIV, JIA, TB, RA, syphilis, toxoplasmosis

Uveitis: investigations

When to investigate

Ideally, one would perform the minimum number of investigations to gain the maximum amount of information. The usefulness of the test will depend on the pre-test probability of the diagnosis and the specificity and sensitivity of the test. Consider also the potential morbidity of certain tests (e.g. in FFA or vitreous biopsy). In general, investigations may be performed for:

- *Diagnosis*: by identifying causative or associated systemic disease; by identifying a definite aetiology (e.g. an organism).
- *Management*: monitoring disease activity/complications (e.g. OCT for macular oedema); monitoring potential side-effects of treatment (e.g. blood tests for some immunosuppressants).

Role of investigations in diagnosis

The aetiology of most uveitis is unknown, although an autoimmune/autoinflammatory cause is often proposed. In most cases a careful history and examination provides the majority if not all of the information need for diagnosis. Some uveitis syndromes, such as FHC, Behçet's, and toxoplasmosis are diagnosed purely on clinical grounds.

Investigations are helpful in identifying uveitis of infective origin (e.g. TB, HSV, etc.) or systemic disease (e.g. lymphoma, sarcoidosis, demyelination). The role of some investigations is controversial, e.g. when to test HLA-B27 status.

Role of investigations in management

Monitoring disease

This is almost entirely by clinical examination; however, in certain situations investigations may be helpful. For example:

- *OCT*: extremely useful in establishing macular causes of worsening vision, particularly where clinical diagnosis is difficult due to imperfect visualization or pre-existing macular disease (e.g. epiretinal membrane, CMO, macular hole, vitreo-macular traction); this has largely replaced FFA for this purpose.
- *FFA*: particularly helpful in assessing retinal vascular involvement (leakage, ischaemia), neovascularization, and optic disc leakage.
- *EDTs*: required for monitoring birdshot retinochoroidopathy.
- *Visual fields*: for monitoring optic nerve damage either due to disease or associated ↑IOP.

Monitoring therapies

Regular BP, weight, BM, and urinalysis are recommended for patients on systemic corticosteroids. Blood tests (e.g. FBC, U+E, LFT) are necessary for some of the other immunosuppressive agents Antimetabolites, calcineurin inhibitors, and cytotoxics 📖 pp.872–873 and Biologics 📖 pp.874–875.

Table 11.9 Suggested investigations in diagnosis of uveitis types

	Investigation	Consider
Base-line	FBC	
	ESR	
	Syphilis serology	Syphilis
	ANA (in children)	
	Urinalysis	TINU (protein), diabetes (glucose)
	CXR	TB, sarcoidosis
Selective	ACE	Sarcoidosis
	ANCA	Wegener's (PR3)
	Toxoplasma serology	Toxoplasmosis
	Toxocara ELISA	Toxocariasis
	Borrelia serology	Lyme disease
	HLA-B27	B27-associated disease
	HLA-A29	Birdshot retinochoroidopathy
	Mantoux test	TB, sarcoidosis
	Fundus fluorescein angiography	
	Electrophysiology	
	Ultrasound B-scan	
	High-resolution CT thorax	Sarcoidosis
	CT orbits	
	MRI head scan	Demyelination, sarcoidosis, lymphoma
	Gallium scan	Sarcoidosis
	Lumbar puncture	Demyelination, lymphoma
	Conjunctival biopsy	Sarcoidosis
	PCR of intraocular fluid	Infection
	Vitreous biopsy	Infection, lymphoma
	Choroidal biopsy	Lymphoma

Uveitis: complications and treatment

Complications

- *Main complications of intraocular inflammation* are: cataract, CMO, and glaucomatous optic neuropathy. These may occur in isolation, but often in combination.
- *Other complications include*: band keratopathy, vitreous debris/vitritis, retinal detachment, non-glaucomatous optic neuropathy, choroidal neovascularization, macular scar, macular hole, epiretinal membrane, retinal scars, subretinal fibrosis.

Treatment

- Treatment of non-infectious uveitis may be medical or surgical, or a combination of both. Medical therapy is primarily corticosteroid and can be given topically, periocularly, intravitreally, and systemically.
- Systemic immunosuppressants (and biologicals) may need to be added in resistant, sight-threatening cases.
- The use of anti-VEGF agents, such as intravitreal bevacizumab may play a part in the treatment of choroidal neovascularization and macular oedema.
- Secondary ↑IOP is normally treated with the many topical therapies that are now available, and they may need to be given in combination.
- Although topical prostaglandin analogues have been implicated in causing uveitis and CMO, they are not contraindicated in uveitis patients.
- *Surgery includes*: cataract, glaucoma, and vitreoretinal procedures.

Acute anterior uveitis

Anterior uveitis accounts for about 75–90% of all cases of uveitis. It represents a wide spectrum of disease; it may be isolated, part of a panuveitis, or part of a systemic disease.

Idiopathic acute anterior uveitis (AAU)

In about 50% of patients with AAU it occurs in isolation (i.e. HLA-B27 negative with no underlying systemic disease). It affects any age (biphasic peaking at 30 and 60yrs), and both sexes equally. It is almost always unilateral but may affect both eyes sequentially.

Recurrences are common; rarely it may become persistent.

Clinical features
- Pain, photophobia, redness, blurred vision.
- Circumlimbal injection, keratic precipitates (especially inferior), AC flare/cells, PS, vitreous cells.

Treatment
Frequent potent topical steroid (e.g. dexamethasone 0.1% or prednisolone acetate 1% up to every 30min initially, titrating according to disease) and dilate (e.g. cyclopentolate 1% 3×/d; atropine 1% 3×/d in severe cases)—this may be the only chance to break the synechiae; if poor dilation consider subconjunctival mydricaine no. 2 (procaine/amethocaine/adrenaline); subconjunctival betamethasone may also be necessary.

NB if not responding after 48h of half-hourly drops may require expert advice (e.g. consideration of oral corticosteroids).

HLA-B27 associated acute anterior uveitis

Up to 50% of patients with AAU are HLA-B27 positive (cf. 8% in the general population). B27-related disease peaks at 30yrs of age, is commoner in males and is associated with a positive family history. It may be associated with ankylosing spondylitis, Reiter's disease, and less commonly, psoriasis or inflammatory bowel disease. It is almost always unilateral but may affect both eyes sequentially ('flip-flop'); rarely may become persistent. Inflammation is often more severe and recurrences more frequent than in idiopathic AAU.

Clinical features
- Pain, photophobia, redness, blurred vision.
- Anterior segment inflammation may be severe: circumlimbal injection, keratic precipitates (especially inferior), AC flare/cells/fibrin (fibrin is a key feature in HLA-B27-associated uveitis) ± hypopyon, PS, vitreous cells.

Treatment
As for idiopathic AAU.

Other causes

Although the vast majority of AAU is idiopathic or HLA-B27-related, it is important to be keep an open mind. 'Atypical' features may suggest an alternative diagnosis requiring different treatment. Important differential diagnoses include:

Herpes viral group (HSV, VZV) anterior uveitis

Consider if: unilateral persistent anterior uveitis with patchy iris atrophy/transillumination defects/semidilated pupil, ↑IOP ± evidence of active/previous keratitis (see 📖 p.392).

Posner–Schlossman syndrome

Consider if: ↑IOP (40–80mmHg), white eye, few keratic precipitates, minimal flare, occasional AC cells, no synechiae (PS or PAS), open angle (see 📖 p.372).

Systemic disease

AAU is associated with a number of systemic diseases, some of which may be undiagnosed at the time of presentation. For example, a fibrinous uveitis in a middle-aged adult may be the first presentation of their diabetes.

Systemic diseases to consider include: diabetes, sarcoidosis, vascular disease (e.g. carotid artery stenosis), and renal disease (e.g. TINU, IgA nephropathy).

Table 11.10 Comparison of HLA-B27 positive vs negative AAU

	HLA-B27 positive	HLA-B27 negative
Age at onset (yrs)	32–35	39–48
Gender	M:F 1.5–2.5:1	1:1
Eye involvement	Unilateral 48–59%	Bilateral 21–64%
	Alternating 29–36%	
Pattern of uveitis	Acute in 80–87%	Chronic in 43–61%
Recurrence	Frequent	Uncommon
Keratic precipitate	Mutton fat keratic precipitate in 0–3%	Mutton fat keratic precipitate in 17–46%
Fibrin in anterior chamber	25–56%	0–10%
Hypopyon	12–15%	0–2%
Associated systemic disease	48–84%	1–13%
Family history	Yes	No
Posterior synechiae	40.4%	18.7%
Cataract	12.9%	13.6%
Ocular hypertension	11.4%	11.4%
Glaucoma	4.4%	6.6%
Cystoid macular oedema	11.7%	1.0%

Table published in Albert & Jakobiec's *Principles and practice of ophthalmology* (3rd edn) by Albert and Miller, p 1139. Copyright Elsevier; reproduced by kind permission.

Uveitis with HLA-B27-related arthropathies

HLA-B27 is a type I major histocompatibility complex (Ch6) molecule: a cell surface polypeptide involved in presenting antigen to the immune system. There are 24 subtypes of HLA-B27, encoded by 26 different alleles. Subtypes vary by ethnic origin, and some are more highly associated with inflammatory disease, notably HLA-B*2705 (the ancestral type), B*2702 (more common in white people), and B*2704 (more common in Asians).

HLA-B27 is present in 8% of the general population, but is seen in up to 50% of patients with AAU and is strongly linked to the seronegative spondyloarthropathies. This is a group of overlapping inflammatory conditions that, as the name suggests, are negative for rheumatoid factor and generally include an axial (spinal) arthritis. They may all be associated with uveitis.

Ankylosing spondylitis

AS is a chronic spondyloarthropathy, predominantly affecting the spine and sacroiliac joints. More common in males, it usually presents in early adulthood. Of those with AS: 95% are HLA-B27 positive; 25% will develop anterior uveitis; of these 80% will have involvement of both eyes, but nearly always sequentially.

Clinical features
- *Ophthalmic*: AAU; unilateral but may affect both eyes sequentially ('flip-flop'); rarely may become persistent.
- *Systemic*: axial arthritis, sacroiliitis, kyphosis, stiffness, enthesitis, aortic regurgitation.

Treatment
- *Ophthalmic*: as for idiopathic AAU (see 📖 p.368).
- *Systemic*: investigation and treatment by rheumatologist. This may include lumbar spinal X-ray (bamboo spine; sacroiliitis) and HLA-B27 status; treatment may include oral NSAIDs; physiotherapy.

Reiter syndrome (reactive arthritis)

Reiter syndrome describes a reactive arthritis, urethritis (or cervicitis), and conjunctivitis occurring after a sexually transmitted or dysenteric infection. Candidates include *Chlamydia, Yersinia, Salmonella*, and *Shigella*. Of those with Reiter syndrome: 70% are HLA-B27 positive; 50% will develop conjunctivitis, and 12% anterior uveitis.

Clinical features
- *Ophthalmic*: bilateral mucopurulent conjunctivitis; acute anterior uveitis; keratitis (punctate epitheliopathy, subepithelial infiltrates).
- *Systemic*: oligoarthritis (typically knees, ankles, sacroiliac joints), enthesitis (incl. plantar fasciitis), aphthous oral ulcers, circinate balanitis, keratoderma blenorrhagica (scaling skin rash on the soles).

Treatment
- *Ophthalmic*: conjunctivitis—self-limiting; AAU—see p.368.
- *Systemic*: investigation and treatment by rheumatologist.

Inflammatory bowel disease

Of those with ulcerative colitis and Crohn's disease, about 5% will develop anterior uveitis.

Clinical features
- *Ophthalmic*: AAU; rarely epi/scleritis or retinal vasculitis.
- *Systemic*: gut inflammation (patchy, transmural, anywhere from mouth to anus in Crohn's; continuous, superficial, colorectal in ulcerative colitis), cholangitis, chronic active hepatitis, arthritis (oligo- or AS-like), rash (erythema nodosum, pyoderma gangrenosum).

Treatment
- *Ophthalmic*: see Idiopathic AAU (🕮 p.368).
- *Systemic*: investigation and treatment by gastroenterologist.

Psoriatic arthritis

Of those with psoriasis, 10% will develop psoriatic arthritis, and of these 10% will develop anterior uveitis.

Clinical features
- *Ophthalmic*: conjunctivitis; AAU; rarely keratitis (peripheral corneal infiltrates).
- *Systemic*: salmon pink lesions with silvery scaling, which may be in isolated plaques (more common on extensor rather than flexor surfaces) or as a pustular rash (soles and palms or, more seriously, generalized); nail changes (pitting, onychlysis, oil-drop); arthritis may be axial (AS-like), oligoarthritis (Reiter's-like), distal interphalangeal joints (OA-like) with nail changes, symmetrical peripheral arthropathy (RA-like), or arthritis mutilans.

Treatment
- *Ophthalmic*: the conjunctivitis is self-limiting; treat anterior uveitis, see Idiopathic AAU 🕮 p.368.
- *Systemic*: investigation and treatment by dermatologist and rheumatologist.

Anterior uveitis syndromes (1)

Fuchs' heterochromic uveitis (syn Fuchs heterochromic cyclitis)

This is an uncommon, 'chronic', 'non-granulomatous' anterior uveitis of unknown cause, although rubella virus has recently been implicated. It typically affects young adults and there is no gender bias. It is unilateral in about 90%.

Clinical features
- Floaters, glare; ↓VA due to cataract ± vitreous opacities; may be asymptomatic.
- White eye, white stellate KPs over whole corneal endothelium, mild flare, few cells, iris atrophy (washed out, moth-eaten), transillumination defects (not sectoral), abnormal iris vessels, iris heterochromia with the affected eye appearing 'bluer', heterochromia difficult to assess in brown irides, iris nodules Koeppe > Busacca are frequently seen; no PS; cataract in about 80% of cases (posterior subcapsular), vitreous opacities are commonly seen, ↑IOP in 10–15% leading to secondary glaucoma in some cases. Iris crystals are infrequently seen.
- *Gonioscopy*: open angle; ± twig-like neovascularization of the angle; these may lead to hyphaema in response to paracentesis (Amsler haemorrhage).

Treatment
- *Of inflammatory process*: not usually necessary, as topical corticosteroid appears ineffective, and mydriatic unnecessary as PS do not form.
- *Of cataract*: conventional phakoemulsification but with careful postoperative control of inflammation 🕮 p.288. Corticosteroid prophylaxis is not required prior to surgery. Excellent visual outcome with 90% patients achieving 6/9 vision. A large Amsler haemorrhage at surgery may result in a poorer visual outcome.
- *Of ↑IOP*: treat as for POAG (see 🕮 p.308), but may require augmented drainage surgery/tube.

Posner–Schlossman syndrome

This is an inflammatory glaucoma syndrome characterized by recurrent unilateral episodes of very high IOP with only mild AC activity. It typically affects young males. The suggested aetiology is of acute trabeculitis, perhaps secondary to herpesvirus, e.g. HSV.

Clinical features
- Blurring of vision, haloes, painless.
- ↑IOP (40–80mmHg), white eye, few keratic precipitates, minimal flare, occasional AC cells, no synechiae (PS or PAS), open angle.

Treatment
- *Of inflammatory process*: topical steroid (e.g. dexamethasone 0.1% or prednisolone acetate 1% 4×/d initially, titrating according to disease).
- *Of ↑IOP*: consider topical (e.g. β-blocker, α-agonist, carbonic anhydrase inhibitor, prostaglandin analogue) or systemic (e.g. acetazolamide) according to IOP level.

Anterior segment ischaemia

This is an uncommon but important cause of anterior uveitis, particularly in the elderly.

Clinical features

- Dull ache, usually unilateral.
- AC significant flare/moderate cells, sluggish pupil; if part of ocular ischaemic syndrome there may also be dilated irregular retinal veins (not tortuous), attenuated retinal arterioles, mid-peripheral retinal haemorrhages, rubeosis, and posterior segment neovascularization.

Investigate: for carotid artery stenosis with carotid Doppler ultrasound and refer to vascular surgeon if indicated.

Schwartz syndrome

This is the uncommon association of anterior segment inflammation (mild) and ↑IOP (with an open angle) arising from a RRD. Detachments most commonly associated with this syndrome were large in area (and macula-off), flat in height, and long in duration. Postulated mechanisms include mechanical blockage by photoreceptor outer segments and trabeculitis.

Refer to a vitreoretinal team for assessment and repair (see 📖 pp.426–429). The ↑IOP and anterior uveitis may be treated medically in the interim but tend to resolve rapidly with surgical repair.

Anterior uveitis syndromes (2)

Tubulointerstitial nephritis with uveitis

This is the rare association of tubulointerstitial nephritis (often presenting as acute renal failure) and uveitis. It typically affects young females (median age 15; F:M 3:1) but can occur at almost any age. It is commonly idiopathic but may be associated with drugs (NSAIDs, penicillin, frusemide) or infection (*Streptococci, Staphylococci*, etc.).

Clinical features

- *Uveitis*: usually anterior (80%), bilateral (77%), and most often presents after the systemic disease (65%); uveitis may recur or follow a persistent course in over 50%. Ocular complications include PS, ↑IOP, and cataract.
- *Renal disease*: usually recovers, but chronic renal impairment occurs in 11%, with dialysis being required in 4%.

Investigations

- *Serum*: ↑creatinine, ↑ESR.
- *Urine*: proteinuria, haematuria, ↑β_2-microglobulin levels, sterile pyuria.
- *Renal biopsy*: required for definitive diagnosis; shows oedema in the renal interstitium with predominantly mononuclear infiltrate of activated T cells, plasma cells, and histiocytes. The glomerular and vascular structures are relatively unaffected.

Treatment

The renal disease is commonly treated with systemic steroids; for treatment of uveitis, *see* Idiopathic AAU (📖 p.368).

IgA nephropathy

This is a relatively common renal disease of children in young adults in which recurrent micro- or macroscopic haematuria may be related to respiratory tract infections. In some patients, episodes are associated with an anterior uveitis—for treatment, *see* Idiopathic AAU (📖 p.368).

Kawasaki disease

This is an uncommon acute vasculitis of children defined as fever (≥5d) with four of the following five criteria: conjunctival injection, rash, desquamation of extremities, cervical lymphadenopathy, and mucosal changes (pharyngeal injection, cracked red lips, strawberry tongue). An anterior uveitis is common in the first week of illness; rarely disc oedema and dilated retinal vessels are seen. Most seriously cardiac abnormalities (notably coronary artery aneurysms) occur in 20%.

Uveitis with juvenile idiopathic arthritis

JIA is the commonest chronic rheumatic disease of childhood. It is a heterogeneous group of disorders characterized by a chronic inflammatory arthritis.

One or more joints are affected with swelling or limited joint range and pain on movement for at least 6wks, with the age at onset being less than 16yrs. JIA is more common in females than males. The incidence is 5–18 per 100 000, with prevalence of approximately 1 per 1000 children although the prevalence may be higher, as many children may be undiagnosed, or incorrectly diagnosed.

JIA is classified using the ILAR (International League of Associations of Rheumatologists) Classification (Box 11.1). The prevalence of uveitis in JIA overall is approximately 8–30%, but in young oligoarticular onset group (i.e. arthritis in which up to 4 joints are involved) it may be as high as 45–57%.

Risk factors for uveitis are: young age at diagnosis, female sex, antinuclear antibody positivity, and the subtype of JIA, in particular the persistent and extended oligoarthritis groups.

Classification

> Box 11.1 Classification of JIA (ILAR)
>
> • Systemic arthritis
> • Oligoarthritis—persistent
> • Oligoarthritis—extended
> • Polyarthritis—RF negative
> • Polyarthritis—RF positive
> • Psoriatic arthritis
> • Enthesitis-related arthritis
> • Undifferentiated arthritis

Clinical features

Ophthalmic

• Asymptomatic; rarely floaters; ↓VA from cataract.
• White eye, band keratopathy, small KPs, AC cells/flare, PS, cataract, secondary glaucoma, vitritis, cystoid macular oedema; other complications include hypotony that may lead to phthisis bulbi.

NB In long-standing uveitis chronic breakdown of the blood aqueous barrier leads to persistent flare; AC cells are therefore a better guide than flare to disease activity.

Screening

Principles

• **Initial screening examination:** Uveitis often starts soon after onset of arthritis but may also start before the arthritis. **The initial screening examination is therefore a clinical priority** and should occur as soon as possible and no later than **6wks** from referral.
• **Symptomatic patients** or patients suspected of cataracts or synechiae should be seen within **1wk** of referral.

Table 11.11 Summary of follow-up for JIA (Guidelines for Screening for Uveitis in JIA by the Royal College of Ophthalmologists and the British Society for Paediatric and Adolescent Rheumatology 2006)

First screening: within 6wks of referral
Subsequent screening
Every 2mths from onset of arthritis for 6mths then every 3–4mths for duration see table
Duration of screening

Disease type/ANA status	Age of onset	Duration
Oligoarticular, psoriatic and enthesitis-related irrespective of ANA status	<3yrs	8yrs
	3–4yrs	6yrs
	5–8yrs	3yrs
Polyarticular, ANA+	9–10yrs	1yr
	<6ys	5yrs
Polyarticular, ANA-	6–9yrs	2yrs
	<7yrs	5yrs

Alternatively all the above groups may be screened until 11–12yrs old. Older patients (>11yrs) should be screened for 1yr.

Treatment

- *Of uveitis:* refer to a tertiary referral centre for advice about specific immunosuppression if (1) complications are present at onset, or (2) if the disease is active after 2yrs of topical treatment. Management of complex cases is optimized in tertiary centres with joint clinics between a paediatric rheumatologist and specialist ophthalmologist. *Treatment options* include topical steroid eye drops mydriatics, sub-tenon injections of steroids, orbital floor injections occasionally systemic steroids (IV methylprednisolone pulses or oral prednisolone) and increasingly with weekly methotrexate. Ciclosporin. Mycophenolate and anti-TNF agents (infliximab, adalimumab) may also be considered.
- *Of ↑IOP:* initially topical therapy, but up to two-thirds may require surgery (commonly an augmented trabeculectomy or a tube procedure).
- *Of cataract:* aim to defer until the eye has been quiet for a minimum of 3mths although weigh against the risk of amblyopia in younger children; there is considerable debate over surgery, including whether to implant a lens or leave aphakic.
- *Of band keratopathy:* chelation with EDTA or excimer phototherapeutic keratectomy.

Intermediate uveitis

The term intermediate uveitis refers to uveitis where the vitreous is the major site of inflammation The term pars planitis may be used where there is snowbank or snowball formation occurring in the absence of an associated infection or systemic disease (i.e. idiopathic).

Intermediate uveitis accounts for about 10% of all cases of uveitis. It is bimodal being commonest in young adults, but with a second peak in the middle aged/elderly. Males and females are equally affected. It is bilateral in 80%, but is often asymmetric.

Clinical features
- Floaters, ↓VA (may indicate macular oedema); may be asymptomatic.
- Vitritis (cells, 'snowballs'), exudation at the ora serrata ('snowbanking', commonly inferior but can be 360°), peripheral periphlebitis, rarely vitreous haemorrhage; some AC activity is common.
- *Complications*: CMO, cataract, secondary glaucoma, cyclitic membrane, tractional retinal detachment, retinal tears, vitreomacular traction, epiretinal membrane, retinal neovascularization.

Investigation
Consider FBC, U&E, ESR, VDRL, TPHA, urinalysis, CXR for all patients; further investigation should be directed by clinical indication (Table 11.12). OCT or FFA may be helpful to confirm CMO.

Table 11.12 Associations of intermediate uveitis

Group	Cause	Consider
Primary ocular	Idiopathic/pars planitis	After exclusion of other associations
Secondary systemic	MS	MRI brain, LP
	Sarcoid	ACE, Ca, CXR, CT thorax
	Inflammatory bowel disease	Bowel studies, biopsy
	CNS/intraocular lymphoma	MRI brain, LP
Secondary infective	*Toxocara*	Serology
	Lyme disease	Serology
	HTLV-1	Serology

Treatment
Observation
If no CMO and VA > 6/12 then monitor only.

Medical therapy
- *Topical*: if significant AC activity control with topical corticosteroids and mydriatics (e.g. cyclopentolate 1% 1–2×/d).
- *Periocular/systemic*: if CMO or visually disabling floaters consider periocular corticosteroid (e.g. orbital floor/subtenons methylprednisolone/triamcinolone 40mg) for unilateral disease or systemic corticosteroids (e.g. prednisolone initially 1mg/kg/d and titrating down or pulsed methylprednisolone 500–1000mg three doses daily or alternate days in severe cases), ± other immunosuppressives (e.g. methotrexate, azathioprine, ciclosporin, mycophenolate mofetil)

normally reserved for bilateral or resistant disease, or failure to get oral corticosteroid dose to <10mg/d, or intolerable corticosteroid side-effects. There may be a role for anti-TNF (infliximab, adalimumab) in highly resistant cases.

- *Intraocular*: intravitreal triamcinolone 4mg—complications similar for periocular therapy, but also ↑IOP and sterile endophthalmitis. Fluocinolone acetonide intravitreal sustained release device (Retisert®) has shown significant reductions in the number of inflammatory episodes and decreased reliance on systemic corticosteroids or other immunomodulatory therapies, but a high incidence of ocular hypertension and glaucoma.

Surgical therapy

- *Vitrectomy*: indications include vitreous opacities, CMO, vitreo-macular traction, epiretinal membrane, retinal detachment. It may be combined with phakoemulsification and intraocular lens implant for visually disabling cataract. Often intravitreal triamcinolone 4mg is given at the end of surgery providing there are no contra-indications (e.g. known steroid induced rise in IOP).
- Cataract surgery is frequently required.
- Glaucoma surgery may be needed if there is a failure of medical therapy.

Retinal vasculitis

Retinal vasculitis (Tables 11.13 and 11.14) comprises inflammation of the retinal vasculature. It may be a primary ocular disease or secondary to either infection or systemic disease.

Clinical features

- ↓VA, floaters, positive scotomata; may be asymptomatic if peripheral.
- Perivascular sheathing of arteries, veins, or capillaries; retinal haemorrhages; vitritis; disc swelling, CMO.
- *Complications*: B/CRVO, neovascularization, vitreous haemorrhage, ischaemic maculopathy, tractional RD.

Investigations

- *FFA*: vessel wall staining, vascular leakage, skip lesions, widespread capillary leakage, new vessel leakage, disc leakage, petalloid macular leakage, enlarged foveal avascular zone (ischaemia), vascular occlusion, capillary 'drop-out'.
- Consider FBC, U&E, ESR, VDRL, TPHA, ANA, ANCA, urinalysis, CXR for all patients; further investigation should be directed by clinical indication (see 🕮 Table 11.13).

Treatment

- Where possible the underlying disease is treated e.g. with antibiotics for infective cases.
- Treatment options are similar to those used for intermediate uveitis (see Intermediate uveitis 🕮 p.378).
- In most instances immunosuppression is required. Corticosteroids are first line and may be periocular, oral (e.g. prednisolone 1–2mg/kg), IV (e.g. pulsed methylprednisolone 500–1000mg three doses daily or alternate days), or intraocular (intravitreal triamcinolone or fluocinolone acetonide intravitreal sustained release device). Ciclosporin and azathioprine tend to be used second line, although methotrexate, mycophenolate, tacrolimus, sirolimus, anti-TNF e.g. infliximab/adalimumab and α-interferon (mainly in Behçet's), and cyclophosphamide (mainly in Wegener's) also have their place.

Table 11.13 Causes of Renal Vasculitis

Group	Cause	Consider
Primary ocular	Intermediate uveitis	Urine, blood glucose
	Birdshot retinochoroidopathy	EDTs
	Eales' disease	PPD skin test, CXR
	VKH	
	Sympathetic ophthalmia	
Secondary infective	CMV	PCR
	HSV	PCR
	VZV	PCR
	HTLV-1	Serology
	HIV	Serology, CD4 count
	Toxoplasmosis	Serology
	Tuberculosis	PPD skin test, CXR
	Lyme disease	Serology
	Cat scratch disease	Serology, PCR
	Syphilis	Serology (VDRL, TPHA)
	Whipple's disease	PCR
Secondary systemic	Leukaemia	FBC LP, bone marrow
	Lymphoma	MRI brain LP
	SLE	ANA, dsDNA
	Behçet's disease	Pathergy
	Sarcoidosis	ACE, Ca, CXR, HRCT thorax
	Wegener's granulomatosis	c-ANCA (PR3)
	PAN	p-ANCA, tissue biopsy
	Antiphospholipid syndrome	Anticardiolipin antibodies

Table 11.14 Diagnostic pointers in retinal vasculitis

Clinical feature	Possible cause of vasculitis
Arteritis	ARN (HSV, VZV)
BRVO	Behçet's disease
RPE changes	TB
	Sarcoidosis
	Lymphoma
Capillary closure	TB
	MS
	Sarcoidosis

Sarcoidosis (1)

This relatively common granulomatous multisystem disorder may be life-threatening. The eye is affected in up to 25% of patients. Of these, anterior uveitis occurs in 60% and posterior segment disease occurs in 25% of patients. Sarcoid affects up to 0.1% of the population, being higher in females and with peaks in the third and sixth decades. It is commoner in African-Caribbeans, Irish, and Scandinavians.

The cause of sarcoidosis is unknown; there is PCR evidence for several agents (including atypical mycobacteria) that may trigger the disease in susceptible individuals. The Th1 response predominates in typical sarcoid granulomas, although it appears that a transition to the Th2 response underlies progressive pulmonary fibrosis.

The presentation may be acute or insidious. An acute presentation, typically with erythema nodosum and bihilar lymphadenopathy, has a better prognosis. The course tends to be self-limiting although steroids may hasten recovery. An insidious presentation is more commonly followed by a relentless progression to pulmonary fibrosis.

Classification

Recently, a number of diagnostic criteria have been proposed for intraocular sarcoidosis (Table 11.15):

Clinical features

Ophthalmic

- *Anterior uveitis* (2/3 are persistent, 1/3 acute; unilateral or bilateral; 'granulomatous'): circumlimbal injection, mutton-fat keratic precipitates, AC flare/cells, PS, vitreous cells; iris granulomas and nodules.
- *Intermediate uveitis*: vitreous cells, snowballs, snowbanking.
- *Posterior uveitis*: CMO (commonest cause of ↓VA), periphlebitis (± patchy sheathing ± 'candle wax dripping'), occluded vessels (especially BRVO), neovascularization, choroidal/retinal/preretinal nodules (probably granulomas), pigment epithelial changes, disc swelling (from inflammatory papillitis, optic nerve granuloma, or papilloedema secondary to CNS disease). Peripheral multifocal chorioretinitis (small punched-out atrophic spots) are highly suggestive of a sarcoidosis.
- *Complications*: cataract, glaucoma (↑risk with duration of active disease), CNV.

Systemic

- *RS*: often asymptomatic despite CXR changes, dry cough, dyspnoea; bihilar lymphadenopathy, parenchymal disease.
- *CVS*: pericarditis, cardiomyopathy, conduction defects, cardiac failure, cor pulmonale.
- *Skin*: erythema nodosum (red, tender, elevated lesions typically on the shins; commonest in younger females); cutaneous granulomas (non-tender, nodules/papules/macules, almost anywhere, including the lids); lupus pernio (uncommon, bluish plaque, typically on the face/ears).
- *Joints*: arthritis (commoner in acute sarcoid); bone cysts (usually in the digits).
- *Glands*: swelling of any of lacrimal, salivary, parotid, and submaxillary glands, lymphadenopathy, hepatosplenomegaly.

- *CNS* (neurosarcoidosis, commoner in patients with posterior uveitis): cranial nerve palsies (most commonly VIIn; can be bilateral), peripheral neuropathy, myopathy, aseptic meningoencephalitis (typically basal leptomeninges); CNS granuloma may mimic a tumour; optic nerve involvement may present as an atypical optic neuritis.

Table 11.15 Proposed diagnostic criteria for intraocular sarcoidosis[*]

All other possible causes of uveitis, in particular tuberculous uveitis, have to be ruled out.	
Definite ocular sarcoidosis	Biopsy supported diagnosis with a compatible uveitis
Presumed ocular sarcoidosis	Biopsy not done; presence of bilateral hilar lymphadenopathy with a compatible uveitis
Probable ocular sarcoidosis	Biopsy not done and bilateral hilar lymphadenopathy negative; presence of three of the suggestive intraocular signs and two positive investigational tests
Possible ocular sarcoidosis	Biopsy negative, four of the suggestive intraocular signs and two of the investigations are positive

[*] First International Workshop on Ocular Sarcoidosis

Sarcoidosis (2)

Investigations

The diagnosis is essentially clinical but may be supported by investigations such as serum ACE, imaging and ideally typical histology. In some cases it may be difficult to distinguish neurosarcoidosis from MS.

- Serum ACE (commonly elevated in active sarcoid due to synthesis by activated macrophages), serum Ca^{2+} (less commonly elevated).
- *CXR*: abnormal in >90% with ocular sarcoid: stage 0 (normal); stage 1 (bilhar lymphadenopathy only); stage 2 (bihilar lymphadenopathy + parenchymal disease); stage 3 (parenchymal disease only).
- *High resolution CT thorax*: high sensitivity and specificity; particularly useful in those with normal CXR.
- MRI brain/optic nerves (ideally fat suppressed, gadolinium enhanced, T1) and LP in suspected neurosarcoid.
- *Gallium67 scan*: typical uptake pattern is lacrimal and parotid glands (panda appearance) or mediastinum (lambda sign).
- *Positron emission tomography–CT scan*: although traditionally used to detect cancers, positron emission tomography captures images of miniscule changes in the body's metabolism caused by the growth of abnormal cells, while CT images simultaneously allows the exact location, size and shape of the diseased tissue to be pinpointed. Essentially, small lesions (e.g. lymph nodes) are detected with positron emission tomography and then precisely located with CT.
- *Biopsy*: transbronchial, endobronchial, or conjunctival biopsy may reveal the typical non-caseating granulomas of whorls of epithelioid cells surrounding multinucleate giant cells. Bronchoalveolar lavage may show lymphocytosis with high CD4+/CD8+ ratio, but low specificity.
- *FFA*: include ischaemia (hypofluorescence), leakage from periphlebitis, new vessels, CMO (hyperfluorescence).
- *ICG*: choroidal stromal vasculitis, early lobular hypofluorescence, late hyperfluorescence (focal or diffuse).

Treatment of ophthalmic disease

- Anterior segment inflammation: see Idiopathic AAU (🕮 p.368).
- Posterior segment inflammation: see Intermediate uveitis (🕮 p.378).
- *Cataract*: conventional surgery but with tight control of inflammation.
- *Glaucoma*: medical ± surgical (augmented trabeculectomy).
- *CNV*: medical treatment, laser, PDT, or surgery. There may be a role for intravitreal anti-VEGF therapy.

Sarcoidosis syndromes

- *Heerfordt syndrome (uveoparotid fever)*: parotid/submandibular gland enlargement, VIIn palsy, uveitis.
- *Lofgren syndrome*: fever, erythema nodosum, bihilar lymphadenopathy.
- *Mickulicz syndrome*: diffuse swelling of lacrimal/salivary glands (most commonly due to sarcoidosis).

Box 11.2 Differential diagnosis of elevated serum ACE

- Child (peaks at 13yrs of age, adult level by 18yrs)
- Sarcoidosis
- Mycobacterial infection (including leprosy and tuberculosis)
- Certain chronic lung diseases (including berylliosis, silicosis, farmer's lung. histoplasmosis, lymphangiomyomatosis)
- Gaucher disease

Behçet's disease

Possibly first recognized by Hippocrates, the modern description of this disease dates from the Greek Adamantiades and the Turk Behçet. It is an idiopathic, chronic multisystem disease characterized by recurrent episodes of acute inflammation. The commonest ophthalmic presentation is of a sight-threatening pan-uveitis and retinal vasculitis.

Prevalence is highest along the traditional Silk Route, peaking in Turkey, where up to 0.4% of the population may be affected. It typically affects young adults. There is some geographical variation of risk factors, including gender, family history (more significant in Middle Eastern countries), and the HLA-B51 allele (more significant in Japan with a relative risk of 6.7).

Clinical features

Ophthalmic

- *Anterior uveitis*: acute anterior non-granulomatous uveitis, typically with hypopyon.
- *Posterior uveitis*: vitritis, macular oedema, retinal infiltrates/haemorrhage/oedema, occlusive periphlebitis ± BRVO/CRVO), neovascularization ± vitreous haemorrhage/tractional retinal detachment, diffuse capillary leakage.
- *Complications*: cataract, glaucoma, end-stage disease (optic atrophy, retinal atrophy with attenuated vessels; often blind).

Systemic

- *Oral ulceration* (aphthous or scarring).
- *Genital ulceration*.
- *Skin lesions*: erythema nodosum, pseudofolliculitis, papulopustules, acneiform rash.
- *Joints*: arthritis (mono/poly).
- *Vascular*: thromboses (venous > arterial) including superficial thrombophlebitis, superior/inferior vena cava obstruction.
- *GI*: nausea, vomiting, abdominal pain, bloody diarrhoea.
- *CNS*: meningoencephalitis, sinus thrombosis ± intracranial hypertension, cranial or peripheral neuropathies, focal CNS signs.

Investigations

- *Positive pathergy test*: sterile pustule appearing 24–48h after oblique insertion of 20-gauge needle.
- *MRI/MRV brain*: if neurological features.

Treatment

- Liaise with physician; systemic corticosteroids (e.g. initially 1–2mg/kg/d prednisolone PO); IV (e.g. pulsed methylprednisolone 500–1000mg 1x/d or alternate days for a total of 3 doses) for an acute flare, consider adding steroid-sparing agents, including ciclosporin, azathioprine, and anti-TNF therapies (infliximab/adalimumab), and α-interferon.

Table 11.16 Criteria for diagnosis of Behçet's disease (International Study Group for Behçet's Disease 1990)

	Classification criteria
Must have:	• Recurrent oral ulceration (minor, major, or herpetiform) ≥ 3× in 12mths
Plus two of:	• Recurrent genital ulceration (aphthous or scarring)
	• Eye lesions: uveitis (anterior, posterior, or cells in the vitreous) or retinal vasculitis
	• Skin lesions: erythema nodosum, pseudofolliculitis, or papulopustular lesions; or acneiform rash (in post-adolescent patient not on corticosteroids)
	• Positive pathergy test

Vogt–Koyanagi–Harada disease

VKH is a multisystem inflammatory disease affecting the eyes (bilateral granulomatous panuveitis), ears, brain, skin, and hair. It is thought to be a T-cell-mediated autoimmune disease directed against melanocyte antigen(s). Prevalence is higher in darker-skinned races, including Asians, native Americans, Hispanics, and those from the Middle and Far East. It is commonest in women in their third and fourth decade, but may occur in either sex at any age. It is associated with HLA-DR4 notably HLA-DRB1*0405, which recognizes various melanocyte proteins. VKH may arise after cutaneous injury, presumably via liberation of melanocyte antigens.

Clinical features

There is often a prodrome of fever, meningism, and auditory symptoms for a few days, before blurring/profound visual loss from the uveitis develops. (See 📖 Table 11.17.)

Ophthalmic

- *Anterior uveitis*: bilateral granulomatous anterior uveitis, PS, iris nodules, AC shallowing.
- *Posterior uveitis*: multifocal choroiditis, multifocal detachments of sensory retina, exudative retinal detachments, choroidal depigmentation 'sunset glow fundus', Dalen–Fuchs nodules (peripheral yellow–white choroidal granulomas), subretinal fibrosis.
- *Complications*: cataract, glaucoma, CNV membrane.

Systemic

- *Cutaneous*: late features—vitiligo, alopecia, poliosis.
- *Auditory*: tinnitus, deafness, vertigo.
- *Neurological*: sterile meningitis (headache, neck stiffness), encephalitis, (convulsions, altered consciousness), cranial neuropathies (including ocular motility disturbance).

Investigations

- *FFA*: focal areas of delay in choroidal perfusion, multifocal areas of pinpoint leakage, large placoid areas of hyperfluorescence, pooling within subretinal fluid, and optic nerve staining.
- *US*: low to medium reflective diffuse choroidal thickening.
- *LP* (not always required): lymphocytic pleocytosis.

Treatment

- Liaise with physician; start high-dose systemic corticosteroids (e.g. 1–2mg/kg/d prednisolone PO or methylprednisolone 1g/d IV for 3d).
- For resistant or recurrent disease consider adding steroid-sparing agents, such as methotrexate, azathioprine, and ciclosporin.

Table 11.17 Diagnostic criteria for Vogt–Koyanagi–Harada disease (AUS criteria)[1]

1 No history of penetrating ocular trauma or surgery preceding initial onset of uveitis
2 No clinical or laboratory evidence suggestive of other ocular disease entities
3 Bilateral ocular involvement:

3 Bilateral ocular involvement:

  a Early:

      (1) diffuse choroiditis (focal subretinal fluid or bullous serous retinal detachments)

      (2) if fundus findings equivocal then there must be characteristic FFA findings (see opposite) AND diffuse choroidal thickening (in the absence of posterior scleritis on US)

  b Late:

      (1) history suggestive of prior presence of early features AND two or more of

      (2) ocular depigmentation (Sunset glow fundus or Sugiura sign)

      (3a) nummular chorioretinal depigmented scars

      (3b) retinal pigment epithelium clumping/migration

      (3c) recurrent or chronic anterior uveitis

4 Neurological/auditory findings

  a meningismus (malaise, fever, headache, nausea, abdominal pain, neck/back stiffness)

  b tinnitus

  c CSF pleocytosis

5 Integumentary findings (not preceding ocular/CNS disease)

  a alopecia

  b poliosis

  c vitiligo

Complete VKH requires all criteria (1 to 5).

Incomplete VKH requires criteria 1 to 3 AND either 4 or 5.

Probable VKH (isolated ocular disease) requires criteria 1 to 3.

[1]. Read RW et al. Revised diagnostic criteria for VKH disease: report of an international commitee on nomenelature. Am J Ophthalmol 2001; **131**:647–52.

Sympathetic ophthalmia

Sympathetic ophthalmia is a rare bilateral granulomatous panuveitis that bears remarkable parallels to VKH, but differs in being causally related to antecedent trauma or surgery. Although this response to injury can occur within a few days or over 60yrs later, it usually arises between 1 and 12mths after injury. It appears to be a T-cell-mediated response to a ocular antigen, presumably liberated during the initial insult. It occurs in 0.1% cases of penetrating ocular trauma and in 0.01% cases of routine vitrectomy. In one prospective study (British Ophthalmic Surveillance Unit) the commonest cause of sympathetic ophthalmia was ocular (particularly vitreoretinal) surgery.

Clinical features

Ophthalmic

- *Anterior*: bilateral granulomatous anterior uveitis with mutton fat keratic precipitates, PS.
- *Posterior*: vitritis, choroidal infiltration, Dalen–Fuchs nodules, macular oedema, exudative retinal detachment; the exciting eye may be phthisical.
- *Complications*: cataract, secondary glaucoma, end-stage disease (optic atrophy, chorioretinal scarring).

Systemic

As for VKH (📖 p.388), but systemic involvement less common.

Prevention

After trauma there is a short window of opportunity (about 10d) in which enucleation would almost certainly prevent sympathetic ophthalmia. This may be the best option for blind painful eyes with no hope of useful vision. However, for the many traumatized eyes with visual potential there is now a strong trend to preserve the eye where possible.

Treatment

Once inflammation has developed, the role of enucleation of the exciting eye is controversial; some suggest that it may favourably modify the disease if performed within 2wks of symptoms.

- *Immunosuppression*: start with high-dose systemic corticosteroids (e.g. 1–2mg/kg/d prednisolone PO or methylprednisolone 1g/d IV for 3d); for resistant/recurrent disease or unacceptable steroid side-effects consider adding steroid-sparing agents, such as methotrexate, azathioprine, ciclosporin, or mycophenolate mofetil. With aggressive treatment 60% may achieve ≥6/18 in the sympathizing eye.

Viral uveitis (1)

Herpes simplex virus

HSV1 (very rarely HSV2) may cause an anterior uveitis which is usually associated with keratitis, but may be isolated.

Clinical features

- *Anterior*: unilateral persistent anterior uveitis with KPs, PS, and patchy iris atrophy (with transillumination defects); semidilated pupil ± corneal scarring/keratitis/↓corneal sensation (see Herpes simplex keratitis 📖 pp.204–207); the uveitis may be 'granulomatous'.
- Glaucoma is common (secondary to trabeculitis or blockage by inflammatory debris).
- *Posterior (rare)*: healthy individuals may get ARN (see below); those with disseminated HSV or HSV encephalitis may get an occlusive vasculitis (usually bilateral) with relatively few haemorrhages but commonly complicated by retinal detachment.

Treatment

- If keratitis then antiviral cover generally required (see Herpes simplex keratitis 📖 pp. 204–207).
- *For isolated anterior uveitis*: titrate topical steroids according to inflammation and taper very slowly (frequency/potency) as highly steroid sensitive and relapses are common; cycloplegia.
- For frequent recurrences consider long-term oral antiviral prophylaxis.

Varicella zoster virus

Primary VZV infection (chickenpox) commonly causes a widespread vesicular rash that may be associated with keratitis (superficial, disciform, or stromal), mild anterior uveitis, and very occasionally necrotizing retinitis. Reactivation (shingles) usually occurs in the elderly or immunosuppressed and frequently affects Va (ophthalmic branch), known as HZO. Of this group, up to 40% have anterior uveitis, with an increased risk if the nasociliary branch is involved (Hutchinson sign: vesicles at side of nose). Typical ocular inflammation (e.g. disciform keratitis with anterior uveitis) may also occur without the rash (HZO sine herpete).

Clinical features

- *Anterior*: unilateral anterior uveitis with KPs, PS, and segmental iris atrophy, (with transillumination defects) ± conjunctivitis, keratitis, epi/scleritis; the uveitis may be 'granulomatous'
- *Glaucoma is common* (up to 40%).
- *Posterior*: ARN or PORN may develop (see Viral uveitis 📖 p.394).

Treatment

- *For isolated anterior uveitis*: titrate topical steroids according to inflammation and taper very slowly (frequency/potency) as highly steroid sensitive and relapses are common with steroid withdrawal; cycloplegia.
- *For HZO*: see (📖 p.208).

Cytomegalovirus

CMV retinitis is the leading cause of visual loss in AIDS, but may also occur in patients who are immunosuppressed due to therapy (e.g. associated with organ transplants) or other disease (e.g. lymphoma). HIV and non-HIV-associated infection behave fairly similarly, both being dependent on the degree of immune system suppression/recovery. Traditionally, HIV associated CMV retinitis required life-long maintenance therapy (cf. non-HIV disease); however, with HAART-induced immune recovery this is no longer always necessary.

Clinical features

- *Anterior uveitis:* unilateral, usually with raised IOP, there may be no obvious iris atrophy (cf. HSV, VZV).
- *Corneal endotheliitis* (appears to be a disease of the oriental race): corneal involvement ranges from small areas of focal endotheliitis (may be coin-shaped) to diffuse bullous keratopathy, stromal corneal oedema, KP (variable appearance), AC inflammation usually mild with no PS, ± diffuse iris atrophy, ↑IOP
- *Posterior:* CMV retinitis (see HIV-associated disease: posterior segment 📖 p.398).

Treatment

For anterior uveitis or corneal endotheliitis: oral valganciclovir.
For CMV retinitis: see HIV-associated disease: posterier segment 📖 p.398.

Other viruses

Other common viruses that may cause an anterior or posterior uveitis include measles (with subacute sclerosing panencephalitis) mumps, rubella, EBV, CMV, and HTLV-1.

Subacute sclerosing panencephalitis

A rare neurodegenerative syndrome following measles infection exhibits a retinitis with focal pigmentary changes in the fovea ± papilloedema or optic atrophy.

Human T-lymphotropic virus type-1 (HTLV-1)

This RNA retrovirus common in Japan and parts of Africa, causes leukaemia and tropical spastic paraparesis; it may cause uveitis in isolation (usually intermediate) or secondary to leukaemia (usually posterior with retinal vasculitis ± secondary infection, e.g. CMV).

Viral uveitis (2)

Acute retinal necrosis

This rare syndrome of necrotizing retinitis is caused by VZV, HSV1, and HSV2 infection (children). It may occur in the immunocompromised and healthy individuals of any age. In the National UK ARN Survey 2001–02 there were 31 cases (22 male, 9 female; aged 13–85yrs, mean 54) of which 28 cases (90.3%) were unilateral. VZV was the commonest cause (identified in 10 patients), followed by HSV-1 (5 patients) and HSV-2 (4 patients). Based on this study, the incidence of ARN in the UK is approximately 1 case per 1.6 to 2.0 million population per year.

Clinical findings
- Usually unilateral ↓VA, floaters, discomfort.
- Predominantly peripheral disease comprising occlusive arteritis, full thickness peripheral necrotizing retinitis (well demarcated, spread circumferentially), marked vitritis ± AC activity.
- *Complications*: retinal detachment (in up to 75%; rhegmatogenous or tractional), ischaemic optic neuropathy.
- *Prognosis*: second eye involvement occurs in about 30% (may occur simultaneously to several years later).

Investigations
AC tap ± vitreous biopsy with PCR to identify viral DNA.

Treatment
- *For all patients*: antiviral (e.g. aciclovir IV dose 10mg/kg 3×/d 2wks then PO dose 6–12wks); consider systemic steroids (vs inflammation), aspirin (vs arterial occlusion), barrier laser photocoagulation (vs retinal breaks) but no clear evidence. Retinal detachment repair is challenging due to the necrotic retina and number of breaks; vitrectomy with silicone oil injection is most commonly used. Recent reports have shown valaciclovir (a prodrug of aciclovir) 1g 3×/d orally to be effective
- *If immunosuppressed*: consider lifelong antiviral treatment.

Progressive outer retinal necrosis

This very rare devastating necrotizing retinitis is caused by VZV infection in the context of immunosuppression (usually HIV with CD4+ T-cell counts <50/mm^3).

Clinical findings
- Uni/bilateral painless rapid ↓VA.
- Rapidly coalescing white areas of outer retinal necrosis (often central as well as peripheral) but with minimal vasculitis, retinitis, or vitritis (cf. ARN).

Treatment
This should be co-ordinated between an ophthalmologist with experience in HIV ocular disease and an HIV physician. Options include IV ganciclovir or foscarnet with additional intravitreal ganciclovir.

The prognosis is very poor, partly due to the extremely high rate of retinal detachment.

Table 11.18 Diagnostic criteria for ARN and PORN[1]

	ARN	PORN
Appearance	One or more foci of full thickness retinal necrosis with disc rete borders	Multiple foci of deep retinal opacification which may be confluent
Location	Peripheral retina (usually adjacent/outside temporal arcades)	Peripheral retina macular involvement
Progression	Rapid (but usually responds to treatment)	Extremely rapid
Direction	Circumferential	No consistent direction
Vessels	Occlusive vasculopathy (arterial)	No vascular inflammation
Inflammation	Prominent AC and vitreous inflammation	Minimal or none
Suggestive features	Optic neuropathy/atrophy Scleritis Pain Perivenular clearing of retinal opacification	

1. Engstrom RE Jr et al. The progressive outer retinal necrosis syndrome. *Ophthalmology* 1994; **101**:1488

HIV-associated disease: anterior segment

The Human Immuno Deficiency Virus (HIV-1 and -2) is an RNA retrovirus that infects CD4+ T cells causing AIDS. Worldwide, about 40 million people are infected with HIV, with about 5 million new infections and 3 million deaths per year (WHO data for 2003). Most infected people live in developing countries (notably sub-Saharan Africa) and under socio-economic deprivation.

Transmission may be via infected blood or other bodily fluids. Major risk factors include unprotected sexual intercourse, IV drug abuse, blood transfusion, and maternal infection (vertical transmission).

The main markers of disease are CD4 level and viral load. The CD4 level is a good indicator of HIV-induced immunocompromise, and correlates with susceptibility to infections (Tables 11.19–11.20). The viral load (i.e. RNA copies/ml) correlates with risk of progression.

Prognosis is greatly improved with highly active antiretroviral therapy (HAART). This regimen involves using at least three antiretroviral drugs, usually two nucleoside reverse transcriptase inhibitors and either a protease inhibitor or a non-nucleoside reverse transcriptase inhibitor.

Management of eye disease should be co-ordinated between an ophthalmologist with experience in HIV and an HIV physician.

Conjunctival microvasculopathy

Microvascular abnormalities of the conjunctiva are common. The mechanism is unclear. Irregular calibre vessels are seen which may be in a corkscrew pattern. Conjunctival microvasculopathy may be associated with abnormalities of the retinal microvasculature (see Viral uveitis, 📖 pp.392–395).

Keratouveitis

- *VZV keratouveitis* is common in HIV, with or without the typical dermatomal rash of HZO. The features include a moderate anterior uveitis, ↑IOP, and iris atrophy. *Treatment* is with systemic antiviral (e.g. aciclovir or famciclovir) (see 📖 p.208).
- *HSV keratouveitis* is less common with probably equal prevalence in the general population. In HIV patients, however, it tends to be limbal, more severe, more recurrences, and dendrites may be larger and less defined. *Treatment* is with topical ± systemic antiviral (e.g. aciclovir) (see 📖 p.204–207).
- *Microsporidial keratouveitis* presents with bilateral irritation and photophobia, punctate keratopathy, often with a follicular conjunctivitis and/or an anterior uveitis.

Anterior uveitis

Anterior uveitis is seen in over half of all patients with HIV. VZV and HSV tend to cause relatively mild inflammation (often with ↑IOP and iris atrophy). However, posterior uveitis associated with toxoplasma or syphilis, may also cause significant AC inflammation. Uveitis may also be caused by concurrent therapy notably rifabutin (anti-atypical mycobacteria) and cidofovir (anti-CMV).

Table 11.19 Ophthalmic complications of HIV infection

	Infective	Tumour	Other
Adnexae	HZO Molluscum contagiosum Preseptal cellulitis	Kaposi sarcoma Squamous cell carcinoma	Conjunctival microvasculopathy
Orbit	Orbital cellulitis	Non-Hodgkin lymphoma	
Anterior Segment	Viral keratitis *(VZV, HSV)* Bacterial keratitis *(S. aureus, S. epidermidis,* *P. aeruginosa)* Protozoan keratitis *(microsporidia)*		Conjunctival microvasculopathy Vortex keratopathy (antivirals, atovaquone) Dry eye Anterior uveitis
Posterior segment	CMV retinitis VZV retinitis *(incl.* *PORN, ARN)* HSV retinitis *(incl. ARN)* Toxoplasma retinochoroiditis Syphilis retinitis Pneumocystis choroiditis Cryptococcus choroiditis Tuberculous choroiditis	Ocular-CNS non-Hodgkin lymphoma	Retinal micro- vasculopathy Ischaemic maculopathy Immune recovery uveitis
Neuro- ophthalmic	Cerebral toxoplasmosis Cryptococcal meningitis Neurosyphilis Progressive multifocal leucoencephalopathy	Ocular-CNS non-Hodgkin lymphoma	Optic neuritis Optic atrophy Ocular motility disorders

Table 11.20 CD4 level and typical diseases relevant to the eye

CD4 count cells/mm³	Ocular disease
250–500	Herpes zoster ophthalmicus Tuberculosis
150–250	Lymphoma Kaposi's sarcoma
50–150	Pneumocystosis Toxoplasmosis Microsporidiosis VZV retinitis
<50	CMV retinitis

HIV-associated disease: posterior segment

Cytomegalovirus retinitis

This may affect up to 40% of patients with AIDS, but usually only when CD4 <50/mm³. Since the advent of HAART there has been a dramatic reduction in CMV retinitis.

Clinical features

- Floaters, ↓VA, and/or field loss.
- *Anterior*: AC inflammation (± distinctive stellate KPs) is usually mild or absent (depending on degree of immunosuppression).
- *Posterior*: vitritis (usually mild/absent) with retinitis, which may be:
  - *haemorrhagic retinitis*: haemorrhage and necrosis with loss of fundal details ('pizza pie' appearance).
  - *granular retinitis*: relatively indolent, with minimal haemorrhage and no vascular sheathing.
  - *perivascular retinitis*: 'frosted branch angiitis' that spreads along the course of the retinal vessels.
- *Complications* include retinal detachment (up to 30%), retinal atrophy and optic nerve disease (5%).

Treatment

- *HAART*: sustaining a CD4 count >50/mm³ is effective prophylaxis against CMV retinitis. Late introduction of HAART to patients with CMV retinitis is still likely to induce an immune recovery; in such patients anti-CMV treatments are required at least until immune recovery occurs.
- *Specific anti-CMV treatment*: this involves 'induction' and 'maintenance' therapy. Commonly used agents include systemic antiviral (e.g. valganciclovir, ganciclovir, foscarnet, or cidofovir), intravitreal implants (ganciclovir) or injections (ganciclovir and/or foscarnet) or a combination. Life-long maintenance treatment is recommended for all patients without immune recovery.

Toxoplasma retinochoroiditis

This is decreasing in frequency due to the toxoplasmacidal effect of pro-phylactic agents actually intended to eliminate *Pneumocystis*-related lung disease. Ocular toxoplasmosis in HIV is more severe, often multifocal (even bilateral), associated with moderate/severe anterior uveitis and vitritis, and is commonly associated with neuro-toxoplasmosis. In contrast to the immunocompetent situation it always requires treatment (and should not be given with corticosteroids, see 📖 p.406).

Pneumocystis carinii choroiditis

This is relatively uncommon, particularly among those on systemic prophy-laxis for *Pneumocystis carinii* pneumonia (co-trimoxazole) as opposed to inhalational (pentamidine). The choroiditis is often bilateral, comprises yellow choroidal patches of 1/4 to 2DD in size around the posterior pole with minimal vitritis. It is often asymptomatic. *Treatment* is with systemic co-trimoxazole or pentamidine.

Cryptococcus choroiditis

This rare condition is usually associated with cryptococcal meningitis, and may be associated with an optic neuropathy or papilloedema. It is characterized by multifocal off-white choroidal lesions, occasionally with a retinitis or endophthalmitis. *Treatment* is with a systemic antifungal (e.g. amphotericin-B or fluconazole).

Immune recovery uveitis

Eyes with inactive CMV retinitis may show a paradoxical worsening of inflammation, as T-cell recovery takes place. *Presentation* includes moderate/severe vitritis, tractional retinal detachment, CMO, and neovascularization.

Syphilis choroiditis/chorioretinitis

Co-infection with syphilis may occur due to sexual transmission. Syphilis may cause protean ocular and systemic manifestations (see 📖 p.404).

HIV microvasculopathy

About 75% of HIV-infected individuals develop microvascular abnormalities of the retina and/or conjunctiva (see 📖 p.396). It is not clear if this is due to HIV-induced thrombotic tendency, an immune phenomenon, or a direct result of HIV infection of the vessels.

Retinal microvasculopathy

In the retina there may be tortuosity of the vessels with CWS, telangiectasia, intraretinal haemorrhages, and venous or arterial occlusions.

Mycobacterial disease (1)

Tuberculosis

Worldwide more than 1 billion people are infected by *Mycobacterium tuberculosis*, a facultative intracellular bacterium. Tuberculosis (primary or post-primary) develops in about 10%, and of these ocular disease develops in about 1%. Widespread chronic inflammation develops with characteristic caseating granulomas. This immune reaction or occasionally direct ocular penetration may lead to uveitis.

Ocular TB may be difficult to diagnose due to its protean manifestations and the frequent absence of any clinical or radiological evidence of respiratory disease.

Clinical features

Ophthalmic

- *External*: lid abscess, conjunctival infiltration/nodules, phlyctenulosis, scleritis (usually anterior necrotizing), interstitial keratitis.
- *Anterior*: typically granulomatous anterior uveitis with mutton fat KPs, iris granulomas, PS, but can be non-granulomatous.
- *Posterior*: vitritis, vasculitis (periphlebitis ± B/CRVO ± ischaemia), macular oedema, choroidal granulomas (usually multifocal around the posterior pole ± inflammatory retinal detachment); optic neuropathy; Eales' disease (retinal vasculitis with neovascularization and high risk of vitreous haemorrhage, typically in young males).

Systemic

- *RS*: pneumonia, pleural effusion, fibrosis.
- *GI*: ileocaecal (may obstruct), peritoneum (ascites).
- *GU*: sterile pyuria, epididymitis, salpingitis + infertility (in females).
- *CNS*: meningitis, CNS tuberculoma (may mimic tumour).
- *Skeletal*: arthritis, osteomyelitis.
- *Skin*: lupus vulgaris.
- *CVS*: constrictive pericarditis, pericardial effusion.
- *Adrenal*: hypoadrenalism (Addison's disease).
- *LN*: lymphadenopathy, scrofula.

Investigation

- *Microbiology*: sputum, early morning urine (acid-fast bacillus, stains with Ziel-Nielsen stain).
- *CXR*: classically apical infiltrates or cavitation; also consolidation, pleural effusion, hilar lymphadenopathy; normal in 50% of cases of ocular TB.
- *Tuberculin testing*: standard testing involves intradermal injection of 0.1ml of 1:1000 strength tuberculin PPD (i.e. 10 tuberculin units) and measuring the induration 72h later. Interpret with caution as the response can be very variable with up to 17% false negatives, and BCG vaccination inducing 'false' positives (but usually only if within 5yrs). A 1:10 000 strength tuberculin PPD may be used if active TB is suspected, as an intense reaction may become necrotic.
- *QuantiFERON-TB Gold (QFT-G) Test*: See 📖 Box 11.4.

> **Box 11.3 Interpretation of Mantoux testing (CDC recommendations 2005)**
>
> - For *high-risk* individuals (immunosuppressed, contacts of active TB, typical CXR changes) the test is considered positive if induration ≥5mm.
> - For *moderate risk* (e.g. health workers, those with chronic disease, children, immigrants from endemic areas) induration must be ≥10mm.
> - For *low risk* the test is only considered positive if induration ≥15mm.

> **Box 11.4 QuantiFERON-TB Gold Test**
>
> *Advantages*
> This is an interferon-γ release assay that measures the release of interferon after stimulation *in vitro* by *Mycobacterium* tuberculosis antigens. The main advantages of this assay vs Mantoux test is:
> - lack of cross-reaction with bacillus Calmette-Guérin and most nontuberculous mycobacteria.
> - no need for patient to return for test reading in 48–72h.
>
> *Specificity and sensitivity*
> In the immunocompromised host and in paediatric populations, studies suggest that the QFT-G better correlates with the risk of TB than the Mantoux test, but data remain inconclusive. It is more specific than the Mantoux test because it is not confounded by previous BCG vaccination. In active tuberculosis, it has similar sensitivity to the Mantoux test. Current cross-sectional evidence suggests that for the diagnosis of latent TB infection (LTBI), the sensitivity is similar to Mantoux testing.

Treatment

Standard unsupervised treatment
If patient compliance is likely to be good, treatment is unsupervised with a daily regimen, usually using combination tablets such as rifater to increase convenience. Initial 2mths rifampicin, isoniazid, pyrazinamide, ethambutol. Continuation 4mths rifampicin and isoniazid only.

Supervised and extended treatment
Otherwise directly observed therapy is instituted, with higher doses of the same drugs given three times per week. Treatment may be prolonged to 9mths if immunosuppressed or disseminated disease.

Additional treatment
For ocular complications such as CMO, retinal vasculitis, and persistent inflammation consider oral corticosteroids but only if on effective anti-TB treatment.

Monitoring
U+E and LFT should be checked before starting treatment with rifampicin, isoniazid, and pyrazinamide. VA should be checked before starting treatment with ethambutol and the patient advised to report any visual disturbance (↓VA, ↓colour vision, ↓visual field).

Mycobacterial disease (2)

Leprosy (Hansen disease)

Worldwide about 15 million people have leprosy, of whom about two-thirds are in Asia. The spectrum of leprosy is cased by the interaction of the obligate intracellular bacterium *Mycobacterium leprae* with the host's immune system. A poor cell-mediated immune response leads to the lepromatous form ,which is generalized and commonly affects the eyes. A strong response leads to tuberculoid leprosy, which is more localized and rarely affects the eye.

Clinical features

Ophthalmic

- *External*: madarosis, trichiasis, lagophthalmos (VIIn palsy), conjunctivitis, epi/scleritis, keratitis (neuropathic/exposure/secondary infection).
- *Anterior*: anterior uveitis usually persistent, less commonly AAU; 'iris pearls' at the pupil margin, which may enlarge and drop into the AC, iris atrophy, miosis.

Systemic

- *Tuberculoid*: thickened/tender nerves associated with hypopigmented anaesthetic patches and muscle atrophy.
- *Lepromatous*: nerve changes less marked but widespread infiltration, including skin, ears, nose (saddle-nose), face (leonine appearance), larynx (hoarse voice).

Investigation and treatment

This should include skin/nasal mucosa smears for non-cultivable acid-fast bacilli. Systemic treatment should be co-ordinated by a specialist centre with multidisciplinary support. Treatment of eye disease is usually with topical steroids.

Spirochaetal and other bacterial uveitis

Syphilis

The spirochaete *Treponema pallidum* is usually transmitted by sexual contact or transplacentally. Acquired syphilis is divided into primary, secondary, and tertiary stages. Congenital syphilis may be divided into early (equivalent to acquired secondary stage) and late (equivalent to acquired third stage).

Clinical features (Tables 11.21 and 11.22)

Anterior uveitis

- This is the commonest ocular feature of both secondary and tertiary syphilis.
- Granulomatous or non-granulomatous; variable severity; ± roseolae (vascular fronds on the iris); ± iris atrophy; nodules on the iris/iridocorneal angle occur in tertiary disease only.

Posterior uveitis

- This may be uni- or bilateral, uni- or multifocal, and choroiditis or chorioretinitis.
- Yellow plaque-like lesions with overlying vitritis ± serous retinal detachment. Resolution of the lesions results in a pigmentary retinopathy.

Investigation (Table 11.23)

- *Non-treponemal serology*: Venereal disease research laboratory (VDRL) tests disease activity; it may become negative in later disease syphilis. Rapid plasma reagin (RPR) is a simple test used in screening.
- Treponemal serology: fluorescent treponemal antibody absorption (FTA-ABS) and haemagglutination tests (TPHA) test previous or current infection. They do not distinguish from other treponematoses (e.g. yaws).
- Dark-ground microscopy of chancre/mucocutaneous lesion.
- LP: consider if active ocular disease, suspected neurosyphilis, or HIV. CSF typically shows raised protein, pleocytosis, and positive VDRL.
- HIV test; coinfection is increasingly observed.

Treatment

Management of syphilitic eye disease should be in conjunction with a genitourinary physician. Treatment requires high-dose penicillin with an extended regimen for late latent and tertiary syphilis. Benzathine penicillin is now the preferred preparation for syphilis in the UK (unlicensed indication)[1]). Spirochaete death may transiently worsen inflammation (Jarish–Herxheimer reaction). Consider topical steroids for interstitial keratitis and anterior uveitis. Systemic steroids must be used with caution but have a role in sight-threatening posterior uveitis or scleritis.

Other bacteria

Other bacteria that may cause uveitis include the spirochaetes *Borrelia burdorferi* (Lyme disease) and *Leptospira interrogans* (Leptospirosis including Weil's disease), the Gram-positive bacillus *Tropheryma whippelii* (Whipple's disease), and the Gram-negative bacilli *Bartonella henselae* (Cat-scratch disease), and *Brucella* (brucellosis).

Table 11.21 Ophthalmic complications of syphilis

Adnexae	Gummata	Madarosis
Anterior Segment	Conjunctival chancre	Interstitial keratitis
	Papillary conjunctivitis	Anterior uveitis
	Epi/scleritis	
Posterior segment	Multi/unifocal choroiditis/	Neuroretinitis
	chorioretinitis	Retinal vasculitis
Neuro-ophthalmic	Argyll Robertson pupils	Perioptic neuritis
	Papilloedema	Ocular motility disorders
	Retrobulbar neuritis	Visual field defects

Table 11.22 Stages of syphilis

Stage	Main features
Congenital	
Early <2yrs of age	Mucocutaneous rash; periostitis and osteochondritis;
	Chorioretinitis and retinal vasculitis producing the characteristic salt-and-pepper fundus
Late >2yrs of age	Saddle nose, frontal bossing, sabre shins, Hutchinson's teeth
	Interstitial keratitis
Acquired	
Primary from 2wks post-infection	Painless ulcer (chancre) with regional lymphadenopathy appears 2–6wks post infection and resolves within a further 6wks
Secondary from 8wks post-infection	Diffuse maculopapular rash (including palms/soles) often with generalized lymphadenopathy, malaise, and fever
	Anterior or posterior uveitis
Tertiary from 5yrs post-infection	Around one-third progress to this stage. Aortitis may cause aortic regurgitation and dissection. Neurosyphilis may cause meningitis, CNS vasculitis and parenchymatous degeneration resulting in the syndromes of tabes dorsalis and generalized paresis of the insane (GPI)
	Anterior or posterior uveitis; interstitial keratitis

Table 11.23 Sereological tests for syphilis

	Primary		Secondary	Tertiary	Treated
	Early	Late			
VDRL	−/+	+	+	+	− or low +
Titre	Rising titre	Titre α activity	Titre may wane	Falling titre	
FTA-ABS	+	+	+	+	+
TPHA	−/+	+	+	+	+

False-positive VDRL may occur in other conditions including EBV, mycoplasma, autoimmune disease, chronic liver disease, and malignancy.

Protozoan uveitis

Toxoplasmosis

The protozoan *Toxoplasma gondii* is an obligate intracellular parasite which is estimated to infect up to 50% of the world's population. Lifetime risk of ocular toxoplasmosis is about 18/100 000 in the UK, but up to 20 times this level in West Africa.

The definitive host is the cat; livestock and humans are only intermediate hosts. Oocysts are excreted in cat faeces, which are ingested by humans/livestock in which they may become encysted (bradyzoite) or actively proliferate (tachyzoite). Human infection arises from contact with cat faeces/contaminated soil, ingestion of undercooked meat (bradyzoites), contaminated water, or transplacentally. In the past most toxoplasmosis was thought to be congenital but acquired disease is increasingly recognized.

The vertical transmission rate (transplacental) increases from 15% in the first trimester to 60% in the third trimester; disease severity is, however, much greater if acquired in early pregnancy.

Clinical features
Ophthalmic
Affects both eyes in 40%, but if simultaneously active suspect immunocompromise:
- Asymptomatic finding, floaters, ↓VA.
- Vitritis (may have 'vitreous precipitates' akin to KPs on posterior surface of PVD), retinitis (white, fluffy area when active; becomes circumscribed and pigmented as it heals; atrophic scar with pigmented border when inactive; satellite lesions adjacent to old scars commonly seen); retinal vasculitis (periphlebitis); may have an anterior uveitis often with ↑IOP.
- *Other presentations include*: scleritis, punctate outer retinitis (with quiet vitreous), large lesions (especially in the elderly), endophthalmitis-like, neuroretinitis, serous retinal detachments, pigmentary retinopathy.
- *Complications*: cataract, glaucoma, CNV membrane.

Systemic
- *Congenital*: the impact of transplacental infection is greatest early in pregnancy; complications include hydrocephalus, cerebral calcification, hepatosplenomegaly, retinochoroiditis (more commonly bilateral and affecting the macula).
- *Acquired*: if immunocompetent is usually asymptomatic, but may have fever and lymphadenopathy; if immunocompromised (usually HIV +ve patients) may have life-threatening disease including encephalitis, intracerebral cysts, hepatitis, myocarditis.

Investigation
This is essentially a clinical diagnosis. Interpret positive serological tests with caution. Many of the adult population are positive for anti-toxoplasma IgG; however, IgM antibodies do suggest recent acquired infection and negative serology in undiluted serum makes the diagnosis unlikely. Matched early and convalescent samples are not required. PCR of intraocular samples may also be used.

Treatment

> **Box 11.5 Indications for treatment**
>
> * Lesions involving disc, macula or papillomacular bundle
> * Lesions threatening a major vessel
> * Marked vitritis
> * Any lesion in an immunocompromised patient

Systemic

≥4wks of prednisolone AND co-trimoxazole OR clindamycin/sulfadiazine OR pyrimethamine/sulfadiazine/folinic acid (weekly FBC required) OR atovaquone. Steroids must not be used without effective anti-toxoplasmosis therapy, and should not be given if immunosuppressed. For maternal infection acquired during pregnancy use spiramycin (named-patient basis) to reduce transplacental spread. Atovaquone may theoretically reduce recurrences, as it is active against bradyzoites as well as tachyzoites.

Prognosis

In immunocompetent patients the disease is self-limiting and hence does not require treatment unless sight-threatening. Recurrence is common; mean number of recurrences is two, but a wide range is seen.

Pregnancy

Education is key (Table 11.24). Some countries perform serial antenatal serological screening to detect active toxoplasmosis in order to permit early initiation of treatment. Treat maternal infection acquired during pregnancy with spiramycin.

Table 11.24 Toxoplasmosis and pregnancy

Advice	Wash all fruit/vegetables
	Avoid unpasteurized goat's milk
	Cook all meat thoroughly
	Avoid handling cat litter (or use rubber gloves)
Risk of transmission	15–60% risk if acquired during pregnancy
	No risk otherwise (even if recurrence of active disease during pregnancy)

Microsporidiosis

Microsporidia are protozoan obligate intracellular parasites of which four genera may cause the human disease, microsporidiosis. This is usually seen in the immunosuppressed (notably in AIDS) where it may present as chronic diarrhoea, respiratory infection, or keratoconjunctivitis. Microsporidial keratoconjunctivitis presents with bilateral irritation and photophobia, punctate keratopathy, often with a follicular conjunctivitis and/or an anterior uveitis.

Nematodal uveitis

Toxocariasis

The ascarid *Toxocara canis* is one of the commonest of all nematode infections, and is a significant cause of visual loss worldwide. The definitive hosts are puppies (or kittens for the less common *T. catis*).

Ova excreted in faeces are inadvertently ingested by humans in whom they develop into larvae. The larvae invade the gut wall and spread haematogenously throughout the body notably to the liver, lung, brain, heart (visceral larva migrans), or the eye (ocular toxocariasis). Larval death causes an intense inflammatory reaction. Infection by *Toxocara* usually occurs <3yrs of age, although some ocular disease may not present until adulthood.

Clinical features
Ophthalmic
Ocular toxocariasis is unilateral. Presentation may vary with age:
- *Diffuse chronic endophthalmitis (age 2–9yrs)*: VA + floaters; white eye with chronic anterior uveitis, PS, vitritis, snowbanking, macular oedema, exudative retinal detachment; complications include tractional retinal detachment, cyclitic membrane, cataract, hypotony.
- *Posterior pole granuloma (age 6–14yrs)*: VA; yellow–white granuloma 1-2DD at the macula/papillomacular bundle with retinal traction and vitreous bands.
- *Peripheral granuloma (age 6–adult)*: usually asymptomatic until significant traction; yellow–white granuloma anterior to the equator with vitreous bands; traction may cause macula heterotopia or retinal detachment (tractional or rhegmatogenous).
- *Less common presentations include*: isolated anterior uveitis, intermediate uveitis, optic papillitis, and vitreous abscess.

Systemic (visceral larva migrans)
- Usually <4yrs of age.
- Fever, pneumonitis + bronchospasm, hepatosplenomegaly, fits, myocarditis, death (rare); eosinophilia.

Investigation
This is essentially a clinical diagnosis although ELISA for serum antibodies may be supportive and B-scan US may help differentiate from other diagnoses.

Treatment
Ocular toxocariasis: systemic or periocular steroids titrated according to disease severity; antihelminthics (e.g. thiabendazole) are of limited use; consider vitrectomy to clear debris, relieve traction, and to repair retinal detachments.

Diffuse unilateral subacute neuroretinitis (DUSN)

An increasingly recognized cause of posterior uveitis in young people in which a solitary nematode persists in the subretinal space for years causing progressive damage. Two unknown nematodes may cause the syndrome. They have different sizes (0.5mm and 1–2mm) and occur in different geographical distributions. Signs include a unilateral vitritis, optic disc swelling, deep retinal grey–white lesions, and sometimes the worm itself.

Treatment is difficult. If directly visualized the worm may be killed by argon laser; if not use antihelminthics (e.g. thiabendazole). Steroids suppress inflammation but do not alter outcome.

Onchocerciasis

Worldwide onchcocerciasis (river blindness) affects about 20 million people, causing visual impairment in 10%. The filarial nematode *Onchocerca volvulus* is spread between humans (definitive host) by bites of the Simulium blackfly (vector). Having entered the subcutaneous tissue the larvae mature into adult worms (up to 80cm long) and mate to produce microfilariae within large subcutaneous nodules. The microfilariae then spread to nearby tissues that may include the eye. The Simulium breed in areas of fast flowing water that also tend to be those regions that are most fertile and heavily farmed.

Ocular disease from the microfilariae includes sclerosing keratitis (with an opaque 'apron' over the inferior cornea), chorioretinitis, sclerosis of the retinal vessels, optic neuritis, and optic atrophy. Microfilariae may best be seen in the AC after face down posturing. Histology may be obtained from skin nodules.

Treatment was traditionally with diethylcarbamazine (which induces the severely itchy Mazzotti reaction), but has now been replaced with ivermectin.

Fungal uveitis

Candidiasis

Candida albicans is a higher fungus of the class blastomycetes. It is yeast-like (i.e. reproduces by budding) and imperfect (i.e. no sexual stage has yet been identified). It is often a commensal of skin, mouth, and vagina, but opportunistic systemic infection may arise from haematogenous spread, notably in IV drug abuse, indwelling venous catheters, and immunosuppression. Uveitis in an IV drug abuser should be considered fungal until proven otherwise.

Clinical features

- *Risk group*: IV drug abuse, indwelling catheters (haemodialysis, parenteral nutrition), immunosuppression (AIDS, steroids, cytotoxics, long-term antibiotics), systemic debilitation (malignancy).
- ↓VA, floaters, pain; often bilateral.
- Multifocal retinitis (yellow–white fluffy lesions ≥1DD in size) ± vitritis (colonies appear as 'cotton balls' that may be joined together forming a 'string of pearls') anterior uveitis.
- *Complications*: retinal necrosis, tractional retinal detachment.

Investigation and treatment

- Vitrectomy (send whole vitrectomy cassette) for microscopy/culture to confirm diagnosis.
- Intravitreal antifungals (e.g. 5µg amphotericin B).
- Systemic antifungals: liaise with microbiology/infectious disease specialist; oral fluconazole (usually 400mg initially then 200mg 2x/d) ± fucytosine is generally effective; consider IV amphotericin B (dose according to preparation) for known systemic involvement or resistant cases; duration of treatment is usually ≥4wks.
- Review frequently; admission may be helpful especially if poor compliance likely or IV treatment necessary.

Aspergillosis

Aspergillus may occasionally cause an endogenous endophthalmitis similar to *Candida*. It generally occurs in those with chronic pulmonary disease who are severely immunosuppressed. It is more aggressive than Candidal infection with pain and rapid visual loss being marked. A confluent yellowish infiltrate is seen in the subretinal space that progresses to a sub-retinal hypopyon. Other features include intraretinal haemorrhages, dense vitritis, and AC hypopyon.

Treatment is similar to *Candida* but usually requires IV amphotericin B. Final VA is usually <6/60.

Histoplasmosis and presumed ocular histoplasmosis syndrome (POHS)

Histoplasma capsulatum is a higher dimorphic fungus that grows as a yeast at 37°C and as a mycelium in soil. It is endemic in southern Europe, southern USA, central America, and Asia.

Ocular disease from direct infection of the globe is rare, usually occurs in the very young or the immunosuppressed and may involve posterior/panuveitis or endophthalmitis.

Treatment is with ketoconazole or amphotericin B.

More commonly *H. capsulatum* is invoked as the possible agent underlying presumed ocular histoplasmosis syndrome (POHS), albeit via an abnormal immune response. The evidence for *H. capsulatum* being the causative agent is, however, inconclusive. Epidemiology indicates that while there is correlation between regions of high prevalence of *H. capsulatum* and POHS, an apparently identical syndrome is seen in non-endemic areas (such as the UK, northern Europe, and northern USA). It is most common in the fourth decade. It is usually bilateral but sequential, with a mean interval of 4yrs between onset of symptoms in each eye.

Clinical features
- Well-demarcated atrophic choroidal scars (≤1DD) around posterior pole/mid periphery ('histo' spots); peripapillary atrophy; peripheral linear atrophic streaks; no significant vitritis.
- *Complications*: choroidal neovascularization (type 2); this is often the presenting feature of otherwise asymptomatic disease.

Investigation and treatment
- Diagnosis is clinical but FFA is required if CNV suspected.
- Antifungals have no benefit.
- Active lesions at the macula are often treated with immunosuppression (commonly corticosteroids).
- For extrafoveal and juxtafoveal memranes, CNV conventional laser photocoagulation is of benefit (MPS: severe vision loss at 5yrs 42% for untreated vs 12% for argon-treated extrafoveal).
- For subfoveal membranes, PDT or submacular surgery (membrane excision or macular rotation) should be considered. Emerging therapies include anti-VEGF treatments.

White dot syndromes (1)

Acute posterior multifocal placoid pigment epitheliopathy (APMPPE)

This is an uncommon condition of young adults that is usually bilateral and may be preceded by a flu-like illness. There appears to be an association with HLA-B7 and HLA-DR2.

Clinical features
- Acute ↓VA sequentially in both eyes (usually after a few days interval).
- Post-equatorial lesions of the RPE (initially grey-white but fades over weeks with irregular depigmentation/pigmentation), mild vitritis.

Investigations and treatment
FFA: early dense hypofluorescence and late staining of lesions. Spontaneous recovery within 2–3mths so treatment is not usually indicated.

Serpiginous choroidopathy

This is a rare bilateral condition of the middle-aged that may superficially resemble acute posterior multifocal placoid pigment epitheliopathy but has a much worse prognosis.

Clinical features
- ↓VA but often asymptomatic until macular involvement.
- Peripapillary lesions at the level of the RPE/inner choroid (grey-white, spread centrifugally from the disc but may 'skip', becomes atrophic over months with irregular depigmentation/pigmentation), mild vitritis.
- Complications: extensive subretinal scarring, CNV membrane (≤30%).

Investigations and treatment
- FFA: early dense hypofluorescence and late staining of lesions.
- Corticosteroids/other immunosuppressives are commonly used in the acute phase, although there is no clear evidence of benefit.
- CNV membranes may be treated by laser, PDT, or surgery.
- There may be a role for intravitreal anti-VEGF therapy.

Birdshot retinochoroidopathy

This is an uncommon bilateral condition of middle-aged Caucasian adults with a slight female preponderance. About 90% are HLA-A29 positive.

Clinical features
- ↓VA, ↓colour vision, floaters, nyctalopia.
- Lesions at the level of the RPE (oval, cream-coloured, radiate from the optic disc to the equator, associated with large choroidal vessels; become atrophic but not pigmented), moderate vitritis, vasculitis, CMO.
- Complications: CNV membrane, optic atrophy.

Investigations and treatment
This is one condition in which treatment should be directed by electrodiagnostic results rather than the clinical picture alone.
- ERG: ↓b wave amplitude and latency; EOG: ↓Arden index.
- HLA testing: HLA-A29 positive in 90%. If HLA-A29 negative consider sarcoid as a differential as this can give a similar picture.

- Corticosteroids/other immunosuppressants are used to treat any CMO, although it is not clear if this improves final outcome. CNV membranes may be treated by laser, PDT, or surgery. There may be a role for intravitreal anti-VEGF therapy.

Table 11.25 Summary of white dot syndromes

Syndrome	Age	Sex	Laterality	Vitritis	Lesion size	Prognosis
PIC	20–40	F>M	Bilateral	–	1/10DD	Guarded
POHS	20–50	M=F	Bilateral	–	1/3DD	Guarded
MEWDS	20–40	>M	Unilateral	+	1/5DD	Good
APMPPE	20–40	M=F	Bilateral	+	1 DD	Good
Serpiginous choroidopathy	30–60	M=F	Bilateral	+		Poor
Birdshot retinochoroidopathy	23–79	F>M	Bilateral	++	1/4–1/2DD	Guarded
Multifocal choroiditis with panuveitis	30–60	F>M	Bilateral	++	1/10DD	Guarded

White dot syndromes (2)

Multifocal choroiditis with panuveitis (MCP) and punctate inner choroidopathy (PIC)

These are uncommon bilateral conditions which may simulate POHS (sometimes called pseudo-POHS). Both are commoner in women, but PIC tends to affect a younger age group. A viral aetiology has been suggested.

Clinical features
- ↓VA, scotomata, photopsia.
- Multifocal choroiditis with panuveitis: choroidal lesions (grey, peripheral + posterior polar), vitritis anterior uveitis, CMO, subretinal fibrosis, CNV membrane.
- PIC: quiet eye (no vitritis) with lesions at the level of the inner choroid/retina (initially yellow–white but become atrophic pigmented scars similar to POHS; posterior polar), serous retinal detachment, CNV membrane.

Investigations and treatment
- FFA: early hypofluorescence and late staining of lesions.
- Corticosteroids are commonly used for acute lesions or CMO.
- CNV membrane: medical treatment, laser, PDT or surgery. There may be a role for intravitreal anti-VEGF therapy.

Multiple evanescent white-dot syndrome (MEWDS)

This is a rare unilateral condition typically of young women that may be preceded by a flu-like illness.

Clinical features
- Acute ↓VA, scotomata ± photopsia.
- Small white dots at level of outer retina/RPE, tiny orange-white dots at the fovea, mild vitritis.

Investigations and treatment
- FFA: early punctate hyperfluorescence and late staining of lesions.
- ERG: ↓a-wave.
- Spontaneous recovery within 2–3mths so treatment is not usually indicated.

Acute zonal occult outer retinopathy (AZOOR)

This may form part of a spectrum of disease comprising MEWDS, multi-focal choroiditis with panuveitis, PIC, and the acute idiopathic blind-spot enlargement syndrome.

It is an uncommon condition affecting one or both eyes, typically in myopic young/middle-aged women after a flu-like illness.

Clinical features
- Acute scotomata, worse in bright light; photopsia.
- Acutely may have vitritis; later may have zonal atrophy/irregular pigmentation (RP-like).

Investigations and treatment
- ERG: variably abnormal in a patchy distribution and often asymmetric.
- Immunosuppression is common during the acute phase but is of no proven benefit.

Chapter 12

Vitreoretinal

Anatomy and physiology

Anatomy

Vitreous

The vitreous makes up 80% of ocular volume or about 4.0ml. It is a transparent gel of which 99% is water. The remainder consists of hyaluronic acid and collagen (types II, IX, and a V/XI hybrid).

Collagen fibrils connect the vitreous to the retinal internal limiting membrane.

The vitreous base is a 3–4mm wide zone overlying the ora serrata.

Retina (see Medical retinal anatomy and physiology 🕮 p.454)

The retina is a transparent light-transforming laminated structure comprising photoreceptors, interneurones, and ganglion cells overlying the retinal pigment epithelium.

Superficial retinal vessels form four major arcades over the surface of the retina. Within the suprachoroidal space are the long posterior ciliary nerves and arteries that can be seen peripherally at 3 and 9 o'clock. Similarly, the vortex ampullae (which drain into the vortex veins) may be seen at all four diagonal quadrants just anterior to the equator.

Vitreoretinal adhesions

- *Normal attachments* are strongest at the disc, the fovea, and, in particular, the ora serrata/vitreous base that remains adherent even when posterior vitreous detachment is otherwise complete.
- *Abnormal attachments* include areas of lattice degeneration (posterior border), white-without-pressure, congenital cystic tufts, pigment clumps, and condensations around vessels.

Physiology

Forces of attachment

The retinal position is maintained by hydrostatic forces and to a lesser extent by the adhesion of the interphotoreceptor matrix. The hydrostatic forces are both active (the RPE pump) and passive (the osmotic gradient).

Forces of detachment

Vitreoretinal traction may be dynamic (due to eye movement) or static (due purely to vitreoretinal interaction, e.g. diabetic fibrovascular proliferation). The direction of static forces may be tangential, bridging, or anteroposterior. Gravitational forces are probably a significant factor in superior breaks.

Vitreous liquefaction

The ageing vitreous becomes progressively liquefied (syneresis) resulting in optically empty fluid filled spaces (lacunae), and a reduction in the shock-absorbing capacity of the vitreous.

Liquefaction occurs earlier in myopia, trauma, inflammation, and many disorders of collagen and connective tissue. A break in the cortical vitreous permits vitreal fluid to flow through into the retrohyaloid space causing separation and collapse of the remaining vitreous (posterior vitreous detachment).

Retinal detachment: assessment

Retinal detachment is a relatively common sight-threatening condition with an incidence of about 1/10 000/yr (Tables 12.1–12.3).

Rhegmatogenous retinal detachment (RRD)

This is usually an ophthalmic emergency, notably in the presence of a U-shaped tear and where the macula is still 'on' (i.e. attached) (see Rhegmatogenous retinal detachment ☐ pp.426–429).

It is the commonest form of retinal detachment and usually arises when PVD causes a break in the retina, although some RRD arise without PVD (e.g. with round holes or with dialysis).

Untreated it almost always leads to a blind eye, but with appropriate early treatment may have an excellent outcome.

Table 12.1 An approach to assessing retinal detachments

Visual symptoms	Asymptomatic; flashes, floaters, distortion, 'curtain' field defect, ↓VA
POH	Refractive error (myopia), surgery (e.g. complicated cataract extraction), laser treatment, trauma
PMH	Connective tissue syndromes (e.g. Stickler), diabetes, anaesthetic history
FH	Retinal problems/detachments, connective tissue syndromes
SH	Driver; occupation
Dx	
Ax	Allergies or relevant drug contraindications
Visual acuity	Best-corrected/pin-hole
Pupils	RAPD (if extensive RD)
Cornea	Clarity (for surgery)
AC	Cells/flare (mild activity is common)
Lens	Cataract
Tonometry	IOP may be low, normal, or high
Vitreous	Haemorrhage, pigment ('tobacco dust', Shafer's Sign)
Fundus	Retinal detachment: location, extent, age (atrophy, intraretinal cysts, pigment demarcation lines), proliferative vitreoretinopathy (vitreous haze, retinal stiffness, retinal folds), retinal break(s): location, associated degeneration
Macula	On, threatened or off
Other eye	Degenerations, breaks, other disease

Indirect fundoscopy with scleral indentation to the ora serrata of both eyes

Tractional and exudative retinal detachment (TRD, ERD)

In these there are usually no causative breaks in the retina; it is either pulled (tractional) or pushed (exudative) from position.

- Tractional detachments (see Tractional retinal detachment 📖 p.430) tend to be slowly progressive but may be static for long periods.
- Exudative detachments (see Exudative retinal detachment 📖 p.432) may fluctuate according to the underlying disease process.

Table 12.2 Differentiating features of retinal detachments

	RRD	ERD	TRD
Vitreous	Pigment ± blood	No pigment ± inflammatory cells	No pigment
Fluid	Fairly static	Dependent shifting fluid	Little fluid, non-shifting
Shape	Convex corrugated	Convex smooth	Concave
Retinal features	Break(s) ± degeneration	Normal or features of underlying disease	Preretinal fibrosis

Table 12.3 Differentiating features of RRD vs retinoschisis

	RRD	Retinoschisis
Dome	Convex corrugated	Convex smooth
Laterality	Unilateral	Usually bilateral
Field defect	Relative	Absolute
Chronic changes	Demarcation line	No demarcation line
Breaks	Present	Absent or small inner leaf holes
Response to laser	No uptake	Good uptake

Peripheral retinal degenerations

Almost all eyes have some abnormality of the peripheral retina. Only about 1 in 40 of the population develop any form of retinal break. Identification of different types of peripheral retinal degeneration permits risk stratification, and selective treatment of those lesions that are likely to progress. (Table 12.4)

It is important to appreciate that prophylactic laser treatment may carry the risk of *causing* retinal breaks.[1]

Lattice degeneration

Lattice degeneration is present in about 6% of the normal population but 30% of all RRDs. It is more common in myopes and connective tissue syndromes (e.g. Stickler).

- Areas of retinal thinning with criss-cross white lines ± small round holes within the lesion; typically circumferential but may be radial (more common in Stickler).
- Retinal tears may occur at posterior margin and at the ends of areas of lattice (due to strong vitreous adhesion) → retinal detachment.
- Clinical retinal detachment occurs in only 1% of patients with lattice degeneration.[2] Prophylactic laser treatment is not usually performed in asymptomatic eyes unless the fellow eye has previously had a detachment.

Snailtrack degeneration

- Snailtrack degeneration is relatively common in myopes and may be an early form of lattice degeneration.[3]
- Long circumferential areas of retinal thinning with a glistening appearance ± large round holes.
- Large round holes within the lesion may lead to retinal detachment.

Peripheral cystoid degeneration

- Peripheral cystoid degeneration increases with age to become almost universal.
- Close-packed tiny cystic spaces at the outer plexiform/inner nuclear level ± retinoschisis.

Retinoschisis (degenerative type)

- Retinoschisis is present in about 5% of the normal population but is more common in hypermetropes. It is usually bilateral. It is asymptomatic unless posterior extension causes a significant field defect.
- Splitting of retina usually at outer plexiform/inner nuclear level leads to inner leaf ballooning into the vitreous cavity; usually inferotemporal and arising in areas of peripheral cystoid degeneration.
- Rarely, a combination of small inner leaf holes and the less common larger outer leaf breaks may lead to retinal detachment.

White without pressure

- This is fairly common in young and heavily pigmented patients. It represents the vitreoretinal interface and is probably of no significance.
- Whitened ring of retina just anterior to the retina and underlying the vitreous base.

Snowflake degeneration
- Snowflake degeneration may represent vitreous attachments to retinal Müller cells. It is probably of no significance; rare familial cases probably reflect a different process.
- Diffuse frosted appearance with white dots.

Pavingstone degeneration
- Pavingstone degeneration is common with increasing age and myopia.
- Irregular patches of absent RPE and choriocapillaris forming windows to the large choroidal vessels and sclera ± mild retinal thinning.

Cobblestone degeneration
- Cobblestone degeneration is commoner with increasing age and is of no significance.
- Small drusen-like bodies with pigment ring at level of Bruch's membrane.

Reticular pigmentary degeneration (honeycomb pigmentation)
- Reticular pigmentary degeneration is commoner with increasing age and is of no significance.
- Honeycomb pattern of peripheral pigmentation.

Meridional folds
- Meridional folds do not increase risk of retinal detachment, but in cases of detachment the hole(s) may be closely related to these folds.
- Small radial fold of retina in axis of dentate process ± small hole at base.

Retinal tufts
- Retinal tufts are common lesions and often associated with holes; however, they are usually within the vitreous base and thus of no significance.
- White inward projections of retina due to abnormal traction ± small holes.

Table 12.4 Peripheral retinal degenerations

Moderate risk	Low risk
Lattice	Peripheral cystoid degeneration
Snail track	Retinoschisis
	White without pressure
	Snowflake degeneration
	Pavingstone degeneration
	Cobblestone degeneration
	Reticular pigmentary degeneration
	Meridional folds
	Retinal tufts

1. Chauhan DS et al. Failure of prophylactic retinopexy in fellow eyes without a posterior vitreous detachment. *Arch Ophthalmol* 2006;**124**:968–71.

2. Byer NE. Long-term natural history of lattice degeneration of the retina. *Ophthalmology* 1989;**96**:1396–402.

3. Shukla M, Ahuja OP. A possible relationship between lattice and snail track degenerations of the retina. *Am J Ophthalmol* 1981;**92**:482–5.

Retinal breaks

Approximately 2.5% of the population have an identifiable full-thickness retinal defect (break).

As progression to retinal detachment is rare and retinopexy (laser or cryotherapy) is not without risk, attempts have been made to identify and treat only the high-risk group. High risk may be a function of the type of break (e.g. fresh symptomatic U-tear associated with acute PVD), the eye (e.g. high myopia), events in the contralateral eye (e.g. giant retinal tear), or the patient as a whole (e.g. Stickler syndrome) (Tables 12.5–12.6).

Retinal hole

This is a full thickness retinal defect due to atrophy without vitreoretinal traction. It may be associated with peripheral retinal degeneration, e.g. lattice or snailtrack.

An operculated hole is used to denote a hole caused by PVD where the operculum has avulsed and is now free floating within the vitreous.

Retinal tear

This is a full thickness U-shaped defect due to PVD. It is associated with abnormal vitreous adhesions, e.g. lattice degeneration.

Ongoing vitreoretinal traction at flap apex causes progression to RRD in at least one-third of cases.

Giant retinal tear

A giant retinal tear is a tear of more than 3 clock-hours in extent. They are normally located in the peripheral retina at the posterior border of the vitreous base. They are associated with PVD, distinguishing a giant retinal tear from a retinal dialysis. The vitreous remains attached to the attached anterior retina They are associated with systemic disease (e.g. Marfan syndrome and Stickler syndrome), trauma, and high myopia.

Dialysis

This is a full thickness circumferential disinsertion of the retina from the ora serrata. It may arise spontaneously or after trauma. It is not related to PVD and usually progresses slowly as the vitreous is attached. It is usually inferotemporal but post-trauma cases may be superonasal.

Treatment of retinal breaks

- Treatment is controversial. Common practice is that all U-tears (especially if symptomatic) should be treated, usually with laser photocoagulation or less commonly cryotherapy. Asymptomatic small round holes are commonly not treated. Dialyses are treated with scleral buckling if there is associated RD or with laser/cryotherapy if no/limited RD.
- Fellow eye treatment is also controversial. In giant retinal tear the fellow eye is often treated, e.g. with 360' cryotherapy or laser[1]. In a case of simple RRD, lattice in the fellow eye is often not treated unless there is an additional risk factor, e.g. high myopia, aphakia, etc.
- A 'retinal detachment warning' should be given in all cases, i.e. advise to seek urgent ophthalmic review if further episodes of new floaters, flashes, a 'curtain' field defect or drop in vision.

Table 12.5 Risk factors for RRD according to type of break

High risk	Low risk
U-tear, large hole, or dialysis	Giant retinal tear in the other eye
Asymptomatic small round holes	Breaks within the vitreous base

Table 12.6 Risk factors for RRD according to other ocular and systemic features

Ocular	General	Trauma (blunt/penetrating)
		Surgery
	Refractive	Myopia
	Lenticular	Aphakia
		Pseudophakia (especially complicated surgery, e.g. vitreous loss)
		Posterior capsulotomy
	Retinal	Lattice degeneration
		Retinoschisis
		Retinal necrosis (CMV, ARN/PORN)
	Other eye	Previous contralateral retinal detachment (especially giant retinal tear)
Systemic		Stickler syndrome
		Marfan syndrome
		Ehlers–Danlos syndrome

1. Wolfensberger TJ, Aylward GW, Leaver PK. Prophylactic 360°∞ cryotherapy in fellow eyes of patients with spontaneous giant retinal tears. *Ophthalmology* 2003;**110**:1175–7.

Posterior vitreous detachment

With age the vitreous becomes progressively liquefied (syneresis). This results in optically empty spaces (lacunae), and a reduction in its shock-absorbing capability. The liquefaction process occurs earlier in myopia, trauma, inflammation, and many disorders of collagen and connective tissue. When a break in the cortical vitreous occurs, vitreal fluid can flow through into the retrohyaloid space, to cause separation of the vitreous and retina, with collapse of the remaining vitreous—posterior vitreous detachment (PVD).

It is of significance because: (1) it is very common; (2) it may be associated with a retinal tear in 10% cases; and (3) the symptoms are similar to retinal detachment.

Clinical features

- Flashes (usually an arc of white light in the temporal field of view), floaters (usually a ring or cobwebs; move or 'wobble' with ocular movement; the less common shower of black specks suggests haemorrhage and is often associated with a retinal tear).
- Vitreous: Weiss ring (indicates detachment at the optic disc), visible posterior hyaloid face; occasionally haemorrhage.
- *Complications*: retinal break(s), vitreous haemorrhage, retinal detachment.

NB It is critical to achieve a complete fundal examination using 360° scleral indentation to rule out any associated retinal breaks. Remember in eyes with retinal breaks, there is more than one break in 50% cases.

Treatment

- *Uncomplicated PVD*: reassure but give 'retinal detachment warning', i.e. advise to seek urgent ophthalmic review if further episodes of new floaters, flashes, a 'curtain' field defect or drop in vision.
- *PVD complicated by vitreous haemorrhage*: clear visualization of whole retina to the ora serrata is necessary to rule out breaks/early RRD; if not possible then use B-scan US (see Table 12.7); follow up frequently as an outpatient until haemorrhage has cleared.

NB US can miss retinal tears: a large fundus-obscuring haemorrhage in a high-risk eye is best treated by early vitrectomy.

- PVD complicated by retinal tear: treat, e.g. by laser photocoagulation (focal argon retinopexy).

Table 12.7 Ultrasonic features of vitreoretinal pathology

PVD	Faintly reflective posterior hyaloid face may appear incomplete except on eye movement
	Eye movement induces staccato movement with 1s after-movement
	Low reflectivity on A-scan
	No blood demonstrated on colour flow mapping
RRD	Highly reflective irregular convex membrane
	Eye movement induces undulating after-movement (unless PVR)
	High reflectivity on A-scan
	Blood demonstrated on colour flow mapping
Tractional retinal detachment	Highly reflective membrane tented into vitreous
	Eye movement induces no after-movement of membrane
	Blood demonstrated on colour flow mapping
Choroidal detachment	Highly reflective regular dome-shaped membrane
	Attached to the vortex ampulla/vein
	Blood demonstrated on colour flow mapping both in retina (6–8cm/s) and choroid (8–10cm/s)
Vitreous haemorrhage	Reflective particulate matter within the vitreous space (indistinguishable from vitritis)
	More detailed examination can usually distinguish the underlying cause, e.g. RRD, CNV, PDR, or C/BRVO

Rhegmatogenous retinal detachment (1) (RRD)

RRD is usually an ophthalmic emergency. Untreated, it usually progresses to blindness and even phthisis. However, with appropriate early treatment it may have an excellent outcome. It is the commonest form of retinal detachment with an incidence of 1/10 000/yr.

RRD occurs when vitreous liquefaction and a break in the retina allows fluid to enter the subretinal space and separate the neural retina from the RPE.

Clinical features

- Flashes (usually temporal, more noticeable in dim conditions), floaters (distinct, e.g. Weiss ring, or particulate, e.g. blood), 'curtain' type field defect, ↓VA (suggests macula involvement).
- *Vitreous*: PVD + vitreal pigment ('tobacco dust') ± blood. These are more obvious on vitreous movement: ask the patient to look up and down while at the slit-lamp.
- *Retinal break(s)*: usually U-tear (occasionally giant, i.e. >3 clock hours); sometimes large round holes or dialysis. The upper temporal quadrant is the commonest location (60%). Identifying the primary break may be assisted by considering the effect of gravity on the subretinal fluid (Box 12.1, modified from Lincoff's rules[1]). However, multiple breaks are common, and meticulous view of the whole peripheral retina is essential.
- *Retinal detachment*: unilateral corrugated convex dome of retina and loss of RPE/choroidal clarity; usually peripheral (subretinal fluid extends to ora serrata) but occasionally posterior polar if secondary to a macular or other posterior hole.
- *Chronic changes*: retinal thinning, demarcation lines from 3mths, intraretinal cysts from 1yr; some develop proliferative vitreoretinopathy. May also have RAPD (if extensive detachment), relative field defect, ↓IOP (but may be normal or ↑ (Schwartz syndrome)), and mild AC activity.

Rhegmatogenous retinal detachment associated with round holes or dialysis
Theses are not associated with a PVD and so do not get associated symptoms of flashes and floaters; these RRD are therefore usually picked up as an asymptomatic finding or when macular involvement → ↓VA.

Box 12.1 Locating the primary retinal break[2]

In superior retinal detachments[1]

- For superonasal or superotemporal detachments the break is usually near the superior border of the detachment
- For symmetric superior detachments crossing the vertical meridian (i.e. superonasal and superotemporal) the break is usually near 12 o'clock

In inferior retinal detachments

- For inferior detachments the break is usually on the side with most fluid (i.e. the higher fluid level) BUT
  - it may be quite inferior (i.e. not related to the superior border) and
  - slower fluid accumulation means that non-midline breaks may still result in symmetrical inferior detachments.
- For bullous inferior detachments the primary break is above the midline.

Table 12.8 Features of a chronic retinal detachment

Retinal thinning
Demarcation lines ('high water marks')
Intraretinal cysts
Proliferative vitreoretinopathy

Table 12.9 Proliferative vitreoretinopathy

Type	A	Vitreous haze/pigment
		Pigment on inner retina
	B	Retinal wrinkling + stiffness
	C	Rigid retinal folds ('starfolds')
Subtypes of C		
Location	Pre vs post- equatorial	Anterior
		Posterior
Extent	1–12	Number of clock-hours
Contraction	Type 1	Focal
	Type 2	Diffuse
	Type 3	Subretinal
	Type 4	Circumferential
	Type 5	Anterior

1. Lincoff H, Gieser R. Finding the hole. *Arch Ophthalmol* 1971;**85**:565–69.

Rhegmatogenous retinal detachment (2)

Investigation
- *Consider US* if unable to adequately visualize (e.g. dense cataract or haemorrhage).
- *B-scan US*: highly reflective irregular convex membrane; eye movement induces undulating after-movement (unless PVR).

Treatment
Urgent vitreoretinal referral
- Macula-on detachments with a U-tear should be referred urgently.
- Once the macula has detached there is some evidence that surgery any time in the next 7d has the same visual outcome.[1]

Posturing
- *Posture so that dependent fluid moves away from macula*: it is mainly useful for upper bullous attachments and giant retinal tears (position so tear is unfolded).
- Traditional posturing for superior detachments would usually involve being flat on one's back with ipsilateral cheek to pillow for temporal detachments (i.e. right cheek for right eye) and contralateral cheek to pillow for nasal detachments (i.e. left cheek for right eye).
- Posturing is not of use in RRD associated with round holes or a dialysis.

Surgery
Scleral buckling and vitrectomy have advantages in different contexts. Vitrectomy is now the more commonly used procedure (about 80% cases) but there is considerable inter-surgeon variation.
- *Scleral buckling (see □ pp.446–447)*: suitable for most simple RRD, and procedure of choice if no pre-existing PVD; segmental (single breaks or multiple breaks within 1 clock-hour) vs encircling (more extensive breaks).
- *Vitrectomy (see □ pp.448–449)*: indicated for retinal detachments with posterior retinal breaks, giant retinal tears, proliferative vitreoretinopathy but also increasingly used for bullous retinal detachments of all types, including those with high-risk features (e.g. aphakia/pseudophakia).

---

1. Ross WH, Kozy DW. Visual recovery in macula-off rhegmatogenous retinal detachments. *Ophthalmology* 1998; **105**:2149–53.

Tractional Retinal Detachment

Tractional retinal detachment

Tractional retinal detachment (Table 12.10) is uncommon. It arises due to a combination of contracting retinal membranes, abnormal vitreoretinal adhesions, and vitreous changes. It is usually seen in the context of diseases that induce a fibrovascular response, e.g. diabetes.

Clinical features
- Often asymptomatic; distortion (if macular involvement).
- *Retinal detachment*: concave tenting of retina that is immobile and usually shallow ± macular ectopia (drag); slowly progressive.
- May also have relative field defect, metamorphopsia on Amsler grid, ↓VA and evidence of underlying disease process (e.g. diabetic retinopathy).
- *Complications*: may detach the macula or may develop a break to become a rapidly progressive combined tractional RRD.

Treatment

Surgery is difficult and thus often deferred until the macula is threatened or detached. It usually requires removal of tractional forces by vitrectomy and membrane peel, or delamination followed by tamponade with either a long-acting gas or oil if needed (retinal break).

Table 12.10 Causes of tractional retinal detachments (selected)

Proliferative diabetic retinopathy
ROP
Sickle cell retinopathy
Vitreomacular traction syndrome
Incontinentia pigmenti
Retinal dysplasia

Exudative retinal detachment

Exudative (serous) retinal detachment (Table 12.11) is relatively rare. It arises from damage to the outer blood–retinal barrier allowing fluid to access the subretinal space and separate retina from RPE.

Clinical features

- Distortion and ↓VA (if macula involved), which may fluctuate; relative field defect; floaters (if vitritis).
- *Retinal detachment*: smooth convex dome that may be shallow or bullous; in bullous exudative retinal detachment the fluid moves rapidly to the most dependent position ('shifting fluid'); the fluid may be clear or cloudy (lipid-rich); no retinal breaks or evidence of traction.
- May also have irregular pigmentation of previously detached areas and evidence of underlying disease (e.g. abnormal Coats' vessels).

Investigation and treatment

- All patients require a full ophthalmic and systemic examination, BP, and urinalysis.
- Consider B-scan US, especially if posterior scleritis suspected.
- Surgery is very rarely indicated and treatment is directed towards the underlying disease process.

Table 12.11 Common causes of exudative retinal detachments

Congenital		Nanophthalmos (→2° Uveal effusion syndrome)
		Mucopolysaccharidoses (II and VI)
		Familial exudative vitreoretinopathy
Acquired	Vascular	Exudative AMD
		Coats' disease
		Central serous chorioretinopathy
		Vasculitis
		Malignant hypertension
		Pre-eclampsia
	Tumours	Choroidal tumours
	Inflammatory	Posterior uveitis (notably Vogt–Koyanagi–Harada syndrome, Sympathetic ophthalmia)
		Posterior scleritis
		Postoperative inflammation
		Extensive PRP
		Orbital cellulitis
		Idiopathic orbital inflammatory disease

Retinoschisis

Retinoschisis is by definition a splitting of the retina. Degenerative retino-schisis is common, being present in about 5% of the normal adult population.

Degenerative retinoschisis

Degenerative retinoschisis (Table 12.12) is more common in hypermetropes and is usually bilateral.

In typical senile retinoschisis the break is at the outer plexiform/inner nuclear level. In the less common reticular type the split is at the nerve fibre layer (i.e. as occurs in X-linked juvenile retinoschisis, see 📖 p.436).

Clinical features

- Asymptomatic (unless very posterior extension); absolute field defect.
- *Retinoschisis*: split retina with inner leaf ballooning into the vitreous cavity; usually inferotemporal; arises in areas of peripheral cystoid degeneration; scleral indentation may cause outer leaf to whiten, sometimes with a reticular appearance.
- *'T-test'*: using the indirect ophthalmoscope, project a T-shape using the head of a scleral indenter onto the retinoschisis. The patient will be unable to see the T-shape due to the absolute scotoma caused by the retinoschisis.

Complications:

- Inner leaf breaks (small/round) and/or outer leaf breaks (less common; large with rolled edges).
- *Retinal detachment*: either low-risk limited type (outer leaf break only with fluid from the schisis cavity causing local retinal elevation) or high-risk rhegmatogenous type (inner and outer leaf breaks with full thickness retinal elevation beyond area of schisis).

Investigations

This is essentially a clinical diagnosis but laser take-up by the posterior leaf or OCT findings can differentiate from retinal detachment.

Treatment

No treatment is necessary unless complicated by retinal detachment.

X-linked juvenile retinoschisis (📖 p.436)

This rare condition is seen in males and may present in childhood with maculopathy. It results in retinal splitting at the nerve fibre layer (cf. typical degenerative retinoschisis). Visual prognosis is poor.

Table 12.12 Differentiating retinoschisis from chronic RRD

	Retinoschisis	**RRD**
Vitreous	Clear	Pigment ± blood
Dome	Convex smooth	Convex corrugated
Laterality	Usually bilateral	Unilateral
Field defect	Absolute	Relative
Signs of chronicity	No demarcation line	Demarcation line
Breaks	Absent or small inner leaf holes	Present
Response to laser	Good uptake	No uptake

Hereditary vitreoretinal degenerations

These are rare, inherited conditions characterized by premature degeneration of vitreous and retina.

Interestingly, the primary abnormality may be vitreal with secondary retinal changes (e.g. Stickler syndrome) or retinal with secondary vitreous abnormalities (e.g. X-linked juvenile retinoschisis).

Stickler syndrome

This condition arises from abnormalities in type II collagen (COL2A1, Ch12q), and is autosomal dominant with complete penetrance but variable expressivity.

Also known as hereditary arthro-ophthalmopathy, it is the commonest of this group of conditions.

Clinical features

- High myopia, optically empty vitreous, perivascular pigmentary changes (lattice-like).
- *Complications*: retinal tears, giant retinal tears, retinal detachments, cataract (comma-shaped cortical opacities), ectopia lentis, glaucoma (open-angle).
- *Systemic*: epiphyseal dysplasia → degeneration of large joints, cleft palate, bifid uvula, midfacial flattening, Pierre–Robin sequence, sensorineural deafness, mitral valve prolapse.

Investigations and treatment

- Essentially a clinical diagnosis, although genetic testing is available.
- Consider annual dilated fundoscopy.
- Unfortunately, retinal detachments are common (up to 50%) and carry a poor prognosis.
- Multidisciplinary care may include genetic counselling.
- Treat myopia early to prevent amblyopia.

X-linked juvenile retinoschisis

This rare condition appears to arise from abnormalities in an intercellular adhesion molecule (located on Xp22), which results in retinal splitting at the nerve fibre layer.

It is seen in males, and may present in early childhood with maculopathy. Visual prognosis is poor.

Clinical features

- Foveal schisis with spoke-like folds separating cystoid spaces (superficially resembles CMO but no leakage on FFA); later non-specific atrophy; peripheral retinal schisis ± inner leaf breaks (may coalesce to leave free-floating retinal vessels).
- *Complications*: vitreous haemorrhage, retinal detachment.

Investigations

- This is essentially a clinical diagnosis.
- Scotopic ERG shows selective loss of B-wave and oscillatory potentials.
- Visual field: absolute visual field loss in schitic areas.

Treatment
Prophylactic treatment of X-Linked retinoschisis is highly controversial and may cause retinal detachment.[1]

Goldmann–Favre syndrome

This very rare condition is similar to juvenile retinoschisis, but is autosomal recessive with more marked peripheral abnormalities (RP-like changes with whitened retinal vessels).

Familial exudative vitreoretinopathy

This rare condition usually shows autosomal dominant inheritance (Ch11q).

Clinical features
- Abrupt cessation of peripheral retinal vessels at the equator (more marked temporally), vitreous bands in the periphery.
- *Complications*: neovascularization, subretinal exudation (akin to Coat's disease), macular ectopia (akin to ROP), retinal detachment.

Other hereditary vitreoretinal degenerations

These include Wagner syndrome, erosive vitreoretinopathy, Knobloch syndrome, autosomal dominant neovascular inflammatory vitreoretinopathy, and autosomal dominant vitreoretinochoroidopthy.

1. Kellner U *et al.* X-linded congenital retinoschisis. Graefes *Arch Clin Exp Ophthalmol* 1990; **228**: 432-7. Combined Schisis detachment requires vitrectomylgas (or oil)/retuiopexy and scleral buckling

Choroidal detachments and uveal effusion syndrome

Choroidal detachments

Choroidal detachments (Tables 12.13 and 12.14) are usually seen in the context of acute hypotony, for example after glaucoma filtration surgery or cyclodestructive procedures. They are usually easily distinguished from retinal detachments.

Clinical features
- Smooth convex dome(s) of normal/slightly dark retinal colour.
- Arises from extreme periphery (may include ciliary body, and ora serrata becomes easily visible) but posterior extension limited by vortex vein adhesions to the scleral canals.
- Choroidal detachments may touch ('kissing choroidals') causing retinal adhesion and retinal detachment.

Treatment
- Management is either by observation (e.g. if this reflects an appropriate post-trabeculectomy fall in IOP) or by treating the underlying disease process.
- Choroidal haemorrhage may require surgical drainage, although this may be best left until the blood has liquefied.

Uveal effusion syndrome

This is a rare syndrome of idiopathic exudative retinal detachments of choroid, ciliary body and retina thought to arise from impaired posterior segment drainage usually associated with scleral thickening.

Idiopathic uveal effusion syndrome usually affects healthy adult men. It is sometimes divided into three types:
- nanophthalmic eyes (type 1);
- non-nanophthalmic eyes with clinically abnormal sclera (type 2); and
- non-nanophthalmic eyes with clinically normal sclera (type 3).

Nanophthalmos and the presence of clinically detectable thickened/rigid sclera is a good predictor both for histologically abnormal sclera and of good response to surgery.[1]

Clinical features
Combined choroidal detachments and exudative retinal detachments.

Treatment
Surgery: scleral windows (± application of mitomycin C) may decompress the vortex veins.

1. Uyama M *et al.* Uveal effusion syndrome: clinical features, surgical treatment, histological examination of the sclera and pathophysiology. *Ophthalmology* 2000;**107**:441–9.

Table 12.13 RRD vs choroidal detachment

	RRD	Choroidal detachment
Colour	Pale	Darker/normal colour
Dome	Convex corrugated	Convex smooth
Breaks	Present	Absent
Ora serrata	Visible with indentation	Easily visible
Maximal extent	*Anterior*: ora serrata	*Anterior*: ciliary body
	Posterior: unlimited	*Posterior*: vortex veins

Table 12.14 Common causes of choroidal detachment

Effusion	Hypotony
	Extensive PRP
	Extensive cryotherapy
	Posterior uveitis
	Uveal effusion syndrome
	Nanophthalmos
Haemorrhage	Intra-operative
	Trauma
	Spontaneous

Epiretinal membranes

Common synonyms for the disease reflect its appearance (macular pucker, cellophane maculopathy) and uncertain pathogenesis (premacular fibrosis, idiopathic premacular gliosis).

The condition is more common with increasing age (present in 6% of those over 50yrs), in females and after retinal insults (Box 12.2).

The membranes are fibrocellular and avascular, and are thought to arise from the proliferation of retinal glial cells that have migrated through defects in the ILM; such defects probably arise most commonly during PVD.

Clinical features

- Asymptomatic, metamorphopsia, ↓VA.
- Membrane may be transparent (look for glistening light reflex), translucent or white; retinal striae; vessels may be tortuous, straightened, or obscured; pseudohole.
NB The features are well demonstrated on red-free light.
- *Complications*: fovea ectopia; tractional macular detachment; CMO; intra/preretinal haemorrhages.

Investigations

- *OCT*: not essential, but confirms diagnosis (may differentiate pseudo- vs true hole) and useful to compare pre- and postoperative status.
- *FFA*: seldom used now due to advent of OCT, but nicely demonstrates vascular abnormalities and any associated CMO.

Treatment

- *Indications*: severely symptomatic membranes; ensure that macular function is not limited by an additional underlying pathology (e.g. ischaemia due to a vein occlusion)
- *Surgery*: vitrectomy/membrane peel; some surgeons assist visualization by staining with various dyes, e.g. indocyanine green, trypan blue, brilliant blue G.
- *Complications*: include cataract (up to 70% rate of significant nuclear sclerosis within 2yrs), retinal tears/detachment, retinal toxicity from dyes, worsened acuity (up to 15%), and symptomatic recurrence (5%).

Prognosis

- The disease is fairly stable with over 75% patients showing no further reduction in VA after diagnosis.
- With surgery, 60–85% patients show visual improvement (≥2 Snellen lines).
- Poor prognostic features are duration of symptoms before surgery, underlying macular pathology and lower pre-operative acuity (but may still show significant improvement).

Box 12.2 Causes of epiretinal membranes (ERM)

Idiopathic
Retinal detachment surgery
Cryotherapy
Photocoagulation
Trauma (blunt or penetrating)
Posterior uveitis
Persistent vitreous haemorrhage
Retinal vascular disease (e.g. BRVO)

Macular hole

The incidence of macular hole is about 1/10 000/yr; it is more common in women (2:1 F:M) and has a mean age of onset of 65yrs.

In some cases a predisposing pathological condition is identified. In the remaining 'idiopathic' cases, abnormal vitreo-macular traction may be observed clinically and with OCT. Release of this traction by vitrectomy ± removal of tangential traction by ILM peeling appears to underlie the success of surgery in treating this condition.

Staging

The developing macular hole may initially be asymptomatic, but can cause a progressive distortion of vision and a drop in acuity to approximately 6/120. Worsening acuity approximately correlates with the pathological stages described by Gass.

Clinical features

- *Stage 1*: no sensory retinal defect.
  - a: small yellow foveolar spot ± loss of foveal contour.
  - b: yellow foveolar ring.
- *Stage 2*: small (100–200µm) full-thickness sensory retinal defect.
- *Stage 3*: larger (350–600µm) full-thickness sensory retinal defect with cuff of subretinal fluid ± yellow deposits in base of hole.
- *Stage 4*: as for stage 3 but with complete vitreous separation.
- Watzke–Allen test (thin beam of light projected across the hole is seen to be thinned centrally or 'broken') may help differentiate from pseudo- or lamellar holes.

Investigations

- *OCT*: may assist diagnosis and staging where required.
- *FFA*: not usually indicated, but usually shows a window defect.

Treatment

- Refer to vitreoretinal surgeon; the chance of successful surgery is highest if performed at less than 6mths and halves if surgery delayed by more than 1yr.[1]
- *Surgery*: vitrectomy, ILM peel, and gas (will require face-down posturing); adjunctive agents such as autologous serum/platelets may be used.
- *Complications*: include cataracts (50% rate of significant nuclear sclerosis within 2yrs), retinal tears/detachment (about 1%), failure (anatomical up to 10%; visual up to 20%), late re-opening of hole (5%) and endophthalmitis.

Prognosis

- Stage 1 holes spontaneously resolve in 50%.
- *Without surgery*, stage 2 holes almost always progress, resulting in final VA of about 6/120.
- *With surgery*, early stage 2 holes show anatomical closure in >90% and visual success (≥2 Snellen lines) in 80%.
- If there is a PVD in the fellow eye, the risk of a macular hole is <1% over 5yrs. If there is no PVD in the fellow eye, the risk is about 10–20% over 5yrs.[2]

Box 12.3 Causes of macular holes

Idiopathic
Trauma
CMO
ERM/vitreomacular traction syndrome
RRD
Laser injury
Pathological myopia (with posterior staphyloma)
Hypertension
Diabetic retinopathy

1. Jaycock PD *et al.* Outcomes of macular hole surgery: implications for surgical management and clinical governance. *Eye* 2005;**19**:879–84.

2. Ezra E *et al.* Incidence of idiopathic full-thickness macular holes in fellow eyes. A 5-year prospective natural history study. *Ophthalmology* 1998;**105**:353–9.

Laser retinopexy and cryopexy for retinal tears

Laser retinopexy (slit-lamp or indirect delivery systems)

Mechanism

Laser light is absorbed by target tissue generating heat and causing local protein denaturation (photocoagulation) adhering the neural retina to the RPE. Green light is mainly absorbed by melanin and haemoglobin.

Indication

- Retinal break with risk of progression to rhegmatogenous retinal detachment (usually U-tears) and without excessive subretinal fluid.
- Equatorial and post-equatorial lesions can be reached with slit-lamp delivery system; more anterior lesions require indirect laser with indentation or cryotherapy.

Method

- *Consent*: explain what the procedure does; likely success rate (about 80%); and possible complications, including need for retreatment (about 20%), detachment despite treatment (9%, half of which are from a different break).
- *Ensure maximal dilation* (e.g. tropicamide 1% + phenylephrine 2.5%) and topical anaesthesia (e.g. oxybuprocaine 0.4%).

Slit-lamp

- *Set laser* (varies according to model): commonly spot size of 500µm, duration 0.1s and low initial power, e.g. 100mW.
- *Position contact lens* (usually a wide field lens, e.g. Transequator or the 3-mirror; both require coupling agent).
- *Focus and fire laser* to generate 2–3 rings of confluent grey–white burns (adjust power appropriately).

Indirect ophthalmoscope

- *Set laser* (varies according to model): commonly duration 0.1s and low power, e.g. 100mW.
- *Insert speculum* and coat cornea with hydroxypropylmethylcellulose or ensure regular irrigation to maintain clarity.
- While *viewing* with indirect ophthalmoscope gently indent to clearly visualize lesion.
- *Focus and fire laser* to generate 2–3 rings of confluent grey–white burns (adjust power appropriately). If the anterior portion of the tear is still out of reach or not visible, then a laser barricade up to the Ora may suffice.
- *Complications*: failure resulting in retinal detachment, retinal/vitreous haemorrhage, epiretinal membrane formation, CMO.

Cryopexy

Mechanism

Freezing causes local protein denaturation adhering the neural retina to the RPE.

Indications
- Retinal break with risk of progression to rhegmatogenous retinal detachment (usually U-tears) and without excessive subretinal fluid.
- Cryotherapy is most suitable for pre-equatorial lesions. It has advantages over laser retinopexy where there is a small pupil or media opacity, but may induce more PVR.

Methods
- *Consent*: explain what the procedure does; likely success rate; and possible complications, including failure/need for retreatment, discomfort, inflammation, and retinal/choroidal detachment.
- *Ensure maximal dilation* (e.g. tropicamide 1% + phenylephrine 2.5%).
- *Give local anaesthesia* (e.g. by subconjunctival injection as this preserves mobility).
- *Insert speculum* and coat cornea with hydroxypropylmethylcellulose or ensure regular irrigation to maintain clarity.
- While *viewing* with indirect ophthalmoscope gently indent with the cryoprobe to clearly visualize lesion.
- *Surround* the break with a single continuous ring of applications. The duration of each application should be just long enough for the retina to whiten. The probe should not be removed until thawing has occurred.
- *Post-procedure*: consider mild topical steroid/antibiotic combination (e.g. Betnesol-N® 4×/d for 1wk).
- *Complications*: inflammation, failure resulting in retinal detachment, retinal/vitreous haemorrhage, epiretinal membrane formation.

Scleral buckling procedures

Scleral buckling

Mechanism

It is suggested that the buckle closes the break by multiple mechanisms, including moving the RPE closer to the retina and moving the retina closer to the posterior vitreous cortex. It is postulated that these may reduce flow through the break (including the amount of fluid pumped through during eye movements) and relieve vitreous traction on flap tears.

Indications

- *Most simple RRD and dialyses:* procedure of choice in situations where there is no pre-existing PVD as a vitrectomy would require the induction of a PVD during surgery (highly difficult manoeuvre).
- *Segmental buckles:* for single breaks or multiple breaks within 1 clock-hour.
- *Encircling bands:* traditionally for extensive/multiple breaks or breaks in the presence of high-risk features (e.g. aphakia/pseudophakia, etc.); however, the majority of these would now have a vitrectomy (and no local buckle or encirclement).

Methods

Consent: explain what the operation does and possible complications, including failure, diplopia, refractive change, inflammation, infection, haemorrhage, explant extrusion, and worsened vision.

Perform appropriate conjunctival peritomy

- *Inspect sclera* for thinning and anomalous vortex veins; place traction sutures around selected rectus muscles to assist positioning.
- *Identify break* by indirect ophthalmoscope and indentation using the cryoprobe (or one of a number of instruments specifically designed for this purpose).
- *Perform cryopexy* by surrounding break(s) with a continuous ring of applications. Each application should last just long enough for the retina to whiten; the probe should not be removed until thawing has occurred. Mark the external position of the break on the sclera using indentation and a marker pen.
- *Select buckle size:* this should cover double the width of the retinal tear; position so that it extends from ora serrata to cover the posterior lip of the break.
- *Place partial-thickness 5-0 non-absorbable sutures* using a spatulated needle. These are usually mattress-type sutures and are placed at least 1mm away from the buckle on either side. (**NB** wider separation of sutures may result in a higher buckle. The number of sutures depends on the size of explant.)
- *Tighten sutures.* **NB** Tighter sutures results in a higher buckle.
- *Confirm buckle position* is correct and that arterial perfusion of the optic nerve is unaffected.
- *Close conjunctiva* (e.g. with 7-0 absorbable suture).

Complications
- *Intraoperative*: scleral perforation, subretinal fluid (SRF) drainage problems (retinal incarceration, choroidal/subretinal haemorrhage).
- *Postoperative*: infection, glaucoma, extrusion, choroidal effusion/detachment, epiretinal membrane, CMO, diplopia, refractive change, diplopia.

Prognosis
Anatomical success >90%, but only about 50% achieve a VA of 6/18 (macula-on detachments).

Options
Choice of buckle

Table 12.15 Buckle options

Material	Solid silicone rubber vs silicone sponge
Orientation	Segmental vs encircling
Size	Wide range available (and can be cut to size)

Drainage procedures
- Trans-scleral drainage of subretinal fluid with a 5-0 spatulated needle is done where there is deep subretinal fluid at the site of the break. Doing this when the IOP is high (e.g. by digital pressure on the globe) reduces risk of haemorrhage.
- Drainage of subretinal fluid is sometimes combined with the injection of intravitreal air in the DACE (drain–air–cryotherapy–explant) procedure.

Vitrectomy: outline

Vitrectomy

Mechanism

Vitrectomy removes dynamic tractional forces exerted on the retina by the vitreous; static tractional forces arising from membranes/fibrovascular proliferation can be removed at the same time.

Vitrectomy also allows surgical access to the retina to permit drainage of subretinal fluid, removal of intraocular membranes, and insertion of tamponade agents.

Indications

Retinal detachments
- *RRD*: traditionally reserved for those with posterior retinal breaks, giant retinal tears, proliferative vitreoretinopathy, or media opacity; now usage widened to include most bullous detachments, and detachments associated with aphakia/pseudophakia (or other higher-risk features).
- Tractional retinal detachment.

Other
- *Diagnostic*: e.g. biopsy for endophthalmitis, lymphoma.
- *Pharmacological*: e.g. administration of antibiotics, steroids.
- *Macular pathology*: macular holes, epiretinal membranes.
- *Trauma*: e.g. removal of FB.
- *Persistent media opacity*: vitreous haemorrhage, inflammatory debris, floaters (severe).
- *Complications of cataract surgery*: dropped nucleus, dislocated IOL.

Method

- *Consent*: explain what the operation does; the presence of a postoperative gas bubble; the importance of posturing; and possible complications, including failure, inflammation, infection, haemorrhage, and worsened vision.
- *Make 3 sclerostomies 4mm (phakic) or 3.5mm (aphakic/pseudophakic)* behind the limbus, placed inferotemporally, superotemporally, and superonasally.
- *Secure the infusion cannula* to the inferotemporal port. The infusion is used both to maintain the globe (so permitting aspiration) and can be used to increase pressure if intraocular bleeding occurs. It is important to visualize the tip of the infusion port before turning on the infusion.
- *Insert the light-pipe and then the vitrector* through the two superior ports under visualization (contact lens or indirect microscope system with inverter).
- *Vitrectomy*: of the posterior vitreous face and extending out to the periphery.
- *Replace the infusion fluid with a tamponade agent if required* (usually gas, sometimes oil for complicated cases).
- *Close the sclerostomies.*
- *Postoperative care*: if intraocular gas tamponade used, advise re posturing, warn against air travel and the use of nitrous oxide (anaesthetic agent) until the intraocular gas resorbed.

Complications
- *Intra-operative*: retinal breaks (posterior, peripheral), choroidal haemorrhage, lens touch.
- *Postoperative*: retinal breaks/RRD, cataract, glaucoma, inflammation, endophthalmitis (1/2000), hypotony, corneal decompensation, sympathetic ophthalmia (0.01% of routine vitrectomy).
- *Tamponade gas-associated*: ↑IOP, posterior subcapsular 'feathering' of the lens (usually temporary), anterior IOL movement (if pseudophakic).
- *Silicone oil-associated*: ↑IOP, hyperoleum ('inverse hypopyon'), adherence to silicone IOL, oil keratopathy (if oil in AC), peri-oil fibrosis.

Prognosis
Anatomical success for simple RRD approximately 90%, chance of anatomical success rises with repeated procedures.

Box 12.4 Vitreoretinal surgery with 23- and 25-gauge systems

Outline
- Increasingly popular alternatives to standard 20-gauge vitreoretinal surgery are the narrow gauge systems.
- In a 23- and 25-gauge vitrectomy, entry site sleeves are inserted transconjunctivally.
- The scleral openings are smaller (usually about 23–24 gauge for a 25-gauge system) and, therefore, usually self-seal, so avoiding the need for scleral or conjunctival sutures.

Proposed advantages
- Reduced operating time
- Improved patient comfort (smaller incisions/no sutures)
- Reduced postoperative inflammation
- More rapid visual recovery

Proposed disadvantages
- Increased risk of endophthalmitis
- Increased risk of hypotony
- Increased rate of cataract

Vitrectomy: heavy liquids and tamponade agents

Perfluorocarbon ('heavy') liquids

Indications: may be useful in
- repositioning of giant retinal tears
- flattening PVR-associated retina
- floating up dislocated lens fragments or IOLs
- assisting haemostasis.

Agents
Perfluoro-*n*-octane is the most commonly used agent.

Tamponade

Indications
- *Simple retinal detachment*: consider air or SF6/air mix.
- *Complicated retinal detachment* (e.g. PVR, giant retinal tear, multiple recurrences): consider C3F8/air mix, silicone oil or 'heavy' silicone oil. Overall, silicone oil and C3F8 are similarly effective in PVR, although silicone oil is associated with better final VA in anterior disease, does not require postoperative posturing and allows easier intraoperative and immediate postoperative visualization. 'Heavy' silicone oils are denser than water and so allow tamponade of the inferior retina. They may be useful when there are inferior breaks, or an inferior retinectomy, especially with PVR.
- Where vitrectomy has been performed for indications other than RD there may be no need for tamponade.

Agents

Table 12.16 Common tamponade agents

Agent	Symbol	Expansion if 100%	Non-expansile concentration (mixed with air)	Duration
Air	Air	Nil	100%	≤1wk
Sulphur hexafluoride	SF6	X 2	20%	1–2wks
Perfluoro-propane	C3F8	X 4	12%	8–10wks
Silicone oil	Si oil	Nil	100%	Until removal

Complications
↑IOP (may be related to overfill), posterior subcapsular 'feathering' of the lens, anterior IOL movement (if pseudophakic).

Posturing
- Postoperative posturing by the patient aims to achieve effective tamponade of the break by the gas bubble and to keep the gas bubble away from the crystalline lens.

- Posturing should start as soon as possible (same day of surgery), for as much of each day as possible (commonly 50min in every hour, and adopt appropriate sleeping posture) and continue for 1–2wks (some variation according to tamponade agent).
- The posture required will depend on the location of the break but aims to move the break as superiorly as possible.
- Advise against flying or the use of nitrous oxide anaesthetic agents until the gas bubble has resolved—these situations can result in blindness due to expansion of the gas bubble and subsequent ↑IOP.

Medical retina

Anatomy and physiology (1)

The retina is a remarkable modification of the embryonic forebrain that gathers light, codes the information as an electrical signal (transduces), and transmits it via the optic nerve to the processing areas of the brain.

Embryologically it is derived from the optic vesicle (neuroectoderm), with an outer wall that becomes the RPE, a potential space (the subretinal space) and an inner wall that becomes the neural retina.

Anatomy

Retinal pigment epithelium (RPE)

The RPE is a continuous hexagonal monolayer of epithelial cells that extends anteriorly from the margins of the optic nerve to the ora serrata, where it is continuous with the pigmented layer of the ciliary body.

The apices form microvilli that envelop the photoreceptor outer segments. Near the apices adjacent RPE cells are joined by numerous tight junctions to form the outer blood–retinal barrier. The base of the RPE is crenellated (to increase surface area) and mitochondrion rich. The basement membrane of the RPE forms the inner layer of Bruch's membrane.

Neural retina

This is a thin (150–400µm) layer of transparent neural tissue, comprising photoreceptors (rods, cones), integrators (bipolar, horizontal, amacrine, ganglion cells), the output pathway (nerve fibre layer), and the support cells (Müller cells). The major vessels of the retinal circulation can be visualized traversing the neural retina. Anteriorly the neural retina is continuous with the non-pigmented layer of the ciliary body.

The macula is defined histologically by a multilayered ganglion cell layer (i.e. more than one cell thick), and approximates to a 5500µm oval centred on the fovea and bordered by the temporal arcades. It is yellowish due to the presence of xanthophyll. The macula is further divided into perifovea (1500µm wide band defined by 6 layers of bipolar cells), parafovea (500µm wide band defined by 7–11 layers of bipolar cells) and fovea (1500µm diameter circular depression).

The fovea comprises a rim, a 22° slope and a central floor, the foveola (350µm diameter, 150µm thin). The umbo is the very centre of the foveola (150µm diameter) with maximal cone density equating to highest acuity.

Blood supply

The neural retina has a dual blood supply that is derived from branches of the ophthalmic artery. These include the central retinal artery, which supplies the retinal circulation, and the three posterior ciliary arteries, which provide the choroidal circulation.

Anatomically, the retinal circulation supports the inner two-thirds of the retina, whereas the choroidal circulation supports the outer third; the watershed is at the outer plexiform layer. Physiologically, this equates to two-thirds of the retina's oxygen/nutrient requirements being supplied by the choroidal circulation.

The retinal circulation comprises a small part of ocular blood flow (5%), but with a high level of oxygen extraction (40% arteriovenous difference), contrasting with figures of 85% and 5% for the choroidal circulation. In the retinal circulation the arterial branches lie in the nerve fibre layer but give rise both to an inner capillary network (ganglion cell layer) and an outer capillary network (inner nuclear layer). However, there are no capillaries in the central 500μm, the foveal avascular zone.

The outer blood–retinal barrier is formed by the tight junctions of the RPE cells, whereas the inner is formed by the non-fenestrated endothelium of the retinal capillaries.

Anatomy and physiology (2)

Physiology

Retinal pigment epithelium

The RPE is vital to the normal function of the neural retina. Functions include:

- the maintenance of the outer blood–retinal barrier and retinal adhesion;
- storage of metabolites and vitamin A;
- nutrient supply to the photoreceptors;
- absorption of scattered light (by melanosomes);
- production and recycling of photopigments;
- phagocytosis of photoreceptor discs (each sheds >100 discs per day).

Neural retina

Photoreceptors

Each human eye contains about 120 million rods and 6.5 million cones. The rods subserve peripheral and low-light (scotopic) vision, whereas the cones permit normal (photopic), central, and colour vision.

The rods reach their highest density at 20° from the fovea, in contrast to blue cones, which are densest in the perifovea, and red and green cones, which are densest (up to 385 000/mm^2) at the umbo.

Light perception is mediated in the outer segments of the photoreceptors by a group of G protein receptors called opsins (rhodopsin in rods, iodopsins in cones), which are bound to a vitamin A derived chromophore 11 *cis* retinal. These transmembrane photopigment molecules undergo *cis–trans* isomerization on absorption of a photon of light (495nm for rods, 440–450nm for blue, 535–555nm for green, and 570–590nm for red cones).

Activation of a single photopigment molecule starts a chemical phototransduction cascade (transducin activates phosphodiesterase, which in turn hydrolyses cGMP) with 100-fold amplification at every stage.

Falling cGMP levels cause closure of Na channels, with photoreceptor hyperpolarization. The resting potential is then restored by the action of recoverin, which activates guanylate cyclase to cGMP and reopens Na channels.

Bipolar and amacrine cells

Rods synapse with 'on' bipolar cells, which in turn synapse with amacrine and ganglion cells. Cones synapse with 'on' and 'off' bipolar cells, which in turn synapse with 'on' and 'off' ganglion cells.

Negative feedback is provided by the laterally interacting horizontal cells (between photoreceptors) and amacrine cells (between bipolar cells and ganglion cells). This contributes to the centre-surround phenomenon exhibited by ganglion cells in which they are activated by stimulation in the centre of their receptive field, but inhibited by stimulation of the surround.

Ganglion cells

Ganglion cell representation is maximal at the fovea where the cone: ganglion cell ratio approaches 1:1.

The ganglion cells can be divided into two main populations.

- The parvocellular system subserves fine VA and colour. These ganglion cells are mainly foveal, have small receptive fields, and show spectral sensitivity.
- The magnocellular system subserves motion detection, and coarser form vision. These ganglion cells are mainly peripheral, have larger receptive fields, have high luminance and contrast (but no spectral) sensitivity, and are very sensitive to motion.

This division is preserved both in the lateral geniculate nucleus (layers 1–2 magnocellular, 3–6 parvocellular) and the visual cortex.

Age-related macular degeneration (1)

Age-related macular degeneration (AMD) is the leading cause of blindness for the 'over-50s' in the Western world. Its prevalence increases with age. Estimates vary according to the exact definition of AMD. One study found visually significant disease (VA ≤ 6/9) in about 1% for 55–65yrs, 6% for 65–75yrs, and 20% for >75yrs. Drusen (not necessarily with ↓VA) are increasingly common with age.

Other risk factors include smoking, gender (female>male), ethnic origin (white >> black), diet, cardiovascular risk, and hypermetropia.

The possible role of cataract surgery in accelerating progression of AMD is controversial, with conflicting reports in the world literature. The risk from genetic variation, such as regulation of complement factor H are being determined.

Non-neovascular (dry) age-related macular degeneration

Accounting for 90% of AMD, this tends to lead to gradual but potentially significant reduction in central vision. It is characterized by drusen (hard or soft) and RPE changes (focal hyperpigmentation or atrophy).

Histology

There is loss of the RPE/photoreceptor layers, thinning of the outer plexiform layer, thickening of Bruch's membrane, and atrophy of choriocapillaris exposing the larger choroidal vessels to view. Drusen are PAS-positive amorphous deposits lying between the RPE membrane and the inner collagenous layer of Bruch's membrane; they may become calcified. Another abnormal deposit, basement membrane deposit, lies between the RPE membrane and the RPE cells; it is not visible clinically.

Clinical features

- ↓VA, metamorphopsia, scotomas; usually gradual in onset.
- Hard drusen (small, well-defined, of limited significance), soft drusen (larger, pale yellow, poorly defined, tendency to coalesce and form 'confluent drusen,' increased risk of CNV), RPE focal hyperpigmentation, RPE atrophy ('geographic atrophy' if well-demarcated).

Investigation

- *FFA* is not usually necessary.
- Newer imaging techniques such as OCT and fundus autofluorescence facilitates the assessment of AMD and other retinal disorders.

Treatment

- *Supportive*: counselling, and linking to support group/social services.
- *Refraction:* with increased near-add; low-vision aid assessment/provision often best arranged in a dedicated low vision clinic.
- *Registration*: should be offered, as it may improve access to services.
- *Amsler grid:* regular use of an Amsler grid allows the patient to detect new or progressive metamorphopsia prompting them to seek ophthalmic review.
- *Lifestyle changes*: vitamin supplementation and smoking cessation may slow progression.

Calculating risk of developing advanced age-related macular degeneration

The Age-Related Eye Disease Study (AREDS) observed a number of factors to be predictive of developing advanced AMD. This can be used to predict a patient's risk of developing advanced AMD (choroidal neovascularization or geographic atrophy of the fovea) as follows: assign to *each eye* one risk factor for the presence of large drusen (>125μm) and one risk factor for pigment abnormality and sum the risk factors (i.e. 0–4 scale).

Where advanced AMD has already developed in one eye, the risk of developing AMD in the second eye can be estimated as follows: the presence of advanced AMD in the affected eye counts as two risk factors and this is added to any risk factors present in the second eye.

The 5yr risk is then estimated as per Table 13.1.

Table 13.1 Predicting risk of developing advanced age-related macular degeneration

Number of factors	5yr risk
Zero factors	0.5%
One factor	3%
Two factor	12%
Three factors	25%
Four factors	50%

Ferris FL, et al. Age-Related Eye Disease Study (AREDS) Research Group. A simplified severity scale for age-related macular degeneration: AREDS Report No. 18. *Arch Ophthalmol* 2005;**123**:1570–4.

Age-related macular degeneration (2)

Neovascular (wet) age-related macular degeneration

Although much less common, neovascular AMD leads to rapid and severe loss of vision. There are about 26 000 new cases of wet AMD in the UK each year and it accounts for up to 90% of blind registration due to AMD.

Recently, exciting advances in the treatment of wet AMD with anti-VEGF therapies have been made.

Histology

New capillaries grow from the choriocapillaris though Bruch's membrane and proliferate in the sub-RPE (type I neovascularization) and/or sub-retinal space (type 2 neovascularization). There may be associated haemorrhage, exudation, retina/RPE detachment, or scar formation. Type I choroidal neovascularization is commoner in AMD; type 2 are commoner in younger patients (e.g. with POHS).

Clinical features

- ↓VA, metamorphopsia, scotoma; may be sudden in onset.
- A grey membrane is sometimes visible; more commonly it is deduced from associated signs including sub-retinal (red) or sub-RPE (grey) haemorrhage, subretinal/sub-RPE exudation, retinal or pigment epithelial detachment, CMO or subretinal fibrosis (disciform scar).

Investigation

- Urgent FFA is vital for diagnosis and assessment for treatment. (Figs. 13.1–13.2).
- OCT has become increasingly helpful in the detection and long-term management of neovascular AMD.
- *Classic CNV*: early well demarcated lacy hyperfluorescence with progressive leakage.
- *Occult CNV type I*: fibrovascular pigment epithelial detachment seen as irregular elevation (on stereoscopic view) with stippled hyperfluorescence at 1–2min post-injection.
- *Occult CNV type II*: late leakage of undetermined source, poorly demarcated hyperfluorescence 5–10min post-injection.

Treatment

*Supportive: d*espite major developments in therapy, many patients will in the long-term require supportive care for significant sight loss. Offer counselling, refraction, registration, Amsler grid, and encourage life-style changes as for non-neovascular AMD.

Anti-vascular endothelial growth factor therapies

Intravitreal anti-VEGF therapy has become the treatment of choice for all subfoveal CNV lesions types (see Anti-vascular endothelial growth factor therapy pp.464–467).

Photodynamic therapy

Although anti-VEGF therapy is the preferred strategy for the treatment of CNV, some patients may choose not to undergo an intravitreal procedure. In these cases PDT remains a therapeutic option. The possible role of PDT in combination with anti-VEGF therapies is also under investigation.

Laser photocoagulation
Historically, the only intervention available for CNV was laser photocoagulation (usually Argon green). Extrafoveal and even juxtafoveal CNV were treated in this way with a recognition of the fact that it would cause an immediate scotoma but would hopefully stabilize the lesion. Fortunately, this destructive strategy has been replaced by PDT and, subsequently, anti-VEGF therapies.

Early phase: well demarcated lacy hyperfluorescence

Late phase: progressive leakage

Fig. 13.1 Fundus fluorescein angiography of classic choroidal neovascular membrane.

Age-related macular degeneration (3)

Differential diagnosis of choroidal neovascular membrane

Table 13.2 Common causes of CNV

Degenerative	AMD
	Pathological myopia (lacquer crack)
	Angioid streaks
Trauma	Choroidal rupture
	Laser
Inflammation	POHS
	Multifocal choroiditis
	Serpiginous choroidopathy
	Bird-shot retinochoroidopathy
	Punctate inner choroidopathy
	VKH
Dystrophies	Best's disease
Other	Chorioretinal scar (any cause)
	Tumour
Idiopathic	

Early phase: stippled hyperfluorescence usually maximal at 1–2min; masking by blood adjacent to disc

Late phase: progressive leakage

Fig. 13.2 Fundus fluorescein angiography of occult choroidal neovascular membrane.

Anti-vascular endothelial growth factor therapy: outline

Vascular endothelial growth factor A (VEGF-A, also referred to as VEGF) is a secreted protein that induces developmental and pathological angiogenesis, vascular permeability, and inflammation. There are 9 isoforms of varying amino acid length. VEGF 165 is the most abundantly expressed, but all isoforms are thought to contribute to neovascular AMD.

All currently available anti-VEGF therapies require multiple intravitreal injections of an anti-VEGF agent. This results in the resolution of intra- and sub-retinal fluid, restoration of the normal retinal anatomy and halts the neovascular process.

Mechanism

Currently, there are 2 licensed drugs: pegaptanib and ranibizumab. The off-label use of bevacizumab is also common practice.
- *Ranibizumab* is a humanized monoclonal antibody fragment that binds to all VEGF-A isoforms thus preventing binding of VEGF-A to receptors VEGFR-1 and VEGFR-2.
- *Pegaptanib* is a pegylated aptamer (i.e. an oligonucleotide with polyethylene glycol covalently attached) that binds to VEGF-165 and inhibits its activity.
- Bevacizumab is derived from the same humanized monoclonal antibody as ranibizumab.

The commonest indication of anti-VEGF therapy is AMD but recently there has been numerous reports of its use in other vascular disorders e.g. diabetic retinopathy, CRVO, myopic CNV, inflammatory CNV, etc.

Evidence for intravitreal anti-vascular endothelial growth factor therapy

Ranibizumab 0.5mg/0.05ml
- MARINA (minimally classic/occult trial of the anti-VEGF antibody ranibizumab in the treatment of neovascular AMD).
  - Ranibizumab vs sham injection.
  - Benefit of ranibizumab: fewer than 15 letters lost in 95% vs 62% at 1yr; gain of at least 15 letters in 34% vs 5% at 1yr, with a mean gain of 7.2 letters.
- ANCHOR (Anti-VEGF antibody for the treatment of predominantly classic choroidal neovascularization in AMD).
  - Ranibizumab vs sham injection +PDT.
  - Benefit of ranibizumab: fewer than 15 letters lost in 96% vs 64% at 1yr; gain of at least 15 letters in 40% vs 6% at 1yr, with a mean gain of 11.3 letters.
- FOCUS (RhuFab V2 Ocular Treatment Combining the Use of Visudyne® to Evaluate Safety).
  - Ranibizumab + PDT vs sham injection + PDT
  - Benefit of ranibizumab + PDT: gain of at least 15 letters in 24% vs 5%.

Pegaptanib 0.3mg/0.09ml:
- VISION (The VEGF inhibition study in ocular neovascularization)—a combination of the results of two randomized controlled trials published together.
  - Pegaptanib vs sham injection.
  - fewer than 15 letters lost in 70% vs 55% at 1yr; gain of at least 15 letters in 6% vs 2% at 1yr with a mean loss of 8 vs 15 letters in usual care group. Benefit maintained in year 2.

Bevacizumab
Bevacizumab is currently being compared with ranibizumab in the head-to-head CATT trial (Comparison of Age-Related Macular Degeneration Treatments Trial).

NICE guidelines

The National Institute for Health and Clinical Excellence (UK) issued its Final Appraisal Determination for the use of anti VEGF therapies for wet AMD in 2008. In summary they recommend:
- Ranibizumab for neovascular AMD if the eye to be treated has:
  - best-corrected VA between 6/12 and 6/96
  - no permanent structural damage to the central fovea
  - lesion size ≤12 disc areas in greatest linear dimension
  - evidence of recent disease progression (recent ↓VA, blood vessel growth, change on fluorescein angiography).

  However, they stipulate that
- the cost of treatment beyond 14 injections in the treated eye should be met by the manufacturer
- treatment should be continued only in people who maintain adequate response to therapy (further ↓VA, anatomical deterioration).

  In this 2008 ruling NICE did not recommend pegaptanib for the treatment of wet AMD, but advised that ongoing treatment may continue until they and their clinician deem appropriate to stop.

Anti-vascular endothelial growth factor therapy: in practice

Intravitreal injection of anti-vascular endothelial growth factor therapies

In advance
- *Discuss procedure and take informed consent*: explain purpose (to maintain current vision and potentially improve acuity), risks, and that multiple injections may be required. (Box 13.1.)
- Additionally, if using bevacizumab it should be explained that this drug is not licensed for AMD and that the exact safety and efficacy are not yet determined.

Intravitreal injections[1]

Setting
Intravitreal injections may be given in theatre or a dedicated clean room in outpatients that meets stringent conditions such as being enclosed, free from interruptions, good illumination, washable floor, and non-particulate ceiling (i.e. dust free). Full gowning is not necessary but hands should be washed and sterile gloves worn.

Preparation
- Confirm consent and correct eye to be injected; measure IOP; ensure adequate dilation; instil topical anaesthesia.
- Set up equipment trolley and ensure all treatments (including post-injection antibiotics) are available.

Procedure
- Wash hands and don sterile gloves.
- Instil 5% povidone iodine on to the ocular surface; clean periocular area with 10% povidone iodine; drape and insert lid speculum.
- Consider whether supplementation of anaesthesia is necessary: subconjunctival or sub-Tenon's (e.g. lidocaine 1%).
- Prepare syringe/needle/drug immediately prior to injection, and ensure any air in the syringe/needle is expelled prior to injection; maintain aseptic technique throughout.
- Note injection site: this should be 3.0–3.5mm (aphakic/pseudophakic) or 3.5–4mm (phakic) posterior to limbus in either superotemporal or inferotemporal quadrants (superotemporal has the advantage that if a break is induced it is more likely to be amenable to pneumoretinopexy).
- Insert needle (27–30 gauge; 1/2–5/8 inch long) perpendicularly, aiming towards the centre of the globe.
- Inject indicated volume of anti-VEGF (ranibizumab 0.05ml; bevacizumab 0.05ml; pegantanib 0.09ml); carefully remove needle; a sterile cotton-tipped applicator can be used as counter pressure and to prevent any reflux.
- Instil topical antibiotic (e.g. chloramphenicol 0.5%); for immediate post-injection use a preservative-free preparation is recommended.

Post-injection
- Test gross VA.
- Check for central retinal artery patency (may not be necessary if acuity satisfactory).
- Check injection site (at the slit-lamp).
- Check IOP.

Follow-up
- Topical antibiotics (e.g. chloramphenicol 0.5% 4×/d) for ≥3d.
- Review in clinic according to treatment: recommended product administration is monthly for ranibizumab and 6-wkly for pegantanib.
- FFA and OCT are useful in the long-term management of these patients; the use of FFA has significantly reduced as the advent of OCT.

Box 13.1 **Summary of patient advice regarding intravitreal injections**

Potential side-effects/complications
- Endophthalmitis <0.1%
- Retinal detachment
- Lens damage/cataract
- Raised IOP
- Conjunctival haemorrhage
- Vitreous floaters
- Intraocular inflammation
- Eye pain
- Visual loss

Contraindications
- Allergy to any of the components
- Ocular and periocular infections

Advice to patient
- Endophthalmitis warning symptoms should be explained
- Advise that floaters post-procedure are to be expected

1. Amaoku W. *RCOphth intravitreal injections procedure guideline* www.rcophth.ac.uk/docs/publications/published-guidelines/IntravitrealInjectionsJuly2006.pdf/

Photodynamic therapy

PDT describes the laser stimulation of a photoactivated dye that results in the destruction of CNV. This technique aims to selectively destroy the membrane while minimizing damage to the retina above or the RPE and choroid below.

The commonest indication has been for AMD but it has also been used for other CNVs, e.g. in myopia, inflammatory membranes, etc.

Its role as a single agent has now been largely replaced by anti-VEGF therapies, but it appears to be finding a new therapeutic niche as a agent to be combined with the anti-VEGF treatments.

Mechanism

Verteporfin is a photoactivated dye that binds to lipoproteins and becomes concentrated in the proliferating vascular bed of the CNV. Laser light of 689nm wavelength is directed on to the CNV activating the dye. The energy level used (600mW/cm^2 × 83s = 50J/cm^2) is too low to cause thermal damage, but is sufficient to activate the dye that catalyses the formation of the free radical 'singlet oxygen'. This causes local endothelial cell death and occlusion of the blood supply to the CNV.

Photodynamic therapy in practice

In advance

Discuss procedure and take informed consent: explain purpose (to slow progression of disease), risks, and practicalities such as what protective clothing to wear (Box 13.2).

On the day

- Calculate spot size (greatest linear diameter + 1000µm).
- Confirm consent: purpose, risks (Box 13.2).
- Ensure safety precautions (hat, long sleeves, resuscitation equipment available).
- IV cannula in large vein (e.g. antecubital fossa).
- Reconstitute 15mg powder with 7ml water for injections to produce a 2mg/ml solution then dilute requisite dose (6mg/m^2 body surface area) with glucose 5% to a final volume of 30ml and give over 10min.
- At 15min since start of infusion start 83s of laser (689nm, variable spot size, 600mW/cm^2).

Follow-up

Review with FFA at 12wks. If recurrent leakage occurs PDT may be performed up to 4 times/yr. If severe ↓VA of ≥4 lines within 1wk of treatment do not retreat unless VA returns to pre-treatment level.

Evidence for photodynamic therapy in subfoveal choroidal neovascular membrane due to age-related macular degeneration

Predominantly classic choroidal neovascular membrane (include classic with no occult)

- Treatment benefit demonstrated in the TAP (the Treatment of AMD with Photodynamic therapy) study:
    - *TAP1*: fewer than 15 letters lost in 67% vs 39% at 1yr (*p*<0.001);
    - *TAP2*: fewer than 15 letters lost in 59% vs 31% at 2yrs (*p*<0.001).

Minimally classic choroidal neovascular membrane

Emerging evidence for treatment benefit in those cases where there is documented progression of lesion (↑ lesion size on FFA or ↓VA).

100% occult choroidal neovascular membrane

Treatment benefit demonstrated (mainly for small lesions or worse VA):
- VIP (The Verteporfin in Photodynamic therapy) study showed overall treatment benefit. TAP study showed trend towards benefit.
  - VIP2: fewer than 15 letters lost in 45% vs 32% at 1yr (p = 0.03); subgroup analysis suggests main benefit is for smaller lesions (<4 disc areas) or worse VA (<6/15).
- TAP2: fewer than 15 letters lost in 56% vs 30% at 2yrs (p = 0.06).

Evidence for photodynamic therapy in subfoveal choroidal neovascular membrane due to myopia

- Treatment benefit overall; most lesions were predominantly classic; unclear whether benefit for minimally classic or occult lesions.
- VIP1: fewer than eight letters lost in 72% vs 44% at 1yr (p < 0.01).

NICE guidelines

In 2006 NICE (UK) made the following recommendations for the use of PDT in the treatment of subfoveal CNV:
- PDT recommended for classic *with no occult* and VA ≥6/60;
- PDT only recommended for predominantly classic *with some occult* as part of clinical studies.

However, the advent of anti-VEGF therapies has significantly impacted on the use of PDT such that its current use is almost entirely in combination with anti-VEGF therapies.

Box 13.2 Summary of patient advice regarding PDT

Side-effects
- Injection-site reactions: inflammation, leakage, hypersensitivity
- Back pain: 2%
- Transient visual disturbances
- Significant visual loss: up to 4%

Contraindications
- Liver failure
- Porphyria
- Allergy to any of the components

Advice to patient
For 48h post-PDT avoid direct sunlight and bright lights (including solaria, halogen or strip-lights, and undraped windows). If it is necessary to go outside during daylight hours (e.g. returning from PDT clinic) wear wide-brimmed hat, sun-glasses, long-sleeved shirt, trousers and socks.

Diabetic eye disease: general

Diabetes mellitus is estimated to affect 200 million people worldwide and by 2030 it is estimated this will rise to over 360 million. It is the commonest cause of blindness in the working population, being associated with a 20-fold increase in blindness.

WHO divides diabetes into type 1 (insulin-dependent) and type 2 (non-insulin-dependent).

- Type 1 is typically of juvenile onset and is characterized by insulin deficiency.
- Type 2 is typically of adult/elderly onset and is characterized by insulin resistance.

Clinical features

Systemic disease

Presentation

- *Type 1*: acutely with diabetic ketoacidosis or subacutely with weight loss, polyuria, polydipsia, fatigue.
- *Type 2*: incidental finding (may have long asymptomatic period); or symptoms of weight loss, polyuria, polydipsia, fatigue; or complications.

Systemic complications

- *Macrovascular*: myocardial infarction (3–5× risk), peripheral vascular disease, stroke (>2× risk).
- *Microvascular*: nephropathy, neuropathy.

Ophthalmic

- *Retinopathy and sequelae*: risk varies according to type of disease (1 vs 2), duration of disease, glycaemic control, hypertension, hypercholesterolaemia, nephropathy, pregnancy, and possibly intraocular surgery.
  - In type 1 diabetes, retinopathy is rare at diagnosis, but present in over 90% after 15yrs.
  - In type 2 disease, retinopathy is present in 20% at diagnosis, but only rises to 60% after 15ys.
- *Diabetic maculopathy* is the main cause for severe sight loss rather than proliferative retinopathy.
- *Cataract*: occurs at a younger age and more progress quickly.
- *Other*: numerous ocular conditions occur more frequently in diabetes, including dry eye, corneal abrasions, anterior uveitis, rubeosis, neovascular glaucoma, ocular ischaemic syndrome, papillitis, AION, orbital infection, and cranial nerve palsies.

Diagnosis

- Venous fasting plasma glucose ≥7mmol/l.
- Oral glucose tolerance test (usually performed by physician) with a 2h value of >11.1mmol/l.

Diabetes Control and Complication Trial (DCCT) and UK Prospective Diabetic Study (UK PDS)

These large multicentre randomized controlled trials have provided a wealth of information about the natural history and the risk factors in type 1 and type 2 diabetes.

- For type 1 disease the *Diabetes Control and Complication Trial* demonstrated that tight control (HbA1c 7.2% vs 9%) was associated with 76% reduction in retinopathy, 60% reduction in neuropathy, and 54% reduction in nephropathy.
- For type 2 disease the *UK Prospective Diabetic Study* demonstrated that tight control (HbA1c 7% vs 7.9%) was associated with 25% reduction in microvascular disease. Additionally, tight BP control (144/82 vs 155/87) was associated with 37% reduction in microvascular disease and 32% reduction in diabetes-related deaths.

Diabetic eye disease: assessment

When assessing the diabetic patient the ophthalmologist aims to: (1) assess risk factors for eye disease (and to a lesser extent other systemic complications); (2) ensure modifiable risk factors are treated; (3) detect and grade eye disease; and (4) institute ophthalmic treatment where necessary.

Table 13.3 An approach to assessing diabetic eye disease

Visual symptoms	Asymptomatic; ↓VA, distortion, floaters
POH	Previous diabetic eye complications; laser treatment; surgery; concurrent eye disease
PMH	Diabetes: age of diagnosis, type and duration; hypertension, hypercholesterolaemia, smoking; pregnancy; ischaemic heart disease, cerebrovascular disease, peripheral vascular disease, nephropathy, neuropathy
SH	Driver; occupation
Dx	Treatment for diabetes (diet, oral hypoglycaemics, insulin types and frequency), hypertension, hypercholesterolaemia; aspirin/antiplatelet agents
Ax	Allergies or relevant drug contraindications
Visual acuity	Best-corrected/pin-hole/near
Cornea	Tear film
Iris	Rubeosis
Lens	Cataract
Tonometry	
Vitreous	Haemorrhage, asteroid hyalosis
Fundus	Retinopathy (microaneurysms, haemorrhages, exudates, intraretinal microvascular abnormalities, venous beading, venous loops, neovascularization), maculopathy (fluid, exudates, retinal thickening), tractional/rhegmatogenous retinal detachment, arterial/venous occlusion, ocular ischaemia
Disc	New vessels, papillitis, AION

Table 13.4 Definitions in diabetic eye disease

Retinopathy[1]	
Background (low risk)	Microaneurysms, small haemorrhages, hard exudates, occasional cotton wool spots
Pre-proliferative (high risk)	Intraretinal microvascular abnormalities, venous beading/loops, clusters of large blot haemorrhages, multiple cotton wool spots
Proliferative	
NVD	New vessels at the disc or within 1DD of the disc
NVE	New vessels elsewhere in the retina
Maculopathy	
Focal	Well circumscribed areas of leakage with oedema and full/part rings of exudates often surrounding a microaneurysm
Diffuse	Generalized leakage with oedema
Ischaemic	↓VA with relatively normal clinical appearance, but macular ischaemia on FFA
Mixed	Combination, e.g. of diffuse and ischaemic
CSMO	Clinically significant macular oedema: <ul><li>Retinal thickening at or within 500µm of the centre of the macula;</li><li>Hard exudates at or within 500µm of the centre of the macula if associated with adjacent retinal thickening;</li><li>Retinal thickening of >1 disc area any part of which is within 1 disc diameter of the centre of the macula</li></ul>

1. The alternative Airlie House classification (as used in the ETDRS) includes the following categories of NPDR:
• Mild NPDR: at least one microaneurysm
• Moderate NPDR: severe retinal haemorrhages in at least one quadrant, or CWS, venous beading or IRMA definitely present
• Severe NPDR: severe retinal haemorrhages in four quadrants; or venous beading in 2 quadrants; or extensive IRMA in one quadrant
• Very severe NPDR: any two of the features of severe NPDR.

Effectively, Background retinopathy corresponds to Mild Non-Proliferative Diabetic Retinopathy whereas Pre-proliferative retinopathy would include the range from Moderate to Very Severe Non-Proliferative retinopathy.

The international (AAO) classification has similarities to a simplified form of the Arlie House criteria. A summary of the equivalence of the different classification systems may be found in the Roual College of Ophthalmologists Diabetic Retinopathy Guidelines at :

http://www.rcophth.ac.uk/docs/publications/published-guidelines/
DiabeticRetinopathyGuidelines2005.pdf

Diabetic eye disease: management

Optimal diabetic care can best be achieved by a multidisciplinary approach. This includes doctors (primary care physician, endocrinologist, and appropriate specialists according to need), specialist nurses, podiatrists, optometrists, and others. Education to encourage the patient in self-management is critical: good glycaemic and BP control will influence retinopathy.

Table 13.5 An approach to diabetic eye disease[1]

Retinopathy	
None Background	Discharge to community screening service for annual review; if significant systemic disease consider review at 9–12mths by hospital eye service
Pre-proliferative	Observe 4–6 monthly
Proliferative (active)	Pan-retinal photocoagulation (1–2 sessions × ≥1000 × 200–500µm × 0.1s); review 3 weekly; anti-VEGF therapies
Proliferative (regressed)	Observe 4–6 monthly
Maculopathy	
Focal leakage	Focal laser photocoagulation (n × 50–100µm × 0.08–0.1s); review at 3–4mths
Diffuse leakage	Grid laser photocoagulation (n × 100–200µm × 0.1s); review at 3–4mths
Ischaemic	FFA to confirm diagnosis
Persistent maculopathy	Intravitreal triamcinolone (4mg under sterile conditions), anti-VEGF therapies
Resolved maculopathy	Observe 4–6 monthly
Rubeosis	
Rubeosis + clear media	Urgent pan-retinal photocoagulation
Rubeosis + vitreous haemorrhage	Vitrectomy + endolaser
Rubeotic glaucoma	Urgent pan-retinal photocoagulation/anti-VEGF therapies ↓IOP with topical medication/cyclodiode/augmented trabeculectomy/tubes
Vitreous haemorrhage	
No view of fundus	Ultrasound to ensure retina flat + review 2–4 weekly until adequate view
Adequate view	Ensure retina flat + pan-retinal photocoagulation
Persistent	Vitrectomy + endolaser + anti-VEGF therapies

1. See also Royal College of Ophthalmologists Diabetic Retinopathy Guidelines 2005 at www.reophth.ac.uk/docs/published-guidelines/DiabeticRethnopathyGuidelines2005.pdf

Treatment: systemic

Glycaemic control
- Aim for an HbA1c 6.5–7%.
- *For type 1 disease*: insulin regimens include (1) twice daily premixed insulins, and (2) ultra-fast or soluble insulins with each meal and long-acting insulin at night.
- *For type 2 disease*: start with diet, followed by metformin and then a sulphonylurea (e.g. gliclazide or glibenclamide); a glitazone (e.g. rosiglitazone) may be used as an alternative to either of these; insulin may be required.

Table 13.6 Insulin types (and examples)

Short-acting	Insulin Aspart (NovoRapid)®
	Insulin Lispro (Humalog)®
	Soluble insulin (Actrapid®, Humulin S®, Velosulin®)
Intermediate	Isophane insulin (Insulatard®, Humulin® I)
Long-acting	Insulin Zn suspension (Ultratard®)
	Insulin glargine (Lantus®)

Blood pressure control
- Aim for BP < 130/80 or <125/75 if proteinuria.
- Effective antihypertensives include ACE inhibitors, AIIR antagonists, β-blockers, or thiazide diuretics.

Cholesterol control
- Aim for lipid lowering if >30% 10yr risk of coronary heart disease (current recommendations, although ideally treat all with risk >15%). This can be calculated from the Framingham equation or the Joint British Societies nomogram (see *BNF*).
- A statin is the drug of choice; fibrates may be helpful if ↑triglyceride and ↓high-density lipoprotein.

Support renal function
- Microalbuminuria is indicative of early nephropathy and is associated with increased risk of macrovascular complications.
- ACE inhibitors or AIIR antagonists are preferred.

Lifestyle
- *Smoking cessation*: smoking greatly increases macrovascular disease, and strategies to assist the patient 'give-up' should be explored.
- *Weight control*: mainly in type II disease, particularly if BMI >25.
- *Exercise >30min/d*: ↓weight, ↓BP, ↑insulin sensitivity, improves lipid profile.

Diabetic eye disease: screening

What is screening?

Screening is the systematic testing of a population (or subgroup) for signs of asymptomatic or ignored disease.

Screening for diabetic eye disease

The classification systems for diabetic retinopathy range from the very detailed Airlie House system (generally for use in trials), to the dichotomous non-proliferative vs proliferative division. In terms of clinical management the traditional background/pre-proliferative/proliferative grading system is the most familiar to primary care physicians and optometrists and has been adopted by the National Screening Committee (UK).

Although screening may be by dilated fundoscopy, quality assurance can be more readily achieved where there is a photographic record. Hence a national programme of digital photographic screening is underway. Photography could potentially be performed by mobile units, by selected primary/secondary care units, or by community optometrists. Grading of the photographs could be performed by the same units (if approved) or the photographs could be sent to an approved centre. National Screening Committee guidelines are available at www.nscretinopathy.org.uk (Table 13.7).

Appropriate referral to the hospital eye service

- *Pre-proliferative retinopathy (R2)*: referral to hospital eye service (target ≤13wks).
- *Proliferative retinopathy (R3)*: fast-track referral (target ≤2wks).
- *Maculopathy fulfilling screening guidelines (M1)*: referral to hospital eye service (target ≤13wks).
- *Time between listing once seen in eye clinic and photocoagulation if new screenee (P1)*: proliferative retinopathy (R3) ≤2wks, maculopathy target ≤10wks.
- *Unclassifiable (U)*: referral to hospital eye service.
- *Other lesions (OL)*: referral to hospital eye service or to primary physician.

Table 13.7 National screening committee recommendations for grading and management of retinopathy

Retinopathy	R0	None	Annual screening
	R1	Background	Annual screening
		Microaneurysm(s)	Inform diabetes care team
		Retinal haemorrhage(s) ± any exudate	
	R2	Pre-proliferative	Refer to Hospital Eye Service (HES)
		Venous beading	
		Venous loop or reduplication	
		Intraretinal microvascular abnormality (IRMA)	
		Multiple deep, round or blot haemorrhages	
		If CWS then look carefully for above features	
	R3	Proliferative	Fast-track referral to HES
		New vessels on disc (NVD)	
		New vessels elsewhere (NVE)	
		Pre-retinal or vitreous haemorrhage	
		Pre-retinal fibrosis ± tractional retinal detachment	
Maculopathy	M0	No Maculopathy	Annual screening
	M1	Exudate within 1 disc diameter (DD) of the centre of the fovea	Refer to HES
		Circinate or group of exudates within the macula	
		Retinal thickening ≤1DD of the centre of the fovea (if stereo available)	
		Any microaneurysm or haemorrhage ≤1DD of the centre of the fovea only if associated with a best VA of ≤6/12 (if no stereo)	
Photo-coagulation	P1	New screenee who has had focal or scatter treatment	Refer to HES
	P2	Quiescent screenee who has been quiescent since focal/scatter treatment	Annual screening
Other	OL	Other lesions	Refer to HES/GP
		Non-diabetic lesions, e.g. AMD	
Unclassifiable	U	Ungradable	Refer to HES
		E.g. If media opacity, poor photographs	

Central serous chorioretinopathy

The aetiology of central serous chorioretinopathy (*syn* central serous retin-opathy) is unknown. Pathological features include hyperpermeability, fluid accumulation, RPE detachment, disruption of outer blood–retinal barrier (RPE tight junctions), and subsequent detachment of the sensory retina.

Risk factors

It typically affects adult men (20–50yrs), and is reportedly associated with type A personalities, psychosocial stress, pregnancy (usually 3rd trimester), Cushing's disease (5% prevalence), and numerous drugs (notably corticos-teroids).

Clinical features

- Unilateral sudden ↓VA, positive scotoma (usually central), metamorphopsia, increased hypermetropia.
- Shallow detachment of the sensory retina at the posterior pole deeper small yellow–grey elevations (RPE detachments); multifocal or diffuse pigmentary changes suggest chronicity; occasionally fluid tracks inferiorly from the posterior pole to cause a bullous non-rhegmatogenous detachment of the inferior peripheral retina.

Investigations

- *FFA (Fig. 13.3)*: one or more points of progressive leakage and pooling classically in a smoke-stack or ink-blot pattern.
- *ICG*: when performed shows bilateral multifocal hyperfluorescence of greater extent than seen clinically or on FFA.
- *OCT*: shows neurosensory retinal detachment and accompanying small detachments of the RPE.

Treatment

- *Conservative*: central serous chorioretinopathy has a high rate of spontaneous remission. Conservative management includes lifestyle counselling and the avoidance glucocorticoid medication.
- *Argon laser treatment*
  - *Indications*: persistence > 6mths, contralateral persistent visual defect from central serous chorioretinopathy, multiple recurrences, occupational needs.
  - *Technique*: mild burns to the leakage site (usually <10 burns, 50–200µm, 0.1s, power adjusted to produce very gentle blanching only).
- *PDT*: recent case-series suggest that half usual dose PDT may be beneficial for those with severe disease who are not amenable to conventional laser treatment, e.g. subfoveal.

Prognosis

In 80% there is spontaneous recovery to near normal VA (≥6/12) within 1–6mths. Subtle metamorphopsia may persist. Chronic (5%) or recurrent episodes (in up to 45%) may be associated with more significant visual loss. A small risk (<2% per year) of CNV is reported.

Pregnancy associated central serous chorioretinopathy usually resolves 1–2mths post-delivery.

Differential diagnosis

Other causes of serous detachments of the sensory retina include optic disc pits, CNV, idiopathic polypoidal choroidal vasculopathy, optic neuritis, papilloedema, VKH, choroidal tumours, macular holes, vitreous traction, posterior scleritis, and hypertensive choroidopathy.

Early phase

Late phase: point of progressive leakage in an ink-blot type pattern

Fig. 13.3 Fundus fluorescein angiography of central serous chorioretinopathy.

Cystoid macular oedema

This important macular disorder is a common pathological response to a wide variety of ocular insults. It is thought that prostaglandin secretion and vascular endothelial damage cause fluid accumulation in the outer plexiform layer. The relatively loose intercellular adhesions of this layer then permit the formation of cystoid spaces. It most commonly arises after cataract surgery (Irvine–Gass syndrome; see Postoperative cystoid macular oedema ☐ p.294) or in association with diabetic maculopathy, retinal vein occlusions, and posterior uveitis (Box 13.3).

Clinical features
- Asymptomatic, ↓VA (may be severe), metamorphopsia, scotomas.
- Loss of foveal contour, retinal thickening, cystoid spaces; central yellow spot, small intraretinal haemorrhages, and telangiectasia (occasional).
- Associated features depend on the underlying cause (e.g. diabetic retinopathy, B/CRVO, uveitis).
- *Complications*: lamellar hole (irreversible ↓VA).

Investigations
- *FFA*: typically dye leakage from the parafovea into the cystoid spaces (petalloid pattern) and from the optic disc.
- *OCT*: detection rate is equal to FFA, and can measure degree of retinal thickening and specific pathology, e.g. vitreomacular traction.

Treatment
Although there may be some variation according to the underlying cause, a step-wise approach is recommended. Review the diagnosis if atypical or slow to respond. One approach is as follows:
1. *Topical*: steroid (e.g. dexamethasone 0.1% 4×/d) + NSAID (e.g. ketorolac 0.3% 3×/d);
Review in 4–6wks; if persisting then:
2. *Periocular* steroid (e.g. orbital floor/subtenons; methylprednisolone/ triamcinolone) and continue topical Rx.
Review in 4–6wks; if persisting then:
3. Consider: repeating periocular or giving intravitreal steroid (triamcinolone 4mg); vitrectomy; systemic steroids (e.g. prednisolone 40 mg 1×/d, titrating over 3wks; or IV methylprednisolone 500mg single dose); oral acetazolamide (500mg/d; limited evidence).

Prognosis
Prognosis varies according to underlying pathology. Most patients with CMO arising after cataract surgery will attain VA ≥6/9 within 3–12mths of their operation.

Box 13.3 Causes of CMO

- Postoperative (cataract/corneal/vitreoretinal surgery)
- Post-cryotherapy
- Post-laser (peripheral iridotomy, panretinal photocoagulation)
- Uveitis (posterior > intermediate > anterior)
- Scleritis
- Retinal vein obstruction
- Diabetic maculopathy
- Ocular ischaemia
- Choroidal neovascular membrane
- Retinal telangiectasia
- Hypertensive retinopathy
- Radiation retinopathy
- Epiretinal membrane
- Retinitis pigmentosa
- Autosomal dominant CMO
- Tumours of the choroid/retina
- Vitreomacular traction
- Medication, e.g. nicotinic acid

Degenerative myopia

Myopia is common and is regarded as physiological if less than –6D. Of those with high myopia (>–6D) there is a subset in whom the axial length may never stabilize (progressive or pathological myopia) and who are at risk of degenerative changes.

The prevalence of progressive myopia varies from 1 to 10%, with geographic variation (highest in Spain and Japan). It is a significant cause of blindness in the developed world and affects the working population. Risk factors include genetic influences (autosomal dominant/recessive, sporadic) and environmental (excessive near work).

Clinical features
- Increasing myopia, ↓VA, metamorphopsia, photopsia (occasional).
- *Fundus*: pale, tessellated with areas of chorioretinal atrophy both centrally and peripherally; breaks in Bruch's membrane ('lacquer cracks') may permit CNV formation, spontaneous macular haemorrhage and subsequent elevated pigmented scar (Förster–Fuchs' spot); posterior staphyloma; lattice degeneration.
- *Disc*: tilted, atrophy temporal to the disc ('temporal crescent').
- Vitreous syneresis; posterior vitreous detachment (at younger age).
- *Other associations*: long axial length, deep AC, zonular dehiscence, pigment dispersion syndrome and glaucoma.
- *Complications*: CNV (myopia is commonest cause of CNV in young patients), macular hole, peripheral retinal tears, rhegmatogenous retinal detachment, posterior retinoschisis.

Investigations
- *Ultrasound*: can confirm a staphyloma and can monitor axial length.
- *FFA*: if CNV is suspected.
- *OCT*: useful if posterior retinoschisis or CNV is suspected.

Treatment
- *Prevent progression*: this is extremely controversial.
- *Choroidal neovascular membranes*
  - Preliminary short-term results for the use of anti-VEGF therapies (*see* Anti VEGF therapies ▢ pp.464–467) are very encouraging for all myopic CNV.
  - Alternative treatments are PDT (*see* PDT ▢ pp.464–467) for subfoveal CNV, and argon laser photocoagulation for extrafoveal CNV. **NB** With time there is often significant creep of the resultant atrophic zone.

Prognosis
- High myopia is the commonest cause of CNV in young patients, accounting for >60% of CNV in those under 50yrs of age.
- Risk factors for CNV development are lacquer cracks (29% develop CNV) and patchy atrophy (20% develop CNV).
- At 5yrs following onset of myopic CNV (untreated) about 90% of patients have a VA ≤6/60. It is hoped that this will be improved by the advent of anti-VEGF therapies, although their long-term efficacy and safety is not yet known.

Table 13.8 Associations of myopia

Stickler syndrome
Marfan syndrome
Ehlers–Danlos
Down syndrome
Gyrate atrophy
Congenital rubella
Albinism

Angioid streaks

Angioid streaks are breaks in an abnormally thickened and calcified Bruch's membrane. This type of brittle Bruch's membrane may result from a number of endocrine, metabolic, and connective tissue abnormalities, but in about half no underlying cause is found.

Clinical features
- Asymptomatic; ↓VA, metamorphopsia.
- *Angioid streaks*: narrow irregular streaks radiating from a peripapillary ring; the colour of the streaks varies from red to dark brown depending on background pigmentation.
- *Associated features*: peripapillary chorioretinal atrophy; local/diffuse RPE mottling ('peau d'orange'; commonest in PXE); disc drusen.
- *Complications*: CNV, choroidal rupture (after minor trauma) subfoveal haemorrhage.

Investigations
FFA: if CNV suspected; angioid streaks show hyperfluorescence due to window defect.

Treatment
- *Conservative*: advise to avoid contact sports/risk of trauma
- *All CNV*: preliminary results suggest intravitreal anti-VEGF therapy may be beneficial.
- *Extrafoveal/juxtafoveal CNV*: consider argon laser photocoagulation: results for juxtafoveal suggest stability with PDT but fails to prevent subfoveal progression.
- *Subfoveal CNV*: results suggest that PDT may be of benefit in the short term, but benefit is lost with a progressive decline in vision by 2yrs.

Table 13.9 Causes of angioid streaks

Pseudoxanthoma elasticum
Ehlers–Danlos syndrome
Paget's disease
Acromegaly
Haemaglobinopathies
Hereditary spherocytosis
Neurofibromatosis
Sturge–Weber
Tuberous sclerosis
Idiopathic (50%)

Choroidal folds

These are corrugations in the choroid and Bruch's membrane that are seen as a series of light and dark lines. They are usually horizontal and lie over the posterior pole, although they can be vertical, oblique, or jigsaw-like. They are distinguished from retinal striae by being deeper and broader.

FFA shows alternating lines of hyperfluorescence (peaks) and hypofluorescence (troughs).

Although they may in themselves cause visual dysfunction, their main significance is to prompt thorough investigation for an underlying disease.

Table 13.10 Causes of choroidal folds

Idiopathic
Hypermetropia
Retrobulbar mass
Posterior scleritis
Uveitis
Idiopathic orbital inflammatory disease
Thyroid eye disease
Choroidal mass
Hypotony
Papilloedema

Toxic retinopathies (1)

A number of prescribed and non-prescribed drugs may cause retinal injury, usually via damage to the RPE layer. A high level of clinical suspicion may be required as these conditions are seen infrequently and use of the drug is often not volunteered.

Be alert to the possibility of toxicity when there is unusual pigmentary disturbance or crystal deposition. Withdrawal of the drug (co-ordinate with the prescribing physician) may lead to halting and even regression of the retinopathy; in some cases, however, it may continue to progress. If macular changes are evident before starting treatment then baseline photos (± fundus autofluorescence) are useful for monitoring.

Chloroquine and hydroxychloroquine

These aminoquinolones are widely used both as antimalarials and immunomodulators (e.g. in RA and SLE).

Doses of >3.5mg/kg/d for chloroquine and >6.5mg/kg/d for hydroxychloroquine may result in retinopathy; risk increases with increasing dose, increasing duration, and reduced renal function.

Clinical features
- Asymptomatic, central/paracentral scotomas, ↓VA.
- Altered foveal reflex ± irregular central macular pigmentation → depigmentation of surrounding zone ('bull's eye maculopathy') → end-stage disease (generalized atrophy, RP-like peripheral pigmentation, arteriolar attenuation, optic atrophy).
- *Associated features:* enhanced Hudson–Stahli line, vortex keratopathy, contact lens intolerance.

Prevention and screening
Current prescribing practice (<3.5mg/kg/d for chloroquine and <6.5mg/kg/d for hydroxychloroquine) very rarely (if ever) causes retinopathy.

Table 13.11 Summary of Royal College of Ophthalmologists recommendations to prescribing physician 2004

Hydroxychloroquine of <5yrs duration	
Pre-treatment	Ask about visual impairment or eye disease and record VA for near. If visual impairment or eye disease, arrange review by optometrist who can refer any abnormality to an ophthalmologist
Treatment	Do not exceed recommended dose (6.5mg/kg/d hydroxychloroquine). Ask about visual symptoms and check near VA at least annually. If abnormality refer to ophthalmologist with a view to stopping treatment
Chloroquine, or hydroxychloroquine of > 5yrs duration	
	Regular ophthalmic review is recommended and this should be negotiated between local ophthalmologists and rheumatologists

Vigabatrin

This anticonvulsant is used in the treatment of complex partial seizures and certain other types of epilepsy, including infantile spasms, especially those secondary to tuberous sclerosis. In about one-third of cases visual field defects develop, but are often unrecognized as patients are asymptomatic and retain good acuity.

Clinical features

- Usually asymptomatic with good central VA.
- May develop optic atrophy.
- *Bilateral visual field defects*: generalized constriction or binasal; generally static once established, with no improvement on withdrawal of treatment.
- Normal retinal appearance.

Prevention and screening

Table 13.12 Summary of Royal College of Ophthalmologists recommendations 2000

Pre-treatment	Perform baseline visual field examination (Humphrey 120 to 45° or Goldmann).
Treatment	Reassess every 6mths for 3yrs
	Reassess annually thereafter

Toxic retinopathies (2)

Thioridazine

This phenothiazine is a second-line treatment in schizophrenia. Doses of >1g/d for just a few weeks may result in retinopathy.

Clinical features

- Asymptomatic, scotomas (paracentral or ring), ↓VA, nyctalopia, brownish visual discoloration.
- Pigmentary disturbance at the posterior pole; geographic areas of chorioretinal atrophy.

Prevention

Current prescribing practice (maintenance <300mg/d) should not lead to retinopathy.

Chlorpromazine

- This phenothiazine is used in schizophrenia and other psychoses.
- Doses of >2g/d for a year may result in retinopathy.

Clinical features

- Usually asymptomatic.
- Pigmentary disturbance.
- *Associated features*: corneal endothelial deposits, anterior lens granules.

Prevention

Current prescribing practice (<300mg/d) should not lead to retinopathy.

Tamoxifen

This oestrogen antagonist is used in the treatment of breast cancer. Retinopathy most commonly occurs after 1yr of therapy when a cumulative dose of >100g has been taken.

Clinical features

- Asymptomatic or mild ↓VA.
- Crystalline maculopathy with fine white refractile deposits in the inner retina centred around the fovea.
- *Associated features*: cystoid macular oedema, vortex keratopathy, optic neuritis.

Prevention

Current prescribing practice (<40mg/d) very rarely leads to retinopathy.

Desferrioxamine (desferrioxamine)

This chelating agent is commonly used to treat overload of iron (e.g. after multiple transfusions in chronic anaemias such as thalassaemia) and aluminium (e.g. dialysis patients). There appears to be no 'safe' dose: retinopathy occurred in one instance after a single administration.

Clinical features

- ↓VA, nyctalopia, abnormal colour vision, scotomas (usually central/centrocaecal).
- Central and peripheral pigmentary disturbance.

Sildenafil

Sildenafil is used in the treatment of erectile dysfunction and ocular side-effects are uncommon. Incidence and severity is dependant on blood concentration, occurring from 15 to 30min after ingestion and peaking at 60min.

Clinical features
• Transient changes in colour perception, blurred vision.
• Increased perception of brightness/photopsia especially on blinking.
• ERG changes.

Didanosine

This antiretroviral is used in the treatment of HIV infection. In children it has occasionally been observed to cause a retinopathy.

Clinical features
• Asymptomatic or mild peripheral field loss.
• Peripheral well-defined areas of retinal/RPE atrophy.

Clofazimine

This antimycobacterial is used in the treatment of leprosy and AIDS-related *Mycobacterium avium* infection.

Clinical features
Unusually extensive bull's-eye maculopathy with irregular pigment and atrophy extending beyond the arcades.

Retinal vein occlusion (1)

Retinal vein occlusions are common, can occur at almost any age and range in severity from the asymptomatic to the painful blind eye. They are divided into branch or central retinal vein occlusions (equating to occlusion anterior or posterior to the cribriform plate), and ischaemic or non-ischaemic types. Most occur in those over 65yrs, but up to 15% may affect patients under 45yrs. BRVO are three times more common than CRVO.

Central retinal vein occlusion

Although the division of non-ischaemic vs ischaemic CRVO is an arbitrary cut-off based on FFA findings, it is a useful predictor of visual outcome and risk of neovascularization. The clinical picture also differs.

Clinical features

Non-ischaemic

- ↓VA (mild–moderate), painless, metamorphopsia.
- Dilated, tortuous retinal veins with retinal haemorrhages in all four quadrants; occasional CWS; mild optic disc oedema.
- *Complications*: CMO.

Ischaemic

- ↓VA (severe); painless (unless neovascular glaucoma has developed).
- As for non-ischaemic but RAPD, deep haemorrhages, widespread CWS (5–10 is borderline; >10 is significant); rarely vitreous haemorrhage, exudative retinal detachment.
- *Chronic*: venous sheathing, resorption of haemorrhages, macular pigment disturbance, collateral vessels (especially at disc).
- *Complications*: CMO, neovascularization (NVI > NVD > NVE), neovascular ('90-day') glaucoma.

Investigations

- *For all patients*: BP, FBC, ESR, U+E, glucose, lipids, protein electrophoresis, TFT, and ECG. Further investigation is directed by clinical indication and may include CRP, serum ACE, anticardiolipin, lupus anticoagulant, autoantibodies (RF, ANA, anti-DNA, ANCA), fasting homocysteine, CXR, and thrombophilia screen (e.g. proteins C and S, antithrombin, factor V).
- *FFA*:
  - *non-ischaemic*: vein wall staining, microaneurysms, dilated optic disc capillaries.
  - *ischaemic*: as for non-ischaemic but capillary closure (5–10 disc areas is borderline; >10 is significantly ischaemic), hypofluorescence (blockage due to extensive haemorrhage), leakage (CMO, NV).
- *OCT*: shows extent of macular oedema and is useful for documenting progression.

Treatment

Although the evidence is lacking, the following are common practice (Table 13.14):

- ↓*IOP*: if elevated (in either eye).
- *Pan-retinal photocoagulation*: if neovascularization or high risk.

- *Treat underlying medical conditions*: liaise with a physician. **NB** In young adults with CRVO a mortality of 12% due to vascular disease has been reported.
- *Consider emerging treatments*: intravitreal triamcinolone for associated CMO, anti-VEGF therapy (off-label use) for associated CMO/ neovascularization and radial optic neurotomy for ischaemic CRVO.

Prognosis
- *Non-ischaemic* recovery to normal VA is <10%.
- *Non-ischaemic* progression to ischaemic: 15% by 4mths, 34% by 3yrs.
- *Ischaemic* progression to rubeosis: 37% by 4mths. Highest risk if VA <6/60 or ≥30 disc areas of non-perfusion on FFA.
- Risk of CRVO in contralateral eye: 7% by 2yrs.

Table 13.13 Associations of CRVO

Atherosclerotic	Hypertension
	Hypercholesterolaemia (including secondary to hypothyroidism)
	Diabetes
	Smoking
	Obesity
Haematological	Protein S, protein C, or antithrombin deficiency
	Activated protein C resistance
	Factor V Leiden
	Myeloma
	Waldenström's macroglobulinaemia
	Antiphospholipid syndrome
Inflammatory	Behçet's disease
	Polyarteritis nodosa
	Sarcoidosis
	Wegener's granulomatosis
	SLE
	Goodpasture syndrome
Ophthalmic	Glaucoma (open or closed angle)
	Trauma
	Optic disc drusen
	Orbital pathology

Retinal vein occlusion (2)

Branch retinal vein occlusion

Clinical features

- Most commonly supertemporal, unilateral in 90%.
- May be asymptomatic; ↓VA, metamorphopsia, visual field defect (usually altitudinal).
- *Acute*: retinal haemorrhages (dot, blot, flame), CWS, oedema in the distribution of a dilated, tortuous vein; superotemporal arcade most commonly affected; usually arise from an arteriovenous crossing.
- *Chronic*: venous sheathing, exudates, pigment disturbance, collateral vessels.
- *Complications*: CMO, neovascularization (NVE > NVD > NVI), recurrent vitreous haemorrhage.

Investigations

- Hypertension is the commonest association with BRVO (up to 75% of patients). BRVO may be investigated similarly to CRVO (see above).
- *FFA*: if uncertain diagnosis or where VA <6/12 at 3mths.
- *OCT*: useful for documenting macular oedema.

Treatment (Table 13.15)

- *Macular grid laser* (after FFA to determine perifoveal capillary perfusion): if macular oedema, VA ≤6/12 and no spontaneous improvement by 3–6mths.
- *Sectoral PRP*: if neovascularization.
- *Fill-in PRP*: if neovascularization progresses or vitreous haemorrhage.
- The possible role of anti-VEGF therapy in both macular oedema and neovascularization in BRVO is under evaluation.

Prognosis

- *Recovery to ≥6/12*: 50%.
- *Risk of macular oedema*: 57% (for temporal BRVO).
- *Risk of retinal neovascularization*: 20%, usually within the first 6–12mths.
- *Risk of neovascularization of disc or iris*: low.
- *Risk of BRVO in contralateral eye*: 6.6% by 4y.

Hemispheric branch vein occlusion

In approximately 20% of eyes the central retinal vein forms posterior to the lamina cribrosa from superior and inferior divisions. These are generally regarded as a variant of CRVO. Ischaemic hemispheric vein occlusions have an intermediate risk of rubeosis (compared with ischaemic BRVO and CRVO) but a greater risk of NVD than either ischaemic BRVO or CRVO. Treatment (in particular the role of laser) is as for BRVO.

Table 13.14 Summary of Royal College of Ophthalmologists recommendations for management of CRVO 2004

Ischaemic with no NV	Examination (including gonioscopy) monthly for first 6mths then every 3mths for 1yr; can be discharged if stable by 24mths
Ischaemic with NVI (angle or iris)	PRP (1500–2000 × 500µm × 0.05–0.1) Follow-up as above
Neovascular glaucoma with visual potential	↓IOP with topical agents or cycloablation
Neovascular glaucoma in blind eye	Keep comfortable with topical steroids and atropine
Non-ischaemic	Every 3mths for first 6mths; can usually be discharged if stable by 24mths

Table 13.15 Summary of Royal College of Ophthalmologists recommendations for management of BRVO 2004

Ischaemia >1 quadrant with no NV	Review at 3mths, then every 3–4mths; if stable can usually be discharged by 24mths
Ischaemia with NVD or NVE	Sectoral PRP (400–500 × 500µm × 0.05–0.1) Follow-up as above
Macular oedema	If VA <6/12 then perform FFA at >3mths and grid laser (20–100 × 100–200µm × 'gentle') at 3–6mths
Non-ischaemic	Review at 3mths, then every 3–6mths; if stable can usually be discharged by 24mths

Retinal artery occlusion (1)

Retinal artery occlusion is an ocular emergency in which rapidly instigated treatment *may* prevent irreversible loss of vision. Central retinal artery occlusion has an estimated incidence 0.85/100 000/yr, with men twice as often affected as women and with a mean age of 60yrs. CRAO causes almost complete hypoxia of the inner retina. Experimental evidence shows that this causes lethal damage to the primate retina after 100min. Acute coagulative necrosis is followed by complete loss of the nerve fibre layer, ganglion cell layer, and inner plexiform layer.

Central retinal artery occlusion

Clinical features
- Sudden painless unilateral ↓VA (usually CF or worse).
- White swollen retina with a cherry-red spot at the macula; arteriolar attenuation + cattle-trucking; RAPD; visible emboli in up to 25%.
- *Variants:* a cilioretinal artery (present in 30%) may protect part of the papillomacular bundle allowing relatively good vision; ophthalmic artery occlusion causes choroidal ischaemia with retinochoroidal whitening (no cherry-red spot) and complete loss of vision (usually NPL).
- *Complications:* neovascularization (NVI in 18%; NVD in 2%); rubeotic glaucoma; optic atrophy; ocular ischaemic syndrome (if ophthalmic artery occlusion).

Investigations
In the acute setting the diagnosis is not usually in doubt so the urgent priority is to rule out underlying disease (such as GCA) that may threaten the contralateral eye. When the presentation is delayed the clinical picture is less specific and may require ancillary tests.

Identify cause
- Most importantly consider GCA (if age >50yrs then ESR, CRP, FBC temporal artery biopsy, see AION ⬚ pp.588–591); more common causes are atherosclerosis (check for ↑BP, diabetes, hypercholesterolaemia, and smoking) and particularly carotid artery disease (may have carotid bruit).
- Further investigation is directed by clinical indication and may include PTT, APTT, thrombophilia screen (e.g. proteins C and S, antithrombin, factor V), antiphospholipid screen, vasculitis autoantibodies (ANA, ANCA, DNA, RF), syphilis serology (VDRL, TPHA), blood cultures, ECG, echocardiography, carotid Doppler scans (Table 13.16).

Treatment
- *Treat affected eye* (if within 24h of presentation):
  - ↓IOP with 500mg IV acetazolamide, ocular massage ± AC paracentesis (all common practice, but no proven benefit); selective ophthalmic artery catheterization with thrombolysis is performed in some centres.
- *Protect other eye:* e.g. treat underlying GCA with systemic steroids immediately (see AION, ⬚ pp.588–591).

Prognosis
- *Visual outcome*: 94% are CF or worse at presentation; about 1/3 show some improvement (with or without treatment).
- *Neovascularization*: neovascularization of the iris occurs in up to 16%; however, disc neovascularization is uncommon.

Table 13.16 Associations of CRAO

Atherosclerotic	Hypertension (60%) Diabetes (25%) Hypercholesterolaemia Smoking
Embolic sources	Carotid artery disease Aortic disease (including dissection) Cardiac valve vegetations (e.g. infective endocarditis) Cardiac or other tumours (e.g. atrial myxoma) Arrhythmias Cardiac septal defects Post-intervention (e.g. angiography/-plasty) Amniotic fluid
Haematological	Protein S, protein C, antithrombin deficiency, activated protein C resistance or factor V Leiden mutation Antiphospholipd syndrome Leukaemia or lymphoma Hyperhomocysteinaemia
Inflammatory	Giant cell arteritis Polyarteritis nodosa Wegener's granulomatosis SLE Kawasaki's disease Pancreatitis Susac's disease
Infective	Toxoplasmosis Mucormycosis Syphilis
Pharmacological	Oral contraceptive pill Cocaine
Ophthalmic	Trauma Optic nerve drusen Migraine

Retinal artery occlusion (2)

Branch retinal arteriolar occlusion

Most BRAO are due to emboli that are often visible clinically. The commonest emboli are:

- *Cholesterol (Hollenhorst plaque)*: small, yellow, refractile.
- *Fibrinoplatelet*: elongated, white, dull.
- *Calcific*: white, non-refractile, proximal to disc.
- Antiphospholipid syndrome is associated with multiple BRAO.

Clinical features

- Sudden painless unilateral altitudinal field defect.
- White swollen retina along a branch retinal arteriole; branch arteriolar attenuation + cattle-trucking; visible emboli common in over 60%.
- *Complications*: neovascularization may occur but is rare.

Investigations and treatment

- Identify underlying cause (as for CRAO). **NB** GCA is extremely rare as a cause of BRAO and does not need investigation in the absence of other supporting evidence.
- There is no proven treatment for BRAO.

Cilioretinal artery occlusion

Present in up to 30% of the population, this branch from the posterior ciliary circulation perfuses the posterior pole. Three distinct patterns of occlusion occur:

- *Isolated*: usually in the young, associated with systemic vasculitis, relatively good prognosis.
- *Combined with CRVO*: usually in the young, possibly a form of papillophlebitis, relatively good prognosis (as for non-ischaemic CRVO).
- *Combined with AION*: usually in the elderly, associated with GCA, very poor prognosis.

Hypertensive retinopathy

Systemic hypertension is one of the commonest diseases of the Western world, where it may affect up to 60% of those aged over 60yrs.

- *Risk factors*: include age, gender (men > women), ethnic origin (African-Caribbean > white people), and society (industrialized > agricultural).
- Exercise is protective.

The majority of hypertension is chronic and of unknown cause ('essential'). It causes sclerosis and narrowing of the arterioles seen both in the retinal and more severely in the choroidal circulation. In about 1% of cases hypertension is acute and severe (accelerated or 'malignant' hypertension). This causes fibrinoid necrosis of arterioles and accelerated end-organ damage.

- This medical emergency requires urgent assessment, treatment and identification of an underlying cause. Untreated, accelerated hypertension carries a 90% mortality at 1yr.

Chronic hypertension

There is no absolutely 'safe' BP and, therefore, no absolute definition of hypertension. However, intervention is currently recommended for BP >140mmHg systolic or >90mmHg diastolic on two separate occasions (Table 13.17).

Clinical features

- *Systemic*: usually asymptomatic. May have evidence of end-organ damage (cardiovascular, cerebrovascular, peripheral vascular, renal disease).
- *Ophthalmic*: narrowing/irregularity of arterioles (copper and silver-wiring), arteriovenous nipping, CWS, blot or flame haemorrhages.
- *Complications*: macroaneurysms, non-arteritic AION, C/BRVO, C/BRAO.

Investigation and treatment

- Alert the primary care physician who will monitor, assess vascular risk, and treat as required (Table 13.17–13.18).
- The target is <140/90 for most patients, <130/80 for those with diabetes, and <125/75 for diabetics with proteinuria.

Accelerated hypertension

Severe ↑BP (e.g. >220mmHg systolic or >120mmHg diastolic) with papilloedema or fundal haemorrhages and exudates.

Clinical features

- *Systemic*
  - headache
  - accelerated end-organ damage (e.g. myocardial infarct, cardiac failure, stroke, encephalopathy, renal failure).
- *Ophthalmic*
  - scotoma, diplopia, photopsia, ↓VA
  - *retinopathy*: focal arteriolar narrowing, CWS, flame haemorrhages
  - *choroidopathy*: infarcts, which may be focal (Elschnig's spots) or linear along choroidal arteries (Siegrist's streaks), serous retinal detachments
  - *optic neuropathy*: disc swelling ± macular star.

Investigation and treatment

Refer to medical team for admission and cautious lowering of BP; too rapid a reduction may be deleterious (e.g. stroke).

Table 13.17 Treatment of hypertension (after Joint British Societies' guidelines[1,2])

Systolic (mmHg)	Diastolic (mmHg)	Management
≥ 220	≥ 120	Admit and treat immediately
180–219	110–119	Treat if sustained over 1–2wks
160–179	100–109	If high risk: treat if sustained over 3–4wks If low risk: modify lifestyle but treat if sustained over 4–12wks
140–159	90–99	If high risk: treat if sustained at up to 12wks If low risk: modify lifestyle, recheck monthly, and treat if cardiovascular risk is ≥20% in 10yrs

High risk = end-organ damage (e.g. renal impairment, LVH), cardiovascular complications or diabetes. **1.** *Heart* 2005;**91** (Suppl V): v1–v52. **2.** BNF 2008.

Table 13.18 Common antihypertensives

Group	Example	Contraindication	Side-effects
Thiazide diuretic	Bendroflu-methiazide	Renal/hepatic failure, persistent $\downarrow K^+$, $\downarrow Na^+$	$\downarrow K^+$, $\downarrow Na^+$, postural hypotension, impotence
β-blocker	Atenolol	Asthma; caution in cardiac failure	Bronchospasm, cardiac failure, lethargy, impotence
ACE-inhibitor	Lisinopril	Renal artery stenosis, aortic stenosis,	Cough, $\uparrow K^+$, renal failure, angioedema
AIIR-antagonist	Losartan	Caution in renal artery stenosis, aortic stenosis	Mild hypotension, $\uparrow K^+$
Ca^{2+}-channel antagonist	Nifedipine	Cardiogenic shock, within 1mth of MI	Dependent oedema, flushing, fatigue
α-blocker	Doxazosin	Aortic stenosis	Dependent oedema, fatigue, postural hypotension

Haematological disease

Haemoglobinopathies

Normal adult haemoglobin (HbA) comprises two α- and two β-globin chains associated with a haem ring. In sickle haemoglobinopathies (Table 13.19) there is a mutant haemoglobin, such as HbS (β-chain residue 6 Glu → Val), which behaves abnormally in response to hypoxia or acidosis. This causes 'sickling' and haemolysis of red blood cells. Many other mutant haemoglobins have been described of which the most common is HbC.

In thalassaemias the problem is one of inadequate production of one or more of the α- or β-chains. Although systemic disease is most severe in sickle-cell disease (HbSS), ocular disease is most severe in HbSC and HbS–Thal disease.

Sickle haemoglobinopathies are seen in Africans and their descendents; thalassaemias are mainly seen in Africans and Mediterranean countries.

Table 13.19 Sickle haemoglobinopathies

Disease	Hb	Prevalence in African-American population
Sickle trait	HbAS	5–10%
Sickle-cell disease	HbSS	0.4%
Haemoglobin SC disease	HbSC	0.2%
Sickle-cell thalassaemia	HbS-Thal	0.5–1.0%; 0.03% severe

Clinical features
• Proliferative retinopathy (Table 13.20).

Table 13.20 Goldberg staging of proliferative retinopathy

Stage 1	Peripheral arteriolar occlusions
Stage 2	Arteriovenous anastamoses
Stage 3	Neovascular proliferation ('sea-fans')
Stage 4	Vitreous haemorrhage
Stage 5	Retinal detachment

• *Non-proliferative retinopathy*: arteriosclerosis, venous tortuosity, equatorial 'salmon patches' (pre-retinal/superficial intraretinal haemorrhages), and 'black sunbursts' (intraretinal haemorrhage disturbing RPE with pigment migration), macular ischaemia, and atrophy ('macular depression sign'); occasional CWS, microaneurysms.
• *Other*: conjunctival 'comma-shaped' capillaries, sectoral iris atrophy.

Investigation
Hb electrophoresis, FBC. **NB** Some patients with HbSC or HbS–Thal may be unaware of their disease.

Treatment
- Observation.
- Consider laser photocoagulation in proliferative sickle retinopathy—controversial as most sea-fans spontaneously regress. The rationale is to remove the drive to neovascularization by ablating the ischaemic retina.
- Consider vitreoretinal surgery for persistent vitreous haemorrhage (e.g. >6mths) and tractional retinal detachment, although the results are generally disappointing, and specialist perioperative care is required.

Anaemia
- Retinal findings increase with severity of anaemia, particularly in the presence of thrombocytopenia.
- The retinopathy is usually an incidental finding, and thus investigation and treatment should already be under way with their haematologist.

Clinical features
- *Retinopathy*: usually asymptomatic; haemorrhages, CWS, venous tortuosity.
- *Other*: subconjunctival haemorrhages, optic neuropathy (if ↓B12).

Leukaemia
- Retinal findings are more common with acute rather than chronic leukaemias.
- Leukaemic complications may be due to direct infiltration or secondary anaemia and hyperviscosity.

Clinical features
- *Retinopathy*: usually asymptomatic; haemorrhages, CWS, venous tortuosity, pigment epitheliopathy ('leopard spot' from choroidal infiltration), neovascularization (rare).
- *Other*: spontaneous haemorrhage (subconjunctival or hyphaema), infiltration (iris → anterior uveitis ± hypopyon; orbit → proptosis; optic nerve → optic neuropathy ± disc swelling).

Hyperviscosity
Hyperviscosity arises from abnormally high levels of:
- blood constituents, either cells (e.g. primary or secondary polycythaemia, leukaemias), or
- protein levels (e.g. multiple myeloma, Waldenström's macroglobulinaemia).

Clinical features
- *Retinopathy*: usually asymptomatic; haemorrhages (may be peripheral), CWS, venous tortuosity, and dilation.
- *Other*: disc swelling in polycythaemia and multiple myeloma, conjunctival/corneal crystals, iris/ciliary body cysts in multiple myeloma.

Retinal telangiectasias

Retinal telangiectasia describe abnormalities of the retinal vasculature usually with irregular dilation of the capillary bed, and segmental dilation of neighbouring venules and arterioles. Most commonly they are acquired secondary to another retinal disorder (e.g. CRVO).

Congenital forms represent a spectrum of disease from the severe and early onset of Coats' disease, to the more limited and later onset of idiopathic juxtafoveal telangiectasia.

Coats' disease

- This uncommon condition is the most severe of the telangiectasias.
- Affects mainly men (M:F 3:1) and the young, although up to 1/3 may be asymptomatic until their 30s.
- Although often considered a unilateral disease, about 10% cases are bilateral.

Clinical features

- May be asymptomatic; ↓VA, strabismus, leucocoria.
- Telangiectatic vessels, 'light bulb' aneurysms, capillary drop-out, exudation (may be massive), scarring.
- *Complications*: exudative retinal detachment, neovascularization, vitreous haemorrhage, rubeosis, glaucoma, cataract.

Investigations

FFA: highlights abnormal vessels, leakage, and areas of capillary drop-out.

Treatment

- Main aim is to control exudation: consider laser photocoagulation (or cryotherapy) of leaking vessels; treat directly rather than a scatter approach.
- Scleral buckling with drainage of subretinal fluid may be performed for significant exudative detachment but carries a guarded prognosis.

Leber's miliary aneurysms

This is essentially a localized, less severe form of Coats' disease presenting in adults with unilateral ↓VA, fusiform and saccular aneurysmic dilation of venules and arterioles, and local exudation. Again direct photocoagulation of abnormal vessels may be beneficial.

Idiopathic juxtafoveal retinal telangiectasia (*syn* idiopathic macular telangiectasia)

This rare condition presents in adulthood with mild ↓VA due to telangiectatic juxtafoveal retinal capillaries with local exudation. The possible role of anti-VEGF therapies for this group of diseases is under investigation.

Described by Gass in 1982; there are two main classifications:

Classification by Gass ('Idiopathic juxtafoveal retinal telangiectasia')

- *Group 1A*: unilateral parafoveal telangiectasia of the temporal macula; early middle-aged men; VA approximately 6/12, focal laser treatment may be effective.

- *Group 1B*: unilateral parafoveal telangiectasia of ≤1 clock hour at the edge of the foveal avascular zone; middle-aged men; VA approximately 6/7, laser treatment not indicated.
- *Group 2*: bilateral symmetrical parafoveal telangiectasia; late middle-age; gradual ↓VA due to foveal atrophy or CNV.
- *Group 3*: bilateral perifoveal occlusive telangiectasia; very rare; adulthood; gradual ↓VA due to capillary occlusion.

Classification by Yannuzzi ('Idiopathic macular telangiectasia')

The more recent classification by Yannuzzi is simpler.

- *Type 1*: aneurysmal telangiectasia (includes Gass groups 1A and 1B).
- *Type 2*: perifoveal telangiectasia (includes Gass group 2).

Table 13.21 Causes of retinal telangiectasias

Primary	Coats' disease
	Leber's miliary aneurysms
	Idiopathic juxtafoveal telangiectasia
	IRVAN syndrome
Secondary	ROP
	RP
	Diabetic retinopathy
	Sickle retinopathy
	Radiation retinopathy
	Hypogammaglobulinaemia
	Eales' disease
	CRVO/BRVO

Other retinal and choroidal vascular anomalies

Macroaneurysm

This is a focal dilatation of a retinal arteriole occurring within the first three orders of the arterial tree. They tend to be 100–250µm in size with a fusiform or saccular shape. Typically, they occur in hypertensive women over the age of 50.

Clinical features
- ↓VA (if macular exudate or vitreous haemorrhage); often asymptomatic.
- Saccular or fusiform dilatation of arterial often near AV crossing; haemorrhage (sub-/intra-/preretinal and vitreal); exudation (often on the temporal arcades with circinates).

Investigations
FFA: immediate complete filling (partial filling suggests thrombosis) with late leakage.

Treatment
- High rate of spontaneous resolution, particularly of the haemorrhagic (rather than exudative) lesions.
- Consider photocoagulation (either direct or to the surrounding capillary bed) if symptomatic due to exudation at the macula.
- Vitrectomy may be required for non-clearing vitreous haemorrhage.

Idiopathic retinal vasculitis, aneurysms, and neuroretinitis (IRVAN syndrome)

This is a rare recently recognized abnormality with distinctive retinal characteristics: retinal vasculitis, arterial aneurysmal dilations, and neuroretinitis. Other features include capillary closure, exudation, and neovascularisation. It is commoner in the young (mean age 32yrs) and women. No systemic associations have been reported.

Treatment with PRP before the development of posterior or anterior segment neovascularization appears to be beneficial. Outlook once neovascularization occurs is poor.

Idiopathic polypoidal choroidal vasculopathy

This is an uncommon but increasingly recognized abnormality of the choroidal vasculature. Risk factors include female sex and hypertension; although originally described in African-Caribbeans it may occur in any race.

The underlying abnormality is of polypoidal aneurismal dilation of abnormal choroidal vasculature usually around the posterior pole. These result in the clinical picture of recurrent multiple serous or haemorrhagic detachments of retina/RPE in the absence of features suggestive of AMD (e.g. drusen) or intraocular inflammation. The choroidal aneurysms can be confirmed on ICG, assisting differentiation from AMD or other neovascular processes.

Prognosis is variable. Early polypoidal choroidal vasculopathy lesions can regress spontaneously. Direct focal photocoagulation to lesion may be successful. Lesions are generally poorly responsive to anti-VEGF treatment, although there may be a role if associated with a CNV.

Radiation retinopathy

Irradiation of the globe, orbit, sinuses, or nasopharynx may lead to retinal damage. This usually occurs after a delay of 6mths–3yrs, which is thought to be the turnover time for endothelial cells of the retinal vasculature. Risk of retinopathy increases with radiation dose.

- 90% of brachytherapy patients receiving a macular dose of ≥7500rad developed maculopathy.
- Over 50% of patients receiving orbital/nasopharyngeal irradiation may develop retinopathy.
- Retinopathy is unlikely after doses of ≤2500rad given in fractions of ≤200rad.

Clinical features

- Focal drop-out and irregular dilatation of the capillary bed at the posterior pole; microaneurysms, telangiectasia, exudation, fine intraretinal haemorrhages.
- *Acute response to high-dose radiation*: ischaemic retinal necrosis with widespread vascular occlusion, CWS, widespread superficial and deep haemorrhages; intraretinal microvascular abnormalities; neovascularization tractional retinal detachment/vitreous haemorrhage.
- *Papillopathy (usually accompanied by retinopathy)*: acute disc hyperaemia, oedema, peripapillary haemorrhage, and CWS; chronic severe optic atrophy.

Treatment

Consider focal photocoagulation for macular exudation and panretinal photocoagulation for proliferative radiation retinopathy, although less intensive treatment is usually required than in diabetic retinopathy.

Retinitis pigmentosa

Retinitis pigmentosa (RP) is the commonest of the retinal dystrophies affecting about 1 in 4000 of the population.

It comprises a spectrum of conditions in which abnormalities of over 50 different genes may cause loss of predominantly rods (rod-cone dystrophy) or cones (cone-rod dystrophy).

It may be sporadic or inherited (autosomal dominant (20%) or recessive (13%), or X-linked (8%)). Autosomal disease is the commonest form (but the least severe), whereas X-linked disease is the least common (but the most severe).

Most RP is isolated (i.e. with no systemic features), but about 25% have associated systemic disease. A number of specific syndromes are also described.

Clinical features
- Nyctalopia, tunnel vision, ↓VA.
- Mid-peripheral 'bone-spicule' retinal pigmentation, waxy pallor of the optic disc, arteriolar attenuation; cataract.
- *Complications*: CMO.

Investigations
- *ERG*: scotopic affected before photopic; b waves affected before a waves. This test can be used to monitor disease.
- EOG is abnormal.
- *Visual fields*: initially may have ring scotomas before developing frank tunnel vision.

Treatment
- *Supportive measures* including counselling, low vision aids, and social services must not be neglected.
- *Medical*: vitamin A palmitate (15 000IU/d) appears to slow disease progression slightly; acetazolamide (250–500mg/d) may be effective in RP-related CMO.
- *Cataract surgery*: reduce operating light levels, prophylactic post-operative acetazolamide.

Variants
RP variants include unusual distributions (sectoral or central RP) and odd patterns, such as retinitis punctata albescens (scattered white dots predating more typical RP changes).

Table 13.22 Associations of retinitis pigmentosa (selected)

Isolated	Sporadic
	Familial (AD, AR, X)
Systemic	Usher syndrome
	Bardet–Biedl syndrome
	Laurence–Moon syndrome
	Kearns–Sayre syndrome
	Batten disease
	Mucopolysaccharidoses I–III
	Abetalipoproteinaemia
	Refsum disease
	Osteopetrosis

Table 13.23 Genes involved in retinitis pigmentosa (selected)

AD RP	Rhodopsin
	Peripherin-RDS
	NRL
	RP1
	FSCN2
	PRPC8
AR RP	PDEB
	PDEA
	CNCG
	Rhodopsin
	RLB1
	TULP1
	ABCR4
	RPE65
	RP12
	USH2A
	CRB1
X-linked RP	RP GTPase regulator (RPGR)
	RP-2 protein RP2
Digenic RP	Mutation in RDS and ROM1

Congenital stationary night blindness

A group of disorders that share the feature of early, but non-progressive, nyctalopia (night blindness). They may be divided into those with normal fundus (with autosomal dominant, autosomal recessive, and X-linked subtypes) and those with fundal abnormalities (Oguchi's disease, fundus albipunctatus).

Autosomal dominant CSNB has been traced back in family pedigrees as far as the 17th century (Nougaret pedigree).

Congenital stationary night blindness with normal fundi

There are a number of different subclassifications based on inheritance, ERG findings, or presence of myopia. Mutations in rhodopsin, rod cGMP-PDE, and rod transducin have all been identified in AD CSNB.

Clinical features
- In general, AD CSNB shows non-progressive nyctalopia alone
- AR and X-linked disease show additional features such as ↓VA, nystagmus, and myopia.

Investigations and treatment
- *ERG*: AD CSNB shows the Riggs ERG abnormality, whereas AR and X-linked CSNB show the Schubert–Bornschein ERG abnormality.
- *Treatment*: supportive, and dependent on the type of disease.

Congenital stationary night blindness with abnormal fundi

Oguchi's disease
This rare autosomal recessive disease may arise from mutations in arrestin (Ch2q) and rhodopsin kinase. The arrestin is more common in Japanese Oguchi's disease and rhodopsin kinase in European Oguchi's disease.

In addition to non-progressive nyctalopia, there is an abnormal golden-yellow fundal reflex that normalizes with dark adaptation (Mizuo phenomenon). There is also a delay in dark adaptation (with normalization of the ERG after several hours).

Fundus albipunctatus
A rare autosomal recessive disease due to mutations in the gene for 11-*cis* retinol dehydrogenase. In addition to non-progressive nyctalopia with delayed dark adaptation there are numerous tiny radially distributed white dots covering most of the fundus except the macula and far-periphery.

Macular dystrophies (1)

A number of retinal dystrophies show a predilection for the macula usually causing loss of photoreceptors and the accumulation of a yellow material around the level of the RPE. This causes varying degrees of central vision loss. There is no effective treatment for any of these conditions. Therefore, the priority of the clinician should be towards effective diagnosis, counselling, and supportive care as required.

Newer imaging techniques such as fundus autofluorescence and electrophysical testing may aid the diagnosis and help predict prognosis.

Stargardt's disease and fundus flavimaculatus

These are two clinical presentations of the same disease, being the commonest of the macular dystrophies at about 7% of all retinal dystrophies. Most is autosomal recessive, due to a mutation in the ATP-binding cassette (ABCA4, Ch1p). Rare dominant disease links to the *ELOVL4* gene, Ch6q.

Histologically, there is accumulation of a lipofuscin (up to 5 times normal) and A2E throughout the RPE; in the ABCA4 knock-out mouse model this has been found to be a toxic *bis*-retinoid.

Clinical features

- *Stargardt's disease*: rapid ↓VA (6/18–6/60) usually in childhood, initially with minimal visible signs (but may have detectable abnormal autofluorescence); then posterior polar changes, including pigmentary disturbance, 'beaten-bronze' atrophy, yellowish flecks.
- *Fundus flavimaculatus*: widespread pisciform flecks throughout the fundus usually occurring in adulthood with relative preservation of vision.

Investigations

- *ERG and EOG*: normal in early disease, mild reduction later.
- *FFA*: classically 'dark choroid' (due to blockage by the abnormal deposit) but this is variable.
- *OCT*: the newer OCTs show characteristic thinning of the photoreceptor layer.

Best's disease

This is a rare condition with very variable expression such that some family members may have the genotype but be completely unaffected. It is autosomal dominant arising from a mutation in the RPE transmembrane protein bestrophin (VMD2, Ch11q). Onset is usually in childhood.

Clinical features

- Usually asymptomatic in early stages; ↓VA may be as low as 6/60 but most individuals retain reading, and even driving, vision in one eye.
- Most easily recognized when yolk-like lesion at the posterior pole; this may later be replaced by non-specific scarring, atrophy, or even CNV formation (Table 13.24).

Investigations

- *EOG*: reduced Arden ratio (<150%).
- *ERG*: near-normal.

Table 13.24 Staging of Best's disease

1	Pre-vitelliform	EOG findings only
2	Vitelliform	Yolk-like macular lesion
3	Pseudohypopyon	Partial absorption leaving level
4	Vitelliruptive	'Scrambled' appearance
5	End-stage	Scarring or atrophy

Adult vitelliform degeneration

Adult vitelliform degeneration (includes adult onset foveomacular vitelliform dystrophy of Gass) describes a vitelliform appearance occurring in minimally symptomatic adults with a near-normal EOG.

There is no clear inheritance pattern, although some cases with mutations of VMD2 and peripherin/RDS have been described.

Familial drusen

This is a rare autosomal dominant condition with variable expression. The different patterns seen have traditionally been described separately as Doynes honeycomb dystrophy and malattia leventinese. However, it is thought that these reflect the varied phenotype of the same condition all arising from mutations in EFEMP1. It appears that these mutations result in abnormal basement membrane formation at the level of the RPE.

Clinical features

Usually only mild symptoms; yellow–white drusen at the posterior pole, often confluent, may be small or large

Investigations
- *ERG*: normal;
- *EOG*: mild abnormality.

Pattern dystrophy

This rare group of conditions show abnormal pigment patterns at the level of the RPE.

Different phenotypes may be seen in the same family, hence they are probably best grouped collectively rather than separately under the traditional descriptive names—butterfly dystrophy, etc.

Inheritance is usually autosomal (recessive > dominant), and is in some cases linked to mutations in the peripherin/RDS gene.

Clinical features

Usually only mild symptoms; abnormal pigment patterns at the posterior pole.

Investigations
- *ERG*: normal;
- *EOG*: mild abnormality.

Macular dystrophies (2)

Dominant cystoid macular oedema

This very rare autosomal dominant disease (Ch7q) appears to selectively affect Muller's cells causing multilobulated cystoid spaces arising from the inner nuclear layer.

Clinically, and on FFA, the appearances are of typical CMO.

Sorsby's macular dystrophy

This very rare autosomal dominant disease arises from mutations in a regulator of extracellular matrix (TIMP3, Ch22q).

Usually causes significant ↓VA from 40yrs, when exudative maculopathy develops with subsequent scarring, atrophy, and even choroidal neovascularization.

North Carolina macular dystrophy

This rare autosomal dominant disease was initially described in North Carolina, but has been identified in a number of families worldwide. It links to MCDR1, Ch6q. Onset is from birth.

The disease is confined to the macular and phenotype varies from 6/6 VA with a few drusen to 6/60 with a macular coloboma or subsequent CNV. Vision is often better than expected from the fundal appearance.

Progressive bifocal chorioretinal atrophy

This rare autosomal dominant disease has only been described in the UK, and, like North Carolina macular dystrophy, links to Ch6q.

This is a bizarre pattern of progressive chorioretinal atrophy that spreads from two foci located just temporal and just nasal to the disc. Onset is from birth, and the visual loss is severe.

Cone degenerations

This group of disorders cause selective loss of cone photoreceptors with ↓VA, colour vision abnormalities, central scotomas, and a variable degree of nystagmus and photophobia. The macula may show only a mild granularity or marked central atrophy.

No specific treatment though supportive measures, e.g. tinted spectacles and low visual, aids can be beneficial.

Central areolar choroidal dystrophy

This rare autosomal dominant disease links to Ch17p and usually presents in young adults.

There is slowly progressive loss of central vision, with central geographic atrophy, including loss of the underlying choriocapillaris.

Choroidal dystrophies

The choroidal dystrophies are inherited, potentially blinding conditions in which the primary clinical abnormality is atrophy of RPE and choroid. In fact the co-dependence of retina and choroid is well demonstrated by the discovery that in choroideraemia the underlying defect is probably in the rod photoreceptors, where 'stop' mutations in the *CHM* gene prevents its normal production of Rab escort protein (REP-1).

Choroideraemia

This rare X-linked recessive condition causes significant disease from childhood in males, but usually only asymptomatic 'moth-eaten' peripheral pigmentary disturbance in female carriers.

Clinical features

- Nyctalopia, visual field loss (e.g. ring scotoma), later ↓VA (usually in middle age).
- RPE/choroidal atrophy: initially mid-peripheral, patchy, and superficial (choriocapillaris); later central, diffuse, and deeper choroidal atrophy to expose the sclera; retinal vessels and optic disc are relatively preserved.
- *Other*: cataract (posterior subcapsular), early vitreous degeneration.

Investigations and treatment

- Reduction in ERG (rod responses affected before cone responses) with prolongation of b-wave implicit time.
- Useful vision is retained until late in disease; supportive treatment and genetic counselling may be offered. Prenatal testing is possible.

Gyrate atrophy

This rare autosomal recessive condition arises from mutations in the *OAT* gene. This encodes for ornithine aminotransferase, which with cofactor B6, catalyses the conversion of ornithine to glutamic-γ-semialdehyde, and thence to proline.

Two clinical subtypes are seen according to whether treatment with B6 lowers plasma ornithine levels. Responders appear to have a milder form of disease. Disease is usually symptomatic from late childhood. It is more common in Finland.

Clinical features

- Nyctalopia, peripheral field loss, later ↓VA.
- *RPE/choroidal atrophy*: well-defined circular patches initially mid-peripheral and superficial (choriocapillaris); later confluent, panfundal (relative sparing of macular, retinal vessels, and optic disc) and deeper choroidal atrophy; ERM, CMO.
- *Other*: high myopia, astigmatism, cataract (posterior subcapsular).

Investigations

- Early reduction in ERG (rod responses affected before cone responses); less marked changes in B6-responsive group.
- *Plasma ornithine*: 10–15× normal level; also elevated in urine and CSF.

Treatment
- *Low-protein diet*: with arginine restriction ornithine levels may be controlled, with control of ocular disease demonstrated at least in the OAT–/– knock-out mouse.
- *Vitamin B6*: reduces ornithine levels in the responsive subgroup, but little evidence for improved control of eye disease.

Other choroidal atrophies

These include diffuse choroidal atrophy and central areolar choroidal dystrophy, which are usually autosomal dominant, may be linked to abnormalities of peripherin/RDS and carry a very poor prognosis.

Albinism

Abnormalities in the synthesis of melanin result in pigment deficiency of the eye alone (ocular albinism) or of the eye, skin, and hair (oculocutaneous albinism). Although there is wide phenotypic variation the VA is generally reduced due to macular hypoplasia. In most patients there also appears to be increased decussation of the temporal fibres at the chiasm.

Ocular albinism

Classic ocular albinism (Nettleship–Falls albinism) represents 10% of all albinism. It is X-linked, the *OA1* gene being implicated in melanosomes function. Ocular features may be severe despite an otherwise normal appearance.

Female carriers may show mild, patchy features of the disease, including a 'mud-splattered' fundus.

Clinical features
- ↓VA, photophobia.
- Nystagmus, strabismus, ametropia, iris hypopigmentation/transillumination, macular hypoplasia, fundus hypopigmentation.

Treatment
- The main priority is to correct ametropia (± tinted lenses for photophobia) and prevent amblyopia.
- Consider surgery for strabismus and some cases of nystagmus.

Oculocutaneous albinism

Oculocutaneous disease is autosomal recessive and accounts for the majority of albinism. It arises from abnormalities in several components of melanogenesis: type I = tyrosinase (Ch11q), type II = *p* product (Ch15q, probably a transporter), and type III = tyrosinase related protein 1 (Ch9p).

Clinical features
- *Ophthalmic*: as for ocular albinism.
- *Systemic*: there is variable hypopigmentation of skin and hair (blond).

Treatment
As for ocular albinism.

Table 13.25 Classification of oculocutaneous albinism

Type I	Tyrosinase	Subtype A	Severe variant
		Subtype B	Yellow variant
		Subtype MP	Minimal pigment
		Subtype TS	Temperature sensitive
Type II	Substance p	Prader–Willi	Learning difficulties, obesity, hypotonia
		Angelmann	Learning difficulties, ataxia, abnormal facies
		Hermansky–Pudlak	Low platelets, pulmonary/renal abnormalities; Puerto-Rican ancestry
		Chediak–Higashi	Immunocompromised secondary to abnormal leucocyte chemotaxis
Type III	TRP1		

Laser procedures

Pan-retinal photocoagulation

Indication
Active proliferative retinopathy, some cases of high-risk pre-proliferative retinopathy.

Method
- *Consent.* Explain:
  - what the procedure does (aims to stop disease progression; further laser treatment may well be required);
  - what the procedure does not do (does not improve vision; is not an alternative to glycaemic control, etc.);
  - what to expect, and possible complications, e.g. pain, loss of peripheral field (with driving implications), scotomas, worsened acuity (e.g. macular decompensation), choroidal or retinal detachment, decreased dark adaptation, and vitreous haemorrhage.
- *Instil topical anaesthetic* (e.g. oxybuprocaine), and position fundus contact lens (e.g. transequator) with coupling agent.
- *Set argon laser* for 200–500μm spot size, 0.1s, and adjust power to produce a gently blanching burn.
  - Consider placing a temporal barrier at least 2–3 disc diameters from fovea, to help demarcate a 'no-go' zone. Then place ≥1000 burns outside the vascular arcades, leaving burn-width intervals between them. A second session of ≥1000 is usually performed a few weeks later.
- *Tips*: the power may need to be adjusted frequently according to variable retinal take-up. If the patient feels pain, consider reducing the duration (e.g. to 0.05s) but increasing the power to maintain burn intensity.
- *Review* 3-weekly ± fill-in PRP until response.

Macular laser (focal or grid)

Indication
Clinically, significant macular oedema (Table 13.4).

Method
- *Consent*: explain what the procedure does (aims to reduce sight loss; further laser treatment may well be required), what to expect and possible complications, e.g. pain, scotomas, worsened acuity, retinal detachment.
- *Instil topical anaesthetic* (e.g. oxybuprocaine), and position fundus contact lens (e.g. area centralis) with coupling agent.
- *Set argon laser* for 50–200μm spot size, 0.08–0.1s, and adjust power to produce a very gently blanching burn. Generally, smaller spot sizes and shorter durations are used for more central burns.
- *For focal treatment*: apply burns to leaking microaneurysms between 500 and 3000μm from the centre of the fovea. Lesions as near as 300μm to the fovea may be treated provided this would not be within the foveal avascular zone.

- *For grid treatment*: place similar burns ≥1 burn-width apart in a grid arrangement around the fovea. They must be at least 500µm from the centre of the fovea and from the disc margin.
- *Review* at 3mths or sooner.

Orbit

Anatomy and physiology

The bony orbit forms a pyramid comprising a medial wall lying anterposteriorly, a lateral wall at 45°, a roof, and a floor. It has a volume of about 30ml and contains most of the globe and associated structures: extraocular muscles (see Anatomy and physiology 📖 p.446), optic nerve (see Anatomy and physiology (1) 📖 p.576), cranial nerves (see Anatomy and physiology (2) 📖 p.578), vascular supply, and lacrimal: system (see Anatomy and physiology 📖 p.150).

Being effectively a rigid box, the only room for expansion is forwards. Most orbital pathology, therefore, presents initially with proptosis, followed by disruption of eye movements.

Table 14.1 Orbital bones

Wall	Bones	Rim	Bones
Roof	Frontal Sphenoid (lesser wing)	Superior	Frontal
Lateral	Sphenoid (greater wing) Zygomatic	Lateral	Zygomatic Frontal
Floor	Zygomatic Maxilla Palatine	Inferior	Zygomatic Maxilla
Medial	Maxilla Lacrimal Ethmoid Sphenoid	Medial	Maxilla Lacrimal

Table 14.2 Orbital apertures

Aperture	Location	Contents
Optic canal	Apex (lesser wing sphenoid)	Optic n, sympathetic fibres Ophthalmic artery
Superior orbital fissure	Apex (greater/lesser wings sphenoid)	III, IV, Va, VI, sympathetic fibres Orbital veins
Inferior orbital fissure	Apex	Zygomatic and infraorbital nerve (Vb) Orbital veins
Zygomaticofacial	Lateral wall	Zygomaticofacial nerve (Vb) and vessels
Zygomaticotemporal	Lateral wall	Zygomaticotemporal nerve (Vb) and vessels
Ethmoidal foramen	Medial wall (frontal/ ethmoidal bones)	Ethmoidal arteries (anterior, posterior)
Nasolacrimal canal	Medial wall (maxilla/ lacrimal)	Nasolacrimal duct

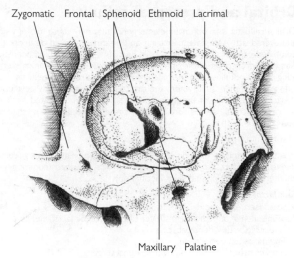

Fig. 14.1 The bones of the orbit.

Orbital and preseptal cellulitis

Orbital cellulitis is an ophthalmic emergency that may cause loss of vision and even death. Assessment, imaging, and treatment should be under the combined care of an ophthalmologist and ENT specialist (and paediatrician in children). Part of the ophthalmologist's role is to assist in differentiating orbital cellulitis from the much more limited preseptal cellulitis.

In younger children in whom the orbital septum is not fully developed there is a high risk of progression and so should be treated similarly to orbital cellulitis. For orbital and preseptal cellulitis in children, (📖 p.702).

Orbital cellulitis

Infective organisms include *Streptococcus pneumoniae*, *Staphylococcus aureus*, *Streptococcus pyogenes*, and *Haemophilus influenza* (commoner in children, but reducing since Hib vaccination).

Risk factors

- *Sinus disease*: ethmoidal sinusitis (common), maxillary sinusitis
  - *infection of other adjacent structures*: preseptal or facial infection, dacryocystitis, dental abscess.
- *Trauma*: septal perforation.
- *Surgical*: orbital, lacrimal, and vitreoretinal surgery.

Clinical features

- Fever, malaise, and peri-ocular pain.
- Inflamed lids (swollen, red, tender, warm) ± chemosis, proptosis, painful restricted eye movements, diplopia, lagophthalmos, optic nerve dysfunction (↓VA, ↓colour vision, RAPD).
- *Complications*: exposure keratopathy, ↑IOP, CRAO, CRVO, inflammation of optic nerve.
- *Systemic*: orbital or periorbital abscess, cavernous sinus thrombosis, meningitis, cerebral abscess.

Investigation

- Temperature.
- FBC, blood culture (but yield is low: range 0–7% in recent studies[1]).
- CT (orbit, sinuses, brain): orbital abscess, diffuse orbital infiltrate, proptosis ± sinus opacity.

Treatment

- Admit for IV antibiotics (e.g. either flucloxacillin 1–2g 4×/d or cefuroxime 750–1500mg 3×/d with metronidazole 500mg 3×/d if history of chronic sinus disease).
- ENT to assess for sinus drainage (required in up to 90% of adults).

Preseptal cellulitis

Preseptal cellulitis is not truly an orbital disease. It is much commoner than orbital cellulitis from which it must be differentiated. It is commoner in children with 80% cases are under 10yrs of age. The main causative organisms are *Staphylococci* and *Streptococci* sp. It is generally a much less severe disease, at least in adults and older children.

Risk factors
- Infection of adjacent structures (dacryocystitis, hordeolum) or systemic (e.g. upper respiratory tract infection).
- *Trauma*: laceration.

Clinical features
- Fever, malaise, painful, swollen lid/periorbita.
- Inflamed lids but no proptosis, normal eye movements, white conjunctiva, normal optic nerve function.

Investigation
Investigation is not usually necessary unless there is concern over possible orbital or sinus involvement.

Treatment
- Daily review until resolution (admit young/unwell children, see Paediatric ophthalmology: Orbital and Preseptal cellulitis 📖 p.526).
- Treat with oral antibiotics (e.g. flucloxacillin 500mg 4×/d for 1wk ± metronidazole 400mg 3×/d for 1wk).

Table 14.3 Orbital vs preseptal cellulitis

	Orbital	Preseptal
Proptosis	Present	Absent
Ocular motility	Painful + restricted	Normal
VA	↓ (in severe cases)	Normal
Colour vision	↓ (in severe cases)	Normal
RAPD	Present (in severe cases)	Absent (i.e. normal)

1. McKinley SH *et al*. Microbiology of pediatric orbital cellulitis. *Am J Ophthalmol* 2007;**144**:497–501.

Mucormycosis (phycomycosis)

This is a rare very aggressive life-threatening fungal infection caused by *Mucor* species or *Rhizopus*. It is a disease of the immunosuppressed, most commonly seen in patients who are also acidotic, such as in diabetic ketoacidosis or renal failure. However, it also occurs in the elderly, malignancy and therapeutic immunosuppression. It represents fungal septic necrosis and infarction of tissues of nasopharynx and orbit.

Clinical features
- Black crusty material in nasopharynx, acute evolving cranial nerve palsies (IIIn, IVn, Vn, VIn, IIn) ± obvious orbital inflammation.

Investigation
- Biopsy: fungal stains show non-septate branching hyphae.
- FBC, U+E, Glu.

Treatment
- Admit and co-ordinate care with microbiologist/infectious disease specialist, ENT specialist, ± physician.
- Correct underlying disease (e.g. diabetic ketoacidosis) where possible; without this the prognosis is extremely poor.
- IV antifungals (as guided by microbiology; e.g. liposomal amphotericin).
- Early and aggressive surgical debridement by ENT specialist ± orbital exenteration (for severe/unresponsive disease).

Thyroid eye disease: general

Thyroid eye disease (TED; *syn* thyroid-associated ophthalmopathy, Graves' ophthalmopathy, dysthyroid eye disease) is an organ-specific autoimmune disease that may be both sight-threatening and disfiguring. Acute progressive disease is an ophthalmic emergency as it may threaten the optic nerve and cornea.

While most patients with TED have clinical and/or biochemical evidence of hyperthyroidism or hypothyroidism, some are euthyroid—at least at the time of presentation. Thyroid dysfunction may precede, be coincident with, or follow TED. Incidence is about 10/100 000/yr. About 40% of patients with Graves' disease develop TED, with the majority having mild features. In a small percentage (4–8%) of patients the orbital inflammation may be very severe and lead to loss of vision and even blindness, if not treated promptly.

Risk factors
- Female sex (F:M 4:1).
- Middle age.
- HLA-DR3, HLA-B8, and the genes for CTLA4 and the TSH receptor.
- Smoking.
- Autoimmune thyroid disease.

Autoimmune thyroid disease
TED is most commonly associated with Graves' disease, but may occur in 3% of Hashimoto's thyroiditis.

Graves' disease
This is the commonest cause of hyperthyroidism. Anti-TSH receptor antibodies cause overproduction of thyroxine (T4) and/or T3.

Classic features include hyperthyroidism, goitre, TED, thyroid acropathy (clubbing), and pretibial myxoedema.

Autoimmune thyroiditis (e.g. Hashimoto's thyroiditis)
This is the commonest cause of hypothyroidism. It may have a transient hyperthyroid stage, before leaving the patient hypothyroid. The associated goitre is usually firm.

Pathogenesis of thyroid eye disease
The cause is unclear. It is probable that the target antigen is shared between the extraocular muscles and the thyroid gland. Activated T cells probably act upon cells of the fibroblast–adipocyte lineage within the orbit; therefore, stimulating adipogenesis, fibroblast proliferation, and glycosaminoglycan synthesis.

Clinical features

Ophthalmic
- Ocular irritation, ache (worse in mornings), red eyes, pain on eye movement, cosmetic changes, diplopia.
- Proptosis (exophthalmos), lid retraction (upper > lower), lid lag (on downgaze), conjunctival and caruncular injection/chemosis, orbital fat prolapse, keratopathy (exposure/superior limbic/keratoconjunctivitis sicca), restrictive myopathy, optic neuropathy.

Table 14.4 Emergencies in thyroid eye disease

Acute progressive optic neuropathy

Optic neuropathy in TED may arise due to compression of the nerve by involved tissues (mainly muscles) or by proptosis-induced stretch

Assess: optic nerve function (VA, colour, visual fields, pupillary reactions).

Treatment

Systemic immunosuppression (liaise with endocrinologist). This is may be oral corticosteroids (e.g. 1mg/kg 1×/d PO prednisolone) or 'pulsed' (e.g. 500mg IV methylprednisolone 1×/d for the first 3d); other immunosuppressives may be added for additional control and as steroid-sparing agents

If this fails then urgent surgical decompression is required. This varies in extent but must decompress the orbital apex where compression is often maximal.

Exposure keratopathy

Exposure keratopathy in TED may arise due to proptosis and lid retraction

Assess: corneal integrity, tear film, lid closure, proptosis

Treatment: lubricants, taping/Frost suture, acute immunosuppression (e.g. systemic corticosteroids) ± orbital decompression.

Systemic

- Systemic signs depend on the thyroid status (over/underactivity) and underlying disease (goitre in Grave's or Hashimoto's; pretibial myxoedema, thyroid acropachy in Grave's).
- There is an increased frequency of other autoimmune diseases, e.g. myasthenia gravis, pernicious anaemia, vitiligo, diabetes mellitus, Addison's disease, etc.

Table 14.5 Common systemic features of thyroid dysfunction

	Hyperthyroidism	Hypothyroidism
Symptoms	Weight loss	Weight gain
	Heat intolerance	Cold intolerance
	Restlessness	Fatigue
	Diarrhoea	Constipation
	Poor libido	Poor libido
	Amenorrhoea	Menorrhagia
	Poor concentration	Poor memory
	Irritability	Depression
Signs	Warm peripheries	Dry coarse skin
	Hair loss	Dry thin hair
	Tachycardia	Bradycardia
	Atrial fibrillation	Pericardial/pleural effusions
	Proximal myopathy	Muscle cramps
	Tremor	Slow relaxing reflexes
	Osteoporosis	Deafness

Thyroid eye disease: assessment

The diagnosis and management of TED depends on accurate clinical assessment. Grading systems aim to formalize this process but generally are not a substitute for careful clinical documentation of disease status (severity and activity). Similarly, while investigations may support a diagnosis of TED they are not diagnostic in their own right.

Rundle's curve

The natural history of TED can be described in terms of an active phase of increasing severity, a regression phase of declining severity, and an inactive plateau phase (Rundle's curve). While specific to each patient these time-courses can be plotted graphically and broadly categorized according to mild, moderate, marked, or severe disease (Rundle a–d).

Assessment of disease severity

Grading systems that attempt to document severity include the NOSPECS classification (Table 14.6). This is now little used by ophthalmologists who generally wish to document disease activity/inflammation in greater detail. It is still widely used by general physicians and endocrinologists.

Table 14.6 NOSPECS disease severity score

0	N	No signs or symptoms
1	O	Only signs, no symptoms
2	S	Soft tissue involvement
3	P	Proptosis
4	E	Extraocular muscle involvement
5	C	Corneal involvement
6	S	Sight loss (↓VA)

On Werner's modified NOSPECS categories II–VI can be further graded as o, a, b, or c (e.g. degree of visual loss for category VI).

Werner SC. Modification of the classification of the eye changes of Graves' disease. *J Clin Endocrinol Metab* 1977;**44**:203–4.

Assessment of disease activity

The most widely used score of clinical activity is the *Mourits* system (Table 14.7) although a standardized protocol based on comparison with clinical photographs has also been devised.

Table 14.7 Mourits et al. clinical activity score (CAS)[1]

Pain	Painful, oppressive feeling on or behind globe	+1
	Pain on eye movement	+1
Redness	Eyelid redness	+1
	Conjunctival redness	+1
Swelling	Swelling of lids	+1
	Chemosis	+1
	Swelling of caruncle	+1
	Increasing proptosis (≥2mm in 1–3mths)	+1
Impaired function	Decreasing eye movement (≥5° in 1–3mths)	+1
	Decreasing vision (≥1 line pinhole VA on Snellen chart in 1–3mths)	+1
Total		/10

1. Mourits MP et al. Clinical criteria for the assessment of disease activity in Graves' ophthalmopathy Br J Ophthalmol 1989;**73**:639–44. Reproduced with permission from BMJ Publishing Group.

Investigation

- *Thyroid function tests* (Table 14.8): usually TSH and free T4, but check free T3 (the active metabolite) if strong clinical suspicion but otherwise normal biochemistry.
- *Thyroid autoantibodies*: anti-TSH receptor, anti-thyroid peroxidase, and anti-thyroglobulin antibodies.
- *Orbital imaging*: CT orbits gives better bony resolution and is preferred for planning decompression; MRI (T2-weighted and STIR) gives better soft tissue resolution and identifies active disease; the bellies of the muscles show enlargement and inflammation, but the tendons are spared.
- *Orthoptic review*: may include field of binocular single vision, field of uniocular fixation, Hess/Lees chart, visual fields.

Table 14.8 Biochemical investigations in thyroid eye disease

Thyroid function tests	Hyperthyroid	Hypothyroid
TSH	↓	↑
Free T4	↑	↓

In subclinical hyper- or hypothyroidism, free T4 will be normal but the TSH will still be ↓ or ↑ respectively.

Table 14.9 Immunological investigations in thyroid eye disease

Autoantibody	Association	
Anti-TSH receptor	>95% Grave's disease	
	40–95% TED	
Anti-thyroid peroxidase	80% Grave's disease	90% Hashimoto's thyroiditis
Anti-thyroglobulin	25% Grave's disease	55% Hashimoto's thyroiditis

Thyroid eye disease: management

Treatment of eye disease

General

- *Multidisciplinary* input from endocrinologist and orthoptist. Meticulous control of thyroid function is associated with reduced severity of TED.
- *Supportive*: counselling, ocular lubricants, tinted glasses, bed-head elevation, prisms for diplopia, support group.

Medical

- Consider immunosuppression in active disease (Clinical Activity Score >3, see ☐ Table 14.7). Early aggressive treatment in the active phase can prevent much of the morbidity associated with TED.
- Treatment is usually with systemic corticosteroids but ciclosporin, methotrexate, azathioprine, and newer agents, such as infliximab (anti-TNF) have all been used.[1]
- Radiotherapy is popular in some centres; it may transiently worsen disease.

Surgical

- *For acute disease*: acute progressive optic neuropathy or corneal exposure may require emergency orbital decompression.
- *For burnt-out disease*. Surgery (usually staged) may improve function and cosmesis. Decompression, motility, or lid surgery are performed as required, and in that order. Decompression can be 1-, 2-, or 3-wall, and by a variety of approaches (e.g. endoscopic, swinging lower-lid flap, etc.) to hide scars.

Prognosis

- A self-limiting disease that usually resolves within 1–5yrs.
- Once stable, dramatic improvements in ocular motility and appearance can be achieved with a staged surgical approach.
- Good long-term vision, however, depends on successfully guarding against sight-threatening complications in the acute phase.

Box 14.1 Poor prognostic factors in TED

- Older age of onset
- Male
- Smoker
- Diabetes
- ↓VA
- Rapid progression at onset
- Longer duration of active disease

Treatment of hyperthyroidism

Carbimazole and propylthiouracil

Carbimazole or propylthiouracil are used to block the production of thyroid hormones. The initial dose (15–40mg for carbimazole; 200–400mg for propylthiouracil) is continued until the patient is euthyroid and then gradually reduced while maintaining normal free T4 levels. Therapy is generally required for 12–18mths.

An alternative regimen is blocking-replacement where higher doses of carbimazole are given simultaneously with thyroxine replacement.

Patients should be warned of the risk of agranulocytosis and to seek medical review (including an FBC) if they develop infections, particularly sore throat.

Radioactive iodine

- A single dose of radioactive sodium iodide (^{131}I) is given. The patient must avoid close contact with others, particularly children, for a period after administration. Subsequent hypothyroidism is common and requires thyroxine replacement.
- There is controversy over the possibility that radioactive iodine worsens TED (or whether this is related to a subsequent hypothyroid dip); it is common practice to give 'prophylactic' oral steroids when administering radioactive iodine in this situation.

Surgical (ablation/thyroidectomy)

This is relatively uncommon but may be used for large goitres; it may be preceded by radioactive iodine to shrink the goitre.

In pregnancy and breast-feeding

- Carbimazole and propylthiouracil cross the placenta and can cause foetal hypothyroidism. Consequently, the lowest dose possible should be used and the blocking-replacement regimen avoided.
- Radioactive iodine is contraindicated in pregnancy.

Treatment of hypothyroidism

Levothyroxine

- Thyroxine replacement is started at a dose of 25–100mcg (50mcg if >50yrs of age; 25mcg if cardiac disease or elderly) and cautiously increased at intervals of 4wks to a maintenance dose of 100–200mcg.
- Treatment is monitored against thyroid function tests (aim to normalize but not suppress TSH) and clinical status.
- Rapid increases or excessive doses may result in angina, arrhythmias, and features of hyperthyroidism.

1. Durrani OM et al. Infliximab, a novel treatment for sight threatening thyroid-associated ophthalmopathy (TAO). *Orbit* 2005;**24**:117–19.

Other orbital inflammations (1)

A number of inflammatory diseases may affect the orbit. These may be purely orbital or related to systemic disease (e.g. TED). The purely orbital diseases may be diffuse (e.g. idiopathic orbital inflammatory disease) or focal (e.g. myositis).

The classification of orbital inflammations is continuing to evolve as our understanding of immunogenetic and clinical features of orbital diseases improves (Table 14.10).

Table 14.10 Inflammatory diseases affecting the orbit (selected)

Isolated	Diffuse	Idiopathic orbital inflammatory disease
		Idiopathic sclerosing inflammation of the orbit
	Focal	Myositis
		Dacryoadenitis
		Tolosa–Hunt syndrome
Systemic		Thyroid eye disease
		Wegener's granulomatosis
		Sarcoidosis

Idiopathic orbital inflammatory disease

This is an uncommon chronic inflammatory process of unknown aetiology. The pattern of inflammation may be predominantly anterior orbit (more common type) or diffuse. It may simulate a neoplastic mass (hence the former term *pseudotumour*) but histology shows a pure inflammatory response with no cellular atypia.

It is a diagnosis of exclusion (Box 14.2), and may in fact represent a number of poorly understood entities. It may occur at almost any age. It is usually unilateral.

Clinical features
- Acute pain, redness, lid swelling, diplopia.
- Conjunctival injection, chemosis, lid oedema, proptosis, restrictive myopathy, orbital mass.

Investigation
- *Orbital imaging*: B-scan (low-medium reflectivity, acoustic homogeneity); MRI (hypointense cf. muscle on T1, hyperintense cf. muscle on T2, moderate enhancement with gadolinium).
- *Biopsy*: required to confirm diagnosis.

Box 14.2 Differential diagnosis of idiopathic orbital inflammatory disease

Orbital cellulitis
Thyroid eye disease
Wegener's granulomatosis
Haemorrhage within a vascular lesion
Rhabdomyosarcoma
Metastatic neuroblastoma
Leukaemic infiltration

Treatment

Immunosuppression: usually systemic corticosteroids, although cytotoxics (e.g. cyclophosphamide) and radiotherapy are sometimes used.

Idiopathic sclerosing inflammation of the orbit

This is a rare relentlessly progressive idiopathic fibrosis akin to retroperitoneal fibrosis.

There is no known cause, no effective treatment, and visual deterioration is common. Differential diagnosis include TED, sarcoid, Wegener's granulomatosus, TB, and malignancy (primary and secondary).

Other orbital inflammations (2)

Myositis

In myositis the inflammatory process is restricted to one or more extraocular muscles, most commonly the superior or lateral rectus. It may occur at almost any age. It is usually unilateral.

Clinical features

Acute pain (especially on movement in the direction of the involved muscle), injection over muscle ± mild proptosis.

Investigations

Orbital imaging: may be diagnosed on CT scan, although MRI gives better soft tissue resolution; the whole of the muscle and tendon shows enlargement and inflammation (cf. TED).

Treatment

- *Immunosuppression*: normally very sensitive to systemic corticosteroids.
- A biopsy will be required if poor response to treatment/persistent symptoms.

Tolosa–Hunt syndrome

- A rare condition; there is focal inflammation of the superior orbital fissure ± orbital apex.
- Presents with orbital pain, multiple cranial nerve palsies, and sometimes proptosis.
- It must be differentiated from other causes of the superior orbital fissure syndrome: carotid–cavernous fistula, cavernous sinus thrombosis, Wegener's granulomatosis, pituitary apoplexy, sarcoidosis, mucormycosis, and other infections.
- It is very sensitive to steroids.

Dacryoadenitis

- Lacrimal gland inflammation may be isolated or occur as part of diffuse idiopathic orbital inflammatory disease.
- Presents with an acutely painful swollen lacrimal gland that is tender to palpation, has reduced tear production and results in a S-shaped deformity to the lid.
- It must be differentiated from infection, tumours of the lacrimal gland and a ruptured dermoid cyst.
- Isolated dacryoadenitis responds well to oral NSAIDS (fluroiprofen 100mg 3x/d.) or oral corticosteroids.
- Complete resolution may take up to 3mths.
- A biopsy is indicated if the inflammation persists.

Wegener's granulomatosis

This is an uncommon necrotizing granulomatous vasculitis that may have ophthalmic involvement in up to 50% of cases and orbital involvement in up to 22%. It is commonest in males (M:F 2:1) and in middle age.

Clinical features

Ophthalmic
- *Orbital disease*: pain, proptosis, restrictive myopathy, disc swelling, and ↓VA.
- *Other ocular disease*: epi/scleritis, peripheral ulcerative keratitis, uveitis, and vasculitis.

Systemic
Pneumonitis, glomerulonephritis, sinusitis, and nasopharyngeal ulceration.

Investigation
- *ANCA*: most cases are c-ANCA positive.
- *CT scan*: obliteration of orbital fat planes by a plaque-like infiltrative mass. Erosion and destruction of sinus and nasal bones.

Treatment
Treatment (co-ordinated by rheumatologist/physician) is usually combined corticosteroids and cyclophosphamide.

Cystic lesions

Dacryops (lacrimal ductal cyst)

These cysts of the lacrimal duct tissue are relatively common, and may arise from any lacrimal tissue (including the accessory lacrimal glands of Krause and Wolfring). Dacryops are often bilateral and protrude into the superior fornix.

Treatment if required is by aspiration.

Dermoid cyst

Dermoids are a type of choristoma (congenital tumours of tissues abnormal to that location). They probably represent surface ectoderm trapped at lines of embryonic closure and suture lines. They are most commonly located on the superotemporal orbital rim, but may extend deceptively far posteriorly. They comprise stratified squamous epithelium (with epidermal structures such as hair follicles and sebaceous glands) surrounding a cavity that may contain keratin and hair.

Clinical features

Superficial dermoids
- Present in infancy.
- Slowly growing firm smooth round non-tender mass.

Deep dermoids
- Present from childhood onwards.
- Gradual proptosis, motility disturbance, ↓VA.
- May extend beyond the orbit into the frontal sinus, temporal fossa, or cranium.

Investigation

Orbital imaging: CT shows well-circumscribed lesion with heterogeneous centre; B-scan US shows well-defined lesion with high internal reflectivity.

Treatment

- They should be excised completely without rupture of the capsule to avoid severe inflammation and recurrence.
- Intracranial spread of deep dermoid cysts requires co-ordination with neurosurgeons.

Mucocele

A mucocele is a slowly expanding collection of secretions due to blockage of the sinus opening. This may be due to a congenital narrowing or arise secondary to infection, inflammation, tumour, or trauma. Over time erosion of the sinus walls permits the mucocele to encroach into the orbit. Orbit-involving mucoceles usually arise from frontal, ethmoidal, or occasionally the maxillary sinus.

Clinical features

Headache, gradual non-axial proptosis or horizontal displacement, fluctuant tender mass in medial or superomedial orbit.

Investigation
Orbital imaging: CT shows opacification of frontal or ethmoidal sinus (+ loss of ethmoidal septae) with a bony defect allowing intraorbital protrusion; B-scan US shows a well-defined lesion with low internal reflectivity.

Treatment
Referral to ENT specialist to excise the mucocele, restore sinus drainage, or obliterate the sinus cavity (in recurrent cases).

Cephalocele

These are developmental malformations resulting in herniation into the orbit of brain (encephalocele), meninges (meningocele), or both (meningoencephalocele). They may be anterior (fronto-ethmoidal bony defects) or posterior (sphenoid dysplasia). Encephaloceles may be associated with other craniofacial or ocular abnormalities; posterior encephaloceles may be associated with neurofibromatosis-1 and morning glory syndrome.

Clinical features
- *Pulsatile proptosis*, which may increase with Valsalva manoeuvre but without a bruit (cf. arteriovenous fistulae).
- *Anterior lesions*: the encephalocele may be visible and proptosis is usually anterotemporal.
- *Posterior lesions*: the encephalocele is not visible and the proptosis is usually antero-inferior.

Investigation
Orbital imaging: CT shows a defect in the orbital wall.

Orbital tumours: lacrimal and neural

Lacrimal gland

Pleomorphic adenoma

The commonest lacrimal neoplasm, and accounts for up to 20% of all lacrimal fossa lesions. They are derived from epithelial and mesenchymal tissue, hence the term benign mixed cell tumour. They may arise from either lobe, most commonly the orbital.

They occur in middle age with a slight male bias (M:F 1.5:1). Malignant transformation occurs in less than 3% in 10yrs and between 10 and 20% in 20yrs.

Clinical features

Gradual painless proptosis (inferonasal), upper lid swelling, choroidal folds, diplopia, palpable mass of the superomedial orbit (orbital lobe tumours may not be palpable).

Investigation

- *US*: round lesion with medium/high reflectivity and regular acoustic structure.
- *CT/MRI*: the classic features of a pleomorphic adenoma are best seen on a CT scan, which shows expansion of the lacrimal fossa, indentations of the globe, and a well circumscribed slightly nodular tumour with calcification present in 30%.

Treatment

- Surgical removal of whole tumour with intact pseudo-capsule without prior biopsy (risk of seeding). This is usually by an anterior (palpebral lobe tumours) or lateral (orbital lobe tumours) orbitotomy.
- Prognosis is excellent with complete excision.

Lacrimal carcinomas

Commonest malignant tumour of the lacrimal gland is the adenoid cystic carcinoma, followed by the mucoepidermoid carcinoma and the pleo-morphic adenocarcinoma. They occur at a similar age to adenomas but cause more rapid proptosis and ophthalmoparesis, and orbital pain from perineural spread is common.

- Imaging shows an irregular poorly defined lesion with bony destruction.
- *Treatment*: seldom curative but consists of exenteration ± radiotherapy.
- Prognosis is very poor.

Neural

Optic nerve glioma

An uncommon slow-growing tumour of astrocytes that usually occurs in children and has a strong association to neurofibromatosis-1.

- Usually present with gradual ↓VA (although this often stabilizes), disc swelling or atrophy, and proptosis.
- Isolated optic nerve involvement occurs in 22%, but most involve the chiasm (72%), often with midbrain and hypothalamic involvement.
- Imaging shows fusiform enlargement of the optic nerve ± chiasmal mass.

- Observation is recommended for patients with isolated optic nerve involvement distant from the chiasm, good vision, and non-disfiguring proptosis.
- Progress is monitored with serial MRI scans.
- Surgical excision is indicated for pain, severe proptosis, or posterior spread threatening the chiasm.
- Chiasmal or midbrain involvement may be an indication for chemotherapy or radiotherapy.
- Prognosis for life is good for optic nerve-restricted tumours but worsens with more posterior involvement.

Optic nerve sheath meningioma

A rare benign tumour of meningothelial cells of the meninges that usually occurs in middle-age and has a slight female bias (F:M 1.5:1). There is an association with neurofibromatosis-2.

- Usually present with gradual ↓VA, disc swelling or atrophy, optociliary shunt vessels (30%), proptosis, and ophthalmoparesis.
- Imaging shows tubular enlargement of the nerve with 'tram-track' enhancement of the sheath ± calcification.
- Observation is recommended if VA is good.
- Surgical excision is indicated for blind eyes, severe proptosis, or threat to the chiasm.
- Prognosis for life is good.

Neurofibroma

Neurofibromas are uncommon benign tumours of peripheral nerves.

- *Plexiform neurofibroma:* presents in childhood and is strongly associated with neurofibromatosis-1. Anterior involvement results in a 'bag-of-worms' mass causing an S-shaped lid deformity. The tumour is poorly defined and not encapsulated. Surgical excision is difficult, and may require repeated debulking.
- *Isolated neurofibroma:* presents in adulthood with gradual proptosis. The tumour is well-circumscribed and surgical excision is usually straight-forward.

Schwannoma

Uncommon slow-growing tumours of peripheral or cranial nerves that are usually benign but may be malignant.

- Usually present in adulthood.
- There is an association with neurofibromatosis.
- It is usually located in the superior orbit and presents as a gradually enlarging non-tender mass (often cystic), with proptosis, ↓VA, and restricted motility.
- Treatment is with complete surgical excision with good prognosis.

Orbital tumours: vascular

Cavernous haemangioma

This is the commonest benign orbital neoplasm of adults. It is a hamartoma but does not usually present until young adulthood, most notably during pregnancy (accelerated growth). It is usually intraconal.

Clinical features

Proptosis (usually axial due to intraconal location); later restricted motility, choroidal folds, and ↓VA.

Investigation

- *US*: well-circumscribed intraconal lesion with high internal reflectivity.
- *CT/MRI*: well-circumscribed intraconal lesion with mild/moderate enhancement.

Treatment

Most may be observed but symptomatic lesions should be completely excised.

Capillary haemangioma

This is a type of hamartoma (congenital tumours of tissues normal to that location). Very large tumours may be consumptive (Kasabach–Merritt syndrome: ↓plt, ↓Hb, ↓clotting factors) or cause high-output cardiac failure.

Superficial lesions ('strawberry naevus')

- Bright red tumours that usually appear before 2mths of age, reach full size by 1yr, and involute by 6yrs.
- May be disfiguring and/or may cause amblyopia by obscuration of the visual axis or associated astigmatism. In these cases treatment (usually intralesional or systemic corticosteroids) may be indicated.

Deep lesions

- May not be visible but cause variable proptosis (worsens with Valsalva manoeuvre/crying).
- With time, partial involution occurs in most of these lesions but large tumours may be treated (corticosteroids or radiotherapy).

Lymphangioma

This is a rare hamartoma of lymph vessels that usually presents in childhood. They increase in size with head-down posture and the Valsalva manoeuvre.

Superficial lesions are visible as cystic spaces of the lid or conjunctiva that may also contain blood. Deep lesions may cause gradual proptosis or present acutely with orbital pain and ↓VA due to haemorrhage ('chocolate cyst'). Most lesions are observed.

If a sight-threatening bleed occurs they may be drained but surgery is difficult.

Orbital tumours: lymphoproliferative

Orbital lymphoid diseases range from benign hyperplasia to malignant lymphomas, the latter being solid tumours that arise from malignant transformation of leucocytes, particularly B lymphocytes (about 85%).

Lymphoproliferative tumours are now classified according to the World Health Organization (WHO) consensus classification system.[1]

Benign reactive lymphoid hyperplasia

An uncommon polyclonal proliferation of lymphoid tissue that usually occurs in the superolateral orbit, often involving the lacrimal gland. It may present with gradual proptosis and/or a palpable firm rubbery mass.

It usually responds to corticosteroids or radiotherapy, although some cases require cytotoxics. Progression to lymphoma occurs in up to 25% by 5yrs.

Atypical lymphoid hyperplasia

This is intermediate between benign reactive hyperplasia and lymphoma, and is characterized by a very homogeneous pattern with larger nuclei.

Malignant orbital lymphoma

An uncommon low-grade proliferation of B cells (non-Hodgkin's type) usually arising in the elderly. The most common subtype is the marginal zone B-cell lymphoma of the mucosa-associated lymphoid tissue (MALT), which accounts for 40–70% of all orbital lymphomas.

About half of orbital B-cell lymphomas are primary tumours (arising solely within orbital structures).[2]

Usually presents with gradual proptosis and/or a palpable firm rubbery mass. Usually unilateral, but bilateral involvement occurs in 25%; systemic involvement is present in up to 40% at diagnosis and in up to 60% within 5yrs.[2,3]

Treatment (radiotherapy or chemotherapy) depends on grade and spread of tumour; a systemic work-up is necessary in all cases.

Langerhans cell histiocytosis

This is a rare proliferative disorder of childhood. It comprises a spectrum of disease from the unifocal, relatively benign eosinophilic granuloma to the disseminated Letterer–Siwe form.

In eosinophilic granuloma orbital involvement is common and presents as rapid proptosis with a superotemporal swelling. Bilateral proptosis may occur in disseminated Langerhans cell histiocytosis.

Surgical excision is usually curative.

1. Jaffe ES et al. WHO classification of tumours—pathology and genetics of tumours of haematopoietic and lymphoid tissues. Lyon: IARC Press, 2001.

2. Coupland SE et al. Lymphoproliferative lesions of the ocular adnexa. Analysis of 112 cases. Ophthalmology 1998;**105**:1430–41.

3. Demirci H et al. Orbital lymphoproliferative tumors analysis of clinical features and systemic involvement in 160 cases. Ophthalmology 2008; **115**: 1626–31.

Orbital tumours: other

Rhabdomyosarcoma

This is the commonest primary orbital malignancy in children. It usually arises in the first decade and has a slight male bias (M:F 1.6:1).

It arises from pluripotent mesenchymal tissue. Histologically, it may be differentiated into embryonal (commonest), alveolar, and pleomorphic types. It is usually intraconal (50%) or within the superior orbit (25%).

Clinical features
Acute/subacute proptosis, ptosis, and orbital inflammation; it may therefore mimic inflammatory conditions such as orbital cellulitis.

Investigation
- *B-scan US*: irregular but well-defined edges, low/medium reflectivity. Colour Doppler shows very high internal flow.
- *CT/MRI*: irregular but well-defined mass ± bony erosion.

Treatment
- A biopsy (to confirm diagnosis) and systemic work-up (to establish spread) is necessary in all cases.
- Surgical excision is possible for well-circumscribed localized tumours.
- Combined radiotherapy and chemotherapy is given for more extensive tumours.

Fibrous histiocytoma

This is an uncommon tumour that may affect middle-aged adults or children who have had orbital radiotherapy. It may be benign or malignant and is usually located superonasally.

It presents with gradual proptosis, ↓VA, and restricted motility. Treatment is by surgical excision, but recurrences are common.

Metastases

Orbital metastases (Table 14.11) are uncommon. In about half of all cases, they precede the diagnosis of the underlying tumour.

Usually present aggressively with fairly rapid proptosis, restricted motility, cranial nerve involvement, and orbital inflammation. Scirrhous tumours (e.g. some breast and gastric tumours) may cause enophthalmos.

Table 14.11 Primary tumours metastasizing to the orbit

Adults	Children
Breast	Neuroblastoma
Lung	Nephroblastoma
Prostate	Ewing sarcoma
Gastrointestinal	

Vascular lesions

Orbital varices

These are congenital venous enlargements that may present from childhood onwards. They are usually unilateral and located in the medial orbit.

Clinical features
- Intermittent proptosis and/or visible varix (worse with increased venous pressure, i.e. Valsalva manoeuvre and in head-down position).
- Occasional thrombosis or haemorrhage.

Treatment
Surgery is difficult, but is indicated if severe or sight-threatening. Incomplete excision is common.

Arteriovenous fistula

These are abnormal anastamoses between the arterial and venous circulation. The *carotid–cavernous fistula* is a high-flow system arising from direct communication between the intracavernous internal carotid artery and the cavernous sinus. The *dural shunt* (also known as indirect carotid–cavernous fistula) is a low-flow system arising from dural arteries (branches of the internal and external carotid arteries) communicating with the cavernous sinus.

Arteriovenous fistulae may be congenital (e.g. Wyburn–Mason syndrome), secondary to trauma (particularly in young adults), or occur spontaneously (most cases in older people).

Clinical features
Carotid–cavernous fistula (direct)
- ↓VA, diplopia, audible bruit.
- Pulsatile proptosis with a bruit, orbital oedema, injected chemotic conjunctiva, ↑IOP, variable ophthalmoparesis (usually VI and III), retinal vein engorgement, RAPD, disc swelling, anterior segment ischaemia.

Dural shunt (indirect carotid–cavernous fistula)
- May be asymptomatic; pain, cosmesis.
- Chemosis, episcleral venous engorgement, ↑IOP.

Investigation
Orbital imaging: B-scan US, CT, MRI show a dilated superior ophthalmic vein and mild thickening of the extraocular muscles.

Treatment
- High-flow carotid–cavernous fistulae may cause visual loss in up to 50% cases and require closure by catheter embolization.
- Low-flow dural shunts spontaneously close by thrombosis in up to 40% cases. Intervention is reserved for cases with glaucoma, ↓VA, diplopia, or severe pain.

Intraocular tumours

Iris tumours

Uveal melanoma

Uveal melanoma is the commonest primary malignant intraocular tumour of Caucasian adults, with a lifetime incidence of about 0.05%. Risk factors include race (light >> dark pigmentation), age (old > young), UV light exposure (possible risk factor), and underlying disorders such as ocular melanocytosis and dysplastic naevus syndrome. It is slightly more common in men than women. Tumours arise from neuroectodermal melanocytes of the choroid, ciliary body, or iris.

Iris melanoma

Compared with the other uveal melanomas, iris tumours are less common (8% of all uveal tumours), present younger (age 40–50yrs), and have a better prognosis. They are more common in females. Histologically, they usually comprise spindle cells alone or spindle cells with benign naevus cells.

Clinical features
- Usually asymptomatic; patient may note a spot or diffuse colour change.
- Iris nodule: most commonly light to dark brown, well-circumscribed, usually inferior iris; may be associated with hyphaema, ↓IOP (tumour or pigment cell blockage of trabecular meshwork), cataract; transpupillary or transcleral illumination may help demarcate posterior extension.

Risk factors for malignancy
Size (>3mm diameter, >1mm thickness), rapid growth, prominent intrinsic vascularity, pigment dispersion, ↑IOP, pupillary peaking, ectropion uveae, iris splinting (uneven dilation).

Investigations
- *Anterior segment US*: assess ciliary body involvement.
- *Biopsy*: consider FNA (simple, safe, but scanty sample with no architecture) or incisional biopsy (corneal/limbal wound, risk of hyphaema).

Treatment
Specialist advice should be sought. Options include:
- *Observation*: in small asymptomatic tumours with no convincing growth intervention may not be necessary.
- *Excision*: consider iridectomy/iridocyclectomy ± cosmetic contact lens (artificial pupil).
- *Radiotherapy*: proton beam radiotherapy.
- *Enucleation*: rarely indicated (non-resectable, extensive aqueous seeding or painful, blind eye).

Prognosis
- Most patients do well and rarely (1–2%) develop metastatic disease.
- Poor prognostic features include large size, ciliary body, or extrascleral extension, and diffuse or annular growth pattern.

Table 15.1 Differential diagnosis of iris mass

Pigmented	Iris melanoma
	Naevus
	ICE syndrome
	Adenoma
	Ciliary body tumours
Non-pigmented	Iris melanoma
	Iris cyst
	Iris granulomas
	IOFB
	Juvenile xanthogranuloma
	Leiomyoma
	Ciliary body tumours
	Iris metastasis

Iris naevus

These common lesions do not require regular ophthalmic observation unless there are suspicious features. Patients will usually detect any worrying change in a lesion themselves.

Clinical features

- Usually asymptomatic; patient may note a spot on the iris.
- Small (<3mm diameter, <0.5mm thick) defined pigmented stromal lesion; pupillary peaking or ectropion uveae occasionally occur in naevi but are suspicious features.

Box 15.1 Suspicious features in an iris naevus

- Size (>3mm diameter, >1mm thickness)
- Rapid growth
- Prominent intrinsic vascularity
- Pigment dispersion
- ↑IOP
- Iris splinting (uneven dilation)
- Pupillary peaking
- Ectropion uveae

Iris metastases

These are typically amelanotic solid tumours that may cause complications such as secondary open angle glaucoma (clogging or infiltration of trabecular meshwork with tumour cells), hyphaema, and pseudohypopyon.

In most cases patients are already known to have a malignancy elsewhere, but in some patients the iris lesion is the presenting feature and requires extensive workup with an oncologist.

Ciliary body tumours

Ciliary body melanoma

These account for about 12% of all uveal melanomas. They most commonly present at about 50–60yrs. In contrast to iris melanomas they usually contain the more anaplastic epithelioid melanoma cells and carry a worse prognosis.

Clinical features
- Usually asymptomatic; occasionally visual symptoms.
- Ciliary body mass (may only be visible with full dilation); dilated episcleral sentinel vessels; anterior extension on to the iris or globe; lens subluxation or secondary cataract; anterior uveitis.

Investigation
- *US* (ocular/anterior segment): size, extension, composition.
- *Biopsy*: consider FNA.

Treatment
Specialist advice should be sought. Options include:
- *Excision*: may be possible for smaller lesions.
- *Radiotherapy*: brachytherapy or proton beam.
- *Enucleation*: for larger lesions or significant extension.

Table 15.2 Differential diagnosis of ciliary body mass

Pigmented	Ciliary body melanoma
	Metastases
	Ciliary body adenoma
Non-pigmented	Ciliary body melanoma
	Ciliary body cyst
	Uveal effusion syndrome
	Medulloepithelioma
	Leiomyoma
	Metastases

Medulloepithelioma

This is a rare slow-growing tumour derived from immature epithelial cells of the embryonic optic cup. It usually arises from the non-pigmented ciliary epithelium, but iris and retinal sites are occasionally seen. They may be benign (1/3) or malignant (2/3), and teratoid (e.g. containing cartilage, brain, bone) or non-teratoid.

Overall, invasion is common but metastasis is rare. Age of onset ranges from congenital to adult, but is usually under the age of 10; both sexes are equally affected.

Clinical features
- Red eye, ↓VA, iris colour change/mass.
- Injection, ciliary body mass (amelanotic, often cystic).
- *Complications*: neovascular glaucoma, lens coloboma/subluxation/ cataract.

Investigation and treatment

Diagnosis may be assisted by US. Iridocyclectomy may be curative for small, well-defined, benign tumours; for most others, enucleation is still required.

Choroidal melanoma

Choroidal melanomas account for 80% of all uveal melanoma. They usually present at about 50–60yrs of age.

They are classified according to size: small (<10mm diameter), medium (10–15mm diameter), and large (>15mm diameter). Histologically, they may comprise spindle cells (types A and B), epithelioid cells, or a mixture (commonest type). Necrosis may prevent cell typing in 5%.

Clinical features

- Often asymptomatic; ↓VA, field loss, 'ball of light' slowly moving across vision.
- Elevated sub-RPE mass: commonly brown, but may be amelanotic; commonly associated with orange pigment (lipofuscin) and exudative retinal detachment; some (20%) may rupture through Bruch's membrane and RPE to form a subretinal 'mushroom'; occasional vitreous haemorrhage, ↑IOP, cataract, uveitis. **NB** The key diagnostic dilemma is to distinguish a malignant melanoma from a benign naevus (see Choroidal naevus 📖 p. 556). Suspicious features are listed in Box 15.2.

> **Box 15.2 Suspicious features suggestive of choroidal melanoma**
>
> Symptomatic
> Juxtapapillary
> Subretinal fluid/retinal detachment
> Lipofuscin on the surface
> Large size (e.g. >2mm thickness)
> Significant growth
> ↑IOP

Investigations

- *US*: solid, acoustically hollow, low internal reflectivity, with choroidal excavation.
- *CT and MRI* may detect extraglobar extension but cannot reliably differentiate between types of tumour.
- *Biopsy*: incisional biopsy should not be performed as it is associated with higher recurrence and metastases; however, FNA may be performed in selected cases.
- *Systemic assessment*: FBC, LFT, liver/abdominal US (or CT, MRI).

At the time of presentation most (98%) do not have detectable metastatic disease.

Treatment

Specialist advice should be sought. Options include:

- *Observation*: for small asymptomatic lesions without suspicious features. COMS (Collaborative Ocular Melanoma Study) showed growth in only 31% of small melanomas by 5yrs.
- *Transpupillary thermotherapy*: consider for small (<10mm diameter, <3mm thick), heavily pigmented lesions that are outside the macula and not touching the optic disc. Relatively high risk of local reoccurrence.

- *Radiotherapy*: plaques (3mm larger in diameter than the lesion; deliver about 80–100Gy to the tumour apex) or proton beam irradiation (usually 50–70Gy in 4–5 fractions). Plaque radiotherapy has fewer local side-effects than proton beam and was shown to be as effective as enucleation for medium-sized melanomas (COMS). Side-effects include radiation retinopathy, cataracts, and neovascular glaucoma.
- *Local resection*: may be suitable for smaller anterior tumours. Unlike enucleation it preserves vision and cosmesis and avoids long-term complications of irradiation. However, surgery is difficult with significant risk of complications (vitreous haemorrhage, retinal detachment, cataract).
- *Enucleation*: usually performed for large tumours (>15mm diameter, 10mm thick), optic nerve involvement, or painful blind eyes. No benefit demonstrated for pre-enucleation radiotherapy.
- *Orbital exenteration*: controversial; occasionally performed for massive orbital extension or recurrence after enucleation.

Prognosis

Poor prognostic features include large size, extrascleral extension, greater age of the patient, epithelioid cell type, and certain mutations (monosomy 3 and partial duplication of 8q).

Table 15.3 Differential diagnosis of choroidal mass

Pigmented	Choroidal melanoma
	Naevus
	CHRPE
	Melanocytoma
	Metastasis
	BDUMP syndrome
Non-pigmented	Choroidal melanoma
	Choroidal granuloma
	Posterior scleritis
	Retinal detachment
	Choroidal detachment
	Choroidal neovascular membrane
	Haematoma (subretinal/sub-RPE/suprachoroidal)
	Choroidal osteoma
	Choroidal haemangioma
	Metastasis

Choroidal naevus

Uveal naevi are benign melanocytic tumours. They may occur in up to 10% of adult caucasians, making them the commonest of all intraocular tumours. Rarely, they may become malignant (1 in 5000).

Their main significance lies in the need to differentiate them from a malignant melanoma. Choroidal naevi are usually incidental findings.

Clinical features

- Asymptomatic, rarely ↓VA.
- Small (<5mm diameter, <1mm thick), homogeneous grey–brown; may have drusen; absence of lipofuscin or subretinal fluid (cf. choroidal melanoma).

Differentiating a naevus from a malignant melanoma

With time a malignant melanoma may declare itself by continued, often rapid, growth. However, it may be possible to identify probable melanomas at the time of presentation due to the presence of suspicious characteristics. Features suggestive of malignancy include:

- **T**hickness (>2mm)
- **F**luid (subretinal)
- **S**ymptoms
- **O**range pigment
- **M**argin touching disc.

In the absence of any of the first five features, a small melanocytic lesion is very unlikely to be a choroidal melanoma (only 3% show significant growth at 5yrs). The presence of one feature increases the risk to 38%, and of two or more to >50%. The following mnemonic has been suggested: TFSOM; 'To Find Small Ocular Melanomas[1]'. Documented growth would also suggest malignancy.

Investigation and treatment

If no suspicious features are present these lesions do not require regular ophthalmic review. The naevus should be photographed and the patient provided with a copy to permit their own optometrist to monitor the lesion (e.g. annually) as part of their routine optometric review.

Melanocytoma of the optic disc

These are comprised of a distinctive cell type—the polyhedral naevus cell. They are heavily pigmented benign tumours involving the optic disc, which may cause axonal compression and consequent visual field defects. Rarely, malignant transformation may occur.

1. Shields CL *et al. Curr Opin Ophthalmol* 2002;**13**:135.

Choroidal haemangiomas

Choroidal haemangiomas are benign vascular hamartomas. Although congenital, they are usually asymptomatic until adulthood when secondary degenerative changes of the overlying RPE and retina, or the development of subretinal fluid may cause visual loss. Two clinical patterns are seen: circumscribed and diffuse.

Histologically they comprise mainly cavernous vascular channels (with normal endothelial cells and supporting fibrous septa), but with some capillary-like vessels (especially in the diffuse form).

Circumscribed choroidal haemangioma

This form is isolated, may be asymptomatic and has no systemic associations. It is usually static but may grow in pregnancy.

Clinical features
- Poorly demarcated, elevated, orange–red choroidal mass; usually 3–7mm diameter, 1–3mm thick; located around the posterior pole (within 2DD of disc or foveola).
- *Complications*: fibrous change of RPE, cystic change, or serous detachment of the retina.

Investigations
- *US*: very high internal reflectivity.
- *FFA*: early hyperfluorescence of intralesional choroidal vessels, followed by hyperfluorescence of the whole lesion.
- *ICG*: early cyanescence of intralesional choroidal vessels, followed by intense cyanescence of the whole lesion and subsequent central fading.

Treatment
Specialist advice should be sought. Options include observation, PDT, transpupillary thermotherapy, or irradiation (usually proton beam).

Diffuse choroidal haemangioma

This form is usually associated with other ocular and systemic abnormalities, forming part of the Sturge–Weber syndrome.

Clinical features
- Deep-red (cf. normal other eye) thickened choroid, particularly at the posterior pole; may have tortuous retinal vessels, fibrous change of RPE, cystic change; or serous detachment of the retina and disc cupping.
- *Complications*: fibrous change of RPE, cystic change or serous detachment of the retina, glaucoma.

Investigations
- *US*: diffuse choroidal thickening with high internal reflectivity.
- *MRI brain*: if CNS haemangioma suspected as part of Sturge–Weber syndrome.

Treatment
- Specialist advice should be sought.
- Options include PDT, transpupillary thermotherapy, or irradiation.
- Liaise with neurologist if cerebral involvement.

Table 15.4 Features of Sturge–Weber syndrome

Ocular	Extraocular
Episcleral haemangioma	Naevus flammeus of the face
Ciliary body/iris haemangioma	CNS haemangioma
Choroidal haemangioma (diffuse)	
Glaucoma	

Other choroidal tumours

Choroidal osteoma

This is a rare benign tumour of the choroid. Originally thought to be a choristoma, it is now felt to be an acquired neoplasm in which mature bone replaces choroid with damage to overlying RPE and retina.

Typically, it is seen in young adult women (F:M 9:1); it may be bilateral in 20%.

Clinical features
- Gradual ↓VA, metamorphopsia.
- Yellow well-defined geographic lesion, usually abutting or surrounding the optic disc; superficial abnormalities include prominent inner choroidal vessels and irregular RPE changes.
- *Complications*: CNV.

Investigations and treatment
- *US*: highly reflective with acoustic shadow.
- *CT*: bone-like signal from posterior globe.
- *FFA*: early mottled hyperfluorescence and late diffuse hyperfluorescence.
- Although treatment of the tumour itself is not indicated, CNV may be treated conventionally.

Choroidal metastases

These are the commonest intraocular malignant neoplasms. Usually, the patients are already known to have a primary tumour, but in about 25% the first clinical manifestation may be an ocular problem.

Although the choroid is the commonest site, metastases may occur in the iris, ciliary body, retina, vitreous, and optic nerve may be involved. Bilateral involvement is seen in about 30%.

Clinical features
- ↓VA, metamorphopsia; may be asymptomatic.
- Yellow–white (breast, bronchus, bowel) ill-defined lesion; usually fairly flat but may have associated exudative retinal detachment.
- *Colour variation*: consider cutaneous malignant melanoma if lesion is black, renal cell carcinoma or follicular thyroid carcinoma if red–orange, and carcinoid if golden–orange.

Investigations
Ocular
- *US*: high internal reflectivity.
- *FFA*: no/few large vessels within the tumour, early hypofluorescence, and late diffuse hyperfluorescence. ICG may show tumours not detected on FFA.
- *FNA*: consider FNA if diagnostic uncertainty and no extraocular tissue available for biopsy.

Systemic

This should be co-ordinated with a general physician or oncologist, and would include a complete examination (including breasts, prostate, lymph nodes, skin) and selected investigations (e.g. CXR, mammography).

Treatment

This will depend on the lesion, the visual status of the eye, and the general health of the patient: options include observation, chemotherapy, radiotherapy (plaque, proton-beam), or occasionally enucleation.

Box 15.3 Commonest primary tumours metastasizing to the eye

Bronchus	Thyroid
Breast	Testis
Bowel	Skin
Kidney	

Retinoblastoma (1)

This is the commonest primary malignant intraocular tumour of childhood. The tumour arises from primitive retinoblasts of the developing retina with loss of function of the Rb tumour suppressor gene (*Ch13q14*).

Lifetime incidence is 1 in 15–20 000, and there is no gender or racial predilection. The median age at presentation is under 12mths in heritable cases, and closer to 24mths in sporadic cases. Presentation after the age of 6yrs is extremely rare.

Genetics

Understanding the genetics of retinoblastoma is critical in planning management. Two separate mutational events, M1 and M2, which result in loss or inactivation of *both* Rb gene copies, are required to initiate the tumour (Knudson's 'two-hit' hypothesis). Recent evidence suggests the occurrence of subsequent mutations (M3–Mn) that determine the progression of tumour. The two hits can occur in one of two situations.

- In the genetic (also referred to as the germline or heritable) form, every cell in the body is missing one copy of the Rb gene, the mutation occurring at the zygote stage. Every photoreceptor cell can potentially give rise to a tumour.
- In the somatic (non-heritable) form, a single developing retinal cell loses one copy of the Rb gene during retinal development (the first hit); the rest of the body cells are normal. The second hit is a random event, and gives rise to a tumour.

Therefore, genetic cases often have multiple tumours in one or both eyes (unilateral multifocal or bilateral), while somatic cases are always unilateral and unifocal.

Inherited vs sporadic retinoblastoma

Retinoblastoma may be inherited or occur sporadically.

- Over 90% cases are sporadic (with no family history). In most of these cases the mutation is somatic and gives rise to isolated unilateral disease.
- A third of the sporadic cases arise from new germline mutations that are heritable (can be passed on to their offspring) but not inherited from the parents.
- 40% of all cases are bilateral (and necessarily germline), and 60% are unilateral (which could be somatic or germline).
- Of the unilateral cases, 15% are germline, and carry the same risks as bilateral germline cases. Germline mutations are highly penetrant.
- Over 90% of children carrying the Rb gene defect will develop retinoblastoma.

Histology

Characteristic histological features include abnormal patterns of retinoblasts such as the Flexner–Wintersteiner rosettes, Homer Wright rosettes, and fleurettes.

Clinical features

- Leucocoria (Box 15.4) (60%), strabismus (20%), ↓VA, acute red eye, orbital inflammation, excess watering.

- White round retinal mass with one of the following growth patterns: endophytic (growth towards vitreous with vitreous seeds), exophytic (growth towards RPE/choroid with subretinal seeds), mixed or diffuse infiltrating (generalized retinal thickening) ± visible calcification.
- Visible calcification on ophthalmoscopy, or detectable on ultrasonography.

Complications (in order of frequency):
- *Optic nerve (± CNS) invasion.*
- *Anterior segment involvement*: glaucoma, ± buphthalmos/corneal oedema, iris invasion manifesting as heterochromia, phthisis bulbi ± pseudohypopyon, rubeosis ± hyphaema.
- *Extraocular spread*: e.g. orbital inflammation.
- *Systemic metastasis*: to bone marrow, liver, and lungs.

Investigations
- *US*: intralesional calcification with high internal reflectivity and acoustic shadow (best detected with low gain setting).
- *CT/MRI*: apart from ultrasonography, routine imaging is not indicated. CT is best avoided as any dose of radiation magnifies the risk of developing secondary malignancies in germline cases. MRI may be useful if there is suspicion of extraocular (particularly intracranial) spread, if the child presents with signs of raised ICP (to look for pineal blastoma–trilateral retinoblastoma) or if the diagnosis is in doubt.
- *Mutation testing*: is an essential investigation, and can be performed on peripheral blood, and tumour tissue if available (from the enucleated eye). The information gained often helps distinguish between germline and somatic cases, which has major implications for determining the risk to unaffected relatives and future siblings and offspring.

Staging
The new international classification has 5 groups A–E of increasing severity, and guides initial management.

Treatment principles
- Retinoblastoma is a unique cancer by virtue of its confinement within the scleral envelope, and has a 95% cure rate with appropriate treatment.
- The diagnosis is clinical, and it is important to avoid any intraocular procedure (e.g. diagnostic biopsy) as it may lead to extraocular spread, which could result in death.
- A combination of treatment modalities, e.g. chemotherapy with laser/cryotherapy/plaque brachytherapy helps minimize adverse effects
- Close monitoring with EUA at decreasing frequency as the child grows older is important for early detection of recurrent or new tumours, with awake exams for older children.
- During active treatment, chemotherapy is given over 4–6 cycles at 3-weekly intervals, with EUAs before each cycle to monitor response and apply local treatment (laser or cryo).
- Local treatment may be continued at further EUAs until all tumours are inactive.

Retinoblastoma (2)

Treatment
This requires significant multidisciplinary input and should be co-ordinated by a specialized centre. Options include:

Laser treatment
- Using green laser (532nM) for photocoagulation or large spot infrared (810nM) laser for transpupillary thermotherapy: suitable for smaller tumours, or larger tumours after they have been shrunk to a treatable size with chemotherapy (chemoreduction).
- Laser treatment is not effective for vitreous seeds.

Cryotherapy
Suitable for larger, peripheral tumours, or localized vitreous disease close to the retina.

Radiotherapy
- External Beam RadioTherapy (teletherapy): once the mainstay of treatment, this is now reserved for diffuse disease in the only remaining eye, or recurrent disease not responsive to all other forms of treatment. **Disadvantages**: large dose of diffuse radiation causing ↑ risk of inducing secondary malignancies (major risk in germline cases), soft tissue/bony atrophy, cataracts, and dry eyes.
- Plaque brachytherapy involves suturing a radioactive plaque on to the sclera for a specified period of a few hours to 3–4d, which delivers a high dose of radiation to a very localized area, with no risk of secondary tumours. It is highly effective against localized vitreous disease and for elevated tumours where laser is ineffective.

Chemotherapy
- The main role of chemotherapy is to shrink the tumour(s) to a size where laser treatment can be effective (chemoreduction). It is also very effective against vitreous and subretinal disease, and invaluable for extraocular involvement and metastases.
- Common regimens include carboplatin, etoposide, and vincristine. Significant short- and long-term side-effects of chemotherapy (e.g. hearing loss with carboplatin, and nephrotoxicity). Usually given over 4–6 sessions at 3-weekly intervals.

Enucleation
- The oldest, and most effective treatment, enucleation is curative for intraocular retinoblastoma and is the treatment of choice for advanced uniocular disease or the worse eye of bilateral cases.
- The eye is removed with a long segment of optic nerve and sent for histology, and tumour DNA studies to identify the mutations; comparison with peripheral blood can then differentiate germline vs somatic cases.
- An orbital implant of 18–22mm diameter (porous polyethylene (Medpor), hydroxyapatite, or bioceramic) is inserted at the same time to restore lost volume; later a cosmetic prosthetic shell (matched to the other eye) is fitted.

Supportive treatment
- *Prosthesis fitting for enucleated eyes*: is an important part of rehabilitation, usually 6wks after surgery.

- *Psychological support for children and families*: to deal with loss of eye, vision, and a chronic illness.
- *Protective eye wear* for the better/remaining eye during contact sport.
- *Long-term oncological surveillance especially for germline cases*: this is best undertaken by the oncologists.
- *Counselling*: genetic counselling (including risk to siblings and offspring) and advice regarding the risk of secondary malignancies (including advice about risk factors, such as smoking, and how to look out for early warning signs). Parents should be counselled soon after diagnosis, and the patients usually when they reach adolescence.
- Cataract surgery if needed should be delayed for at least 1–2 years after active treatment.

Screening for retinoblastoma

Screening close relatives of retinoblastoma patients is invaluable in early detection and treatment, saving eyes and lives. If the mutation for the index case is known, mutation testing (see Retinoblastoma (1) 📖 p.563) can be offered to relatives to determine if they are at risk of suffering/ passing on the disease.

Screening is offered if (1) mutation positive, or (2) if the mutation is not known for the index case and risk cannot be excluded. Screening is not needed if the relative tests negative for the mutation. This approach helps avoid unnecessary screening, and saves resources.

Prognosis

Most untreated tumours proceed to local invasion and metastasis, causing death within 2yrs. Occasionally, however, the tumour may spontaneously stop growing to form a retinoma, or necrose to cause phthisis bulbi.

Most small/medium tumours without vitreous seeding can be successfully treated while preserving useful vision. Overall, there is a 95% survival rate (in the developed world). *Poor prognostic factors include*: size of tumour, optic nerve involvement, extraocular spread, and older age of child.

Patients with germinal mutations are at increased risk of pineoblastoma (trilateral retinoblastoma), ectopic intracranial retinoblastoma, and osteogenic or soft tissue sarcomas. This risk is increased with radiation exposure.

Box 15.4 **Differential diagnosis of leucocoria**

- Retinoblastoma
- Cataract
- Persistent faetal vasculature syndrome
- Inflammatory cyclitic membrane
- Coats' disease
- ROP
- Toxocara
- Incontinentia pigmenti
- Familial exudative vitreoretinopathy
- Retinal dysplasia (e.g. Norrie disease, Patau syndrome, Edward syndrome)
- Other posterior segment tumours (e.g. combined hamartoma of RPE and retina)

Retinal haemangiomas

Capillary haemangioma

This is an uncommon benign hamartoma of the retinal (or optic disc) vasculature consisting of capillary-like vessels. It may present at any age but is most commonly diagnosed in young adults. Isolated capillary haemangiomas are usually not related to systemic disease but most multiple/bilateral tumours are seen in the context of von Hippel–Lindau symdrome (VHL) (Table 15.5).

Histologically, there are endothelial cells, pericytes, and stromal cells. The VHL mutation may be restricted to the stromal cells, suggesting that despite their innocent appearance they are the underlying neoplastic cell.

Clinical features

- ↓VA; asymptomatic (may be diagnosed on family screening).
- Red nodular lesion with tortuosity and dilatation (often irregular) of feeding artery and draining vein ± exudation, exudative retinal detachment, rubeosis/neovascular glaucoma, epiretinal membranes, tractional retinal detachment, vitreous haemorrhage.
- Optic disc haemangiomas are less well-defined and do not have obvious feeder vessels.

Investigation

FFA: rapid sequential filling of artery, haemangioma, and vein, with extensive late leakage; leakage into vitreous may make late images hazy.

Treatment

- *Systemic disease*: if VHL is suspected, multidisciplinary care with physician and clinical geneticist is required.
- *Ocular disease*:
  - *photocoagulation*: for small (<3mm diameter) tumours; requires confluent white burns covering the entire tumour ± feeder vessel; multiple treatment sessions are usually required;
  - *cryotherapy*: for peripheral or larger tumours; usually double freeze–thaw technique; multiple treatment sessions are usually required;
  - radiotherapy;
  - excision.

Table 15.5 Features of von Hippel–Lindau syndrome

Ocular	Extraocular
Retinal capillary haemangioma	Haemangioblastoma of cerebellum, spinal cord, or brainstem
	Renal cell carcinoma
	Phaeochromocytoma
	Islet cell carcinoma
	Epididymal cysts/adenomas
	Visceral cysts

Cavernous haemangioma

This is an uncommon benign hamartoma of the retinal (or optic disc) vasculature consisting of large-calibre thin-walled vessels. It is usually isolated but familial bilateral cases do occur.

Clinical features

- Usually asymptomatic; occasional ↓VA or floaters.
- Cluster of intraretinal blood-filled saccules (a plasma level may separate out due to the slow flow); otherwise normal retinal vasculature; ± vitreous haemorrhage.

Investigation and treatment

- *FFA*: slow filling, remain hyperfluorescent, no leakage.
- Treatment is not usually necessary.

Racemose haemangioma

These are rare retinal AVMs and are therefore not true tumours. Although congenital they progress with age and are usually detected in early adulthood. These may be isolated or associated with ipsilateral AVMs of the CNS (Wyburn–Mason syndrome, Table 15.6).

Clinical features

- Usually asymptomatic; occasional ↓VA.
- Enlarged tortuous vascular abnormality with direct connection between arterial and venous circulations with similar colour throughout.

Investigation and treatment

- This is usually a clinical diagnosis.
- There is no effective treatment for retinal AVMs although intracranial AVMs have been successfully treated by surgery, radiotherapy, and embolization.

Table 15.6 Features of Wyburn–Mason syndrome

Ocular	Extraocular
Retinal AVM	Cerebral/brain stem AVM
Orbital/periorbital AVM	

Other retinal tumours

Astrocytoma

This is a rare benign tumour of the neurosensory retina composed of astrocytes. There is debate as to whether it is acquired or is actually a hamartoma.

Typically, it presents in childhood/adolescence; both sexes are equally affected. Isolated astrocytomas are usually not associated with systemic disease but most multiple/bilateral tumours are seen in the context of tuberous sclerosis. An association with neurofibromatosis (type 1) is also suggested.

Clinical features
- ↓VA, but often asymptomatic.
- Superficial white well-defined lesion (translucent to calcified 'mulberry' type; flat or nodular) ± exudative retinal detachment.

Investigation and treatment
Further evaluation is not usually required other than ruling out possible syndromic associations.

Table 15.7 Features of tuberous sclerosis

Ocular	Extraocular
Retinal astrocytoma	Adenoma sebaceum
	Ash leaf spots
	Shagreen patches
	Subungual fibromas
	Cerebral astrocytomas (with epilepsy and ↓IQ)
	Visceral hamartomas (e.g. renal angiomyolipoma, cardiac rhabdomyoma)
	Visceral cysts
	Pulmonary lymphangioleiomyomatosis

Retinal pigment epithelium tumours

Congenital hypertrophy of the retinal pigment epithelium

This is a common benign congenital proliferation of the RPE occurring in about 1% of the population (typical form). The typical form is unilateral and either solitary or, more commonly, grouped ('bear tracks'). They are unrelated to systemic disease. The atypical form is bilateral and multifocal, and is associated both with familial adenomatous polyposis (Table 15.8), and its variants.

Histologically the RPE cells are of increased height with increased numbers of melanin granules.

Clinical features

Typical CHRPE
- *Solitary*: black, well-defined, flat, round lesion, often with depigmented 'lacunae' within it, deep to the neurosensory retina; usually 2–5mm.
- *Grouped*: similar smaller lesions, grouped to form 'bear tracks'; usually <2mm.

Atypical CHRPE
- Bilateral, multiple, widely separated, black oval lesions with irregular depigmentation; usually <2mm.

Investigation and treatment

Typical CHRPE does not require investigation. Atypical CHRPE should prompt an investigation of family history and consideration of referral to a gastroenterologist. If familial adenomatous polyposis is diagnosed (by a gastroenterologist), prophylactic colectomy is recommended. In untreated familial adenomatous polyposis the development of colonic carcinoma is almost universal.

Table 15.8 Features of familial adenomatous polyposis

Ocular	Extraocular
Atypical CHRPE	Colonic polyps and carcinoma
	Gardner's variant: bone cysts, hamartomas, soft tissue tumours
	Turcot's variant: CNS neuroepithelial tumours

Combined hamartoma of the retinal pigment epithelium and retina

This is a rare benign hamartoma of the RPE, retinal astrocytes, and retinal vasculature. It is usually not related to systemic disease but may be associated with neurofibromatosis type 2 and rarely type 1.

Clinical features
- ↓VA, floaters, leucocoria.
- Elevated lesion with whitish sheen superficially (epiretinal membranes and intraretinal gliosis), tortuous vessels, and variable deeper pigmentation; usually juxtapapillary but may be peripheral; usually 4–6mm in diameter.

Investigation and treatment

Assess for the possibility of underlying neurofibromatosis.

Table 15.9 Features of neurofibromatosis-1

Ocular	Extraocular
Optic glioma	**Café-au-lait spots (≥6; each >0.5cm pre-puberty or >1.5cm post-puberty)**
Lisch nodules (≥2)	**Axillary/inguinal freckling**
Lid neurofibroma	**Neurofibromas (≥1 plexiform type or ≥2 any type)**
Choroidal naevi	**Characteristic bony lesion (sphenoid dysplasia, which may →pulsatile proptosis; long bone cortex thinning/dysplasia)**
Retinal astrocytoma	**First-degree relative with NF-1**

Diagnosis requires two or more of the features in bold.

Table 15.10 Features of neurofibromatosis-2

Ocular	Extraocular
Early-onset posterior subcapsular or cortical cataracts	Acoustic neuroma
	Meningioma
Combined hamartoma of the RPE and retina	Glioma
	Schwannoma
	1st-degree relative with NF-2

Definite NF-2:
- Bilateral acoustic neuroma, OR
- First-degree relative with NF-2 AND either unilateral acoustic neuroma (at <30yrs) or two of the other diagnostic features

Probable NF-2:
- Unilateral acoustic neuroma (at <30yrs) AND one of the other diagnostic features; OR
- Multiple meningiomas AND one of the other diagnostic features

Lymphoma (1)

Although this is an uncommon tumour of the eye, ocular lymphoma is increasing in incidence.

- It is both sight-threatening and life-threatening, and is easily missed as it may masquerade as a number of other conditions, such as uveitis.
- Risk factors include immunosuppression (e.g. therapeutic, AIDS, etc.).

Classification

Lymphoma is divided into Hodgkin lymphoma (*syn* Hodgkin's disease) and non-Hodgkin lymphoma.

Hodgkin lymphoma

Hodgkin lymphoma is characterized by the Reed–Sternberg cell (thought to be an abnormal B cell) and accounts for 20% of lymphomas (about 1500 new cases/yr in the UK).

Non-Hodgkin lymphoma

This comprises all other lymphomas (80%; about 9700 new cases/yr in the UK). It is usually subclassified according to cell type. Most non-Hodgkin lymphomas are B-cell lymphomas but some are T-cell lymphomas.

In the ophthalmic context non-Hodgkin lymphoma is frequently described in terms of its anatomical distribution (ocular-CNS type vs systemic) or traditionally in terms of its type of ophthalmic presentation ('vitreoretinal' vs 'uveal').

B-cell non-Hodgkin lymphoma: The commonest types of B-cell lymphoma are diffuse large B-cell lymphoma and follicular lymphoma; other types include Burkitt lymphoma, MALToma (extranodal marginal zone B-cell lymphoma), nodal marginal zone B-cell lymphoma, mantle cell lymphoma, mediastinal large B-cell lymphoma, small lymphocytic lymphoma and Waldenström's macroglobulinaemia.

T-cell non-Hodgkin lymphoma: T-cell lymphomas include cutaneous lymphoma (mycosis fungoides; Sezáry syndrome), peripheral T-cell lymphoma, anaplastic large cell lymphoma, and lymphoblastic lymphoma.

Ocular-CNS type intraocular lymphoma

Ocular-CNS non-Hodgkin lymphoma (or 'primary CNS lymphoma) with ocular involvement' or primary intraocular lymphoma) is the commonest type of intraocular lymphoma.

Histology

This is usually an intermediate/high-grade diffuse large B-cell lymphoma.

Disease distribution and presentation

Disease distribution: bilateral ophthalmic disease occurs in 90%; coexistent intracranial disease occurs in up to 85% of patients with primary intraocular disease; conversely up to 20% who present with primary CNS lymphoma develop concurrent ocular disease.

Disease presentation: the ocular disease is the presenting feature in 50–65% (and can precede CNS disease by months or years), whereas in 35–50% it is found concurrent with or after presentation of CNS disease.

Risk factors

- May occur in both immunocompetent and immunocompromised individuals.
- In patients on immunosuppressive drugs, risk is related to degree and duration of immunosuppression.
- In patients with HIV it is normally associated with CD4+ counts of <30/mm^3; EBV is strongly associated with ocular-CNS lymphoma in AIDS patients.

Clinical features

Typically, ocular-CNS non-Hodgkin lymphoma presents with a 'vitreo-retinal' pattern of disease, sometimes being described as a uveitis 'masquerade' syndrome.

Ophthalmic features

- *Typical*: 'vitritis' (cellular infiltrate), yellowish sub-RPE plaques with overlying pigment clumping, usually bilateral; may be misdiagnosed as a refractory 'uveitis' (although corticosteroid treatment may initially be successful).
- *Atypical*: exudative retinal detachment; retinitis, which may mimic diseases seen with CMV, ARN, sarcoidosis, TB, and syphilis; neovascular glaucoma.

CNS features

- *Typical*: progressive focal symptoms indicative of a space-occupying lesion ± seizures, mental state change.
- *Atypical presentations*: meningeal (may present with headache, isolated cranial neuropathy, spinal nerve root problems); progressive dementia; intravascular malignant lymphomatosis (multiple stroke-like episodes); neurolymphomatosis (CNS lymphoma with peripheral nerve infiltration); relapsing-remitting form.

Investigation

Ophthalmic: consider mechanical vitrectomy, fine-needle vitreous aspiration (25-gauge needle) or even incisional biopsy (if chorioretinal involvement) to obtain cytology/histology. Multiple vitreous biopsies may be needed to make the diagnosis. The vitreous specimen requires careful handling and should be spun down. Levels of interleukin 10 are generally elevated. In one study of 159 patients (51 with intraocular lymphoma), elevated interleukin 10 was a useful predictor of intraocular lymphoma: for the AqH interleukin 10 >50pg/ml (sensitivity 0.89; specificity 0.93) and for the vitreous interleukin 10 >400pg/ml (sensitivity 0.8; specificity 0.99). Alternatively, an interleukin 10:interleukin 6 ratio of >1.0 has been used. Clonal bcl-2/IgH translocations may be detected by PCR in up to two-thirds of cases.

Systemic: assessment and treatment should be co-ordinated by an oncologist and would usually include MRI brain ± LP (for ocular-CNS type) and abdominal-pelvis imaging (for systemic involvement).

Treatment

Treatment options include radiotherapy (external beam or plaque) and chemotherapy (systemic or intravitreal). CNS involvement may require aggressive treatment with combined intrathecal and intravenous chemotherapy and radiotherapy.

Lymphoma (2)

Systemic type intraocular lymphoma

Secondary intraocular involvement may occur with systemic lymphoma. This is less common, typically has a 'uveal' pattern of disease and may be associated with involvement of other orbital structures.

Histology

The most common systemic lymphoma type to involve the eye is diffuse large cell B-cell lymphoma, multiple myeloma and Waldenström's macro-globulinaemia. It carries a better prognosis than the ocular-CNS type.

Clinical features

- *Typical*: more diffuse yellowish choroidal thickening (may be multi focal), with minimal if any vitritis.
- *Atypical*: may mimic melanoma (or other choroidal tumours), posterior scleritis, uni/multifocal choroiditis.

Investigation

Ophthalmic: in most cases, tissue diagnosis of lymphoma has already been made from non-ocular tissue, although ocular fluid/tissue may be obtained as described for primary intraocular disease. Orbital imaging (US/MRI) may be helpful in assessing extent of disease.

Systemic: assessment and treatment should be co-ordinated by an oncologist. It is likely to include extensive imaging (e.g. abdomen-pelvis) with a view to assessing extent of disease and identifying suitable tissue for biopsy. MRI brain and LP (suspected CNS involvement).

Treatment

Treatment options include radiotherapy and chemotherapy as directed by histological grade of lymphoma and extent of systemic and intraocular disease.

Coupland SE *et al*. Lymphomas involving the eye and the ocular adnexa. *Curr Opin Ophthalmol* 2006;**17**:523–31.

Neuro-ophthalmology

Anatomy and physiology (1)

Within the retina, photoreceptors transduce photons into electrical impulses, which are relayed via bipolar cells to the retinal ganglion cell.

The ganglion cells can be divided into two populations: parvocellular system for fine visual acuity and colour, and the magnocellular system for motion detection and coarser form vision. This division is preserved both in the lateral geniculate nucleus and the visual cortex.

Optic nerve

The optic nerve is about 50mm long, carries 1.2 million axons, and runs from the optic disc to the chiasm. It may be divided into:

- *Intraocular part (1mm long)*: unmyelinated axons pass through the channels of the lamina cribrosa to become myelinated, so doubling in diameter (1.5mm prelaminar to 3.0mm retrolaminar).
- *Intraorbital part (25mm long)*: this portion has a full meningeal sheath of tough outer dura (continuous with sclera anteriorly and periosteum of sphenoid posteriorly), arachnoid, subarachnoid space, and inner pia mater. It has about 8mm of 'slack' permitting free ocular motility.
- *Intracanalicular part (5–9mm long)*: the nerve enters the optic foramen to travel through the optic canal within the lesser wing of the sphenoid.
- *Intracranial part (12–16mm long; 4.5mm diameter)*: the nerve runs up, posteriorly and medially to form the chiasm. Neighbouring structures include the frontal lobes superiorly, the ICA laterally, and the ophthalmic artery inferolaterally.

Blood supply

The ophthalmic artery originates from the ICA. It lies inferolaterally to the intracranial optic nerve, inferiorly to the intracanalicular part, and perforates the intraorbital part 8–12mm behind the globe to become the central retinal artery. The intracranial, intracanalicular, and intraorbital portions of the optic nerve are supplied by the pial plexus fed by branches of the ophthalmic artery and, most posteriorly, by the superior hypophyseal artery. The intraocular part (the optic nerve head) is supplied by the circle of Zinn–Haller, an anastomosis fed mainly by the short posterior ciliary arteries.

Optic chiasm

The optic chiasm (8mm long, 12mm wide) represents the joining of both optic nerves, the hemidecussation of the nasal fibres, and the emergence of the optic tracts. The chiasm usually lies directly above the pituitary gland (80%), but may be relatively anterior (prefixed) or posterior (postfixed). The pituitary itself lies within the sella turcica of the sphenoid, roofed by the diaphragma sellae, a sheet of dura between anterior and posterior clinoids. Neighbouring structures include the cavernous sinus and ICA inferolaterally and the third ventricle lying posteriorly.

Within the chiasm fibres from superonasal retina are found to decussate relatively posteriorly while inferonasal fibres decussate more anteriorly; some of these inferonasal fibres appear to loop so far forward as to join the contralateral optic nerve to form Wilbrand's knee. Macular fibres decussate in the central and posterior chiasm.

Optic tract and lateral geniculate nucleus

The optic tract runs from the chiasm to the LGN, during which axons from corresponding locations of each retina start to become associated. Within the tract parvocellular fibres run centrally with magnocellular fibres on the outside. The LGN is organized into six layers: contralateral fibres synapse with 1 (magnocellular), 4 and 6 (parvocellular); ipsilateral fibres with 2 (magnocellular), 3 and 5 (parvocellular). There may be other modifying pathways (akin to K cells in primates) located between these layers. Axons from the superior retina synapse medially, inferior retina laterally. Macular fibres synapse in the central and posterior LGN. Blood supply is from branches of the middle cerebral artery and thalamogeniculate branches of the posterior cerebral artery.

Optic radiation

Axons of the optic radiation project from the LGN to the visual cortex.

Fibres from the superior retina project posteriorly through the parietal lobe. Fibres from the inferior retina project through the temporal lobe but deviate laterally round the inferior horn of the lateral ventricle to form Meyer's loop. Macular fibres generally lie between these two courses.

The blood supply is from the internal carotid, middle, and posterior cerebral arteries.

Visual cortex

The primary visual cortex (V1, Brodmann area 17, striate cortex) is located on the medial surfaces of both occipital lobes on either side of the calcarine sulcus.

V1 is organized into six layers: optic tracts synapse mainly with layer IV; layers II and III project to secondary visual cortex; layer IV to superior colliculus; and layer VI back to LGN.

Superior retina is represented superiorly, inferior retina inferiorly, macula most posteriorly, and extreme temporal periphery (temporal crescent) anteriorly. Blood supply is mainly from the posterior cerebral artery but with middle cerebral artery contributions at the anterior and lateral margins.

The visual cortex cells are arranged into basic processing units representing discrete areas of the visual field. These hypercolumns comprise right and left ocular dominance columns, and orientation columns. The orientation columns are divided into blobs (colour) and interblobs (orientation). Cell types range in complexity. Least discriminatory are the circularly symmetrical cells that respond to small central stimulus regardless of orientation and movement. Simple cells require a centrally located single contrast stimulus that must be correctly orientated and moving in the correct direction. Complex cells are similar but do not require the stimulus to be centrally located. Hypercomplex cells require that the stimulus is also of a particular length.

Further processing occurs in the visual association areas, which may also integrate information from nuclei involved with head and eye movement. Subspecialization occurs in V3 (depth perception, dynamic form), V4 (colour), and V5 (motion, maintenance of fixation).

Anatomy and physiology (2)

Ocular motor nerves (Fig. 16.1)

Third nerve (oculomotor nerve)

The III nucleus lies in the midbrain anterior to the periaqueductal grey matter at the level of the superior colliculus. It consists of a single central nucleus innervating both LPS muscles, and separate subnuclei for each superior rectus (contralateral innervation), medial rectus, IR, and IO (all ipsilateral innervation).

The IIIn fasciculus travels anteriorly through the MLF, the red nucleus, and the cerebral peduncle. On leaving the midbrain it emerges within the interpeduncular fossa and passes anteriorly beneath the posterior cerebral artery, above the superior cerebellar artery and lateral to the posterior communicating artery. It travels within the lateral wall of the cavernous sinus, dividing into superior and inferior branches that enter the orbit via the superior orbital fissure and annulus of Zinn. The superior branch innervates LPS and SR, whereas the inferior branch innervates MR, IR, IO, and the pupillary sphincter.

Parasympathetic fibres from the Edinger–Westphal nucleus travel in the IO branch as far as the ciliary ganglion and then in the short ciliary nerves to the globe where they innervate the ciliary muscle and pupillary sphincter.

Fourth nerve (trochlear nerve)

The IV nucleus lies just below the III nucleus in the lower midbrain at the level of inferior colliculus.

The fasciculus decussates within the anterior medullary velum and exits the midbrain posteriorly. It then curves round the midbrain, passes anteriorly between the posterior cerebral and superior cerebellar arteries, travels within the lateral wall of the cavernous sinus (inferolateral to III, superior to Va). It then enters the orbit through the superior orbital fissure (but superior to the annulus of Zinn) and terminates in the superior oblique.

Sixth nerve (abducens nerve)

The VI nucleus lies in the lower pons anterior to the fourth ventricle at the level of the facial colliculus. Although most axons innervate the ipsilateral LR, about 40% of axons project via the MLF to the contralateral MR subnucleus.

The fasciculus travels anteriorly through the medial leminiscus and corticospinal tract, just medial to the trigeminal nuclear complex and vestibular nuclei. After emerging at the pontomedullary junction it ascends in the subarachnoid space between the pons and the clivus, before turning anterior over the petrous apex of the temporal bone and under the petroclinoid ligament to enter the cavernous sinus. Here it runs within the sinus itself just lateral to the internal carotid artery and inferomedial to III, IV, and Va, which run in the sinus wall. It then enters the orbit via the superior orbital fissure and annulus of Zinn to terminate in LR.

Posterior communicating artery

III nerve

VI nerve

IV nerve

Fig. 16.1 Cranial nerves III, IV, and VI.

Anatomy and physiology (3)

Seventh nerve (facial nerve)

The facial nerve nuclei are located in the lower pons below the level of the fourth ventricle. There are three nuclei: (1) the main motor nucleus; (2) the parasympathetic superior salivatory and lacrimal nuclei (nucleus salivatorius superior); and (3) the sensory nucleus (nucleus of tractus solitarius). Fibres from the later 2 nuclei form the nervus intermedius.

The main motor nucleus is bilaterally innervated by the cerebral cortex and the neurons pass around the VI nerve nuclei, before emerging anteriorly from the brain stem with the nervus intermedius, at the lower border of the pons. Passing above the VIII nerve they pass over the cerebellopontine angle into the internal auditory canal. It transverse the petrous temporal bone and exits behind the stylomastoid process through the stylomastoid foramen. It terminates in the temporal, zygomatic, buccal, mandibular, and cervical branches.

- *Motor functions*: muscles of facial expression and movement; superficial platysma muscles of the neck and the stapedius ear muscles.
- *Sensory and secretory functions* (nerve intermedius and geniculate ganglion): lacrimal gland (via the greater superficial petrosal nerve) and salivary glands (via the chorda tympani, mediating taste for the anterior two-thirds of the tongue).

Autonomic supply

Sympathetic

The *first-order neurones* originate in the posterior hypothalamus, descend through the brainstem to synapse in the spinal cord at the ciliospinal centre of Budge (C8–T2).

The *second-order neurones* emerge anteriorly in the ventral root (close to the lung apex) and then ascend in the sympathetic chain to synapse at the superior cervical ganglion.

The *third-order neurones* ascend along the internal carotid artery to the cavernous sinus, and then via the nasociliary branch of Va into the orbit, and subsequently the long ciliary nerves to terminate in the dilator pupillae.

Parasympathetic

The light and near reflexes are both mediated by the parasympathetic supply from the Edinger–Westphal nucleus. The afferent arm for the light reflex is by (1) retinal ganglion cells that synapse in the ipsilateral pretectal nucleus, and then (2) interneurones that innervate bilateral Edinger–Westphal nuclei. The inputs for the near reflex are less well-defined, but probably include cortical influences (frontal and occipital lobes) mediated by a midbrain centre (anterior to the pretectal nucleus).

The efferent arm for both reflexes comprise (1) preganglionic neurones from the Edinger–Westphal nucleus, which travel in III then inferior division of III then nerve to IO before synapsing at the ciliary ganglion, and (2) postganglionic neurones, which run via the short ciliary nerves to terminate in the constrictor pupillae and ciliary muscle.

Cerebrospinal fluid

CSF is produced by the choroid plexus in the lateral ventricles and the third ventricle. It flows from the lateral ventricles via the foramen of Munro to the third ventricle, and then via the aqueduct of Sylvius to the fourth ventricle. From there it leaves either via the lateral foramina of Luschka or the medial foramen of Magendie to bathe the spinal cord and cerebral hemispheres in the subarachnoid space. It is then absorbed into the cerebral venous system by the arachnoid granulations.

The subarachnoid space is continuous with the optic nerve sheath.

Optic neuropathy: assessment

The optic nerve is vulnerable to injury from numerous local and systemic diseases. Clinical features often include ↓VA, relative/complete afferent pupillary defect, ↓light sensitivity, ↓colour vision, visual field defects, and optic disc abnormalities, such as pallor.

Table 16.1 An approach to assessing optic nerve disease

Visual symptoms	Blurring, 'wash out' of colours, 'blind spots'; may be asymptomatic; check duration, speed of onset/ recovery, precipitants, associations (diplopia, proptosis, red eye)
POH	Previous/current eye disease; refractive error
PMH	Vascular risk factors and disease; neurological disease (e.g. MS); connective tissue disease (e.g. SLE, RA); granulomatous disease (e.g. sarcoid, TB)
SR	Detailed review of all systems; particularly any headache or abnormalities of sensation/motor system/ speech/balance/ hearing
SH	Driver; profession; diet, tobacco consumption, alcohol intake, toxin exposure(e.g. lead, tin, or carbon monoxide)
FH	Family members with visual problems
Dx	Previous/current toxic drugs (e.g. anti-TB)
Ax	Allergies or relevant drug contraindications
Visual acuity	Best-corrected/pin-hole/near
Retinoscopy	Rule out refractive error
Visual function	Check for RAPD, colour vision, red desaturation, visual fields (formal perimetry)
Orbit	Proptosis
AS	Features suggestive of glaucoma, uveitis, CCF
Tonometry	Intraocular pressure
Optic disc	Size, cup, colour, oedema, congenital abnormalities, flat/ elevated/tilted, crowding, peripapillary oedema or haemorrhages, retinociliary collateral vessels, spontaneous venous pulsations
Macula	Abnormalities which may cause central scotoma
Fundus	Abnormalities (e.g. retinoschisis) that may cause peripheral field loss; posterior uveitis; or vasculitis
Vessels	Arteriosclerosis, hypertensive changes, occlusions and emboli
CNS/PNS	Cranial nerves (incl. ocular motility), sensory, motor, cerebellar function, speech, mental state
CVS	Pulse, heart sounds, carotid bruits
Systemic review	Including respiratory, GI, GU, ENT systems

Diagnosis is more difficult in early symmetric disease where there may be no objective signs. Electrodiagnostic tests may be helpful in such cases. Also typical 'optic neuropathy' features may be seen in other diseases (e.g. central scotoma, ↓colour vision, or secondary optic atrophy in retinal disorders). The challenge is thus first to recognize the optic neuropathy and then elucidate the cause (Tables 16.2 and 16.3).

Unexplained optic neuropathy requires urgent investigation (see Optic neuritis (2) 📖 p.586) to elucidate the cause and rule out serious disease, such as compression secondary to a tumour.

Table 16.2 Clinical features of optic nerve vs macular disease

	Optic neuropathy	Macular disease
History		
Main complaint	Grey/darkness	Distortion
Scotoma	Negative	Positive
Associated symptoms	May have retrobulbar pain, e.g. on eye movement	May have micropsia, hyperopic shift
Examination		
VA	Variable ↓	↓↓
Colour vision[1]	↓ or ↓↓	Normal or mild ↓
RAPD	+	–
Testing		
Perimetry	Central, centrocaecal, arcuate, or altitudinal defects	Central scotoma
Amsler chart	Scotoma	Metamorphopsia
VEP latency	↑	Normal or mild ↑

Classically optic neuropathies preferentially affect the red–green axis and macular disease the blue–yellow axis, but there are many exceptions to this (e.g. glaucoma preferentially affects the blue–yellow axis).

Optic neuritis (1)

Inflammation of the optic nerve may be divided into papillitis (where the disc is swollen), retrobulbar neuritis (where the disc is spared), and neuroretinitis (with retinal involvement, 'macular star').

The most common cause of optic neuritis is demyelination, although a number of important differential diagnoses must be considered.

Acute demyelinating optic neuritis

Incidence within the general population is about 5/100 000/yr, but occurs in up to 70% of patients with known MS. The majority is female (F:M 3:1), and are usually aged 20–50. The disease is usually unilateral, although bilateral involvement may be seen in children.

Clinical features

- Rapid ↓VA over hours/days (rarely become NPL); recovery starts within 2wks and may continue for a few months; ↓contrast sensitivity, ↓colour vision, field loss (variable pattern), retrobulbar pain (present in 90%; often worse on eye movement, may be very severe, usually precedes ↓VA), photopsia.
- RAPD (may be absent if pre-existing contralateral disease), disc swelling (only 1/3 of cases); disc should not be pale in the acute stages of a first episode; may have few haemorrhages, retinal exudates, and mild vitritis.

Investigations

- If episode is entirely typical (Box 16.1) the diagnosis may be made on clinical grounds alone.
- If episode is atypical investigate to rule out a progressive optic neuropathy (see atypical optic neuritis).

> **Box 16.1 Features of typical optic neuritis (Optic Neuritis Treatment Trial)**
>
> Age 20–50
> Unilateral
> Worsens over hours/days
> Recovery starts within 2wks
> Retrobulbar pain (may be worse on eye movement)
> ↓Colour vision
> RAPD

Treatment

This remains controversial. IV methylprednisolone hastens visual recovery but does not affect final visual acuity (ONTT: Optic Neuritis Treatment Trial[1]). There is no conclusive evidence that corticosteroids (IV or oral) are beneficial in terms of recovery to normal VA, visual field, or contrast sensitivity.[2] On this basis it may be offered to those with poor vision in the other eye or with severe pain.

Other disease-modifying agents

- *Interferon* β: compared with placebo interferon β significantly lowers the risk of converting from a clinically isolated event to clinically definite MS.[3] In the UK interferon β is often reserved for those who have suffered >2 significant relapses within the last 2yrs (CHAMPS,[4] ETOMS[5]).

- *Mitoxantrone:* this is an anthracenedione that is moderately effective in reducing frequency of relapses and disease progression.[6]
- *Glatiramer acetate:* evidence is not supportive for use in MS.[7]
- *Diet:* polyunsaturated fatty acids and vitamins currently lack evidence for disease modification.[8]

Prognosis

- *Visual recovery:* all patients will have some improvement, with >90% attaining 6/9 in the affected eye. However, even if RAPD resolves and VA recovers to ≥6/6 abnormalities of colour perception, contrast sensitivity, stereopsis, or field may persist. About a third have a further episode (either eye) within 5yrs. On MRI poor visual prognosis is associated with length of optic nerve involvement and intracanalicular segment involvement.
- *Probability of developing MS:* Risk factors are female sex, multiple white matter lesions on MRI, and CSF oligoclonal bands.
- 15yr probability of MS increases from 25% if normal MRI at baseline to 72% if >1 white matter lesion.[9]

Neuromyelitis optica (Devic's disease)

This is an idiopathic, severe, demyelinating disease of the CNS.

Revised diagnostic criteria include optic neuritis and acute myelitis, with two supportive criteria: negative brain MRI at onset; MRI evidence of contiguous spinal cord lesion 3 or more vertebral segments in length; initial brain MRI non-diagnostic for MS or NMO-IgG seropositivity[10].

1. Beck RW, Cleary PA, Anderson MM Jr, Keltner JL, *et al.* A randomized, controlled trial of corticosteroids in the treatment of acute optic neuritis. The Optic Neuritis Study Group. *N Engl J Med.* 1992;**326**(9):581–8.

2. Vedula SS, Brodney-Folse S, Gal RL, Beck R. Corticosteroids for treating optic neuritis. *Cochrane Database of Syst Rev* 2007, Issue 1. Art. No.: CD001430. DOI: 10.1002/14651858.CD001430.pub2.

3. Clerico M, Faggiano F, Palace J, Rice G, *et al.* Recombinant interferon beta or glatiramer acetate for delaying conversion of the first demyelinating event to multiple sclerosis. Cochrane Database of Syst Rev 2008, Issue 2. Art. No.: CD005278. DOI: 10.1002/14651858.CD005278.pub3.

4. Galetta SL, The controlled high risk Avonex multiple sclerosis trial (CHAMPS Study).: *J Neuroophthalmol.* 2001; **21**(4):292–5

5. G.Comi, M. Filippi, F. Barkhof, L. Durelli, *et al.* Hommes and the early treatment of MS study group. Effect of early interferon treatment on conversion to definite multiple sclerosis; a randomised study. *Lancet* 2001; **357**: 1576–82.

6. Martinelli Boneschi F, Rovaris M, Capra R, Comi G. Mitoxantrone for multiple sclerosis. *Cochrane Database of Syst Rev* 2005, Issue 4. Art. No.: CD002127. DOI: 10.1002/14651858.CD002127.pub2.

7. Munari L, Lovati R, Boiko A. Therapy with glatiramer acetate for multiple sclerosis. *Cochrane Database of Syst Rev* 2003, Issue 4. Art.No.: CD004678. DOI: 10.1002/14651858.CD004678.

8. Farinotti M, Simi S, Di Pietrantonj C, McDowell N, *et al.* Dietary interventions for multiple sclerosis. *Cochrane Database of Syst Rev* 2007, Issue 1. Art. No.: CD004192. DOI: 10.1002/14651858.CD004192.pub2.

9. Optic Neuritis Study Group. Visual function 15 years after optic neuritis: a final followup report from the Optic Neuritis Treatment Trial. *Ophthalmology.* 2008 Jun; **115**(6):1079-1082.e5.

10. Wingerchuk DM, Lennon VA, Pittock SJ, Lucchinetti CF, *et al.* Revised diagnostic criteria for neuromyelitis optica. *Neurology* 2006 May 23;**66**(10):1485–9.

Optic neuritis (2)

'Atypical optic neuritis'

If an acute optic neuropathy does not fulfil the criteria for typical optical neuritis (e.g. not improving at 2wks) then it must be investigated further to exclude a compressive lesion or other serious pathology (Table 16.3).

Investigations may include: MRI (gadolinium enhanced), CXR, FBC, ESR, CRP, U+E, Glu, LFT, ACE, ANA, ANCA, Syphilis serology, LHON, LP (CSF analysis for microscopy, protein, glucose, oligoclonal bands, and cytology).

A diagnosis of demyelinating disease is supported by typical white matter plaques on MRI and oligoclonal bands in CSF (but not in serum).

Table 16.3 Differential diagnosis of acute/subacute optic neuropathy

Optic neuritis (typical)	Age 20–50, unilateral, ↓VA over hours/days, recovery starts within 2wks, retrobulbar pain
Compressive	Progressive ↓VA, disc pallor ± pain, involvement of other local structures
Sphenoid sinus disease	Persistent severe pain, pyrexia, history of sinusitis; consider fungal disease in the immunosuppressed, in diabetic ketoacidosis or in the elderly; **NB** Can present silently in non-pyrexial individuals
Sarcoidosis	Progressive ↓VA ± uveitis, symptoms or signs of sarcoidosis, very steroid-sensitive
Vasculitis (e.g. SLE)	Progressive ↓VA ± uveitis, symptoms or signs of vasculitis
Syphilis	Progressive ↓VA, disc swelling, ± uveitis; leucocytosis in CSF; symptoms or signs of syphilis; may be HIV+
AION	Sudden painless ↓VA, altitudinal field loss, swollen disc (may be segmental), usually older age group; features of arteritic or non-arteritic disease
Toxic or nutritional	Slowly progressive symmetrical ↓VA with central scotomas; relevant nutritional, therapeutic, or toxic history
LHON	Severe sequential ↓VA over weeks/months, telangiectatic vessels around disc (acutely); usually young adult males; family history
Postviral demyelination	Often bilateral ↓VA few weeks postviral or postvaccination, usually in children/young adults; ± acute disseminated encephalomyelitis

Anterior ischaemic optic neuropathy (1)

This is a significant cause of acute visual loss in the elderly population, affecting up to 10/100 000/yr of those over 50yrs. In 5–10% the aetiology is arteritic (GCA); in 90–95% it is non-arteritic.

GCA is an ophthalmic emergency requiring immediate assessment and appropriate institution of systemic steroid treatment.

Arteritic anterior ischaemic optic neuropathy

In arteritic AION, short posterior ciliary artery vasculitis leads to ischaemic necrosis of the optic nerve head.

Clinical features

- Sudden ↓VA (<6/60 in 76%); headache, scalp tenderness, jaw claudication, weight loss, night sweats, myalgia (association with polymyalgia rheumatica); may have a warning episode of transient ↓VA (short obscurations or longer amaurosis fugax-like episodes).
- RAPD, swollen disc (typically pale; rarely segmental), ± peripapillary haemorrhages and cotton wool spots, abnormal temporal arteries (thickened, tender, non-pulsatile).
- *Associations*: CRAO, BRAO, cilioretinal artery occlusion, III, IV, VI palsy.

Investigations

Immediate ESR, CRP, FBC: ↑ESR, ↑CRP, and ↑Plt are all supportive of GCA. Consider urgent temporal artery biopsy (aim for within a few days, although positive results may be obtained up to 7d after treatment. ESR should be interpreted in context (Box 16.2).

Box 16.2 Interpretation of ESR results

The upper limit of normal for ESR has traditionally been approximated to age/2 for men and (age +10)/2 for women. However, it is increasingly thought that this upper limit may in fact be rather 'generous': a lower upper limit may need to be considered.

ESR will be lower in the presence of polycythaemia, haemoglobin-opathies, hereditary spherocytosis, congestive cardiac failure, and anti-inflammatory medications.

ESR will be elevated by anaemia, malignancy, infection, and inflammation.

Treatment

- Immediate adequate steroid treatment (e.g. 1g methylprednisolone IV 1×/d for 1–3d) followed by oral prednisolone 1–2mg/kg 1×/d). Aspirin may have additional benefit. Once disease is controlled steroids may be titrated according to symptoms and inflammatory markers (CRP responds more quickly than ESR).
- Treatment lasts several years so osteoporosis prophylaxis is important.
- Side-effects of steroids (see Systemic corficosteroids [1] p.868).

Prognosis

The risk of second eye involvement ranges from 10% (if treated) to 95% (untreated). Other complications of GCA include: TIA, stroke, myocardial infarcts, neuropathies, mesenteric artery occlusion, thoracic artery aneurysms, and death.

Box 16.3 American College of Rheumatology (ACR) Traditional Criteria 1990 for the diagnosis of giant cell arteritis

- Age ≥50yrs at disease onset
- New onset of localized headache
- Temporal artery tenderness or decreased pulse
- ESR ≥50mm/h
- Arterial biopsy with necrotizing arteritis with a predominance of mononuclear cell infiltrates or granulomatous process with multinuclear giant cells

The presence of three or more of five of the above criteria was associated with 93.5% sensitivity and 91.2% specificity.

Table 16.4 Investigations in GCA

	Sensitivity	Specificity
Histological		
Temporal artery biopsy	80–90% (unilateral Bx)	≤100%
	95–97% (bilateral Bx)	
Haematological		
Bx proven GCA vs normal controls (Hayreh[1])		
↑ ESR	92%	94%
↑ CRP	100%	
↑ ESR + ↑ CRP		97%
Bx positive vs negative patients with clinical suspicion of GCA (Foroozan[2])		
↑ ESR + ↑ Plt	51%	91%
Imaging		
Duplex US:		
Characteristic 'halo rings' = oedematous wall swellings (Karassa[3])		
US compared with Bx proven GCA	69%	82%
US compared with the ACR Criteria	55%	94%
High resolution MRI (Bley[4])		
MRI compared with the ACR Criteria	80.6%	97%

1. Hayreh SS, Podhajsky PA, Raman R, Zimmerman B. Giant cell arteritis: validity and reliability of various diagnostic criteria. *Am J Ophthalmol* 1997 Mar;**123**(3):285–96.

2. Foroozan R, Danesh-Meyer H, Savino PJ, Gamble G, *et al.* Thrombocytosis in patients with biopsy-proven giant cell arteritis. *Ophthalmology.* 2002 Jul;**109**(7): 1267–71.

3. Karassa FB, Matsagas MI, Schmidt WA, Ioannidis JP. Meta-analysis: test performance of ultrasonography for giant-cell arteritis. *Ann Intern Med.* 2005 Mar 1;**142**(5):359–69.

4. Bley TA, Uhl M, Carew J, Markl M, Schmidt D, Peter HH, Langer M, Wieben O.

Diagnostic value of high-resolution MR imaging in giant cell arteritis. *AJNR Am J Neuroradiol.* 2007 Oct; **28**(9): 1722–7. Epub 2007 Sep 20.

Anterior ischaemic optic neuropathy (2)

Non-arteritic anterior ischaemic optic neuropathy

Non-arteritic AION comprises 90–95% of AION. Although the exact mechanism is unclear, there is perfusion insufficiency in the short posterior ciliary arteries, which leads to infarction of the retrolaminar portion of the disc.

Identified vascular risk factors should be modified to try to prevent further ophthalmic and systemic complications.

Risk factors

These are multiple and include: diabetes, atherosclerosis, disc morphology ('disc at risk'—crowded disc with a small cup), hypertension hyperlipidaemia, hypotension, haemoconcentration, haemodilution, and hypercoagulable states.

Clinical features

- ↓VA (usually sudden, but can be progressive; VA >6/60 in 61%; ≥6/12 in 18%); commonly occur overnight; occasional pain.
- RAPD, field loss (45% inferior altitudinal; 15% superior altitudinal), swollen disc (typically hyperaemic, ± segmental, telangiectasia).
- *Associations*: 'disc at risk' in fellow eye.

Investigations

- First rule out GCA (assessment, see AION (1) 📖 p.588).
- If non-arteritic then: BP, glucose, lipids, FBC. If patient <50yrs then consider also vasculitis screen.

Treatment

- No proven benefit for any treatment (including steroids, optic nerve sheath defenestration, hyperbaric oxygen, dopamine, and aspirin); however, aspirin (e.g. 75mg/d) is commonly prescribed.
- Refer to physician for vascular assessment and treatment.

Prognosis

The risk of second eye involvement is about 19% over 5yrs, with an increased risk after cataract surgery. Additionally, cardiovascular and cerebrovascular diseases are more common, possibly with increased mortality.

Posterior ischaemic optic neuropathy

This rare condition describes ischaemia of the more posterior (retrolaminar) optic nerve. It appears to result from watershed infarction, associated with hypotension or low haematocrit. Clinically, there is sudden visual loss with an RAPD (if unilateral) but normal optic disc; bilateral involvement is common.

Table 16.5 Arteritic and non-arteritic AION

	Arteritic AION	Non-arteritic AION
Incidence	1/100 000/yr	10/100 000/yr
Cause/possible associations	GCA	*Major:* diabetes, hypertension, disc morphology
		Minor: smoking, hyperlipidaemia, hypotension, anaemia, hypermetropia, obstructive sleep apnoea
Age (mean)	70yrs	60yrs
VA + field	Sudden ↓	Sudden ↓
	Usually <6/60	Usually >6/60
		Often altitudinal field loss
Associated symptoms	Scalp tenderness, jaw claudication, headache	Usually none
Disc	Swollen	Swollen (often sectoral)
	Commonly pale	Commonly hyperaemic
		Predisposed (small + crowded)
ESR	↑↑ (mean = 70mmHg)	Normal
CRP	↑↑	Normal
Plt	↑	Normal
Risk to fellow eye	10% (if treated) to ≤95% (unteated)	
Prognosis	Up to 15% improve	40% improve (by ≥2 Snellen lines)

Perioperative visual loss

A very rare but devastating complication following non-ocular surgery. Presumed mechanism is ischaemic optic neuropathy with AION more commonly reported following cardiac procedures and PION reported following prolonged spinal surgery in the prone position. The exact aetiology is not known. Most have bilateral simultaneous involvement usually associated with very poor visual function. This complication warrants senior review and careful medical documentation. Owing to the serious implications of this diagnosis, this aetiology should not be postulated until due consideration of the evidence.[1]

1. American Society of Anesthesiologists Task Force on Perioperative Blindness. Practice advisory for perioperative visual loss associated with spine surgery: a report by the American Society of Anesthesiologists Task Force on Perioperative Blindness. *Anesthesiology* 2006 Jun; 104(6):1319–28.

Other optic neuropathies/atrophies

Leber's hereditary optic neuropathy

This rare condition is maternally inherited, arising from point mutations in mitochondrial DNA. It may present at almost any age but typically in young adult males (M:F 3:1). Family history is present in around 50%. The mutations identified are 11 778 (the commonest comprising 95%), 3460 and 14 484, all of which affect complex I of the respiratory chain. LHON has some similarities to nutritional and toxic neuropathies and indeed the presentation of LHON may be precipitated by a toxic insult.

Clinical features
- Sudden painless sequential ↓VA (usually affects second eye within 2mths; typically 6/60 HM).
- Large dense centrocaecal scotoma, ↓colour vision; disc may show peripapillary telangiectasia and peripapillary nerve fibre layer swelling (early) and temporal pallor (late); **NB** pupillary reactions are usually normal.

Investigations and treatment
Mitochondrial DNA analysis for LHON mutations (peripheral blood); consider also screening for differential diagnosis, including toxins/deficiencies. There is no effective treatment. The majority has a poor visual prognosis, although some spontaneous recovery is seen with the uncommon 14 484 mutation.

Nutritional and toxic optic neuropathies

These uncommon acquired optic neuropathies all behave in a similar manner, probably due to a common disruption of mitochondrial oxidative phosphorylation.

Tobacco–alcohol amblyopia may represent a combination of toxin (cyanide in tobacco smoke) and nutritional deficiency (low B12 associated with alcohol excess). Numerous other agents have been identified (Table 16.6).

Clinical features
- Subacute painless bilateral ↓VA (typically 6/9–6/60).
- Small central/centrocaecal scotomas, ↓colour vision; ± swelling of disc/peripapillary nerve fibre layer (early) and temporal pallor (late).

Investigations and treatment
- A detailed history may reveal the cause.
- *Consider*: B1, B2, B12, folic acid levels (peripheral blood), and heavy metal screening (including 24h urine).
- Treat deficiency with oral supplementation, other than B12 (IM and must be given with folate). In alcoholics, consider prophylactic vitamin supplementation.
- Identify and prevent route of toxin exposure (may affect others, e.g. family members).

Inherited optic atrophy

Autosomal dominant
Kjer syndrome is the commonest isolated optic atrophy, and is due to a mutation in 3q. Bilateral symmetrical ↓VA (usually 6/9–6/36) occurs insidiously in mid/late childhood.

Autosomal recessive

- *Isolated*: this is rare, severe, and presents early (age <4yrs).
- *Behr syndrome*: optic atrophy ± nystagmus, ataxia, spasticity, ↓IQ.
- *Wolfram syndrome* (DIDMOAD): diabetes insipidus, diabetes mellitus, optic atrophy, deafness.

Table 16.6 Causes of optic atrophy

Inherited		Kjer syndrome Behr syndrome Wolfram syndrome LHON
Compression	Extrinsic tumour	Pituitary Craniopharyngioma Meningioma Metastasis
	Intrinsic tumour	ON glioma ON sheath meningioma
	Other	Aneurysm Mucocele
Vascular		CRAO AION or PION
Inflammatory		Acute demyelinating optic neuritis Sarcoidosis Vasculitis (e.g. SLE, PAN)
Infection		Bacterial (e.g. TB, syphilis) Rickettsial (e.g. Lyme disease) Viral (e.g. measles, mumps, varicella) Fungal (e.g. *Aspergillus*)
Nutritional		B1 (thiamine) deficiency B2 (riboflavin) deficiency B6 deficiency B12 deficiency Folate deficiency
Toxic		Amiodarone Ethambutol Methanol Carbon monoxide Cyanide Isoniazid Lead Triethyl tin
Other		Trauma Disc oedema (e.g. papilloedema) Retinal disease (e.g. RP)

Papilloedema

Papilloedema describes optic disc swelling (usually bilateral) arising from raised intracranial pressure (ICP); the term should not be used to describe other causes of disc oedema. Raised ICP is transmitted from the subarachnoid space via the optic nerve sheath to cause axoplasmic hold-up and consequent disc oedema.

The urgent priority is to rule out an intracranial mass (e.g. tumour, abscess, haemorrhage); however, the commonest cause of papilloedema is idiopathic intracranial hypertension.

Clinical features

- Visual obscurations (transient ↓VA, few seconds duration, up to 30×/d, uni/bilateral, may be precipitated by posture/straining, etc.); diplopia; field defects (usually enlarged blind spot); sustained ↓VA is a serious sign of irreversible damage—it may occur early in aggressive disease or late in chronic papilloedema.
- ↑ICP leads to headache (often worse lying down/straining), nausea, vomiting, pulsatile tinnitus.
- Disc swelling: usually bilateral; however, swelling may not occur in an already abnormal disc/nerve sheath (e.g. congenital anomaly, optic atrophy, high myopia).

Staging of papilloedema

- *Early*: hyperaemic, blurred + elevated margin, subtle peripapillary nerve fibre layer oedema, dilated disc capillaries, distended retinal veins, absent SVP. Paton's lines are circumferential retino-choroidal folds that can be sometimes seen around the disc.
- *Acute*: as above + peripapillary haemorrhages, cotton wool spots, increased nerve fibre layer oedema (may obscure retinal vessels).
- *Chronic*: ↓hyperaemia, ↓CWS/haemorrhages, variable swelling, usually still elevated; ± drusen-like deposits and opto-ciliary shunt vessels at the disc (in which case sometimes called vintage papilloedema).
- *Atrophic/late*: pale atrophic disc, ↓ swelling, attenuated arterioles.

Investigation

Urgent neuroimaging (preferably MRI with gadolinium enhancement): may reveal primary pathology, hydrocephalus, or empty sella. *Consider*:

- *MRV* to check cerebral venous sinuses.
- *LP*: check opening pressure (normal <20cmH$_2$O or <25cmH$_2$O in the obese), glucose, protein, protein electrophoresis, microscopy, culture.
- *FFA* (if diagnostic uncertainty): late leakage from dilated disc capillaries.

Treatment

- Intervention depends on the underlying cause and severity and may range from weight loss to extensive neurosurgery.
- Shared care with another specialty (neurosurgery, neurology, oncology, medicine) is often necessary.
- Regular ophthalmic assessment of acuity, colour vision, fields, and disc status is invaluable to preserving vision.

Table 16.7 Causes of raised intracranial pressure

Mass effect	Tumour
	Haemorrhage
	Trauma (haematoma/oedema)
Increased CSF production	Choroid plexus tumour
Reduced CSF drainage	Stenosis of foramen/aqueduct (congenital or secondary to tumour, cyst, infection, etc.)
	Damage to arachnoid granulations (meningitis, subarachnoid haemorrhage)
	Idiopathic intracranial hypertension
Other	Malignant hypertension

Table 16.8 Conditions that cause intracranial hypertension[1]

Drugs	Tetracycline
	Corticosteroid withdrawal
	OCP
	Vitamin A derivatives
	Nalidixic acid
	Lithium
	Growth hormone
	Indometacin
	Cimetidine
Systemic disorders	Hypoparathyroidism
	Adrenal adenomas
	Renal failure
	Addison's disease
	Obstructive sleep apnoea syndrome
	Chronic obstructive pulmonary disease
Habitus	Obesity
Haematological	Cerebral venous sinus thrombosis

1. Digre KB, Corbett JJ. *Neurologist* 2001;**7**:2–67.

Idiopathic intracranial hypertension

Idiopathic intracranial hypertension (formerly known as benign intracranial hypertension and pseudotumour cerebri) is the commonest cause of papilloedema. It is a diagnosis of exclusion made in the presence of normal neuroimaging and CSF analysis, but with an elevated CSF opening pressure (Table 16.9). The prevalence is about 0.9/100 000 in the general population but up to 19/100 000 in obese young women.

Risk factors

It typically affects obese young women, but there is a wide age range of presentation. The strongest risk factors are obesity and recent weight gain.

Clinical features

- Visual obscurations (transient ↓VA, few seconds duration, uni/bilateral, up to 30×/d, may be precipitated by posture/straining, etc.); diplopia; field defects (usually enlarged blind spot); sustained ↓VA may be early in aggressive disease (usually an indication for shunting).
- Headache (in 94%; often worse lying down/straining), retrobulbar pain, pulsatile tinnitus.
- Disc swelling (usually bilateral; 📖 p.594).

Investigations

- *MRI with gadolinium enhancement and MRV*: aim to rule out all other causes of ↑ICP.
- *LP* (only proceed to LP if MRI/CT shows no intracranial mass): check opening pressure, glucose, protein, protein electrophoresis, microscopy, culture. Normal opening pressure in adults is usually <20cm H_2O, or <25cm H_2O in the obese; in children lower levels are normal.

Table 16.9 Diagnostic criteria for idiopathic intracranial hypertension[1]

Symptoms and signs of raised intracranial hypertension
Raised ICP as measured on lumbar puncture in the lateral decubitus position
CSF composition is normal
Neuroimaging with no evidence of hydrocephalus, mass, structural, or vascular lesion
No other cause of intracranial hypertension found (see Table 16.8)

1. Friedman DI, Jacobson DM. *Neurology* 2002;**59**:1492–9533.

Treatment

A Cochrane review in 2005 found no randomized controlled trials for treatment of idiopathic intracranial hypertensions.[2] Current management may include:

- *Weight loss*.
- *Medical*: acetazolamide (up to 500mg 4×/d) or consider furosemide.
- *Surgical*: optic nerve sheath fenestration.
- *Neurosurgical*: CSF diversions using a lumboperitoneal or ventriculoperitoneal shunting (but significant complications).

Titrate treatment against symptoms and risk of visual loss (monitor VA, colour vision, fields, discs). *If pregnant*: acetazolamide appears to be safe after 20wks gestation; weight loss is not advised.

Prognosis
- In the majority this is good. In the UK, a British Ophthalmic Surveillance Unit study found the incidence of blindness was 1–2%, which is lower than previously thought.
- Idiopathic intracranial hypertension can recur at any time after the original episode has resolved.

1. Friedman DI, Jacobson DM. Diagnostic criteria for idiopathic intracranial hypertension. *Neurology.* 2002 Nov 26;**59**(10):1492–5.

2. Lueck C, McIlwaine G. Interventions for idiopathic intracranial hypertension. Cochrane Database of Syst Rev 2005, Issue 3. Art. No.: CD003434. DOI:10.1002/14651858.CD003434.pub2.

Pseudopapilloedema

A number of disc anomalies may resemble papilloedema.

Clinical features
- Usually seen on a routine examination in an asymptomatic patient, whereas papilloedema is often accompanied with clinical symptoms and signs.
- Spontaneous venous pulsation: the central retinal vein can be seen to pulsate in about 80% of normal patients.

Differential diagnosis
- *Disc drusen*: may cause most diagnostic confusion as they may not be clinically obvious (buried) and may cause visual loss. Their prevalence is about 0.5% in caucasians. They may be inherited (autosomal dominant). They are usually bilateral, and become more obvious throughout life. The disc has a lumpy appearance, absent cup and the vessels emerge centrally and then show abnormal branching (trifurcation); opto-ciliary shunt vessels may be present. VA is usually normal but field defects occur in 75% (arcuate, blind spot enlargement, generalized constriction). They are associated with CNV. Their presence may be demonstrated by their autofluorescence, or on B-scan US or CT.
- *Hypermetropic* discs may appear crowded and elevated. *Myopic* discs are often elevated nasally and may show leakage on FFA. *Tilted* discs are usually elevated superotemporally.

Table 16.10 Causes of apparent disc swelling

True disc swelling	Papilloedema	↑ICP	Tumours, etc. (Table 16.7)
	Local disc swelling	Inflammatory	Optic neuritis
			Uveitis
			Scleritis
		Granulomatus	Tuberculosis
			Sarcoid
		Infiltrative	Leukaemia
			Lymphoma
		Vascular	AION
			CRVO
			Diabetic papillitis
		Tumours	Of optic nerve (meningioma, glioma)
			Of orbit
		Hereditary	LHON
No true disc swelling	Pseudo-papilloedema	Structural	Disc drusen
			Tilted discs
			Hypermetropic discs
			Myopic discs
			Myelinated peripapillary nerve fibres

Congenital optic disc anomalies

Congenital optic disc anomalies range from common variations with minimal sequelae (e.g. tilted discs) to severe abnormalities associated with poor vision and CNS abnormalities (e.g. morning glory anomaly).

Tilted disc

In this common bilateral but often asymmetric condition the optic nerves insert obliquely into the globe. It is often associated with myopia and oblique astigmatism.

The bitemporal field defects are unlike chiasmal lesions: they do not respect the vertical midline, they are static and in some cases may be resolved with refractive correction.

Clinical features

- Normal VA; may have superotemporal field defects.
- Disc usually orientated inferonasally with elevation of the superotemporal rim, thinning of the inferonasal RPE/choroid, and situs inversus of the retinal blood vessels.

Optic disc pit

This rare, usually unilateral, condition may cause significant visual problems. Its origin is unclear but it represents a herniation of neuroectodermal tissue into a depression within the optic nerve.

Clinical features

- Often asymptomatic; ↓VA if complications; field defects (commonly paracentral arcuate scotoma).
- Grey pit usually in the temporal part of the disc; disc itself is larger than in the unaffected eye.
- *Complications*: macular retinoschisis and subsequent serous retinal detachment may occur in up to 45%; this can be treated with vitrectomy and gas tamponade.

Optic nerve hypoplasia

This describes a reduced number of axons within the optic nerve. It is a significant cause of poor vision in childhood. It may be isolated or be associated with a range of CNS abnormalities (Table 16.11).

Clinical features

- Variable VA (normal to NPL), field defects, colour vision, pupil reactions.
- Small grey disc surrounded by an inner yellow ring of chorioretinal atrophy and an outer pigment ring (double-ring sign).
- Other features may include aniridia, microphthalmos, strabismus, nystagmus.

Table 16.11 Associations of optic disc hypoplasia

Syndromic	De Morsier syndrome (septo-optic dysplasia)
Non-syndromic	Isolated midline CNS abnormalities
	Endocrine abnormalities

Optic disc coloboma

This rare condition arises from incomplete closure of the embryonic fissure (inferonasal), with variable involvement of the adjacent retina and choroid. It may be sporadic or autosomal dominant, and may be isolated, part of a syndrome, or occasionally associated with trans-sphenoidal encephalocele (Table 16.12).

Clinical features

- ↓VA (according to severity of coloboma), superior field defect.
- Glistening white bowl-shaped excavation within the disc (inferior part predominantly affected) ± chorioretinal/ciliary body/iris colobomas.

Table 16.12 Associations of optic disc coloboma

Chromosomal	Patau syndrome (trisomy 13)
	Edward syndrome (trisomy 18)
	Cat-eye syndrome (trisomy 22)
Other syndromes	Aicardi syndrome
	CHARGE syndrome
	Walker–Warburg syndrome
	Goltz syndrome
	Goldenhar syndrome
	Meckel–Gruber syndrome

Morning glory anomaly

This very rare condition describes a usually unilateral excavation of the posterior globe that includes the optic disc and may even include the macula ('macula capture').

Clinical features

- Severe ↓VA.
- Enlarged pink disc located within the excavation and surrounded by an elevated and irregularly pigmented annular zone; vessels are abnormally straight with arteries and veins being of similar appearance.
- *Complications*: serous retinal detachments may occur in 30%.
- *Associations*: include a syndrome of trans-sphenoidal encephalocele with hyertelorism, flat nasal bridge, midline cleft lip/palate, and often panhypo-pituitarism.

Megalopapilla

Megalopapilla describes an unusually large but essentially normal disc. They have a high cup:disc ratio that may be confused with glaucomatous change.

Chiasmal disorders

The chiasm permits the hemidecussation of visual information from the temporal fields so that information from the right visual field of both eyes is processed in the left visual cortex and vice versa. It lies in an anatomically crowded region so chiasmal syndromes may be accompanied by other neurological or endocrine abnormalities.

The commonest and best known disorder of the chiasm is a pituitary adenoma causing bitemporal hemianopia; however, a wide range of other lesions and clinical presentations may be seen (Table 16.13).

Clinical features

- Often asymptomatic unless central (↓VA) or advanced peripheral field loss; in advanced cases a pre-existing phoria may lead to hemifield slide due to loss of overlap between the 2 eyes (can also cause diplopia); during close work an object placed just beyond fixation may disappear (postfixation blindness).
- *Field loss*: classically bitemporal but often asymmetric and dependent on exact site of lesion (Table 16.14).
- Headache (usually frontal).

Associated features

Involvement of III, IV, Va, Vb, VI, and sympathetic nerve fibres: may result in abnormalities of pupils (including Horner syndrome), ocular motility, and facial sensation. Rarely see-saw nystagmus may occur.

- ↑*ICP*: may cause nausea, vomiting, pulsatile tinnitus, and papilloedema; hydrocephalus (blockage of foramen of Munro from posterior chiasmal lesions) may cause abnormal gait, urinary incontinence, drowsiness, and Parinaud syndrome.
- *Functioning pituitary tumours*: may cause acromegaly or gigantism (↑growth hormone; large hands/feet and coarsening of features or abnormal height), Cushing syndrome (↑ adrenocorticotrophic hormone; moon face, truncal obesity, hypertension), hyperprolactinaemia (impotence and galactorrhoea).
- Pituitary destruction causes hypopituitarism with loss of luteinizing hormone/follicle-stimulating hormone (↓libido, amenorrhoea; may present as primary infertility), growth hormone (silent unless pubertal), TSH (hypothyroidism), and adrenocorticotrophic hormone (secondary hypoadrenalism with collapse). Hypothalamic involvement may cause diabetes insipidus (↓anti-diuretic hormone; polydipsia, polyuria).

Investigations

- Accurate field testing and interpretation is vital.
- *Urgent neuroimaging*: MRI (gadolinium enhanced) is preferred, although CT is better at detecting bony involvement.
- Consider endocrinological assessment and LP for CSF analysis.

Treatment

The ophthalmologist's role is first to diagnose, second to refer for appropriate treatment (e.g. to endocrinology, neurosurgery, or often to a multi-specialty pituitary team), and third to monitor the patient's vision long-term (VA, colour vision, visual fields). Late loss of vision may represent tumour recurrence or may be as a result of treatment (radiotherapy).

Table 16.13 Causes of chiasmal syndromes

Pituitary	Adenoma (functioning or non-functioning)
	Apoplexy (e.g. Sheehan syndrome—very rare)
	Lymphocytic hypophysitis
Suprasellar	Meningioma
	Craniopharyngioma
Chiasm	Optic glioma
	Chiasmatic neuritis
Other	ICA aneurysm
	AVM (e.g. Wyburn–Mason syndrome)
	Cavernous haemangioma
	Germinoma
	Lymphoma
	Sarcoidosis
	Langerhans cell histiocytosis
	Metastasis
	Radionecrosis

Table 16.14 Localization by field defect

Superior bitemporal loss	Inferior lesion, e.g. pituitary adenoma
Inferior bitemporal loss	Superior lesion, e.g. craniopharyngioma
Junctional (central scotoma with superotemporal field loss in contralateral eye)	Anterior chiasmal lesion to side of central scotoma, e.g. sphenoid meningioma
Bitemporal central hemianopic scotomas	Posterior chiasmal lesion, e.g. hydrocephalus
Nasal loss	Lateral lesion, e.g. ectasia of the ICA

Table 16.15 Treatment options for chiasmal lesions

Pituitary adenoma	Medical (cabergoline or bromocriptine if prolactin secreting; octreotide if growth hormone secreting)
	Surgical resection (e.g. trans-sphenoidal route)
	Radiotherapy
Pituitary apoplexy	Hormone replacement (including high-dose corticosteroids)
	Trans-sphenoidal decompression
Meningioma	Surgical resection ± radiotherapy
Craniopharyngioma	Surgical resection ± radiotherapy
Optic glioma	Controversial (conservative vs surgery vs radiotherapy)

Retrochiasmal disorders

Most retrochiasmal disorders are associated with significant additional neurological morbidity, and hence such patients tend to have already been assessed, investigated, and started on treatment/rehabilitation before seeing an ophthalmologist. However, lesions that are otherwise clinically silent (e.g. some occipital pathology) may present first to the ophthalmologist.

The patient will usually be vague as to the problem with their vision, and even a dense hemianopia may be missed unless visual fields are routinely assessed (e.g. by confrontational testing).

Clinical features

Optic tracts

Incongruous homonymous hemianopia, optic atrophy, contralateral RAPD, larger pupil on the side of the hemianopia (Behr pupil), pupillary hemiakinesia (Wernicke's pupil).

Lateral geniculate nucleus

Incongruous homonymous hemianopia, normal pupils; often associated with thalamic and corticospinal signs (mild hemiparesis).

Optic radiations

- *Parietal lesions*: inferior incongruous homonymous defect, usually sparing fixation (macula fibres pass between parietal and temporal lobes); may be associated with damage to the posterior limb of the internal capsule (contralateral hemiparesis + hemianaesthesia), injury to the pursuit pathways (fails to pursue to the side of the lesion; cannot follow an OKN drum rotated to the side of the lesion), and Gerstmann syndrome (dominant parietal lobe only).
- *Temporal lesions*: superior incongruous homonymous defect ('pie in sky'), usually sparing central vision; may be associated with memory loss, hallucinations (olfactory, gustatory, auditory), and receptive dysphasia.
- *Calcarine cortex (occipital) lesions*: congruous homonymous defect; variants include sparing of the temporal crescent (represented anteriorly), sparing of the macula (represented posteriorly), or a congruous homonymous macular lesion (selective injury to the occipital tip); may be associated with visual hallucinations (usually in the hemianopic field) and denial of blindness (Anton syndrome).

Investigations

- *Urgent neuroimaging*: MRI (gadolinium enhanced) is preferable although CT may be adequate for many lesions and may be advantageous in the presence of extensive haemorrhage.
- Further investigations will be directed by the nature of the lesion found.

Treatment

After diagnosis the main role of the ophthalmologist is to refer for appropriate treatment of the underlying cause (e.g. to stroke unit, neurosurgery, oncology). A secondary role is in co-ordinating visual rehabilitation/support (may include visual impairment registration).

Primary headache disorders

Migraine is a very common recurrent headache disorder that may be severely disabling. Its prevalence is estimated as up to 20% for men and 40% for women. About 25% cases present before the age of 10yrs, and 90% before the age of 40yrs. Overall, it is commoner in women but under 12yrs of age is slightly more common in boys. A first-degree relative confers a relative risk of 3.8 for classic migraine and 1.9 for common migraine.

The mechanism is uncertain: migraineurs appear to have an inherited susceptibility to environmental factors that trigger noradrenaline and serotonin release. These cause constriction of cortical vessels (spreading neuronal depression → aura) and dilation of extracranial vasculature (perivascular pain receptors → headache).

Clinical features

Migraine without aura (Box 16.4)
- *Prodrome*: mood/autonomic system disturbance (e.g. fatigue, hunger, irritability).
- *Headache*: unilateral (may generalize), throbbing, moderate-severe intensity, worsens over 1–2h, usually subsides over 4–8h but may last 1–3d; may be associated with nausea, photophobia, and sensitivity to noise ('phonophobia').
- *Termination and postdrome phase*: recovery stages marked by fatigue.

Box 16.4 Diagnostic criteria for migraine without aura (IHS)[1]

At least 5 attacks fulfilling the following criteria:
1 Headache attacks lasting 4–72h (untreated or unsuccessfully treated)
2 Headache has at least 2 of the following:
   1. unilateral location
   2. pulsating quality
   3. moderate or severe pain intensity
   4. aggravated by or causing avoidance of routine physical activity (e.g. walking or climbing stairs).
3 During headache at least one of the following:
   1. nausea and/or vomiting
   2. photophobia and phonophobia
4 No other cause found

1. Headache Classification Subcommittee of the International Headache Society. The International Classification of Headache Disorders (2nd edn). *Cephalalgia*. 2004;**24**:9–160.

Migraine with aura (Box 16.5)
This is characterized by an aura that usually precedes the headache phase, but may coincide with or follow it. The aura is most often visual but may be somatosensory, motor, or speech.
- *Visual* (99% of migraineurs): typically starts paracentrally and expands temporally; the advancing edge forms a positive scotoma (flickering/shimmering/zigzag/multicoloured lights), whereas the trailing edge is negatively scotomatous; other visual phenomena include foggy vision, 'heat waves', tunnel vision, and complete loss of vision.
- *Somatosensory* (40%): hemisensory paraesthesia/anaesthesia.
- *Motor* (18%): hemiparesis.
- *Speech* (20%): dysphasia.

At least 2 attacks fulfilling the criteria of clinical symptoms of either typical aura with migraine; typical aura with non-migraine; typical aura without headache; familial hemiplegic migraine; sporadic hemiplegic migraine or a basilar type migraine. With no other cause found.

1. Headache Classification Subcommittee of the International Headache Society. The International Classification of Headache Disorders 2nd edn. *Cephalalgia*. 2004;**24**:9–160.

Retinal migraine (Box 16.6)
Repeated attacks of monocular visual disturbance, such as scintillations, scotomas or blindness, associated with migraine headache.

At least 2 attacks of a fully reversible monocular positive and/or negative visual phenomena (e.g., scintillations, scotomas or blindness) confirmed by examination during an attack or from the patient history.

The headache must fulfil the criteria 1–4 in Box 16.4 and migraine without aura begins during the visual symptoms or follows them within 60min.

A normal ophthalmology exam between attacks and not attributed to another disorder.

1. Headache Classification Subcommittee of the International Headache Society. The International Classification of Headache Disorders 2nd edn. *Cephalalgia*. 2004;**24**:9–160.

Investigation
Migraine (with or without aura) may be diagnosed on the basis of a typical history in the presence of a normal neurological examination. Atypical features in the history (e.g. age >55yrs, occipitobasal headache) or persistent neurological deficits require further assessment by a neurologist (may include neuroimaging, carotid Doppler scan, ECG, echocardiography, vasculitis screen).

Treatment
- *Prophylactic*: avoid trigger factors (e.g. cheese, chocolate, coffee, citrus, cola, Chinese food, contraceptive pill); medical treatment is considered if ≥2 disabling attacks/month (e.g. propranolol, amitriptyline, sodium valproate).
- *Therapeutic*: relax in a dark quiet room; aspirin, NSAIDs, or combination analgesics; consider 5HT1 agonist (e.g. sumatriptan 50mg PO or 10mg nasally stat) for more severe attacks.

Supranuclear eye movement disorders (1)

Eye movements serve to either bring an object of interest on to the fovea (saccades, quick phase of nystagmus) or maintain it there (vestibular, optokinetic, pursuit, vergences). (See Fig. 16.2.)

Movement of the globe requires sufficient contraction of the extraocular muscles to first overcome orbital viscosity and then to sustain the new position against the elastic restoring force. The ocular motor neurones (originating from III, IV, VI nuclei) achieve this by pulse-step innervation whereby they generate first a phasic and then a tonic stimulus. For example, in saccades a high-frequency signal from excitatory burst neurones excites the ocular motor nucleus directly (resulting in a 'pulse') but also indirectly via neural integrators (which mathematically integrate the signal to give a 'step'). Pause cells act as dampers to prevent unwanted saccadic activity. Supranuclear pathways control this activity. Horizontal conjugate gaze requires the VI nucleus to simultaneously drive ipsilateral LR, drive contralateral MR (via the MLF to contralateral III nucleus), and to inhibit the contralateral LR (via inhibitory burst cells to contralateral VI nucleus). Saccades originate in the contralateral FEF.

Pursuit eye movements originate in the ipsilateral parieto-occipito-temporal junction. Vestibular input (e.g. for vestibulo-ocular reflex) is from the contralateral vestibular nucleus complex. Convergence input is directly to both III nucleus, avoiding the MLF. Control of vertical eye movements are more complex as the system is effectively a torsional one that has been subverted to permit vertical movements.

Disorders of horizontal gaze

Horizontal gaze palsy
Lesions of the PPRF or VI nucleus result in failure to move the eyes beyond the midline to the side of the lesion; the vestibulo-ocular reflex, is preserved in a PPRF lesion, but lost in a VI nucleus lesion.

Internuclear ophthalmoplegia
Lesions of the MLF (connecting the III and contralateral VI nerve nuclei) result in failure of ipsilateral adduction and overshoot of the contralateral eye ('ataxic nystagmus'), which are best demonstrated on saccadic movements; may be associated with upbeat and torsional nystagmus, loss of vertical smooth pursuit, abnormal vestibulo-ocular reflex, and skew deviation. Convergence is preserved.

One and a half syndrome
Lesion of the MLF and the PPRF (or VI nucleus) on the same side result in an ipsilateral gaze palsy and an ipsilateral internuclear ophthalmoplegia. There is loss of horizontal movements other than abduction of the contralateral eye.

Tonic gaze deviation
Destructive lesions of the FEF (e.g. acute strokes) cause loss of gaze initiation to the contralateral side with the result that the eyes deviate to the side of the lesion. Irritative lesions (e.g. trauma, tumour) cause transient deviations to the contralateral side.

Locked in syndrome

Large lesions of the ventral pons may destroy bilateral PPRF and the corticospinal pathways resulting in loss of all voluntary motor activity except lid movements and vertical eye movements (cf. coma where all voluntary movements are lost).

Selective loss of pursuits

Lesions of the parieto-occipito-temporal junction cause failure of pursuit to the side of the lesion. This can also be demonstrated by inability to follow an OKN drum rotated to the side of the lesion. It is often associated with a contralateral homonymous field defect (usually superior).

Selective loss of saccades

Selective saccadic loss may occur in congenital or acquired ocular motor apraxia. In the congenital form the child learns after a few months to compensate by 'head thrusts' (± blinks) beyond the target; these become less noticeable with age. In the acquired form head thrusts are not a major feature; it may occur in bilateral frontoparietal injuries or diffuse cerebral disease.

Fig. 16.2 Supranuclear inputs for horizontal eye movements.

Connections are shown for eye movements to the left (including saccades from frontal eye fields (FEF), smooth pursuit from the parieto-occipito-temporal junction (POT), and vestibulo-ocular reflex from vestibular nucleus). For convergence movements the III nuclei are innervated directly to drive both MR. For further explanation see text. PPRF, paramedian pontine reticular formation. L, lateral rectus; M, medial rectus.

Supranuclear eye movement disorders (2)

Vertical gaze palsies

Parinaud dorsal midbrain syndrome

Lesions of the posterior commissure and pretectal area result in supra-nuclear upgaze palsy (saccades affected first, then pursuits, and finally vestibulo-ocular reflex), light–near dissociation, lid retraction, and convergence retraction nystagmus.

Causes include hydrocephalus, tumour, trauma, AVMs, CVA, demyelination.

Progressive supranuclear palsy (Steele–Richardson–Olszewski syndrome)

PSP is a rare progressive neurodegenerative disease caused by abnormal accumulation of tau proteins (microtubule-binding proteins) proteins. Age of onset is >40yrs.

Clinical features include: vertical supranuclear palsy, with slowing of vertical saccades(ultimately involves horizontal eye movements). Lid apraxia is a very early sign and may lead to corneal exposure from failure of lid closure. Other useful signs include frequent or continuous square wave jerks, abnormal vertical OKN and reduced blink rate. There is prominent postural instability, usually within the first year and early cognitive impairment.

There is no effective treatment at present.

Other supranuclear gaze palsies

Selective upgaze palsy may occur in Wilson's disease. Selective downgaze palsy with athetosis and ataxia occurs in Niemann–Pick's disease type C.

Tonic gaze deviation

Raised ICP or thalamic haemorrhage may cause forced downgaze ('sunset sign'), although it may occur as a transient phenomenon in healthy neonates.

Selective loss of saccades

In Huntington's disease there is selective loss of saccades (vertical more so than horizontal), which may be compensated for by head thrusts and blinks.

Skew deviation

This is a vertical deviation that is usually concomitant and associated with torsion. Dysfunctions of the vertical vestibulo-ocular reflex pathways are usually caused by lesions of the pons or lateral medulla (e.g. CVA, demyelination). Incomitant skews may be confused with IVn (or IIIn) palsies.

Table 16.16 Location of ocular premotor and motor neurones

Pause cell	Nucleus raphe interpositus
Horizontal burst cell	Paramedian pontine reticular formation
Horizontal inhibitory burst cell	Nucleus paragigantocellularis dorsalis
Horizontal integrator	Medial vestibular nucleus Nucleus prepositus hypoglossi
Horizontal ocular motor nucleus	VIn nucleus
Vertical burst cell	Rostral interstitial nucleus of MLF
Vertical inhibitory burst cell	Rostral interstitial nucleus of MLF (probable)
Vertical integrator	Interstitial nucleus of Cajal
Vertical ocular motor nuclei	III nucleus, IV nucleus

Third nerve disorders

A third nerve palsy may be the first sign of an aneurysm of the posterior communicating artery. Unfortunately, it may also be the last sign before the aneurysm ruptures causing subarachnoid haemorrhage and often death.

Diagnosis may be difficult: a partial palsy may simulate a number of other conditions. Classical teaching associates painful, pupil-involving, progressive lesions with compressive disease (e.g. an expanding aneurysm). However, the differentiation of a compressive from an ischaemic third nerve palsy may not be possible on clinical grounds alone.

Anatomy
See Anatomy and physiology (📖 p.578).

Classification
Accurate localization greatly assists diagnosis. Identify whether it is:
- Complete vs partial (including aberrant regeneration).
- Pupil-sparing vs pupil-involving.
- Nuclear, fascicular, or peripheral (nerve palsy).
- Isolated vs complex (other neurological defects).

Clinical features
- Variable presentation according to extent of loss of third nerve function. May include: pain, diplopia (due to horizontal and/or vertical ophthalmoplegia), ptosis, and pupil dilation.

What is the character of the pain/headache?
- A severe headache ('worst pain in my life', 'like someone kicked me in the back of the head') in this context should be assumed to be due to subarachnoid haemorrhage until proven otherwise; pain is classically associated with compressive lesions but may also occur in ischaemia.

Is it complete or partial?
- *Complete*: diplopia (horizontal and often vertical); complete ptosis, eye abducted, and usually depressed.
- *Partial*: any of the above features from near-complete involvement to isolated ptosis or single muscle paresis (rare).
- Aberrant regeneration is usually associated with long-standing compressive lesions. In lid-gaze dyskinesia there is lid elevation on adduction ('inverse Duane's') or on depression ('pseudo von Graefe'). In pupil-gaze dyskinesia there is pupil constriction on adduction or depression. Pure eye movement dyskinesias may also occur (e.g. elevation when trying to adduct).

Is it pupil involving or pupil sparing?
- *Pupil involving*: mydriasis (no light or near response), difficulty focusing.

Is it nuclear, fascicular, or peripheral (nerve palsy)?
- Certain patterns of IIIn disorder are localizing (Table 16.17).

Is it isolated or complex?
- Check for involvement of all other cranial nerves including IIn (especially fields, discs), VIn (abduction), IVn (intorsion), cerebellum, and peripheral nervous system. Other neurological signs may be local (e.g. compressive lesion) or disseminated (e.g. demyelination).

Investigation

- *Pupil-involving or partial IIIn palsies* (often compressive): emergency neuroimaging (MRI with MRA or high resolution CTA). If normal consider further investigation such as LP (CSF for oligoclonal bands, glucose, protein, xanthochromia, MC&S, cytology).
- *Pupil-sparing complete IIIn palsies* (usually ischaemic): assess vascular risk factors (atherosclerosis or arteritis; BP, glu, lipids, ESR, CRP, FBC) and monitor closely for first week (e.g. every 2d) to ensure no developing pupil involvement. Likelihood of ischaemic cause increased if age >40yrs, known vasculopath, acute onset, non-progressive, and no other neurological abnormality. If no recovery at 3mths then investigate further (including MRI). Monitor in conjunction with orthoptists (including Hess /Lees charts and fields of BSV).

Treatment

This is dependent on the underlying cause. Posterior communicating artery aneurysms require immediate transfer to neurosurgical unit for open (clips) or endovascular (coils, balloons) treatment. Other pathologies may require referral to neurology, neurosurgery, oncology, or medicine. Diplopia may be relieved by intrinsic ptosis or occlusion (patch or contact lens).

Surgery is dictated by any residual function and may comprise staged lid and muscle procedures. While this may improve cosmesis, its effect on the field of BSV is less predictable; it may even worsen diplopia.

Prognosis

Untreated posterior communicating artery aneurysms rupture in two-third cases, of which half are fatal. Treatment reduces mortality rate to <5%.

After surgery compressive IIIn palsies usually recover (at least partially) over 6mths. Ischaemic IIIn palsies usually spontaneously recover over 4mths.

Box 16.7 Causes of IIIn palsy

- Aneurysms (usually of the posterior communicating artery)
- Microvascular ischaemia
- Tumour (e.g. parasellar)
- Trauma
- Demyelination
- Vasculitis
- Congenital

Table 16.17 Nuclear and fascicular IIIn syndromes

Nuclear	
Definitely nuclear	Unilateral palsy with contralateral SR paresis and bilateral partial ptosis
	Bilateral palsy without ptosis
Fascicular	
Red nucleus (paramedian midbrain)	Ipsilateral IIIn palsy
	Contralateral intention tremor + ataxia ± contralateral anaesthesia (*Benedikt syndrome*)
Cerebral peduncle (anterior midbrain)	Ipsilateral IIIn palsy
	Contralateral hemiparesis (*Weber syndrome*)

Fourth nerve disorders

Superior oblique weakness secondary to IVn palsy is a common cause of vertical strabismus. A third of cases are congenital, but may not present until adulthood. Acquired cases are commonly traumatic or due to microvascular infarction (Box 16.8). Bilateral IVn palsy is most commonly due to head injury.

Anatomy

See Anatomy and physiology (🕮 p.578).

Clinical features

- Diplopia (vertical and torsional; worse on downgaze), head tilt (to opposite side), aesthenopia.
- Ipsilateral hypertropia/phoria worse on down gaze or on ipsilateral head tilt; compensatory head tilt to opposite side; limited depression in adduction; extorsion (examine fundus: normal foveal position is level with lower third of disc; measure angle with double Maddox rod); may have V pattern.
- See Parks–Bielschewsky 3-step test (🕮 Ocular motility examination p. 31).

Is it congenital or acquired?

A large vertical prism fusion range and high concomitance suggests that the paresis is either congenital or, if acquired, a long-standing lesion.

Is it unilateral or bilateral?

Superior oblique palsy may be bilateral (particularly after head injury) but may be asymmetric. Typically, there is a reversing hypertropia with L/R on right gaze and R/L on left gaze, a prominent V pattern, and significant excyclotorsion (>10°). (See Box 16.9).

Is it isolated or complex?

Check for involvement of all other cranial nerves, including IIn (especially fields, discs), IIIn, Vn, and VIn, pupils (Horner, RAPD), cerebellum, and peripheral nervous system. Other neurological signs may be local (e.g. orbital apex lesion) or disseminated (e.g. demyelination).

Investigation

A history of abnormal head posture (check old photographs) or recent trauma may identify the cause. Assess vascular risk factors (atherosclerosis or arteritis; BP, glu, lipids, ESR, CRP, FBC). Likelihood of ischaemic cause increased if age >40yrs, known vasculopath, acute onset, non-progressive, and no other neurological abnormality.

If aetiology unclear or no recovery at 3mths then investigate further (including MRI). Monitor in conjunction with orthoptists (including Hess/Lees charts and fields of BSV).

Treatment

Orthoptic intervention with a vertical prism (or occlusion) may satisfactorily control diplopia.

Surgical options include ipsilateral IO weakening (myectomy or recession), contralateral IR recession, SO tuck and the Fells modified Harada–Ito procedure. SO tuck carries a significant risk of inducing an iatrogenic Brown syndrome.

Box 16.8 Causes of IVn palsy

- Congenital
- Trauma
- Presumed microvascular ischaemia
- Idiopathic
- Iatrogenic (following ENT, neuro- or ophthalmic surgery)
- Tumour (e.g. pinealoma, tentorial meningioma)
- Demyelination
- Vasculitis
- Meningitis
- Cavernous sinus lesions
- Tolosa–Hunt syndrome
- Herpes zoster ophthalmicus

Box 16.9 Features suggestive of bilateral IVn palsy

- Chin-down head posture (without much tilt)
- Reversing hyperdeviation
- Excyclotorsion >10°
- Prominent V pattern
- Bilateral failure of adduction in depression

Table 16.18 Nuclear and fascicular IVn syndromes

Sympathetic pathways	Ipsilateral Horner syndrome Contralateral SO palsy
MLF	Ipsilateral INO Contralateral SO palsy
Superior cerebellar peduncle	Ipsilateral ataxia, intention tremor Contralateral SO palsy

Sixth nerve disorders

Sixth nerve palsy is the commonest cause of neurogenic strabismus. Although VIn palsy results in an easily recognized abduction deficit, other pathologies may give a similar picture notably Duane syndrome, medial wall orbital fracture, and thyroid eye disease.

Anatomy
See Anatomy and physiology (📖 p.578).

Clinical features
- *Diplopia* (horizontal; worse for distance and on looking to the side of the lesion), head turn (to same side).
- *Esophoria/tropia* (worse for distance and on ipsilateral gaze); ipsilateral abduction deficit (ranges from saccadic slowing only, to complete loss of all movement beyond the midline).

Isolated or complex?
Check for involvement of all other cranial nerves, including IIn (especially fields, discs), IIIn, IVn, Vn, and VIIn, pupils (Horner), cerebellum, and peripheral nervous system. Other neurological signs may be local (e.g. the now very rare Gradenigo syndrome), disseminated (e.g. demyelination), or reflect ↑ICP (if the VIn palsy is a false localizing sign).

Investigation
Assess vascular risk factors (atherosclerosis or arteritis; BP, glu, lipids, ESR, CRP, FBC). Likelihood of ischaemic cause increased if age >40yrs, known vasculopath, acute onset, non-progressive, and no other neurological abnormality.

If aetiology unclear or no recovery at 3mths then investigate further (including MRI). Monitor in conjunction with orthoptists (including prism cover test, Hess charts, and fields of BSV).

Treatment
- Orthoptic intervention with a base-out prism (or occlusion) may satisfactorily control diplopia. Botulinum toxin injection into ipsilateral MR has both a therapeutic and diagnostic role. It may restore BSV, and if only temporary may be repeated. In any event it reveals any residual VIn function that might be augmented by a LR resection/MR recession.
- If there is no residual function then vertical muscle transposition would be required.
- If there is residual LR function transposition surgery will cause exotropia and should be avoided.

Box 16.10 Causes of VIn palsy

- Idiopathic
- Microvascular ischaemia
- Tumour (e.g. clivus, cerebellopontine angle, pituitary, nasopharyngeal)
- ↑ICP
- Trauma (basal skull fracture)
- Demyelination
- Vasculitis
- Meningitis
- Cavernous sinus thrombosis
- Carotid–cavernous fistula
- Congenital

Box 16.11 Differential diagnosis of abduction deficit

- Duane syndrome
- Convergence spasm
- Thyroid eye disease
- Myasthenia
- Myositis
- Medial wall fracture
- Distance esotropia of high myopia

Table 16.19 Nuclear and fascicular VIn syndromes

Nuclear	
PPRF (dorsal pons)	Ipsilateral gaze palsy
PPRF + MLF (dorsomedial pons)	Ipsilateral gaze palsy Ipsilateral INO (*One and a half syndrome*)
AICA territory (dorsolateral pons)	Ipsilateral gaze palsy Ipsilateral VIIn palsy Ipsilateral Vn palsy Contralateral hemianaesthesia (*Foville syndrome*)
Fascicular	
Corticospinal tract (ventral pons)	Ipsilateral VIn palsy
Facial colliculus (dorsal pons)	Contralateral hemiparesis (*Raymond syndrome*)
	Ipsilateral VIn palsy Ipsilateral VIIn palsy (*Millard–Gubler syndrome*)

AICA: anterior inferior cerebellar artery.

Seventh nerve disorders

The seventh or facial nerve has a number of important motor, sensory, and secretory functions. Of these it is the facial nerve's ability to close the eyelids (i.e. innervation of orbicularis oculi) that make it so important to the ophthalmologist.

Facial nerve palsy should not be underestimated. Do not automatically assume that every facial nerve palsy is a 'Bell's palsy', and be alert to its capacity to cause blinding exposure keratopathy.

Anatomy
See Anatomy and physiology (📖 p.578).

Function
- *Motor*: muscles of facial expression and movement; superficial platysma muscles of the neck and the stapedius ear muscles.
- *Sensory and secretory functions* (nerve intermedius and geniculate ganglion): lacrimal gland (via the greater superficial petrosal nerve) and salivary glands (via the chorda tympani, mediating taste for the anterior two-thirds of the tongue).

Clinical features
- Weakness of one side of the face/facial asymmetry (if unilateral).
- Lagophthalmos with or without lower lid ectropion.
- Corneal surface exposure.

NB Specifically assess orbicularis strength, Bell's phenomenon, and for signs of exposure keratopathy.

Is it isolated or complex?
Check for involvement of all other cranial nerves, including V nerve (cerebellopontine lesions), VI nerve (lesion in pons), and VII (cerebello-pontine angle lesions). Check for alteration of taste, salivation, and lacri-mation.

Is it an upper motor neurone or lower motor neurone lesion?
- In upper motor neurone lesions, the upper facial muscles still function (e.g. can still raise eyebrows) due to the bilateral innervation (see Anatomy, 📖 p.578). In lower motor neurone lesions both upper and lower facial muscles are involved.

Investigation
ENT or neurology referral to establish a cause for all new onset facial nerve palsies. All recurrent facial nerve palsy should undergo neuroimaging to exclude inflammatory or neoplastic causes.

Treatment

Box 16.12 Treatment of exposure keratopathy

- *Mild*: regular artificial tears ± ointment lubricant at night
- *Moderate*: intensive preservative free artificial tears; ointment lubrication at night with lids taped. Consider a temporary tarsorrhaphy.
- *Severe*: temporary or permanent tarsorrhaphy. Consider eyelid gold weight in chronic cases.

Box 16.13 Aetiology of VIIn palsy

- Bell's palsy (see Table 16.20)
- Ramsay–Hunt syndrome (VZV)
- Cerebellopontine angle lesions
- Trauma
- Otitis
- Neurofibroma (neurofibromatosis type 2)
- Parotid gland mass
- Congenital causes (Moebius syndrome)
- Guillain–Barré syndrome[1]
- Lyme disease[1]
- Sarcoidosis[1]
- Meningitis[1]

1. Tend to present with bilateral VII nerve weakness.

Table 16.20 Bell's palsy (Idiopathic facial paralysis)

Although the majority of facial nerve palsy (up to 70%) are idiopathic, this is a diagnosis of exclusion.

Natural history:

Can affect any age group (peak 40yrs)

Male Female

Common in diabetes and pregnancy

Symptoms reach their peak at 48h; most start recover at 2wks and 70–80% will spontaneously recover within 3–6mths

Immediate treatment:

Treat corneal exposure

Oral steroids: no significant benefit shown, larger studies required[1]

Oral aciclovir or valaciclovir: more studies, with follow-up of longer than 12mths required to determine benefit[1]

Exercises (EMG biofeedback ± mirror training): Further larger studies required to determine whether should be recommended in clinical practice[2]

Acupuncture: more studies are required to determine benefit[3]

Subsequent management:

Surgical treatment can improve facial function and cosmesis to some degree. Options include facial nerve repair, nerve substitution and muscle transposition

1. *Cochrane Database Syst Rev* 2004.

2. Cardoso JR et al. *Otol Neurotol* 2008.

3. *Cochrane Database Syst Rev* 2007.

Anisocoria

Assessing unequal pupils begins with a detailed history, including when and who noticed the difference in the pupil size; whether there are associated ophthalmic or neurological symptoms; any previous ophthalmic history and systemic history (see Anisocoria 📖 p.782).

Differential diagnosis of unequal pupils
- Physiological ansocoria.
- Iris pathology.
- Pharmacological.
- Sympathetic chain pathology (see 📖 Anisocoria: sympathetic chain p.622).
- Parasympathetic chain pathology (see 📖 Anisocoria: parasympathetic chain p.624).

Investigations
- See Pupils examination (📖 pp.26, 27).

Physiological anisocoria

This is a common cause of unequal pupils, affecting 15–20% of the normal population. As involutional ptosis (from LPS disinsertion) is also common, it is not infrequent to see the two conditions coexist, so mimicking a Horner syndrome.

Clinical features
- Classically the patient is asymptomatic.
- Pupils have brisk response to light.
- Pupils have brisk response to accommodation.
- Pupils briskly re-dilate after testing with light and accommodation.
- Clinically isolated with no associated ptosis or ocular motility problems.
- *Prognosis*: reassure patient.

Iris pathology

Secondary to intraocular surgery or trauma.

Pharmacological anisocoria

This is due to local instillation/inoculation (inadvertent or intentional).

Clinical features
- Fixed large (parasympathetic agents) or fixed small pupils.
- Unreactive to light or accommodation.
- Clinically isolated with no associated ptosis or ocular motility problems.

Table 16.21 Aetiology of pharmacological anisocoria

Dilated pupils	
Atropine	
Scopolamine (hyoscine)	Used in antiemtics (particularly motion sickness and postoperative nausea preparations)
Anticholinergic nasal sprays	
Ipratropium bromide	(e.g. nebulized ipratropium)
Solanaceae plants	Nightshades/belladonna and Datura/ Jimsom weed
Constricted pupils	
Organophosphate agents	(pesticides, nerve agents)
Opiates	
Pilocarpine	

Investigation
- *Dilated pupils*: 1% pilocarpine, wait for 45min. Pharmacological anisocoria is confirmed when there is refusal to fully constrict.
- *Constricted pupils*: 1% tropicamide, wait 45min. Pharmacological anisocoria is confirmed when there is refusal to fully dilate.

Sympathetic chain and parasympathetic chain pathology

For anisocoria arising from disorders of the sympathetic and parasympathetic chains, see Anisocoria: sympathetic chain (📖 pp.622–623) and Anisocoria: parasympathetic chain (📖 p.624).

Anisocoria: sympathetic chain

Horner syndrome

The ocular sympathetic supply may be damaged anywhere along its route. The extent of sympathetic dysfunction, associated neurological signs, and pharmacological tests help to identify the level of the injury.

Clinical features

- Pupil is miotic with normal light and near reaction.
- Anisocoria is most marked in dim conditions.
- Also ptosis, apparent enophthalmos (due to 1–2mm upper lid ptosis and 1mm elevation of lower lid), ↓IOP, conjunctival injection; facial anhydrosis suggests lesion of the 1st- or 2nd-order neuron; iris hypochromia suggests a congenital lesion (also in long-standing acquired lesions).

Is it isolated or complex?

Check for involvement of all other cranial nerves, including IIn (especially fields, discs), IIIn, IVn, Vn, and VIn, cerebellum, and peripheral nervous system. Other neurological signs may be local (e.g. cavernous sinus pathology) or disseminated (e.g. demyelination).

Also check for history of pain (headache, neck pain, arm pain), trauma or surgery, and any other physical signs, e.g. scars and masses (lung apices, neck, thyroid).

Investigation

- *Confirm diagnosis*: 4% cocaine to BE; repeat at 1min. At 0 and 60min measure pupil sizes when fixing on a distant target in identical ambient lighting conditions (bright and dim). Positive for Horner if no/poor dilation to cocaine (blocks reuptake of NorA at the dilator pupillae neuromuscular junction).
- *Identify level*: 1% hydroxyamphetamine to BE. If 1st- or 2nd-order neuron lesion there will be normal dilation; if 3rd-order neuron lesion then there will be no/poor dilation. This test is seldom performed in clinical practice. Topical hydroxyamphetamine is expensive and may not be readily available. The test is not reliable if performed within 48h of cocaine test.
- *Identify cause*: further investigation is directed by the likely cause and level of lesion (Tables 16.22 and 16.23).
- *Identify if congenital or acquired*: old photographs may show changes to be long-standing (view with a 20D to see pupils); also look for additional clinical features (as below).

Treatment and prognosis

- This is dependent on the underlying cause and may involve urgent referral to other specialities. Any recovery of a Horner also depends on the underlying cause and treatment.
- In cases associated with cluster headaches (Raeder syndrome) recovery may occur within a few hours.
- Other causes (e.g. invasive tumours) may cause relentless irreversible progression.

Congenital Horner syndrome

Usually idiopathic, but can be secondary to birth trauma (such as forceps delivery).

Clinical features
- Miosis, ptosis, and apparent enophthalmos, as described above.
- *Heterochromia*: lighter iris pigmentation on ipsilateral side.
- Facial flushing ('harlequin' sign), particularly seen on cycloplegic refraction or crying, due to ipsilateral anhydrosis. Generally the affected side is pale.

Caution
Acquired Horner syndrome in childhood, should be investigated for neuroblastoma.

Table 16.22 Investigations of Horner syndrome

Lesion type	Investigations
Central	MRI brain/spinal cord
Preganglionic	CXR CT thorax Carotid Doppler MRI/A head/neck LN biopsy
Postganglionic	Carotid Doppler MRI/A head/neck MRI orbits ENT assessment

Table 16.23 Aetiology of Horner syndrome

Lesion type	Location	Cause
Central	Brainstem	CVA Tumour Demyelination
	Spinal cord	Tumour Syringomyelia Trauma
Preganglionic	Lung apex	Pancoast tumour Trauma
	Neck	Trauma Surgery Tumour (thyroid, cervical LN) CCA dissection
Postganglionic	ICA	ICA dissection
	Middle ear	Otitis media Herpes zoster
	Cavernous sinus	Thrombosis Tumour
	Orbit	Tolosa–Hunt Tumour Cluster headache

NB Many acquired and congenital cases are idiopathic. CCA: common carotid artery; ICA: internal carotid artery; LN: lymph node

Anisocoria: parasympathetic chain

Adie's tonic pupil

In Adie's pupil the parasympathetic supply from the ciliary ganglion to the iris and ciliary muscle is abnormal. It is thought that this arises due to acute viral denervation and aberrant regeneration.

It is most commonly unilateral (80%) occurring in otherwise healthy young women.

Clinical features

- Classically, pupil is mydriatic, poor response to light with vermiform movements seen at the slit-lamp and exaggerated but slow and sustained (tonic) response to near; light–near dissociation.
- *Variants*: early lesions may show no response to light or near; late lesions are usually miotic; segmental lesions are common; there may be additional absence of deep tendon reflexes (Holmes–Adie syndrome) or patchy hypohidrosis (Ross syndrome); with time the pupil becomes miotic.

Investigations

- *Confirm diagnosis*: 0.125% pilocarpine to BE. At 0 and 30min measure pupil size when fixing on a distant target in identical dim lighting conditions.
- In Adie's the response is greater in the affected eye (denervation hypersensitivity of sphincter pupillae).

Treatment

- Reassure patient.
- Weak strength pilocarpine (e.g. 0.1% as often as required) may help treat mydriatic blurring and accommodative problems.
- Mydriasis may also be helped by a painted contact lens acting as an artificial pupil.
- Reading glasses may also help with the accommodative dysfunction.

Idiopathic intermittent unilateral mydriasis

One pupil transiently becomes large, lasting between 15min to hours. Patients complain of blurred vision, ocular pain, and photosensitivity. On examination the large pupil is clinically isolated. More commonly occurs in women and is associated with migraine, with nearly 50% have history of migraines.

Aetiology is either parasympathetic insufficiency of the iris sphincter, or sympathetic hyperactivity of the iris dilator.[1]

---

1. Jacobson DM. Benign episodic unilateral mydriasis. Clinical characteristics. *Ophthalmology* 1995;**102**:1623–7.

Argyll Robertson pupils

Argyll Robertson pupils present in the tertiary stage of neurosyphilis are now uncommon due to the introduction of penicillin.

Clinical features
- Initially unilateral, then bilateral irregular, miosed pupils.
- React poorly to light.
- Light–near dissociation.
- Iris can be atrophic on slit-lamp examination.

Investigations
- Fluorescent treponemal antibody absorption test (FTA-ABS), treponemal antibody haemagglutination test (MHA-TP) detect antibodies towards *Treponema pallidum* and will remain positive once infected.
- The rapid plasma reagin (RPR), venereal disease research laboratory (VDRL) test, and the automated regain test (ART) are all useful as ongoing measures of disease activity and response to treatment.

Treatment
- Liaise with GU team.
- IM injection of penicillin (dose is dependent on stage; benzathine penicillin is now the preferred preparation for syphilis in the UK (unlicensed indication)[1]).
- Spirochaete death may transiently worsen inflammation (Jarish–Herxheimer reaction).

> **Box 16.14 Differential diagnosis of light near dissociation**
>
> - Optic neuropathy or severe retinopathy
> - Argyll Robertson pupils
> - Long-standing Adie's tonic pupil
> - Mid-brain pathology
> - Diabetes
> - Amyloidosis

---

1. *British National Formulary* **56** (Sept. 2008). BMJ publishing group.

Nystagmus (1)

Nystagmus, oscillations, and saccadic intrusions are a group of involuntary abnormalities of fixation.

- In nystagmus there is an abnormal slow movement away from fixation that is then corrected by a fast movement (jerk nystagmus) or by another slow movement (pendular nystagmus).
- In oscillations and intrusions there is an abnormal saccade away from fixation followed by a corrective saccade, i.e. both movements are fast.
- The corrective saccade may be immediate (oscillation) or delayed (intrusion).

Classification

Analyse the movement disorder in a logical manner.

- *History*: early or late onset; presence of oscillopsia.
- *Abnormal movement away from fixation*: slow or fast.
- *Corrective movement*: slow or fast.
- *Direction*: horizontal, vertical, or rotatory.
- *Symmetry*: conjugate or disconjugate.
- *Effect on direction/amplitude of*: time, direction of gaze, fixation, head position.
- *VA*.
- *Associated involuntary movements*: palate, head, and neck.

Nystagmus with onset in infancy

This is not usually associated with oscillopsia; however, a minority of patients do get oscillopsia especially when looking in the direction of greatest nystagmus.

Idiopathic infantile nystagmus (idiopathic congenital nystagmus)

- Conjugate horizontal (usually) jerk nystagmus, worsens with fixation but improves within 'null zone' and on convergence. The null zone is a direction of gaze in which the nystagmus is damped down.
- It has a very early onset (usually by 2mths of age) and may initially be pendular.
- It can occasionally be vertical or rotatory.
- There is usually only mild ↓VA; strabismus is common.
- It may be inherited (AD, AR, X-linked).

Nystagmus associated with retinal disease (sensory deprivation)

Erratic waveform ± roving eye movements; moderate/severe ↓VA due to ocular or anterior visual pathway disease.

Box 16.15 Common retinal conditions associated with nystagmus in infancy

- Albinism
- Congenital stationary night blindness
- Colour blindness
- Cone-rod dystrophy
- Leber congenital amaurosis

Latent/manifest latent nystagmus
- Conjugate horizontal jerk nystagmus with fast phase towards fixing eye, worsens with occlusion of non-fixing eye, and with gaze towards fast phase but improves with gaze towards slow phase.
- It alternates if opposite eye takes up fixation; often associated with infantile esotropia.

Table 16.24 Early onset nystagmus

Waveform	Effect of occlusion	Nystagmus type
Horizontal jerk	Already evident	Idiopathic congenital
	Becomes manifest	Manifest latent
Erratic ± roving	No effect	Sensory deprivation

Nystagmus (2)

Acquired nystagmus: conjugate

Late onset or acquired nystagmus is usually associated with oscillopsia, and is often associated with other neurological abnormalities.

Gaze-evoked nystagmus

- Conjugate horizontal (usually) jerk nystagmus on eccentric gaze with fast phase towards direction of gaze; it occurs at smaller angles than physiological end-point nystagmus, i.e. <45°.
- Asymmetric gaze evoked nystagmus usually indicates failure of ipsilateral neural integrator/cerebellar dysfunction (*see* Supranuclear eye movement disorders 📖 p.608); symmetric gaze-evoked nystagmus may be due to CNS depression (fatigue, alcohol, anticonvulsants, barbiturates) or structural pathology (e.g. brainstem, cerebellum).

Periodic alternating nystagmus

- Conjugate horizontal jerk nystagmus present in primary position with waxing–waning nystagmus lasting for 90s in each direction with a 10s gap or 'null' period.
- Periodic alternating nystagmus is usually due to vestibulocerebellar disease (e.g. demyelination, Arnold–Chiara malformation). An alternating nystagmus without such regular periodicity may also be seen in severe ↓VA.

NB Periodic alternating nystagmus is easily missed if too brief an assessment of the pattern of nystagmus is made.

Peripheral vestibular nystagmus

- Conjugate horizontal jerk nystagmus, improves with fixation and with time since injury, worsens with gaze towards fast phase (Alexander's law) or change in head position.
- Nystagmus with fast phase away from the lesion is associated with destructive lesions of the vestibular system (e.g. labyrinthitis, vestibular neuritis), whereas nystagmus to the same side may be seen in irritative lesions (e.g. Ménière's disease). It may be associated with vertigo, deafness, or tinnitus.

Central vestibular/cerebellar/brainstem nystagmus

- Conjugate jerk (usually) nystagmus that may be horizontal, vertical, or torsional and that does not improve with fixation.
  - *Horizontal central vestibular nystagmus* is usually due to lesions of the vestibular nuclei, the cerebellum, or their connections.
  - *Upbeat nystagmus in primary position* is usually due to cerebellar or lower brainstem pathology (e.g. demyelination, infarction, tumour, encephalitis, Wernicke syndrome).
  - *Downbeat nystagmus in primary position* is usually due to pathology of the craniocervical junction (e.g. Arnold–Chiari malformation, spinocerebellar degenerations, infarction, tumour, demyelination) or drug induced.

Box 16.16 Pharmacological agents that can induce nystagmus

- Carbamazepine
- Lithium carbonate
- Phenytoin
- Amiodarone
- Morphine
- Fomepizole
- Ketamine abuse
- Nutmeg

Table 16.25 Late onset nystagmus—conjugate

Effect of gaze	Effect of time	Direction	Effect of fixation	Nystagmus type
Present in primary position	Sustained	Horizontal	Improves	Peripheral vestibular
			Worsens	Central vestibular
		Vertical	N/A	Upbeat
				Downbeat
	Periodic	Horizontal	N/A	Periodic alternating
Only present in eccentric gaze	N/A	Usually horizontal	N/A	Gaze evoked

Nystagmus (3)

Acquired nystagmus: disconjugate

Acquired pendular nystagmus
- Usually disconjugate with horizontal, vertical, and torsional components.
- It is associated with brainstem and cerebellar disease, including toluene abuse.
- It may be associated with involuntary repetitive movement of palate, pharynx, and face (oculopalatal myoclonus).

Superior oblique myokymia
- Unilateral high-frequency low-amplitude torsional nystagmus.
- This movement is so small that it may only be detectable at the slit-lamp.
- SO myokymia may cause occasional diplopia.
- It is rarely associated with underlying disease, although it has been reported after SO palsy, and associated with MS and pontine tumours.

Internuclear ophthalmoplegia
- Nystagmus of the abducting (and occasionally adducting) eye.
- The mechanism is uncertain, possibly being due to gaze paresis or ataxia.

See-saw nystagmus
- Vertical and torsional components with one eye elevating and intorting while the other depresses and extorts.
- It is usually a slow pendular waveform, although a jerk see-saw nystagmus may also be seen. In the congenital form the torsional element is reversed, i.e. the elevating eye extorts.

Table 16.26 Late onset nystagmus—disconjugate

Extent	Waveform	Nystagmus type
Unilateral	Torsional	Superior oblique myokymia
	Horizontal in abducting eye	Internuclear ophthalmoplegia associated
Bilateral	Pendular	Acquired pendular
	See-saw	See-saw

Treatment
- Treatment is difficult and often disappointing.
- Treatment options depend on visual potential, presence of visual symptoms (oscillopsia), and the location of a null position.
- *Drug treatment* includes GABA-ergics (e.g. gabapentin), anticholinergics (e.g. scopolamine) and memantine (anti-glutamatergic, anti-serotonergic, and anti-cholinergic).
- *Optical devices* aim to stabilize (e.g. high plus spectacle lens with high minus contact lens) or optimize the null position (e.g. prisms to move null position towards the primary position).
- *Surgical procedures* may generally stabilize (e.g. bilateral weakening procedures—usually only a transient benefit) or move the null position

and reduce the corrective head posture (horizontal, vertical or torsional Kestenbaum procedures).
- *Retrobulbar botulinum toxin* causes general dampening of ipsilateral nystagmus; however, it is associated with ptosis, diplopia, and vertigo (hence may not be suitable for ambulatory patients).

Saccadic oscillations and intrusions

In oscillations and intrusions there is an abnormal saccade away from fixation followed by a corrective saccade, i.e. both movements are fast. The corrective saccade may be immediate (oscillation) or delayed (intrusion).

Saccadic oscillations

Ocular flutter
- Bursts of moderate-amplitude horizontal saccades without intersaccadic interval.
- It is associated with cerebellar and brainstem disease.

Opsoclonus
- Bursts of large-amplitude multidirectional saccades without intersaccadic interval.
- It is associated with loss of pause cell activity that may be caused by viruses, myoclonic encephalopathy, paraneoplastic syndromes (neuroblastoma in children, small cell lung cancer in adults), and demyelination.

Saccadic intrusions

Small infrequent square-wave jerks may be physiological. However, other intrusions are usually pathological, most commonly due to cerebellar disease.

Square-wave jerks and macrosquare-wave jerks
Horizontal 1–5° (square wave) or 10–40° (macro) excursions from fixation and back again.

Macrosaccadic oscillations
Series of hypermetric saccades attempting to narrow in on the target; 'ocular past-pointing'.

Coma-associated eye movements

Ocular bobbing
- Conjugate fast downward movements with slow drift upward.
- Ocular bobbing may be caused by large lesions of the pons, metabolic encephalopathies, or hydrocephalus.

Ocular dipping
- Conjugate slow downward movements with fast saccade upward.
- This and other variants of ocular bobbing are fairly non-specific.

Ping pong gaze
- Conjugate horizontal movements alternating side every few seconds.
- This is associated with bilateral cerebral hemispheric lesions.

Myasthenia gravis

Myasthenia gravis (MG) is an uncommon autoimmune disease characterized by weakness and fatiguability of skeletal muscle. Antibodies against postsynaptic ACh receptors cause loss of receptors and structural abnormalities of the neuromuscular junction.

Its prevalence is estimated as up to 1 in 10 000. It may occur at any age but has a bimodal distribution with peaks at about 20yrs and 60yrs. In the younger group it is more common in females, but in the older group it is more common in males.

It may be associated with thymic hyperplasia, and other autoimmune disease (e.g. Graves' disease in 4–10%).

Clinical features

MG is a great mimic. Consider it when confronted with ocular motility abnormalities that 'do not fit', particularly when these seem to be highly variable.

Ocular signs are the presenting feature in 70% and are present at some point in 90% of MG. Ocular MG becomes generalized in 80% of patients (usually within 2yrs).

Ocular

- Variable diplopia or ptosis (usually worsening towards evening/with exercise).
- Variable and fatiguable ptosis or ocular motility disturbance (any pattern); sustained eccentric gaze of ≥1min or repeated saccades demonstrates fatigue, e.g. attempted prolonged upward gaze demonstrates fatigue of LPS and elevators; Cogan's twitch (ask patient to look down for 20s and then at object in the primary position: positive if lid 'overshoots'); spontaneous twitching is a sign of severe fatigue.

Systemic

- Fatiguable weakness of limbs, speech, chewing, swallowing, breathing; choking, fluids going up nose when swallowing.

NB MG is potentially fatal due to respiratory failure or choking. Take breathlessness or any choking episodes seriously.

Investigations

- *Ice-pack test*: measure ptosis; place ice wrapped in a towel/glove on the closed eyelid for 2min; remeasure ptosis; test significantly positive if ≥2mm.
- *Tensilon® (edrophonium) test*: ensure that IV atropine (0.5–1mg), resuscitation equipment, and trained staff are on hand. Cardiac monitoring essential. Give 2mg edrophonium IV (test dose); if no ill effects at 30s give further 8mg edrophonium IV (slow injection). Compare pre- and post-test ptosis or motility disturbance (consider Hess chart). The objectivity of this test may be improved by having a second syringe of 0.9% saline and using an independent observer who is unaware of which agent is being administered, to comment on the effects of each.
- *Serum antibodies*: anti-ACh receptor is present in ≤95% patients with generalized myasthenia, but only 50% of ocular myasthenia; anti-skeletal muscle is present in 85% of patients with thymoma; antithyroid antibodies and ANA may detect associated disease.

- *EMG*: repetitive supramaximal stimuli demonstrate reduction in action potential amplitude; also jitter (the EMG equivalent of twitch).

Treatment

- Liaise with a neurologist to assess systemic involvement and to optimize care.
- *Anticholinesterases*: pyridostigmine: start 30–60mg PO 1–2×/d, gradually increasing if required to maximum of 450mg/d. Gastrointestinal disturbance may occur, but can be treated by propantheline.
- *Immunosuppression*: if generalized disease, refer to a physician for further assessment and immunosuppression; this may include corticosteroids, azathioprine, intravenous gammaglobulin, plasmaphoresis, and thymectomy.
- Thymectomy is associated with remission of MG in 80% of non-thymoma patients but only 10% of patients with thymoma.

Prognosis

- Fatal cardiorespiratory failure may rarely occur, usually during the first year of disease. Death may also occur from choking episodes. At-risk patients should be nursed sitting upright and require a nasogastric tube.
- Prognosis is worse for those with thymoma, and with a late onset of disease.
- Most patients are well controlled on treatment; some spontaneously remit.

Other disorders of the neuromuscular junction

Congenital myasthenia syndromes

Heterogeneous group of disorders that can occur throughout childhood. They are usually caused by presynaptic, synaptic or postsynaptic defects of the ACh receptor. Commonly have purely ocular disease.

Lambert–Eaton myasthenic syndrome

A disorder of the presynaptic calcium channels causing impaired release of ACh. It is usually associated with malignancy (e.g. small cell lung cancer) but may be an isolated autoimmune disorder. The main ocular feature is decreased lacrimation, although ocular motility abnormalities and tonic pupils may occur. In contrast to MG repeated or sustained testing may cause improvement in any abnormalities.

Toxins

Toxins may act presynaptically to either impair ACh release (botulism, tick paralysis) or increase its release (black widow spider, scorpion bite). Organophosphates (fertilizers, nerve gas) act within the cleft to inhibit acetylcholinesterase. Treatment includes supportive measures, antitoxin (if available) and, for the excitatory syndromes, atropine blockade.

Table 16.27 Neuromuscular junction disorders

Syndrome	Pathogenesis	Ocular features	Systemic features
Inhibitory syndromes			
MG	Antibodies to postsynaptic AChR	Fatiguable ptosis, abnormal motility	Fatigue of limbs, bulbar function, respiratory failure
LEMS	Paraneoplastic presynaptic ↓ACh release	↓Lacrimation, tonic pupils, abnormal motility	Proximal weakness Autonomic dysfunction
Botulism	Toxin presynaptic ↓ACh release	Ptosis, tonic pupils, abnormal motility	Weakness of bulbar function Autonomic dysfunction
Excitatory syndromes			
Organo-phosphate	Toxin inhibits ACh-esterase	Miosis	Respiratory failure Fasciculation Paralysis
Scorpion toxin	Toxin Presynaptic ↑ACh release	↓VA, abnormal motility	Respiratory failure Mental disturbance

Myopathies

Inherited myopathies are rare, insidious, and easily missed in their early stages. Diplopia is uncommon and patients may adopt exaggerated head movements. It is important to consider the diagnosis in all patients with bilateral ptosis partly because a more cautious approach to lid surgery is necessary.

Acquired myopathies due to orbital inflammation or infiltration (e.g. thyroid eye disease and myositis, see Thyroid eye disease 📖 pp. 530–535) are much more common. Florid cases are easily recognized but early cases may cause a non-specific restrictive pattern.

Chronic progressive external ophthalmoplegia

This is a rare group of conditions in which there is progressive failure of eye movement. Mutations of mitochondrial DNA lead to abnormalities of oxidative phosphorylation and consequent muscle and CNS injury.

Clinical features

Bilateral ptosis, ↓smooth pursuits/saccades/reflex eye movements (downgaze usually affected last; diplopia uncommon); weakness of orbicularis oculi and facial muscles

Variants

- *Kearns–Sayre syndrome*: CPEO, pigmentary retinopathy (granular pigmentation, peripapillary atrophy), and heart block; usually presents before 20yrs.
- *MELAS syndrome*: mitochondrial encephalopathy, lactic acidosis, stroke-like episodes; also CPEO, hemianopia, cortical blindness.

Investigations

- *ECG*: check for conduction abnormalities.
- Consider skeletal muscle biopsy (ragged red fibres with peripheral concentration of mitochondria); peripheral blood (mitochondrial DNA analysis: fasting sample for glucose, lactate, pyruvate, pH); MRI, EMG (to rule out other diagnoses).

Treatment

Management of CPEO may involve liaison with neurologists (who may perform the muscle biopsies), clinical geneticists, and cardiologists. Symptomatic ptosis or diplopia may be relieved by cautious surgery (beware weak orbicularis oculi and poor Bell's phenomenon). Conduction abnormalities may require pacemaker insertion. Coenzyme Q10 has some benefit on the systemic features of Kearns–Sayre syndrome.

Oculopharyngeal dystrophy

This rare autosomal dominant (occasionally sporadic) condition is associated with an expanded GCG repeat in the poly(A) binding protein 2 gene. It typically presents in the sixth decade, and has been identified in a large French Canadian pedigree. It is a form of myotonia, i.e. there is a delay in muscle relaxation post-contraction. The condition progresses from dysphagia to bilateral ptosis to external ophthalmoplegia and orbicularis weakness.

Myotonic dystrophy

This uncommon autosomal dominant dystrophy arises due to an expanded CTG repeat in the Dystrophica Myotonica Protein Kinase (DMPK) gene (Ch19q). 'Anticipation' occurs whereby the triplet expansion increases in successive generations leading to earlier and more severe disease. Prevalence is estimated at about 5/100 000, being highest among French Canadians. It is characterized by a failure of muscle relaxation after contraction.

Clinical features

- *Ocular:* bilateral ptosis, cataracts (polychromatic 'Christmas tree cataracts' or posterior subcapsular), orbicularis oculi weakness; rarely pigmentary retinopathy ('butterfly' pigmentation centrally, reticular at mid-periphery, and atrophic far periphery), and myotonia of extraocular muscles.
- *Systemic:* 'mournful' facies, dysphasia, dysphagia, muscle weakness with delayed relaxation ('myotonic grip'), testicular atrophy, frontal baldness, ↓IQ, cardiac myopathy, and conduction abnormalities (may lead to fatal cardiac failure).

Investigations

- *DNA analysis:* confirm diagnosis.
- *ECG:* should be performed annually for conduction abnormalities; these may occur in otherwise minimally affected individuals.

Treatment

- Multidisciplinary management may include neurology, cardiology, physiotherapy, occupational therapy, and speech therapy.
- Offer genetic counselling, annual influenza vaccination, and cataract surgery (when symptomatic).
- **NB** General anesthesia may unmask subclinical respiratory failure leading to problems of ventilatory weaning.

Blepharospasm and other dystonias

Blepharospasm is a relatively common condition, which, in its severe form, can be very disabling both in terms of vision and social function. It is more common in women (F:M 2:1) and increases with age. It is a type of focal dystonia in which there is tonic spasm of the orbicularis oculi. It may be idiopathic (essential blepharospasm) or secondary to ocular or periocular disease. Blepharospasm may be associated with dystonias involving other facial muscles.

Essential blepharospasm

Clinical features

- Bilateral involuntary lid closure, ↑ frequency of lid closure (normal is about 10–20×/min); may be precipitated by stress, fatigue, social interactions; may be relieved by relaxation or 'distraction', e.g. touching face or whistling; often marked fluctuations from day-to-day, but generally worsens over years.
- Associated ocular disease may include underlying precipitants (particularly lid and ocular surface) and secondary anatomical changes of the lid (ptosis or entropion) or brow (brow-ptosis or dermatochalasis).

Investigations

- Typical isolated blepharospasm does not usually require investigation.
- If atypical (e.g. associated weakness or any other neurological abnormality) liaise with a neurologist and consider imaging (e.g. MRI) and other tests (e.g. EMG).

Treatment

- Botulinum toxin (A): this is usually given as multiple injections of the upper and lower lid; it has high rate of success in the short term (up to 98%) but generally only lasts for 3mths; complications include ptosis, epiphora, keratitis, dry eyes, and ocular motility disorders (diplopia).
- Treat any underlying ocular disease.
- Other treatment options include medical (e.g. benzodiazepines) and surgical (myectomy or chemomyectomy with doxorubicin).

Table 16.28 Causes of blepharospasm

Type	Cause
Essential	Idiopathic
Secondary	**Common**
	Blepharitis
	Trichiasis
	Dry eyes/keratoconjunctivitis sicca
	Other chronic lid disease
	Other chronic ocular surface disease
	Rare
	Glaucoma
	Uveitis

Other dystonias of the face and neck

- *Meige syndrome*: blepharospasm with midfacial spasm; regarded as a 'spill-over' of essential blepharospasm to involve the midfacial musculature; may compromise speech and eating/drinking.
- *Torticollis*: tonic spasm of sternocleidomastoid causes sudden sustained movement of the head to one side.

Other involuntary facial movement disorders

- *Hemifacial spasm*: tonic-clonic spasm of facial musculature, which unlike blepharospasm or Meige syndrome is unilateral, may occur during sleep and typically affects a younger age group. It suggests irritation of the root of the VIIn by a compressive lesion (usually an abnormal vessel, but needs imaging to rule out a posterior fossa tumour).
- *Facial myokymia*: fleeting movements of facial musculature that may be associated with caffeine, stress, MS, or rarely tumours of the brainstem.
- *Facial tic*: brief, repetitive stereotypic movements, which are suppressible (at least initially); may be associated with Gilles de la Tourette syndrome.

Lid 'apraxia'

Normal blinking requires both the inhibition of levator palpebrae superioris (LPS) and the activation of orbicularis oculi. In lid opening 'apraxia' there is total inhibition of LPS with no activation of orbicularis oculi. This results in sustained lid closure with difficulty in initiating lid opening.

It is associated with extrapyramidal diseases (e.g. Parkinson's disease, progressive supranuclear palsy, Huntington's disease, Wilson's disease).

Lid retraction and poor initiation of lid closure may also be seen in Parkinson's disease, progressive supranuclear palsy, and Parinaud syndrome.

Functional visual loss

Functional visual loss (*syn.* non-organic visual loss, psychogenic visual impairment) is a diagnosis of exclusion. It can often coexist with genuine pathology.

Suspecting functional visual loss

Consider this diagnosis when the patient reports poor vision but some of the following features are present:

Visual function and history

- Visual functioning obviously does not correlate with history, e.g. reported blindness but able to easily navigate around the waiting room; however, be cautious as some patients with low vision due to organic visual loss *can* navigate surprisingly well.
- Patient cannot perform tasks that he/she may consider to be visual, but actually are not, e.g. signing name.
- Recent stressful event elicited in history, e.g. impending exams.

Normal examination

- No apparent pathology after *detailed* examination.
- Absence of RAPD in the context of profound reported asymmetrical visual loss. **NB** Bilateral symmetrical pathology may give slow ('sluggish') pupillary light responses but no RAPD.
- Retinoscopy and subjective refraction shows absence of uncorrected refractive error.
- Optokinetic nystagmus is demonstrable using field stimulus which patient reports not to be able to discern.

Inconsistent abnormalities in the examination

- *Goldmann perimetry features*: 'Spiralling' isopters regress towards fixation as test progresses; crossed isopters show that a dimmer or smaller target is surprisingly seen further in the periphery than a brighter or larger target; crowded isopters show that targets of greatly differing size or brightness are suddenly seen when they reach about the same eccentricity within the visual field.
- *Ishihara plates*: patient may give inconsistent responses, e.g. recognize '12' but no other numbers, yet repeatedly trace the plates correctly. It is important to exclude defective colour vision in the 'normal eye' in order to validate RAPD observations.

Diagnosing functional visual loss

Diagnose functional visual loss only when the patient has demonstrated normal vision. This requires an encouraging, empathic approach and a slick examination. *Consider*:

Tests of stereoacuity

Normal stereoacuity implies normal visual acuity.

The 'crossed cylinder technique'

- Fog good eye with +6D lens in trial frame, +0.25 before 'blind' eye.
- Rotate a crossed +3D cyl before a −3.0 cyl.
- See if patient can be encouraged to read with the 'blind' eye when the cylinders are superimposed to negate each other.

Tests of reading vision

In some cases normal reading vision can be demonstrated proving normal visual potential despite apparently impaired Snellen acuities.

Tests of colour vision

If the patient gives normal Ishihara plate responses then their visual acuity is at least 6/24. For those with congenital red–green colour blindness the presence of a red filter should enable them to read the plates provided they have an acuity of at least 6/24.

Causes

- *Conversion disorder*: visual loss may be a manifestation of psychological or social difficulties.
- *Malingering*: feigned visual loss for other (usually material) benefit.

Management

- Patients suspected of functional visual loss will often need encouragement, reassurance, and follow up.
- If the diagnosis remains uncertain use a term such as *visual loss of unknown cause* in the notes.
- Referral to a ophthalmologist familiar with unexplained visual loss (e.g. neuro-ophthalmologist or paediatric ophthalmologist) may avoid unnecessary investigations.

Investigations

Investigation is mandatory when there is diagnostic uncertainty. *Consider*:

- EDTs: normal VEP results support reasonable vision but abnormal results can be found in the absence of genuine pathology; EDTs may identify early Stargardt's disease or cone dystrophy.
- Neuro-imaging, e.g. contrast enhanced MRI of visual pathway.
- Investigation as a chronic optic neuropathy of unknown cause, e.g. for Leber's mutations.
- In exceptional circumstances (when cortical injury is suspected) positron emission tomography can reveal organic disease when other imaging techniques give normal results.

Treatment

- When functional visual loss is diagnosed the patient should be counselled carefully. The physician faces the unusual situation of contesting the patient's symptoms. However, an adversarial scenario can be both disagreeable and entirely counter-productive. The patient can be reassured that they have healthy eyes and that the return of normal visual functioning is expected.
- With support, patience, and reassurance the patient can be allowed to resolve their visual functioning.
- The underlying problem may be far beyond the scope of most ophthalmologist's expertise. In some cases a clinical psychologist may be helpful.

Strabismus

Anatomy and physiology (1)

Extraocular muscles

The orbit forms a pyramid in which the lateral and medial walls are at 45° to each other, and the central axis thus at 22.5° (approximated to 23°). The four rectus muscles originate from the annulus of Zinn. (Figs 17.1 and 17.2.)

The superior oblique (like the levator palpebrae superioris) originates from the orbital apex outside the annulus; in contrast the inferior oblique arises from the nasal orbital floor. The obliques lie inferior to their corresponding rectus muscle, i.e. SO lies inferior to SR and IO inferior to IR. The spiral of Tillaux describes the way the recti insert increasingly posterior to the limbus (MR, IR, LR, then SR). Innervation is by IIIn for SR, MR, IR, IO; by IVn for SO; and by VIn for LR.

Table 17.1 Anatomy of extraocular muscles

	Origin	Muscle length	Tendon length	Insertion (mm from limbus)
MR	Annulus of Zinn	40mm	3.6mm	5.5mm
LR	Annulus of Zinn	40mm	8.4mm	6.9mm
SR	Annulus of Zinn	41mm	5.4mm	7.7mm
IR	Annulus of Zinn	40mm	5.0mm	6.5mm
SO	Sphenoid	32mm	From 10mm pre-trochlea	Posterior superotemporal
IO	Orbital floor	34mm	Minimal	Posterior temporal

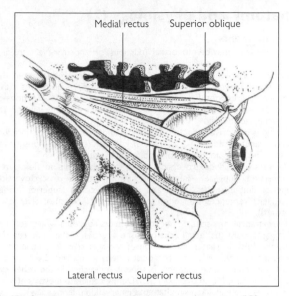

Fig. 17.1 Superior view of the right globe showing muscle insertions (LPS removed).

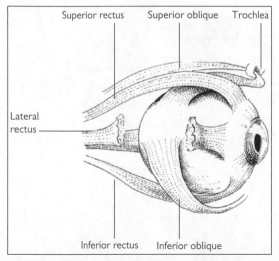

Fig. 17.2 Lateral view of the right globe showing muscle insertions (LR partly removed).

Anatomy and physiology (2)

Eye movements

Eye movements may be monocular (ductions) or binocular (versions and vergences).

Versions are conjugate eye movements, i.e. both eyes move in the same direction, whereas vergences are disconjugate, i.e. both eyes move in opposing directions. Eye movements may be described as rotations of the globe around horizontal (x), anteroposterior (y), and vertical (z) axes—the axes of Fick.

Ductions comprise abduction (outward), adduction (inward), supraduction (upward), infraduction (downward), intorsion (superior limbus moves inward), and extorsion (superior limbus moves outward).

Versions include dextroversion (right gaze), laevoversion (left gaze), supraversion (upgaze), infraversion (downgaze), dextrocycloversion (superior limbus moves right), and laevocycloversion (superior limbus moves left). Vergences are limited to convergence (inward) or divergence (outward).

The extraocular muscles do not act in isolation. Thus each agonist (e.g. LR) has an antagonist that acts in the opposite direction in the same eye (i.e. ipsilateral MR). Increased innervation of the agonist is accompanied by decreased innervation of its antagonist (Sherrington's law). Each agonist also has a yoke muscle that acts in the same direction in the other eye (i.e. contralateral MR in this example). During conjugate movement yoke muscles receive equal and simultaneous innervation (Hering's law).

Table 17.2 Actions of extraocular muscles

	In primary position (subsidiary actions)	In abduction	In adduction
MR	Adduction	Adduction	Adduction
LR	Abduction	Abduction	Abduction
SR	Elevation (intorsion, adduction)	Elevation (isolated at 23° abduction)	Intorsion (isolated at 67° adduction)
IR	Depression (extorsion, adduction)	Depression (isolated at 23° abduction)	Extorsion (isolated at 67° adduction)
SO	Intorsion (depression, abduction)	Intorsion (isolated at 39° abduction)	Depression (isolated at 51° adduction)
IO	Extorsion (elevation, abduction)	Extorsion (isolated at 39° abduction)	Elevation (isolated at 51° adduction)

Fig. 17.3 The six cardinal positions of gaze (from observer's perspective).

Amblyopia

Amblyopia is a developmental defect of central visual processing leading to reduced visual form sense. In essence, during the first 6yrs of life our capacity for high-level vision is vulnerable. Anything less than perfect, balanced foveal images from both eyes can lead to loss of vision in one/both eyes. With increasing age this is harder to reverse and by about 7–8yrs of age is usually permanent.

Causes of amblyopia

No/reduced image

Stimulus-deprivation amblyopia: constant monocular occlusion for >1wk/yr of life is very likely to lead to amblyopia in those <6yrs.

Significant unilateral congenital cataracts require urgent removal with optical correction in the first few weeks of life; significant bilateral congenital cataracts should be removed in the first 6wks of life.

Image blurring from refractive error

- *Anisometropic amblyopia*: high risk if difference of refraction of >2.5D, but may be significant with differences as low as 1D; increased risk if present >2yrs; this is a highly amblyogenic stimulus.
- *Ametropic amblyopia*: very variable; however, refractive error greater than +5.00DS or −10.00DS likely to confer significant risk; bilateral amblyopia may occur if uncorrected.
- *Astigmatic/meridional amblyopia*: significant risk if >0.75D cylinder; risk is increased if different axis and/or magnitude between the two eyes.

Abnormal binocular interaction

Strabismic amblyopia: significant risk if one eye preferred for fixation; if freely alternating then low risk; more common in esotropia than exotropia.

Clinical features

- Reduced visual acuity in the absence of an organic cause and despite correction of refraction.
- Exaggeration of the crowding phenomenon (scores better with single optotypes).
- Tolerance of a neutral density filter. Classically in amblyopia, VA is reduced less by the addition of neutral density filters than in other causes of ↓VA. However, while this may be observed in strabismic amblyopia, it is not seen in anisometropic amblyopia.

Treatment

The critical period during which visual development may be influenced is up to 8yrs. At younger ages there is more rapid reversal of amblyopia but increased risk of inducing occlusion amblyopia in the covered eye.

The general approach is spectacle adaptation first and then either patching or atropine penalization.

Occlusion

Adjust for age, acuity, and social factors. Practice is very variable, but in general longer episodes (time per day) and longer treatment (weeks of patching) have been used for older patients and those with worse VA. There is some evidence that there is little excess benefit in patching for >4h per day and this is used as an upper limit in some centres.

Penalization

Atropinization is gaining an increased role. It may reduce the VA in the better eye to about 6/18 so is really only effective if the amblyopic eye has VA >6/18.

Binocular single vision

In essence, BSV is the ability to view the world with two eyes, form two separate images (one for each eye) and yet fuse these centrally to create a single perception. The development of BSV depends on correct alignment and similar image clarity of both eyes from the neonatal period. Thus a pre-requisite for high-quality BSV is *normal retinal correspondence* in which an image will stimulate anatomically corresponding points of each retina and subsequent stimulation of functionally corresponding points in the occipital cortex to produce a single perception. The points in space that project on to these corresponding retinal points lie on an imaginary plane, the *horopter*. *Panum's fusional area* is the narrow region around the horopter in which, despite disparity, points will be seen as single.

Levels of binocular single vision

Binocular vision may be graded as:
1. *Simultaneous perception*: perception of a single image due to simulta-neous formation of an image on each retina.
2. *Fusion*: stimulation of corresponding points in each retina allows central fusion of image.
3. *Stereopsis*: disparity in fused images gives a perception of depth.

Fusion has sensory and motor components. Whereas sensory fusion generates a single image from corresponding points, motor fusion adjusts eye position to maintain sensory fusion. Fusional reserves indicate the level at which these mechanisms break down (usually seen as diplopia).

Table 17.3 Normal fusional reserves (approximate values)

Horizontal	Near	Convergent	32Δ	BO
		Divergent	16Δ	BI
	Distance	Convergent	16Δ	BO
		Divergent	8Δ	BI
Vertical			4Δ	

Abnormalities of binocular single vision

Confusion and diplopia

These are abnormalities of simultaneous perception.
- *Confusion* is the stimulation of corresponding points by dissimilar images, i.e. two images appear to be on top of each other.
- *Diplopia* is the stimulation of non-corresponding points by the same image, i.e. double vision.

Adaptive mechanisms

Adaptive mechanisms include suppression, abnormal retinal correspondence, and abnormal head posture.

- *Suppression*: a cortical mechanism to ignore one of the images causing confusion (central suppression at the fovea) or diplopia (peripheral suppression). Monocular suppression leads to amblyopia if not treated; alternating suppression (between the two eyes) does not. The size and density of the suppression scotoma is also variable.
- *ARC*: a cortical mechanism to remap anatomically non-corresponding points of each retina to stimulate functionally corresponding points in the occipital cortex to produce a single perception. It permits a degree of BSV despite a manifest deviation.
- *Abnormal head posture*: a behavioural mechanism that brings the field of single vision to a more central location.

Microtropia

The advantages of these adaptive mechanisms are seen in a microtropia. This is a small manifest deviation with a degree of BSV permitted by variable combinations of ARC, eccentric fixation, and central suppression scotoma.

There is usually no movement on cover test (microtropia with identity), unless the eccentric fixation is not absolute (microtropia without identity).

Strabismus: assessment

Although the patient's (or parents') primary concern is likely to be the 'squint', it is imperative to step back and consider the whole child, their visual development, and their ophthalmic status. Assessment requires taking a history (visual/birth/developmental), appropriate measurement of vision, refraction and ophthalmic examination, and consideration of any amblyopic risk. A 'squint' may be the first presentation of serious ocular pathology (e.g. retinoblastoma, cataract) and thus careful ophthalmic examination (including dilated fundoscopy) is essential.

Your general 'ophthalmic' approach to examining the child (see Ophthalmic assesment 📖 pp.680–683) must be adapted to include orthoptic examination and refraction. Turn the examination into a game wher ever possible. Efficient examination helps reduce patient (and examiner) fatigue. Where there is concern over possible systemic abnormalities refer the child to a paediatrician.

The individual tests are discussed as part of clinical methods (see Ocular motility examination (1) 📖 pp.28–31).

History

Table 17.4 An approach to assessing strabismus—history

Visual symptoms	Duration, variability and direction of squint, precipitants, fatiguability, associations (VA/development, diplopia, abnormal head position)
POH	Previous/current eye disease; refractive error
PMH	Obstetric/perinatal history; developmental history
SR	Any other systemic (especially CNS) abnormalities
SH	Family support (for children)
FH	Family history of strabismus/other visual problems
Dx	Drugs
Ax	Allergies

Examination

Table 17.5 An approach to assessing strabismus—examination

Observation	Whole patient (e.g. dysmorphic features, use of limbs, gait), face (e.g. asymmetry), abnormal head posture, globes (e.g. proptosis), lids (e.g. ptosis)
VA	Use age-appropriate test (see Assessment of vision 📖 p.8)
	where quantitative not possible grade ability to fix and follow (i.e. is it central, steady, and maintained?)
Visual function	Check for RAPD
Corneal reflexes	Check for normal position and symmetry
Cover test	Near/distance/far distance
Deviation	Measure with prism cover test or estimate with Krimsky or Hirschberg test; may be measured with synoptophore
Fusional reserves	Measure prism (horizontal and vertical) tolerated before diplopia/blurring
Motility	Ductions/versions (9-positions of gaze). convergence saccades doll's eye movements
Accommodation	
Fixation	Fixation behaviour, normal vs eccentric, visuscope
Binocularity	Check for simultaneous perception with Worth 4-dot test or Bagolini glasses
Suppression	Detect with Worth 4-dot test, 4Δ base-out prism test, or Bagolini glasses
Correspondence	Detect anomalous retinal correspondence with Worth 4-dot, Bagolini glasses, or after-image test
Stereopsis	Measure level with Titmus, TNO, Lang or Frisby tests, or synoptophore,
Refraction	Cycloplegic refraction (for children)
Ophthalmic	This should include dilated fundoscopy. Identify any cause of ↓ VA or associated abnormalities
Systemic review	Notably cranial nerves, sensory/motor/cerebellar function, speech, mental state

Strabismus: outline

Esodeviations: the 'in-turning' eye

Is there a deviation?

Abnormalities of the face, globe, or retina may simulate an esodeviation. Angle kappa (the difference between the pupillary axis and the optical axis) is usually slightly positive. A negative angle occurs due to abnormal nasal positioning of the fovea (high myopia, traction, etc.). This simulates esodeviation.

Table 17.6 Causes of pseudo-esotropia

Specific	Epicanthic folds
	Narrow interpupillary distance
	Negative angle kappa
General	Face—asymmetry
	Globe—proptosis/enophthalmos
	Pupils—miosis/mydriasis/heterochromia

Esophoria vs esotropia

Phorias are latent deviations that are held in position by fusion. In certain circumstances (specific visual tasks, fatigue, illness, etc.) fusion can no longer be maintained and they decompensate. Tropias are manifest deviations. Some individuals may be phoric in one situation (e.g. for distance) and tropic in another (e.g. for near).

Table 17.7 Esotropia

Primary			
Accommodative	Varies with accommodation	Normal AC:A ratio Resolves with hypermetropic correction	*Fully accommodative esotropia*
		Normal AC:A ratio Improves with hypermetropic correction	*Partially accommodative esotropia*
		High AC:A ratio	*Convergence excess esotropia*
Non-accommodative	Constant	Starting <6mths	*Infantile esotropia*
		Starting >6mths	*Basic esotropia*
	Varies with fixation distance despite relief of accommodation	Near fixation only	*Near esotropia (non-accommodative convergence excess)*
		Distance fixation only	*Distance esotropia (divergence insufficiency)*
	Varies with time	Cyclic	*Cyclic esotropia*
Secondary		Organic ↓VA (e.g. media opacities)	*Secondary esotropia(sensory)*
Post-exo		Previous surgery for exotropia	*Consecutive esotropia*

Exodeviations: the diverging eye

Is there a deviation?

As with esodeviations structural abnormalities may simulate an exodeviation. As noted earlier angle kappa is usually slightly positive; an abnormally large positive angle kappa simulates an exodeviation.

Table 17.8 Causes of pseudo-exotropia

Specific	Wide interpupillary distance
	Positive angle kappa
General	Face—asymmetry
	Globe—proptosis/enophthalmos
	Pupils—miosis/mydriasis/heterochromia

Exophoria vs exotropia

Exophorias are latent deviations that are generally asymptomatic. However, when fusion can no longer be maintained they decompensate with symptoms of asthenopia, blurred vision, or diplopia.

Exotropias are manifest deviations that may be variable or constant. Fusion often allows control at one viewing distance with a manifest deviation at a different viewing distance (i.e. simulated distance exotropia).

Table 17.9 Exotropia

Primary	Constant	Starting <6mths	*Infantile exotropia*
		Starting >6mths	*Basic exotropia*
	Variable	Worse for near	*Near exotropia*
		Worse for distance High AC: A ratio	*Simulated distance exotropia*
		Worse for distance Normal AC: A ratio	*True distance exotropia*
Secondary		Organic VA (e.g. media opacities)	*Secondary exotropia*
Post-eso		Develops with time in absence of fusion	*Consecutive exotropia*

Concomitant strabismus: esotropia

Esotropia is a manifest inward deviation of the visual axes. It is the most common form of strabismus. It may be primary, secondary (most commonly due to poor vision), or consecutive (after surgery for an exodeviation). Primary esotropias are classified as accommodative or non-accommodative.

As with all strabismus the assessment should include refraction, full ophthalmic examination, and addressing of amblyopic risk. It is essential to detect/rule-out underlying pathology (e.g. intraocular tumour or cataract) at the outset.

Accommodative esotropia

Accommodative esotropia usually presents between 1 and 5yrs of age. It may be refractive or non-refractive. If there is a refractive element, increased convergence is associated with accommodation (normal or increased accommodative convergence:accommodation (AC:A)) to overcome uncorrected hypermetropia. In the non-refractive group there is an abnormally high AC/A ratio. There may, however, be overlap between these groups.

Refractive: fully accommodative esotropia
Esotropia fully corrected for distance and near by hypermetropic (usually +2 to +7D) correction; normal AC:A ratio; normal BSV if corrected; often intermittent initially (e.g. with fatigue, illness).

Treatment
Full hypermetropic correction; treat any associated amblyopia.

Refractive: partially accommodative esotropia
Esotropia only partially corrected by full hypermetropic correction; BSV absent, or limited with ARC; ± bilateral IO overaction.

Treatment
Full hypermetropic correction; treat amblyopia; consider surgery if potential for BSV or for cosmesis (if cosmetically unacceptable despite glasses).

Non-refractive: convergence excess esotropia
Esotropia for near due to high AC:A ratio; ortho/esophoric for distance; ↓ BSV for near, normal BSV for distance; usually hypermetropic.

Treatment
Treat any associated hypermetropia or amblyopia; consider orthoptic exercises, executive bifocal glasses, surgery (bilateral MR recession posterior fixation sutures) or miotics.

Non-accommodative

The commonest esotropia is the non-accommodative 'infantile esotropia' (*syn.* congenital esotropia). This is a large angle alternating esotropia presenting before 6mths, with poor BSV potential and near normal refraction. Other non-accommodative esotropias usually present later, i.e. after 6mths of age.

Infantile esotropia

Esotropia presenting before 6mths, large angle (>30Δ), alternating fixation (so low risk of amblyopia), poor BSV potential; often emmetropia/mild hypermetropia; ± apparent inferior oblique overaction, ± dissociated vertical deviation (DVD: slow upward deviation on dissociation (i.e. covering one eye) with recovery on removal of cover and no movement of other eye); ± manifest latent nystagmus (see Nystagmas (1) 📖 p.627).

Treatment

- Treat any associated amblyopia (e.g. occlusion of better eye if not freely alternating); correct hypermetropia if >2D; surgery aims for ocular alignment by 18mths (with better potential BSV) and usually comprises symmetrical MR recessions (± LR resection).
- Additional surgery for significant IO overaction may be required.

Other non-accommodative esotropias

- *Basic esotropia*: constant esotropia for near and distance; treat surgically.
- *Near esotropia (non-accommodative convergence excess)*: esotropia for near, ortho/esophoria for distance but with normal AC:A ratio. *Treatment*, if any, is surgical (medial recti > lateral recti).
- *Distance esotropia (divergence insufficiency)*: esophoria (or small esotropia) for near, larger esotropia for distance; associated with poor fusional divergence. **NB** rule out bilateral VIn palsies. Treat with orthoptic exercises initially.
- *Cyclic esotropia*: rare, periodic (e.g. alternate days), may proceed to constant esotropia.

Secondary esotropias

Esotropia may arise secondary to ↓VA and thus full ocular examination is vital in all cases. Some esotropic syndromes may arise secondary to intracranial pathology.

- *Sensory deprivation*: secondary to unilateral/bilateral ↓VA.
- *Divergence paralysis*: secondary to tumour, trauma, or stroke. Unlike a bilateral VI palsy the esodeviation remains constant or even decreases on lateral gaze.
- *Convergence spasm*. Usually intermittent and associated with blurred vision (psuedomyopia due to associated accommodation) and pupillary miosis. If encouraged, ductions (in the absence of miosis) will be normal. In children upper midbrain pathology must be excluded; however, this condition is often non-organic in origin. Attempt treatment with cycloplegia.

Pseudoesotropia

Various conditions may mimic an esotropia (Table 17.6).

Concomitant strabismus: exotropia

Exotropia is a manifest outward deviation of the visual axes. It may be primary, secondary (associated with poor vision), or consecutive (may follow an esotropia with time or after surgical correction). Primary exotropias may be constant or intermittent.

As with all strabismus the assessment should include refraction, full ophthalmic examination, and addressing of amblyopic risk. It is essential to detect/rule-out underlying pathology (e.g. intraocular tumour, cataract) at the outset.

Constant exotropia

Infantile (or congenital) exotropia

- Constant large angle exotropia presenting at 2–6mths of age; often associated with ocular/CNS abnormalities; rarely exotropia is present at birth (congenital exotropia).
- *Treatment* is usually surgical (e.g. bilateral LR recessions ± MR resection).

Basic exotropia

- Constant exotropia for near and distance presenting after 6mths of age.
- *Treatment* is usually surgical.

Intermittent exotropia

This is the commonest form of exotropia, and usually presents at 2–5yrs of age.

True distance exotropia

- Exotropia worse for distance, with normal AC:A ratio; rare.

Simulated distance exotropia

Exotropia worse for distance as an ↑AC:A ratio and/or fusional reserves fully or partially corrects for near; much more common than true distance exotropia.

Treatment

- Myopic correction; treat amblyopia; orthoptic exercises; consider prisms, minus lenses, botulinum toxin, or surgery for more severe cases.
- Surgery is generally performed before 5yrs of age.
- Unilateral LR recession and MR resection for simulated will give a functional result.
- Bilateral LR recession is reserved for true distance exotropia.

Near exotropia

Exotropia worse for near, often exophoric for distance; more common in young adults who report aesthenopia or diplopia for reading; may be associated with myopia.

Treatment

- Full myopic correction
- Orthoptic exercises if poor fusional amplitudes
- Consider surgical treatment (e.g. bimedial MR resection).

Convergence insufficiency
- This is not an exotropia but is considered here as an important differential diagnosis.
- Near point of convergence greater than age normal; no manifest deviation but may be exophoric for near; more common in teenagers who report asthenopia.

Treatment
Full myopic correction; convergence exercises (e.g. pencil push-ups); consider prisms, botulinum toxin, or surgery for more severe cases.

Secondary exotropia

Exotropia is the most common strabismic outcome of ipsilateral ↓VA, although sensory esotropia may occur in young children (see Concomitant strabismus esotropia 📖 p.658). Full ocular examination is vital in all cases.

Consecutive exotropia

With time an esotropia in which fusion has not been established may become an exotropia. Surgical correction may also cause a consecutive exotropia.

Pseudoexotropia

Various conditions may mimic an exotropia (Table 17.8).

Incomitant strabismus

In incomitant strabismus the angle between the visual axes changes according to the direction of gaze. Incomitant strabismus is often grouped into neurogenic or mechanical types; however, the abnormality may occur in the brainstem, nerve, neuromuscular junction, muscle, or orbit.

In assessing incomitant strabismus the aims are to identify the pattern and cause of the strabismus and address any actual or potential complications such as amblyopia, diplopia, or poor cosmesis.

Neurogenic strabismus

Underaction with slowing of saccades in the field of action of paretic muscle (underaction may be more marked for versions than ductions); may develop full sequelae with time.

Investigations

- *Hess chart*: inner and outer fields are equally affected; full sequelae if long-standing.
- *Forced duction test*: full passive movement, unless chronic contracture of antagonist.
- *Further investigation and treatment*: according to cause (see Third nerve palsy ⬚ p. 612; Fourth nerve palsy ⬚ p. 614; Sixth nerve palsy ⬚ p. 616).

Mechanical strabismus

Limitation in direction away from restricted muscle (equal for ductions and versions); saccades of normal speed, but sudden early stop due to restriction; IOP increase in direction of limitation often with globe retraction.

Investigations

- *Hess chart*: inner and outer fields are compressed in direction of limitation; outer affected more than inner; sequelae limited to overaction of contralateral synergist.
- *Forced duction test*: reduced passive movement in direction of limitation.
- *Further investigation and treatment*: according to cause (see Thyroid eye disease ⬚ pp. 530–535; Orbital fracture ⬚ pp. 104–107; Duane and other restrictive syndromes ⬚ pp. 664–665).

Myasthenic strabismus

Variable and fatiguable ocular motility disturbance (any pattern) often associated with ptosis; sustained eccentric gaze of ≥1 min or repeated saccades demonstrates fatigue; Cogan's twitch (ask patient to look down for 20s and then at object in the primary position: positive if lid 'overshoots'); may have systemic involvement (e.g. speech, breathing).

Investigations

- *Hess chart*: range from normal to highly variable/frustrating for operator.
- *Forced duction test*: full passive movement.

- *Ice-pack test*: measure ptosis; place ice wrapped in a towel/glove on the closed eyelid for 2min; remeasure ptosis; test significantly positive if ≥2mm improvement.
- *Further investigation* (including Tensilon® test, serum antibodies, and EMG) *and treatment* (see Myasthenia gravis 📖 p.634).

Myopathic strabismus

Gradual, symmetrical non-fatiguable loss of movement associated with ptosis is seen in the inherited myopathies (e.g. CPEO group). Acquired myopathies (e.g. thyroid eye disease and myositis) may be regarded as causing a mechanical strabismus pattern.

Investigations

- *Hess chart*: symmetrical and proportional reduction in inner and outer fields.
- *Further investigation and treatment*: according to cause (see Myopathies p.638.)

Table 17.10 Features of neurogenic and mechanical incomitant strabismus

	Neurogenic	Mechanical
Ductions/versions	Ductions > versions	Ductions = versions; May be painful
Saccades	Slow in paretic direction	Normal speed with sudden stop
Sequelae	Full sequelae with time	Sequelae limited to overaction of contralateral synergist
IOP change	IOP ± constant	IOP increases in the direction of limitation
Globe	No change	May retract on movement in direction of limitation
Hess	Inner and outer fields are proportional. The smaller field is of the affected eye (but sequelae reduce this effect with time)	Inner and outer fields are compressed in direction of limitation.
Forced duction testing	Full passive movement (but antagonist contracture with time)	Reduced passive movement in direction of limitation

Restriction syndromes

Syndromic patterns of mechanical restriction are uncommon causes of strabismus. They are usually congenital although later presentations may occur.

Duane syndrome

This is thought to arise due to aberrant co-innervation of LR and MR by the IIIn, which may be associated with VI nucleus hypoplasia. It is usually sporadic but may be autosomal dominant. The most common form (type I) preferentially affects girls (60%) and the left eye (60%). It is bilateral (usually asymmetric) in at least 20%.

Clinical features

- Retraction of globe (with reduction in palpebral aperture) on attempted adduction; ± up/downshoots or attempted adduction; additional features according to type (Table 17.11).
- Systemic associations (30%): deafness, Goldenhar syndrome, Klippel–Feil syndrome, Wilderwank syndrome (Duane, Klippel–Feil, and deafness).

Classification

Types of Duane syndrome can be described according to the Huber classification (Table 17.11), which was originally based on electromyography, or the Brown classification, which was based on clinical features alone (Table 17.12)

Table 17.11 Huber classification of Duane syndrome

Type	Frequency	Primary position	Primary feature	Globe retraction
I	85%	Eso or ortho	↓ Abduction	Mild
II	14%	Exo or ortho	↓ Adduction	Severe
III	1%	Eso or ortho	↓ Abduction and ↓ Adduction	Moderate

Table 17.12 Brown classification of Duane syndrome

Type	Key features
A	Limited abduction and adduction—adduction less limited than abduction
B	Limited abduction only
C	Limited abduction and adduction—adduction more limited than abduction

Treatment

Assess and treat for refractive error and potential amblyopia; reassure if managing well with minimal/mild compensatory head posture; most require no further intervention; consider prisms for comfort or to improve head position; consider surgery to improve BSV and improve head position.

Usual practice is uni/bilateral MR recession for esotropic Duane's and uni/bilateral LR recession (± MR resection) for exotropic Duane's. Avoid LR resection as it increases retraction more than improving abduction.

Brown syndrome

This is a mechanical restriction syndrome that Brown attributed to the superior oblique tendon sheath. It appears to arise from structural or developmental abnormalities of the SO muscle/tendon or the trochlea leading to limitation in the direction of its antagonist (IO). In most cases it is congenital (or at least infantile) and usually improves or resolves by 12yrs of age. Acquired cases may arise due to trauma, surgery (e.g. SO tuck, buckling, orbital), or inflammation (e.g. RA, sinusitis).

Clinical features

Limited elevation in adduction ± pain/click ('click' often occurs during resolution); limited sequelae (i.e. overaction of contralateral SR only); V pattern; may downshoot in adduction; positive forced duction test.

Treatment

Reassure if managing well with minimal/mild compensatory head posture: it usually improves with age and upgaze is less of an issue with increased height. Consider surgery if significant abnormal head posture or if strabismus in primary position. The aim is to release the restriction, e.g. with SO tenotomy until a repeated traction test demonstrates free rotation of the globe. Complications include SO palsy and results are often disappointing.

Möbius syndrome

This rare sporadic congenital syndrome includes bilateral VI and VII nerves palsies and often other neurological abnormalities. It is included here as it may be associated with bilateral tight MR causing restriction in addition to the horizontal gaze palsy.

Clinical features

- Bilateral failure of abduction; may be pure gaze palsy or bilateral tight MR can lead to esotropia and positive forced duction test.
- Systemic associations: bilateral VII palsy (expressionless face), bilateral XII palsy (atrophic tongue), ↓IQ, digital abnormalities.

Congenital fibrosis of the extraocular muscles

This rare congenital syndrome probably arises due to abnormal development of the oculomotor nuclei. Classic CFEOM (CFEOM1) is autosomal dominant Ch12q. There is bilateral restrictive ophthalmoplegia and ptosis, with an inability to elevate the globes above the midline. CFEOM2 is autosomal recessive Ch11q. There is bilateral ptosis, wide angle exotropia, and severe limitation of horizontal and vertical movements. In CFEOM3 Ch16q there are more variable motility defects.

Strabismus fixus

In this very rare sporadic congenital syndrome the eyes are firmly fixed in adduction or occasionally in abduction. The eyes appear to be anchored both by fibrosis of the rectus muscles and additional fibrous cords.

Alphabet patterns

Horizontal deviations may vary in size according to vertical position. The deviation is measured at 30° upgaze, primary position, and 30°downgaze while fixing on a distance target. Significant incomitance is described according to the following alphabet patterns (Table 17.13).

V pattern

This is defined as a horizontal deviation, which is 15Δ more divergent (or less convergent) in upgaze than in downgaze.

Clinical features
- V-pattern esotropia usually arises from IO overaction or SO palsy; it is also associated with antimongoloid palpebral fissures (perhaps altering the recti insertions). Patients may adopt a chin-down posture.
- V-pattern exotropia usually arises from IO overaction. Patients adopt a chin-up posture.

Treatment
Surgical treatment for significant V patterns may require IO weakening (if overacting), vertical translations of the horizontal recti (when operating on paired recti upward for LR, downward for MR), and correction of the horizontal component (e.g. MR recession for esotropia; LR recession for exotropia). For both A and V patterns the acronym *MALE* identifies the direction of vertical translation: *MR* to *A*pex, *LR* to *E*nds.

A pattern

This is defined as a horizontal deviation, which is 10Δ less divergent (or more convergent) in upgaze than in downgaze.

Clinical features
- A-pattern esotropia usually arises from SO overaction; it may also be associated with mongoloid palpebral fissures. Patients may adopt a chin-up posture.
- A-pattern exotropia usually arises from SO overaction. Patients adopt a chin-down posture.

Treatment
Surgical treatment for significant A-patterns may require posterior SO disinsertion (if overacting), vertical translations of the horizontal recti (when operating on paired recti upward for MR, downward for LR), and correction of the horizontal component (e.g. MR recession for esotropia; LR recession for exotropia).

Other patterns

Y-pattern
Exotropia in upgaze only. It is usually due to IO overaction in which case it can be treated by IO weakening alone.

λ-pattern
Exotropia in downgaze only. It may be treated by downward translation of both LR.

X-pattern
Exotropia in upgaze and downgaze but straight in the primary position. It usually arises in a long-standing exotropia with overaction of all four oblique muscles or is iatrogenic.

Table 17.13 Causes of alphabet patterns

A pattern	Overaction of SO
	Underaction of IO, IR, LR
V pattern	Brown syndrome
	Overaction of IO, SR, or LR
	Underaction of SO

Strabismus surgery: general

Surgery should only be performed after full assessment and treatment of causative factors (e.g. refractive error) and consideration of non-surgical alternatives (e.g. orthoptic exercises, prisms, botulinum toxin).

The main role for surgery is where significant deviation remains despite appropriate refraction, where the deviation is stable over time and where further improvement is not anticipated.

Surgical options involve weakening, strengthening, or transposing the extraocular muscles. These procedures adjust the effective pull of the muscle (by changing stretch and torque) and/or direction of action. The aim is to produce eyes that are straight in the primary position and down-gaze while keeping the largest possible field of BSV. It may be necessary to sacrifice BSV in lower priority gaze positions (e.g. upgaze) to achieve this.

General principles

- Identify: (1) direction of overaction; (2) any incomitance; and (3) any oblique muscle dysfunction.
- Weaken overacting muscle and strengthen its antagonist.
- Balance these procedures to prevent induced incomitance.
- Treat pre-existing incomitance.
- Reduce oblique muscle overaction.

Adjustable sutures

Surgical results may be improved by the use of adjustable sutures. These can be used in conjunction with recessions, resections, and advancements. They are of particular value in redo operations, mechanical strabismus, and where there is a significant risk of postoperative diplopia.

Complications

Complications include suture granuloma, scleral perforation (0.5%), slipped or lost muscle, anterior segment ischaemia, consecutive strabismus, and postoperative diplopia.

Table 17.14 Overview of common strabismus operations

Operation	Muscles	Procedure
Weakening		
Recession	Recti or IO	Moves insertion closer to origin
Disinsertion	IO	Remove muscle at its insertion
Myotomy/myectomy	IO	Divide muscle (myototmy) or remove a portion of it (myectomy)
'Z' Myotomy	Recti	Two alternate incisions of about 80% width weakens muscle without changing insertion
Faden procedure	SR or MR (very rarely IR)	Post-equatorial fixation suture (non-absorbable) weakens action of muscle without affecting primary position
Strengthening		
Resection	Recti	Shortens/stretches muscle
Advancement	Recti/SO	Moves insertion anteriorly (often of previously recessed muscle)
Tuck	SO	Loop of lax tendon sutured to sclera
Transposition		
To improve abduction (particularly in complete VI N palsy)		
Toxin Transposition	Toxin to MR then SR and IR	Complete transposition of SR and IR to superior and inferior border of LR after toxin injection into MR.
Hummelsheim	SR and IR	Lateral half of SR, and IR disinserted and attached to LR; MR may also be weakened
Jensen	LR, SR, and IR	Split LR, SR, and IR; suture neighbouring parts of LR + SR, and LR + IR together
To improve elevation		
Knapp	LR and MR	LR and MR disinserted and attached adjacent to SR insertion
To improve depression		
Inverse Knapp	LR and MR	LR and MR disinserted and attached adjacent to IR insertion
To improve intorsion		
Fells modification of Harado-Ito	SO	Disinsert anterior half of SO Tendon; advance to the superior margin of LR

Strabismus surgery: horizontal

The most common deviations (esotropia and exotropia) are horizontal and are therefore generally amenable to surgery on the horizontal recti. The most common procedure is a unilateral 'recess/resect', although the options range from single muscle procedures to bilateral (simultaneous or staged) surgery involving multiple muscles.

'Recess/resect'

An MR recession/LR resection will turn the visual angles away from each other, whereas an LR recession/MR resection will turn them towards each other. Estimation of the amount of surgical correction (in mm) required for the size of strabismus (in Δ) may be assisted by surgical tables. However, such tables are only a guide and should be modified by each surgeon according to their own outcomes.

Table 17.15 Outline of horizontal muscle surgery

Recession	Local conjunctival peritomy
	Identify and expose muscle
	Free muscle from Tenon's layer
	Place two locking bites of an absorbable suture through the outer thirds of the muscle
	Disinsert tendon and measure recession
	Suture in new position: either directly to adjacent sclera or to the insertion (hang back technique)
	Close conjunctiva
Resection	Local conjunctival peritomy
	Identify and expose muscle
	Free muscle from Tenon's layer
	Measure and place two locking bites of an absorbable suture posterior to intended resection
	Resect desired length of muscle
	Suture remaining muscle to insertion
	Close conjunctiva

Table 17.16 Absolute maximum surgical adjustments for rectus muscles

	Resect	Recess
LR	10mm	8–12mm
MR	8mm	8mm
SR	5mm	5mm
IR	5mm	5mm

Paediatric ophthalmology

Embryology (1)

The normal eye forms from an outpouching of the embryonic forebrain (neuroectoderm) with contributions from neural crest cells, surface ectoderm, and to a lesser extent mesoderm. The interactions between these layers are complex and failure may result in serious developmental abnormalities (see Developmental abnormalities 📖 pp.722–727).

General

The developing embryo comprises three germinal layers: ectoderm, mesoderm, and endoderm. The ectoderm differentiates into outer surface ectoderm and inner neuroectoderm. The neuroectoderm continues to develop forming first a ridge (neural crest), then a cylinder (neural tube), and finally vesicles within the cranial part of the tube to form the fore-, mid-, and hindbrain (prosencephalon, mesencephalon, telencephalon). The neural crest cells also migrate to contribute widely to ocular and orbital structures.

The globe

The optic vesicle develops as a neuroectodermal protrusion of the prosencephalon. It induces the overlying surface ectoderm to thicken into the lens placode. Then (*wk4*) both these structures invaginate to form a double-layered optic cup and lens vesicle respectively. The cup is not complete but retains a deep inferior groove (optic fissure) in which mesodermal elements develop into the hyaloid and other vessels. Closure starts at the equator (*wk5*) and proceeds anteroposteriorly; failure of closure results in colobomas.

Anterior segment

Lens

As discussed above, the lens placode forms from surface ectoderm and invaginates to form the lens vesicle (*wk5*). At this point it is a unicellular layer surrounded by a basement membrane (the future capsule). This layer continues to divide throughout life. The posterior cells elongate and differentiate into primary lens fibres. The anterior cells migrate to the equator and elongate forming the secondary lens fibres. These meet at the lens sutures.

Cornea

After separation of the lens vesicle, the surface ectoderm reforms as an epithelial bilayer with basement membrane. It is joined by three waves of migrating neural crest cells: the first (*wk6*) forms the corneal and trabecular endothelium; the second (*wk7*) forms the stroma; the third (*also wk7*) forms the iridopupillary membrane. This process is strongly influenced by the interplay between the genes *PITX2* (4q25) and *FOXC1* (6p25).

Sclera

The sclera develops from a condensation of mesenchymal tissue situated at the anterior rim of the optic cup. This forms first at the limbus (*wk7*) and proceeds posteriorly to surround the optic nerve (*wk12*).

Iris, trabecular meshwork, and angle

The optic cup grows around the developing lens such that the cup rims meet the iridopupillary membrane. The optic cup rims give rise to the epithelial layers of the iris that are therefore continuous with the ciliary body and retina/RPE layers. The mesenchymal iridopupillary membrane develops into the iris stroma. The dilator and sphincter muscles are both neuroectodermal. The trabecular meshwork and Schlemm's canal arises from 'first wave' neural crest tissue located in the angle (*wk5*).

Ciliary body

The ciliary body forms as a kink in the optic cup rim (contributing an epithelial bilayer) and associated neural crest tissue (ciliary muscles and vasculature). The longitudinal musculature appears first (*m3*); the circular musculature continues to develop after birth (*y1 postnatal*).

Embryology (2)

Posterior segment

Retina

All retinal tissues develop from the optic cup (neuroectoderm). The inner layer of the cup divides into two zones: a superficial non-nucleated 'marginal zone' and a deeper nucleated 'primitive zone'. Mitosis and migration from the primitive zone leads to the formation of an inner neuroblastic layer (giving rise to Muller cells, ganglion cells, and amacrine cells) and an outer neuroblastic layer (giving rise to bipolar cells, horizontal cells and primitive photoreceptor cells).

Familiar retinal organization starts with the formation of the ganglion cell layer and continues at the deeper levels with both cellular and acellular zones (nuclear and plexiform layers). This wave of retinal development starts at the posterior pole and proceeds anteriorly.

The photoreceptors arise from the outermost cells of the inner layer. Originally ciliated, these are replaced by distinctive outer segments. Cones develop first (m4–6), rods later (m7–). These photoreceptor cells project towards the outer layer of the cup. The outer layer (the retinal pigment epithelium) thins to become one cell thick and becomes pigmented, the first structure in the body to do so.

Retinal vasculature arises from the hyaloid circulation and spreads in an anterior wave reaching the nasal periphery before the temporal periphery (m9); it may therefore not be fully developed in premature infants.

Choroid

This vascular layer arises from: endothelial blood spaces around the optic cup; the extension of posterior ciliary arteries to join the primitive choroidal vasculature; and the consolidation of venous networks to form the four vortex veins.

Optic nerve

Vacuolization of cells within the optic stalk allows ganglion cell axons to grow through from the retina. The appearance of crossed and uncrossed fibres results in the formation of the chiasm (m2–4). Myelination proceeds anteriorly from the LGN (m5) to the lamina cribrosa (m1 postnatal). The inner layer of the stalk gives rise to supportive glial cells; the outer layer contributes to the lamina cribrosa.

Vitreous

The primary vitreous (wk5) forms in the retrolental space. It contains collagen fibrils, mesenchymal elements, and the hyaloid vasculature (which forms the tunica vasculosa lentis). Later (wk6) this is surrounded by the secondary vitreous, and effectively forms Cloquet's canal.

The secondary vitreous is avascular, transparent, and is composed of very fine organized fibres. Failure of the vascular system to regress causes Mittendorf's dot, Bergmeister's papilla, persistent hyaloid artery, and persistent fetal vasculature (formerly known as persistent hyperplastic primary vitreous).

Traditionally, 'tertiary vitreous' was used to describe a relatively anterior condensation associated with the formation of lens zonules (which in fact arise from the ciliary body).

Nasolacrimal drainage system

This arises from a cord of surface ectoderm that is met by proliferating cords of cells both from the lids above and from the nasal fossa below. Cannulation of the cord may be delayed distally causing congenital obstruction. More commonly there is simply an imperforate mucus membrane at the valve of Hasna that disappears within the first year.

Table 18.1 Summary of germinal layers

Ectoderm	Neuroectoderm	Iris epithelium
		Iris sphincter/dilator
		Ciliary body epithelium
		Neural retina
		RPE
		Optic nerve
	Neural crest	Corneal stroma
		Corneal endothelium
		Trabecular meshwork
		Ciliary musculature
		Sclera
		Choroidal stroma
	Surface ectoderm	Skin/lids
		Conjunctival epithelium
		Corneal epithelium
		Lacrimal gland
		Nasolacrimal duct
		Lens
Mesoderm		Extraocular muscles
		Ocular vasculature

Genetics

Genetic disorders may arise from an abnormal karyotype (abnormal number of chromosomes, e.g. trisomies), from an abnormal region of the chromosome (e.g. deletions, duplications), from abnormal gene(s) at a single locus (autosomal or X-linked), from abnormal mitochondrial DNA, or from the interaction of a number of genes with the environment. Single gene autosomal disorders obey the laws of segregation and independent assortment noted by Mendel. This results in predictable patterns of inheritance. More complex patterns arise from X-linked and mitochondrial disease. Most common conditions appear to be polygenic with additional contributions from environmental factors.

Even for single gene disorders the pattern of disease may be unpredictable. Such conditions may have incomplete *penetrance* (i.e. genotype present without the phenotype) or variable *expressivity* (i.e. wide range within the phenotype). In some conditions *anticipation* may occur where succeeding generations develop earlier and more severe disease. This is due to 'triplet repeats' in which the number of repeats of a particular codon (e.g. GCT in the myotonic dystrophy gene) increases from generation to generation.

Inheritance patterns

Table 18.2 Inheritance patterns for single gene defect with 100% penetrance

Autosomal dominant	One parent carries the mutation (and usually has the phenotype);
	50% chance of inheriting the gene and of developing the phenotype
Autosomal recessive	Both parents carry the mutation, but neither has the phenotype
	50% chance of inheriting one copy of gene (i.e. carrier without the phenotype)
	25% chance of inheriting two copies of gene and of developing the phenotype
X-linked	*If mother carries the mutation:*
	50% chance of inheriting the gene and developing the phenotype for a son
	50% chance of inheriting the gene and becoming a carrier for a daughter
	If father carries the mutation:
	100% chance of inheriting the gene and becoming a carrier for a daughter
	0% chance of inheriting the gene for a son
Mitochondrial	The mother carries the mutation
	Variable probability of inheritance dependant on proportion of abnormal mitochondria in the oocyte that becomes fertilized (heteroplasmy)

Table 18.3 Chromosomal locations of genes involved in ophthalmic disease (selected)

1	Schnyder dystrophy
	Stargardt's/fundus flavimaculatus (ABCR4)
	Leber's congenital amaurosis, RP (RPE65)
2	Oguchi disease (arrestin)
	Wardenburg syndrome (PAX3)
3	VHL (*VHL* gene)
	CSNB1(transducin (α))
4	Anterior segment dysgenesis (PITX2)
5	Reis–Bucklers, Thiel–Behnke, Granular, Lattice I (keratoepithelin, BIGH3)
6	Tritanopia (S opsin)
	Anterior segment dysgenesis (FOXC1)
7	
8	RP (RP1, and numerous others)
9	Tuberous sclerosis (TSC1, harmartin)
	Oculocutaneous albinism (OCA III, TRP1)
10	Gyrate atrophy (OAT)
11	Best's, nanophthalmos, AD vitreochoroidopathy (VMD2)
	Aniridia, Peter's anomaly (PAX6)
	Oculocutaneous albinism (OCA1,tyrosinase)
12	Meesman (K3, keratin)
	Chronic fibrosis of extraocular muscles (CFEOM1)
13	Wilson's disease
	Retinoblastoma (RB1)
14	
15	Marfan syndrome (FBN1, fibrillin)
	Oculocutaneous albinism (OCAII, p)
16	Tuberous sclerosis (TSC2, tuberin)
17	Neurofibromatosis-1 (NF1, neurofibromin)
	Meesman (K12, keratin)
18	
19	Myotonic dystrophy (DMPK)
20	
21	Homocystinuria type 1 (cystathionine synthetase)
22	Neurofibromatosis-2 (NF2, merlin)
	Sorsby's (TIMP)
X	Ocular albinism (OA1)
	X-linked RP (RP2)
	X-linked juvenile retinoschisis
	Choroideraemia (REP1)

Ophthalmic assessment in a child (1)

The assessment of children requires a flexible and often undignified approach. The aim is to keep everyone—patient, parents, extended family—on side. Without this it is near impossible to achieve an adequate clinical assessment and completely impossible to institute treatment.

The awake child

Try to entertain the child during recording their history (e.g. with a toy) and as far as possible turn the examination into a game. Explain what you are about to do (e.g. with drops) and why. Examine opportunistically and be patient. Surprisingly, young children may be happy to be examined at the slit-lamp (standing, kneeling on the chair, or sitting on carer's knee). If this is impossible consider a portable slit-lamp for the anterior segment, the indirect ophthalmoscope for the fundus, and the direct ophthalmoscope for higher magnification of the macula and disc. Applanation tonometry and gonioscopy may only be possible by examination under anaesthetic (EUA). Rebound tonometry gives the advantage of not requiring topical anaesthesia.

Keeping the child happy usually keeps the adults happy. Good communication is essential. Restraining the child to examine them, i.e. physically holding them still, is rarely indicated and should only be done after a detailed discussion with the parents and gaining their consent. The relationship between the child and their ophthalmologist may need to last for many years. This can be destroyed by one overzealous, frightening examination.

The anaesthetized child

An EUA may be indicated if detailed examination is impossible with the child awake. It may be possible to perform this when the child is being anaesthetized for a different procedure, so liaison with other specialists involved with the child is essential. The anaesthetist should have appropriate experience of paediatric anaesthesia.

The presence of the speculum may affect IOP and refraction. It is, therefore, recommended that tonometry (Tonopen or Perkins) and retinoscopy are performed early in the examination and before insertion of the speculum.

Inhalational anaesthesia can affect IOP measurements to a greater degree than ketamine sedation. Examine the anterior segment with the portable slit-lamp, the operating microscope, and gonioscope. Examine the posterior segment with the direct and indirect ophthalmoscope. Consider A and B-scan ultrasonography.

Table 18.4 Visual milestones

6wks	Can fix and follow a light source, smiling responsively.
3mths	Can fix and follow a slow target, and converge
6mths	Reaches out accurately for toys
2yrs	Picture matching
3yrs	Letter matching of single letters (e.g. Sheridan Gardiner)
5yrs	Snellen chart by matching or naming

Table 18.5 Taking an ophthalmic history in a child

History	
Visual symptoms	History of poor visual behaviour for their age, strabismus, nystagmus, head nodding, red eye, epiphora, photophobia, asymmetry of pupils/corneas/ globes/ red reflexes—sometimes first noted in photographs
POH	Previous/current eye disease; refractive error
PMH	Obstetric/perinatal history; developmental history
SR	Any other systemic (especially CNS including hearing[1]) abnormalities
SH	Family support
FH	Family history of strabismus/other visual problems
Dx	Drugs
Ax	Allergies

1. Up to 50% children with moderate/severe sensorineural deafness have an associated ophthalmic problem.

Ophthalmic assessment in a child (2)

Table 18.6 An approach to an ophthalmic examination in a child

Examination	
Visual acuity	Select test according to age (see Assessment of vision 🕮 p.8); where quantitative not possible grade ability to fix and follow (i.e. is it central, steady, and maintained?)
Visual function	Check for RAPD, binocularity, stereopsis, suppression and retinal correspondence (see Assessment of vision 🕮 p.8)
Cover test	Near/distance/prism cover test
Motility	Ductions, versions, convergence, saccades, doll's eye movements
Accommodation	
BSV	Level of BSV
Fixation	Fixation behaviour, visuscope
Refraction	Cycloplegic refraction
Orbit	Proptosis, inflammation, masses
Lids	Ptosis, skin crease, lid lag, additional skin folds, puncta
Conjunctiva	Inflammation, adhesions
Cornea	Diameter, thickness, opacity, staining, 'brightness of reflex'
AC	Flare, cells, hypopyon, hyphaema
Gonioscopy	(may require EUA) angle, dysgenesis
Iris	Coloboma, anisocoria, polycoria, corectopia
Lens	Lens opacity, shape, position
Tonometry	Applanation (may require EUA); digital
Vitreous	Hyaloid remnants, inflammation, empty
Optic disc	Size, cup, congenital anomaly, oedema, pallor
Fundus	Macula, vessels, retina (e.g. tumours, inflammation, dystrophies, exudation)
Systemic review	For dysmorphic features (including face, ears, teeth, hair) or any other systemic abnormalities

The child who does not see

Worldwide there are over 1.5 million children who are blind or severely visually impaired. Only 6.5% live in the more affluent regions of the world. Major causes include inherited abnormalities (e.g. cataracts, glaucoma, retinal dystrophies), intrauterine insults (e.g. infection), and acquired problems (e.g. retinopathy of prematurity, trauma).

The ophthalmologist's primary aim—best possible vision for the child—must be seen in the context of the child's overall health, quality of life, and family support. Likewise the ophthalmologist's contribution should be seen in the context of the multidisciplinary team, which may include paediatricians, optometrists, orthoptists, primary care physicians, specialist nurses, social workers, and teachers. The challenge to provide best possible care for the child (and family) will depend on the following factors.

Disability

Is the visual impairment the only problem, or are there associated disabilities? These may range from mild developmental delay (e.g. motor, speech, social) to profound neurological or systemic abnormalities. In some severe diseases life expectancy may also be considerably reduced. Such children require the full benefit of the multidisciplinary team, usually co-ordinated by a paediatrician.

Treatment

What treatment might be possible now or in the future? Be realistic about what is and what is not currently possible. Ensure best visual potential with refraction, visual aids, and other supportive measures. Where more invasive treatment is indicated ensure that the parents are fully aware of the risks, realistic outcome, and the extent of care that they will need to give in the perioperative period (e.g. drops, occlusion, CL, frequent clinic visits, etc.).

Equipment

What equipment will help the child function best at home and at school? Reading may require Braille or large print books (usually beneficial if reading vision worse than N10). Normal-sized print may be read by closed circuit television (CCTV) magnification or by a scanner attached to a computer, which has a magnified display facility or which has optical character recognition with a speech synthesizer. The ease of use of standard computer systems has been revolutionized since accessibility options became a standard feature of computer operating systems (e.g. Windows®).

Schooling

Will the child manage best in a specialist school (for the blind or partially sighted) or in a mainstream school (with specialist teacher support)? This is usually determined by the level of visual impairment, any associated disabilities, and the availability of resources locally. In the UK, the 1981 Education Act signalled the start of a trend to encourage mainstream schooling where possible.

Resources

How much help (practical and financial) are the family and/or state able to provide? Social workers should ensure that the parents are receiving appropriate financial benefits. Community paediatricians may be invaluable in co-ordinating local resources. Support organizations often provide help, including advice and emotional support for the parents.

Social

Is the disability accepted by the family/community? The diagnosis may stretch family relationships to breaking-point. Siblings may become jealous of the extra attention the child needs. In some communities blindness is regarded as a stigma. This may adversely affect family dynamics and hinder the child's wider social interactions.

Implications

Are other family members or future siblings at risk of developing the disease, or of being carriers? Genetic disease may be emotive and counselling requires time, patience, and often multiple consultations. The parents may feel guilty about 'passing on' an inherited disease to their child.

Prognosis

Is the visual impairment stationary or progressive? Parents may want to know the probable impact on navigation, education, work, and driving. Where possible, balance the negative (what they won't be able to do) with the positive (what they will be able to do). Stress that our knowledge is limited and that such prognoses are a 'best guess'.

Child abuse

You have a legal duty of care towards any child you see. This means that if you have any concern or suspicion of possible abuse, it is your responsibility to act.

Concern might relate to injuries that are inconsistent with the mobility of the child or with the reported mechanism, histories that are inconsistent with each other or evolve with time, or an unusual relationship between carer and child. Appropriate action may include discussion with a senior ophthalmologist, referral for a paediatric opinion, direct referral to social services, or liaison with the child's health visitor. It is not acceptable to ignore concerns, or to assume 'someone else' will act.

On occasion the ophthalmologist may be asked to examine a child as part of child protection investigations. This should be performed by the most senior ophthalmologist available. It is important to complete as full an examination as possible and for it to be carefully documented.

Photographs may be helpful: if a digital system is used, an unmodified print-out should be made at the time and signed by two witnesses. If a report is required this should be phrased in terms comprehensible to an educated lay public, and include your full name, qualifications, and the situation in which you saw the child.

Retinal haemorrhages and shaken baby syndrome

Shaken baby syndrome

Retinal haemorrhages in the absence of bony injury or external eye injury may arise from severe shaking of young children (shaken baby syndrome). They are not diagnostic of abuse and must be taken in the context of the whole child.

Alternative mechanisms

The Child Abuse Working Party of the Royal College of Ophthalmologists[1] have considered other putative mechanisms of retinal and intracranial haemorrhage. They conclude:

- *Normal handling (e.g. vigorous play):* 'it is highly unlikely that the forces required to produce retinal haemorrhage in a child less than 2yrs of age would be generated by a reasonable person during the course of (even rough) play, or in an attempt to rouse a sleeping or unconscious child.'
- *Short-distance falls:* 'in a child with retinal haemorrhages and subdural haemorrhages who has not sustained a high velocity injury and in whom other recognised causes of such haemorrhages have been excluded, child abuse is much the most likely explanation. ... 'Rarely accidental trauma may give rise to a similar picture.'
- *High cervical injuries:* cervical injuries alone do not result in retinal bleeding, unless combined with circulatory collapse.
- *Hypoxia:* acute hypoxia from transient apnoea has not been shown to result in the SBS picture, unless combined with circulatory collapse.
- *Intracranial bleeding:* Terson syndrome (retinal haemorrhages secondary to intracranial bleeding) is rare in children and any haemorrhages tend to be concentrated around the disc.

1. Child Abuse Working Party *Eye* 2004; **18**: 795–8; also Child Abuse Working Party. *Eye* 1999;**13**:3–10.

Common clinical presentations: vision and movement

The following pages outline common reasons for parents to seek ophthalmic advice. The underlying diseases range from the innocuous to the blinding and/or fatal. A complete ophthalmic (and usually systemic) examination should be performed in all cases. Tables 18.7–18.19 indicate the main causes of these clinical presentations, their key features, and/or a cross reference to further information.

The child who does not see

Unilateral visual loss may not be noticed by parents until picked up at screening or during investigation for an associated abnormality (usually strabismus). Bilateral visual loss will be apparent in the child's visual behaviour. In addition, children who have bilateral poor vision from an early age often have nystagmus or roving eye movements, although this does not occur in patients with retrochiasmal lesions.

Examination: orthoptic, refractive, ophthalmic, neurological ± systemic (as indicated).

Table 18.7 Poor vision: outline of causes

General	Specific
Refractive	Myopia, hypermetropia, astigmatism
Cornea	Opacity, oedema, abnormal curvature, or size
Lens	Cataract, subluxation, lenticonus
Vitreous	Persistent fetal vasculature, inflammation, haemorrhage
Retina	Coloboma, ROP, detachment, dysplasia, dystrophy, albinism
Macula	Hypoplasia, dystrophy, oedema, inflammation, scarring, traction
Optic nerve	Inherited optic atrophy, compression, infiltration, inflammation
CNS	Hypoxia, inflammation, hydrocephalus, compression, delayed visual maturation
Other	Amblyopia, delayed visual maturation, functional

Abnormal eye alignment

Strabismus is common, affecting about 2% of children. While many cases are detected by parents, significant deviations may be missed due to their size, intermittent nature, or compensatory head posture. Conversely, a number of factors may give the appearance of a squint in a perfectly orthophoric child—'pseudostrabismus'.

Examination: refractive, ophthalmic, neurological ± systemic (as indicated).

Abnormal eye movements

Table 18.8 Abnormal ocular alignment: outline of causes and key features

Strabismus (see Assessment ▢ p.654)	Intermittent or manifest misalignment of eyes that may be horizontal, vertical, or torsional
Pseudostrabismus	Consider epicanthal folds, asymmetry of face, globes (proptosis/ enophthalmos), or pupils, abnormal interpupillary distance or abnormal angle kappa

Abnormal supplementary eye movements may occur as an isolated phenomenon or secondary to ocular or systemic disease (usually CNS pathology). They may be broadly divided into nystagmus or saccadic abnormalities.
Examination: refractive, ophthalmic, neurological ± systemic (as indicated).

Table 18.9 Abnormal eye movements: outline of causes and key features

Nystagmus (▢ p.626)	Slow movement away from fixation corrected by fast movement (jerk nystagmus) or another slow movement (pendular nystagmus)
Saccadic abnormalities (▢ p.632)	Fast movement away from fixation, corrected by fast movement immediately (oscillation, e.g. opsoclonus, ocular flutter) or after delay (intrusion)

Common clinical presentations: red eye, watering, and photophobia

Red (Table 18.10) or watering eyes (Table 18.11) are among the commonest ocular presentations in primary care. Often these are relatively benign conditions, many of which may be successfully treated by GPs. However, in the presence of atypical features (particularly visual symptoms) more serious diagnoses should be considered. The presence of photophobia (also see Table 18.12) is usually an indication of more severe ocular pathology.

Examination: ophthalmic ± refractive, neurological, systemic (as indicated).

Red eye(s)

Table 18.10 Red eye: causes and key features

Normal VA	
Conjunctivitis (infective, allergic, chemical)	Gritty, often itchy, discharge, diffuse superficial injection, ± lid papillae/follicles
FB	FB sensation, FB visible or in fornix/subtarsal, local injection, corneal lacerations (if subtarsal FB)
Episcleritis	Mild local pain, sectoral superficial injection (constricted by phenylephrine)
Scleritis	Severe pain, deep often diffuse injection; complications may lead to ↓VA
Vascular malformation	Abnormal conjunctival blood vessels, usually chronic, ± systemic vascular abnormalities
↓VA	
Corneal abrasion/ erosion	Photophobia, watering, sectoral/circumlimbal injection, epithelial defect
Keratitis	Photophobia watering, circumlimbal injection, corneal infiltrate ± epithelial defect ± AC activity
Glaucoma (acute ↑IOP)	Photophobia, watering, corneal oedema, ↑IOP anterior segment/angle abnormalities
Anterior uveitis (acute)	Photophobia, watering, keratic precipitates, AC activity, ± posterior synechiae
Endophthalmitis	Pain, floaters, watering, diffuse deep injection, inflammation (vitreous > AC), hypopyon, chorioretinitis

Watering eyes

Table 18.11 Watering eye: causes and key features

Increased tears	
Blepharitis (posterior)	Chronic gritty, irritable eyes, poor tear film quality, meibomianitis
Conjunctivitis (infective, allergic, chemical)	Gritty, often itchy, discharge may be sticky, diffuse superficial injection, ± lid papillae/follicles
Foreign body	FB sensation, FB visible or in fornix/subtarsal, local injection, corneal lacerations (if subtarsal FB)
Corneal abrasion/ erosion	Photophobia, sectoral/circumlimbal injection, epithelial defect
Keratitis	Photophobia, sectoral/circumlimbal injection, corneal infiltrate ± epithelial defect ± AC activity
Glaucoma (acute ↑IOP)	Photophobia, injection, corneal oedema, ↑IOP ± anterior segment/angle abnormalities
Anterior uveitis	Photophobia, circumlimbal injection, keratic precipitates, AC activity, ± posterior synechiae
Decreased drainage	
Nasolacrimal duct obstruction	Chronic watering (may have sticky discharge) without other ocular signs ± lacrimal sac swelling

Photophobia

Table 18.12 Photophobia: causes and key features

Anterior segment disease	
Corneal abrasion/ erosion	Watering, sectoral/circumlimbal injection, epithelial defect
Keratitis	Watering, circumlimbal injection, corneal infiltrate epithelial defect ± AC activity
Anterior uveitis (acute)	Watering, circumlimbal injection, keratic precipitates, AC activity, ± posterior synechiae
Glaucoma (acute ↑IOP)	Watering, injection, corneal oedema, ↑IOP ± anterior segment/angle abnormalities
Inadequate iris sphincter	Complete/partial absence of tissue (e.g. aniridia, coloboma), mydriasis, or non-pigmentation (albinism)
Posterior segment disease	
Endophthalmitis	Pain, floaters, watering, diffuse deep injection, inflammation (vitreous > AC), chorioretinitis, hypopyon
Retinal dystrophies	Cone deficiencies (achromatopsia, blue cone monochromatism) or later onset dystrophies
CNS disease	
Meningitis/encephalitis	Fever, headache, neck stiffness, altered mental state, neurological dysfunction, normal ocular examination

Common clinical presentations: proptosis and globe size

Abnormalities of the whole globe are usually congenital and represent developmental abnormalities. Abnormal protrusion of the eye (proptosis, Table 18.13) usually represents an acquired, progressive disease.

Proptosis

Abnormal protrusion of the eye (proptosis) is uncommon, but usually signifies severe orbital pathology. An acute onset in a systemically unwell child may represent orbital cellulitis, an ophthalmic emergency. Orbital tumours usually present with more gradual proptosis, although rhabdomyosarcoma is well-known to present acutely, mimicking orbital cellulitis.

Table 18.13 Proptosis: causes and key features

Infection	
Orbital cellulitis	Febrile, systemically unwell, with acute pain, lid swelling, restricted eye movements, VA
Inflammation	
Idiopathic orbital inflammatory disease	Acute pain, lid swelling, conjunctival injection intraocular inflammation and ↓VA; diffuse orbital disease vs localized (e.g. myositis or dacroadenitis)
Thyroid eye disease	Pain, conjunctival injection, lid retraction, restrictive myopathy, ↓VA; usually older children
Vasculitis	Usually present acutely and be systemically unwell (e.g. Wegener's, PAN)
Tumours	
Acquired e.g. rhabdomyosarcoma	Proptosis ± pain, ↓VA, abnormal eye movements; usually gradual onset but some (e.g. rhabdomyosarcoma) may present acutely
Congenital e.g. dermoid cysts	Superficial lesions present early as a round lump, deep lesions may cause pain and gradual proptosis
Vascular anomalies	
Congenital orbital varices	Intermittent proptosis exaggerated by Valsalva manoeuvre or forward posture
Carotid-cavernous fistula	Arterialized conjunctival vessels, chemosis, ± bruit; usually traumatic in children
Bony anomalies	
Sphenoid dysplasia	Pulsatile proptosis, encephalocele, associated with neurofibromatosis-1
Craniosynostosis	Premature fusion of sutures resulting in characteristic skull abnormalities
Other	
Pseudoproptosis	Consider ipsilateral large globe or lid retraction, contralateral enophthalmos or ptosis, facial asymmetry, shallow orbits

Table 18.14 Orbital tumours of childhood (selected)

Congenital	
Choristoma	e.g. dermoid cysts
Acquired	
Optic nerve	e.g. glioma
Vascular	e.g. capillary haemangioma, lymphangioma
Infiltrative	e.g. myeloid leukaemia, histiocytosis
Other	e.g. rhabdomyosarcoma, teratoma
Metastases	e.g. neuroblastoma, nephroblastoma, Ewing's sarcoma

Abnormal eye size

Abnormalities of globe size usually result from abnormalities of development, although it may arise secondary to ocular disease (e.g. buphthalmos in glaucoma). While severe forms may be obvious from simple observation, milder isolated aberrations of size may only be obvious as an axial refractive error.

Table 18.15 Abnormal eye size: causes and key features

Abnormally large eye	
Axial myopia	Mild (physiological) to severe and progressive (pathological) ↑length; ± other ocular abnormalities
Buphthalmos	Diffusely large eye (with megalocornea) associated with glaucoma
Megalophthalmos	Diffusely large eye (with megalocornea) without glaucoma; ± other ocular abnormalities
'Pseudo-large eye'	Consider proptosis or abnormally small contralateral eye
Abnormally small eye	
Microphthalmos	Diffusely small eye (axial length 2SD < normal) ± ocular/systemic anomalies
Nanophthalmos	Microphthalmos with microcornea, normal-sized lens, and abnormally thick sclera
Phthsis bulbi	Acquired shrinkage of the eye due to chronic ocular disease
'Pseudo-small eye'	Consider ipsilateral ptosis or enophthalmos, or abnormally large contralateral eye

Common clinical presentations: cloudy cornea and leucocoria

Opacification of the cornea, lens, or posterior structures is usually associated with poor vision and may indicate serious, even life-threatening, pathology.

Cloudy cornea

Corneal opacities may be focal (either central or peripheral) or diffuse. They may be an isolated finding, associated with other ocular abnormalities or part of an inherited syndrome. In terms of onset, they may be congenital, acquired at birth, or develop during childhood.

Table 18.16 Corneal opacities: causes and key features

Diffuse	
Birth trauma	Forceps injury may induce ruptures in Descemet's membrane (usually unilateral with vertical break)
Glaucoma (acute ↑IOP)	Corneal oedema, ↑IOP, watering, injection, ± anterior segment/angle abnormalities
Keratitis (infective, allergic, exposure)	Photophobia, watering, circumlimbal injection, corneal infiltrate ± epithelial defect ± AC activity
Corneal dystrophies	Clinical pattern varies but may be evident from birth (e.g. congenital hereditary endothelial dysfunction)
Metabolic	Bilateral corneal clouding with systemic abnormalities in some mucopolysaccharidoses
Central	
Peter's anomaly	Congenital, usually bilateral central opacities adhesions to iris or lens
Peripheral	
Sclerocornea	Bilateral (often asymmetric), peripheral opacification with vascularization ± other corneal/angle anomalies
Limbal dermoid	Solid white mass that may involve peripheral cornea; rarely bilateral and 360° round limbi
Posterior embryotoxon	Peripheral opacity due to anteriorly displaced Schwalbe's line ± other angle/ocular abnormalities

Leucocoria

All patients with leucocoria must be assessed for the possibility of retinoblastoma. Congenital cataracts are generally easily identified. Other conditions may be less readily differentiated from retinoblastoma, most commonly persistent fetal vasculature syndrome, Coats' disease, toxocara infection, and ROP.

Table 18.17 Leucocoria: causes and key features

Lens	
Cataract	Lens opacity: stationary or progressive; isolated, or associated with other ocular/systemic abnormalities
Vitreous	
Persistent fetal vasculature syndrome	Variable persistence of fetal vasculature/hyaloid remnants; often microphthalmic; usually unilateral
Inflammatory cyclitic membrane	Fibrous membrane behind the lens arising from the ciliary body due to chronic intraocular inflammation
Retina	
Retinoblastoma	Retinal mass of endophytic, exophytic, or infiltrating type; may spread to anterior segment, orbit, etc.
Coloboma	Developmental defect resulting in variably sized defect involving disc, choroid, and retina
Coats' disease	Retinal telangiectasia with exudation ± exudative retinal detachment
ROP	Early cessation of peripheral retinal vascularization due to prematurity causes fibrovascular proliferation
Familial exudative retinopathy	Early cessation of peripheral retinal vascularization due to inherited defect causes ROP-like picture
Incontinentia pigmenti	Abnormal peripheral retinal vascularization due to inherited defect causes ROP-like picture
Retinal dysplasia	Grey vascularized mass from extensive gliosis (e.g. Norries' disease, Patau syndrome, etc.)
Infection	
Toxocara	Unilateral granuloma or endophthalmitis

Intrauterine infections: toxoplasmosis, rubella, and other

Congenital infections have a variable effect on morbidity and mortality dependent on the infecting organism and the stage of gestation of the fetus. Overall, however, ocular morbidity is common. Likely organisms are screened for by the 'TORCH' screen looking for maternal antibodies to toxoplasma, other (e.g. syphilis, lymphocytic choriomeningitis virus, West Nile virus), rubella, CMV, herpes family (i.e. simplex and VZV). Elevated neonatal IgM antibody or an IgG level higher than the mother's are indicative of intrauterine infection.

Congenital toxoplasmosis

The impact of transplacental infection by toxoplasma is greatest early in pregnancy. The spectrum of disease ranges from an asymptomatic peripheral patch of retinochoroiditis (often an incidental finding years later) to a blinding endophthalmitis. Seronegative women may decrease their risk during pregnancy by reducing their exposure to cats and careful washing of fruit and vegetables.

Table 18.18 Clinical features of congenital toxoplasmosis

Ocular	Retinochoroiditis (more commonly bilateral and affecting the macula than in acquired disease) Cataract, microphthalmos, strabismus
Systemic	Hydrocephalus, intracranial calcification, hepatosplenomegaly

Congenital rubella

Rubella has declined since the advent of the rubella vaccination in 1969. The virus is well known for its teratogenic effects (especially with early infection). It also has remarkable ongoing pathogenicity with interstitial pneumonitis and pancreatic inflammation within the first year, virus shedding up to 2yrs of age and panencephalitis as late as 12yrs of age. Virus within the lens may explain the intense uveitis that can follow cataract surgery.

Table 18.19 Clinical features of congenital rubella

Ocular	Pigmentary retinopathy with normal electrodiagnostics (commonest feature), retinitis, nuclear cataract, microphthalmos, glaucoma (congenital or infantile), corneal clouding (keratitis and/or raised IOP)
Systemic (early/ late)	Congenital heart disease, sensorineural deafness, anaemia, thrombocytopenia, bone abnormalities, hepatitis, CNS abnormalities (e.g. encephalitis)

Congenital syphilis

Having been in decline, syphilis has made a comeback in recent years. The early stage is characterized by inflammation. Many of the later manifestations are direct sequelae of this process. Others (such as interstitial keratitis) may be an immunological phenomenon.

Table 18.20 Clinical features of congenital syphilis

Early disease (<2yrs of age)	
Ocular	Chorioretinitis and retinal vasculitis (results in the characteristic salt-and-pepper fundus)
	Conjunctivitis
Systemic	Mucocutaneous rash; periostitis and osteochondritis;
Late disease (>2yrs of age)	
Ocular	Interstitial keratitis' (usually presents at 5–20yrs of age)
	Optic atrophy
Systemic	Saddle nose, frontal bossing, sabre shins, Hutchinson's teeth[1], scoliosis, hard palate perforation, sensorineural hearing loss[1]

1. Hutchinson's triad.

Congenital lymphocytic choriomeningitis virus

Very likely underdiagnosed as congenital cases only recently recognized (1993). An arena virus with house mice as reservoir causing outbreaks of disease in which pet hamsters may act as vector.

Table 18.21 Clinical features of congenital lymphocytic choriomeningitis virus

Ocular	Retinochoroiditis, optic atrophy, nystagmus, strabismus, cataract, microphthalmos
Systemic	Features at birth rare (meningitis, hepatosplenomegaly), later mental retardation, seizures.

Intrauterine infections: herpes family

Congenital cytomegalovirus (Table 18.22)

Although commonly asymptomatic, congenital infection with CMV may cause severe systemic disease. Retinitis tends to be unifocal, more akin to toxoplasmosis than adult CMV retinitis.

Table 18.22 Clinical features of congenital CMV

Ocular	Retinitis (focal), keratitis, cataracts, microphthalmos, optic atrophy
Systemic	IUGR, microcephaly, hydrocephalus, intracranial calcification, hepatosplenomegaly, thrombocytopenia, deafness (which may be progressive)

Congenital herpes simplex virus (Table 18.23)

It is rare for HSV to be acquired at the intrauterine stage; more commonly HSV is acquired at birth from maternal genital lesions. HSV-2 > HSV-1. **NB** Systemic aciclovir for ocular surface disease in neonates limits dissemination. Untreated neonatal infection has a high mortality rate.

Table 18.23 Clinical features of congenital HSV

Ocular	Rash involving lids, dendritic keratitis, chorioretinitis
Systemic	Vesicular rash, microcephaly, intracranial calcification

Congenital varicella zoster virus (Table 18.24)

Primary varicella infection in the first trimester rarely causes embryopathay. Unusually, the rate of congenital disease is higher if maternal disease is in the second trimester.

Table 18.24 Clinical features of congenital VZV

Ocular	Chorioretinitis (similar to toxoplasmosis), cataracts, microophthalmia, unilateral Horner syndrome
Systemic	Neuropathic bladder

Ophthalmia neonatorum

Ophthalmia neonatorum is defined as a conjunctivitis occurring within the first month of life. Organisms are commonly acquired from the birth canal. The main risk factor is therefore the presence of sexually transmitted disease in the mother. Ophthalmia neonatorum affects up to 12% of neonates in the Western world and up to 23% in developing countries. It is potentially sight-threatening and may cause systemic complications. In some countries (including the UK) it is a notifiable disease.

Gonococcal neonatal conjunctivitis

Clinical features

Hyperacute (within 1–3d of birth), with severe purulent discharge, lid oedema, chemosis, ± pseudomembrane, ± keratitis.

Investigation

Pre-wet swab or conjunctival scrapings: immediate Gram stain (Gram-negative diplococci), culture (chocolate agar), and sensitivities.

Treatment

- Ceftriaxone 50mg/kg IV 1×/d 1wk; frequent saline irrigation of discharge until eliminated.
- After counselling refer mother (with partner) to genitourinary physician.

Chlamydial neonatal conjunctivitis

This is the commonest cause of neonatal conjunctivitis. A papillary rather than follicular reaction is seen due to delayed development of palpebral lymphoid tissue.

Clinical features

- Subacute onset (4–28d after birth), mucopurulent discharge, papillae, ± preseptal cellulitis.
- Systemic (uncommon): rhinitis, otitis, pneumonitis.

Investigation

- *Prewet swabs*: usually for immunofluorescent staining, but cell culture, PCR, and ELISA may be used.
- *Conjunctival scrapings*: Giemsa stain.

Treatment

- Erythromycin 25mg/kg 2×/d for 2wk.
- After counselling refer mother (with partner) to genitourinary physician.

Other bacterial neonatal conjunctivitis

Other bacterial causes include *Staphylococcus aureus*, *Streptococcus pneumoniae* (which require topical antibiotics only), and *Haemophilus* and *Pseudomonas* (which require additional systemic antibiotics to prevent systemic complications).

Clinical features

Subacute onset (4–28d after birth), purulent discharge, lid oedema, chemosis, ± keratitis (*Pseudomonas*).

Investigation
Prewet swab or conjunctival scrapings: Gram stain, culture, and sensitivities.

Treatment
- *Gram-positive organisms*: topical (e.g. chloramphenicol oc 4×/d or erythromycin oc 4×/d); adjust according to sensitivities.
- *Gram-negative organisms*: topical (e.g. tobramycin oc 4×/d); adjust according to sensitivities.

Herpes simplex virus neonatal conjunctivitis

Although viral causes of neonatal conjunctivitis are uncommon, they may cause serious ocular morbidity and systemic disease.

Clinical features
- Acute onset (1–14d), vesicular lid lesions, mucoid discharge ± keratitis (e.g. microdendrities), anterior uveitis, cataract, retinitis, optic neuritis (rare).
- *Systemic* (uncommon but may be fatal): jaundice, hepatosplenomegaly, pneumonitis, meningoencephalitis, disseminated intravascular coagulopathy (DIC).

Investigation
Swab or conjunctival scrapings transported in viral culture medium; PCR.

Treatment
Aciclovir oc 5×/d for 1wk ± aciclovir IV 10mg/kg 3×/d for 10d.

Chemical conjunctivitis

Silver nitrate drops are commonly used in some parts of the world as a protective measure against ophthalmia neonatorum. While effective against gonococcal disease they are of limited use against other bacteria and are of no use against chlamydia or viruses. In the majority of neonates the drops cause red watering eyes from 12 to 48h after instillation.

Table 18.25 Timing of onset of ophthalmia neonatorum by cause

Chemical	<2d
Gonococcal	1–3d
Other bacteria	2–5d
HSV	1–14d
Chlamydia	4–28d

Conjunctivitis in the older child

Children are commonly affected by both infective and allergic conjunctivitis. In the older child it behaves in a more similar manner to adult disease: viral (see 🕮 p.166), bacterial (see 🕮 p.162–165), chlamydial (see 🕮 p.168), allergic (see 🕮 p.170).

Orbital and preseptal cellulitis

Orbital cellulitis may cause blindness and even death. It requires emergency assessment, imaging, and treatment under the joint care of an ophthalmologist, ENT specialist, and paediatrician. Part of the ophthalmologist's role is to assist in differentiating orbital cellulitis from the much more limited preseptal cellulitis.

Orbital cellulitis

Infective organisms include *Streptococcus pneumoniae*, *Staphylococcus aureus*, *Streptococcus pyogenes,* and *Haemophilus influenza* (previously common in younger children, but less likely if Hib vaccinated).

Risk factors
- *Gender:* M:F 2:1.[1]
- *Sinus disease:* ethmoidal sinusitis (common), maxillary sinusitis.
- *Infection of other adjacent structures:* preseptal or facial infection, dacrocystitis, dental abscess.
- *Trauma:* septal perforation.
- *Surgical:* orbital, lacrimal, and vitreoretinal surgery.

Clinical features
- Fever, malaise, painful, swollen orbit.
- Inflamed lids (swollen, red, tender, warm), proptosis, painful restricted eye movements ± optic nerve dysfunction (↓VA, ↓colour vision, ± RAPD).
- *Complications:* optic nerve compromise is the most important; also exposure keratopathy, ↑IOP, CRAO, CRVO.
- *Systemic:* meningitis, cerebral abscess, cavernous sinus thrombosis, orbital or periorbital abscess.

Investigation
- Temperature.
- FBC, blood culture (low yield: generally <7% from recent studies).
- CT (orbit, sinuses, brain): diffuse orbital infiltrate, proptosis ± sinus opacity, orbital abscess.

Treatment
- Admit for IV antibiotics (e.g. either flucloxacillin 25mg/kg 4×/d or cefuroxime 50mg/kg 4×/d with metronidazole 7.5mg/kg 3×/d).
- ENT to assess for sinus drainage (required in up to 50%).

Preseptal cellulitis

Preseptal infection is much commoner than orbital cellulitis. The majority of cases are under 5yrs of age, and 80% of all cases of preseptal cellulitis are under 10yrs. The main causative organisms are once again *Staphylococci* and *Streptococci*. It is generally a much less severe disease, at least in adults and older children. In younger children in whom the orbital septum is not fully developed there is a high risk of progression and so should be treated similarly to orbital cellulitis.

Clinical features
- Fever, malaise, painful, swollen lid/periorbita.
- Inflamed lids but no proptosis, normal eye movements, normal optic nerve function.

Investigation

Investigation is not usually necessary unless there is concern over possible orbital or sinus involvement.

Treatment

- Admit young or unwell children; otherwise daily review until resolution.
- Treat with oral antibiotics (e.g. flucloxacillin).

Table 18.26 Differentiating features of orbital vs preseptal cellulitis

	Orbital	Preseptal
Proptosis	Present	Absent
Ocular motility	Painful + restricted	Normal
VA	↓ (in severe cases)	Normal
Colour vision	↓ (in severe cases)	Normal
RAPD	Present (in severe cases)	Absent (normal)

Table 18.27 Development of paranasal sinuses

Sinus	Onset of development	Onset of adult configuration
Maxillary	In utero	Late childhood (12yrs)
Sphenoidal	In utero	Puberty
Ethmoidal	In utero	Puberty
Frontal	Postnatal	Adulthood

1. Nageswaran S et al. Orbital cellulitis in children. *Pediatr Infect Dis J* 2006;**25**:695–9.

2. McKinley SH et al. Microbiology of pediatric orbital cellulitis. *Am J Ophthalmol* 2007;144:497–501.

Congenital cataract: assessment

Congenital cataract affects up to 1 in 4000 live births. Worldwide about 200 000 children are estimated to be blind from cataracts.

As amblyopia is likely to limit final visual outcome, this condition requires urgent expert assessment, with a view to early surgery.

Assessment

- *History*: observed visual function, intrauterine exposure (infections, drugs, toxins, radiation), medical history (e.g. syndromes), family history.
- *Visual function*: clinical tests appropriate to age. Poor fixation, strabismus and nystagmus suggest severe visual impairment.
- *Cataract density*: indicated by red reflex pre/post-dilation, and quality of fundal view with a direct/indirect ophthalmoscope. Risk to vision is worse if cataract is posterior, dense, confluent, axial, and >3mm diameter.
- *Cataract morphology*: may suggest underlying cause.
- *Rest of the eye*: visual potential (check pupil reactions, and optic nerve and retina as possible), associated ocular abnormalities (may require treatment, influence surgery, or suggest underlying cause).
- *Rest of the child*: numerous systemic conditions are associated with congenital cataracts (Table 18.28). Clinical examination will direct appropriate investigation.

Investigation

- Extensive investigations are not always required (e.g. in unilateral cataracts with a known family history).
- Co-ordinate with a paediatrician but consider:
  - urinalysis (reducing substances and amino acids).
  - serology—'TORCH' screen (toxoplasma, other (e.g. syphilis), rubella, CMV, HSV1 and 2).
  - biochemical profile—including glucose, calcium, phosphate.
  - erythrocyte enzyme analysis—including galactokinase, G1PUT.
  - karyotyping and clinical geneticist referral—e.g. if child dysmorphic.

Table 18.28 Causes of congenital/pre-senile cataracts

Isolated		AD, AR, XR
Chromosomal	Trisomies	Down (21), Edward (18), Patau (13) syndromes
	Monosomies	Turner syndrome
	Deletions	5p (Cri-du-chat syndrome), 18p, 18q
	Microdeletion	16p13– (Rubinstein–Taybi syndrome)
	Duplications	3q, 10q , 20p
Syndromic	Craniosynostosis	Apert syndrome
		Crouzon syndrome
	Craniofacial defects	Smith–Lemli–Opitz syndrome
		Hallerman–Streiff–Francois syndrome
	Dermatological	Cockayne syndrome, Incontinentia pigmenti
		Hypohidrotic ectodermal dysplasia, Ichthyosis, naevoid basal cell carcinoma syndrome, Rothmund–Thomson syndrome
	Neuromuscular	Alstrom disease, Myotonic dystrophy, Marinesco–Sjögren syndrome,
	Connective tissue	Marfan syndrome
		Alport syndrome
		Conradi syndrome
		Spondyloepiphyseal dysplasia
	AS dysgenesis	Peters anomaly
		Rieger syndrome
Metabolic	Carbohydrate	Hypoglycaemia
		Galactokinase deficiency
		Galactosaemia,
		Mannosidosis
	Lipids	Abetalipoproteinaemia
	Amino acid	Lowe syndrome
		Homocysteinuria
	Sphingolipidoses	Niemann–Pick disease
		Fabry disease
	Minerals	Wilson disease
		Hypocalcaemia
	Phytanic acid	Refsum disease
Endocrine		Diabetes mellitus
		Hypoparathyroidism
Infective		Toxoplasma
		Rubella
		Herpes group (CMV, HSV1&2, VZV)
		Syphilis
		Measles
		Poliomyelitis
		Influenza
Other		Trauma
		Drugs (steroids)
		Eczema
		Radiation

Congenital cataract: surgery

Timing of surgery

Remove visually significant cataracts (Table 18.29) as early as possible. Significant unilateral congenital cataracts require urgent removal with optical correction in the first few weeks of life; significant bilateral congenital cataracts should be removed in the first 6wks of life. If bilateral, remove within a few days of each other.

Earlier surgery results in better visual results (acuity and fixation stability) but carries awn increased risk of glaucoma and a less predictable final refractive outcome.

Table 18.29 Factors that indicate visual significance of cataract

Cataract qualities	Obscures undilated red reflex (use direct ophthalmoscope\)
	Greater than 3mm diameter
	Central, posterior and confluent
Visual function evaluation	Disrupted fixation and re-fixation
	Nystagmus
	Decreased forced choice preferential looking (FPL) performance
	Pattern or sweep VEP decreased estimated acuity

Cataract surgery in children places great demands upon their parents and family. Parents must make an informed choice and know what they are signing up to. They should understand that the results of surgery depend enormously on their compliance with unpopular treatments, and they must be prepared that functional visual improvement may be fairly modest, particularly in unilateral cases.

Procedure

Debate continues over the procedure of choice, and when to use implantable lenses (Table 18.30). The current trend is towards implantation.

Table 18.30 Rationale for postoperative aphakia vs IOL implantation

Advantages of aphakia	Advantages of IOL implantation
Technically easier	Reduced postoperative glaucoma
Fewer secondary procedures	Reduced postoperative strabismus
Less visual axis opacification	Reduced amblyogenic anisometropia (in monocular cases)
No IOL long-term safety issues	Reduced refractive error; reduced need for aphakic glasses and/or contact lenses and related problems.

In younger children (<2yrs), it is most common to perform a mechanical lensectomy–vitrectomy. In older children, an anterior continuous curvilinear capsulorhexis may be performed with a view to implanting a lens. Posterior capsular opacification is universal, so perform a posterior capsulorhexis and shallow anterior vitrectomy (anterior or pars plana approach). Suture (absorbable) to close.

Refractive target for intraocular lens implantation

There is considerable debate over the estimation of IOL power in children undergoing cataract surgery. Problems include: (1) accurately estimating axial length and corneal curvature in children; (2) uncertain reliability of the IOL prediction formulae (such as the SRK I/II, Holladay, etc.), which are based on adult eyes; (3) prediction of how much myopic shift to anticipate with normal eye development; and (4) disagreement as to the optimal postoperative refraction to aim for. Most surgeons target emmetropia in older children (>5yrs), but in younger children there is no consensus: some target hypermetropia (to account for myopic shift), others emmetropia or even mild myopia (to reduce amblyopic risk). In unilateral cataracts, IOL choice may also need to be adjusted to reduce anisometropia to <3D.[1]

Postoperative care

Good postoperative care requires highly motivated parents, co-ordinated orthoptists/ophthalmologists, and regularly updated refractions.

CL have optical and cosmetic advantages (particularly in aphakia) but may be problematic, particularly in younger children. Increasing implantation of IOLs results in smaller refractive errors that can be easily corrected by spectacles. Older children (≥3yrs) benefit from bifocal lenses with an 'add' of +3.00 for near.

In unilateral cases patching of the unaffected eye is essential. Aggressive patching improves the visual outcome in the operated eye but increases the amblyopic risk to the normal eye. Close monitoring is a priority whichever regimen is used.

Parental education pre- and post-surgery is essential.

1. Eibschitz-Tsimhoni M. *et al* Intraocular lens power calculation in children *Surv Opthalmol.* 2007;**52:**474–82.

Congenital cataract: complications

Postoperative complications

Cataract surgery in children is more challenging and more subject to complications than in adults. A good result is more likely to be achieved with careful case selection, well planned surgery and meticulous postoperative care (Table 18.31).

Table 18.31 Postoperative complications and strategies for their management

Complication	Management strategy
Intraocular inflammation (may lead to seclusio pupillae, angle closure, and visual axis opacification)	Steroid (intraoperative periorbital, topical and sometimes systemic).
	Cycloplegia
	Iridectomy (especially if corneal diameter <10mm), laser iridotomy
	Heparin in irrigation fluid
	Tissue plasminogen activator into AC
Visual axis opacification	Primary anterior vitrectomy and posterior capsulotomy
	Acrylic IOL
	Laser membranotomy
	Surgical membranotomy (pars plana approach)
	Meticulous postoperative inflammation control (see above)
Glaucoma	Primary placement of intracapsular IOL
	Secondary surgery: augmented trabeculectomy or tube surgery (where medical treatment fails)
	Cyclodestructive therapies
	NB central corneal thickness is often increased in childhood aphakia
Strabismus	Squint surgery
Amblyopia	Penalization
Premature presbyopia	CL/spectacles aiming for +2 to 3
	Bifocals with add of +3 if over 2–3yrs old
Increased macula exposure to short wavelength light	'Yellow' (blue filter) IOL
Retinal detachment (may occur years later)	Vitreoretinal repair
Contact lens problems	📖 See Contact lenses: complications 📖 pp.765–767

Uveitis in children

Although uveitis is much less common in children than in adults it is still a significant cause of ocular morbidity. This is most marked in the context of the 'silent' anterior uveitis of JIA, which accounts for up to 80% of all childhood uveitis. However, it is important to recognize that most other types of uveitis may also affect children.

Juvenile idiopathic arthritis

JIA is the commonest chronic rheumatic disease of childhood. The prevalence of uveitis in JIA overall is approximately 8–30%, but in young oligoarticular onset group (i.e. arthritis in which up to 4 joints are involved) it may be as high as 45–57%. Its classification, screening, and treatment are discussed in more detail elsewhere (see Uveitis with JIA pp.376–377).

Clinical features

Ophthalmic

- Asymptomatic; rarely floaters; ↓VA from cataract.
- White eye, band keratopathy, small KPs, AC cells/flare, posterior synechiae, cataract, secondary glaucoma, vitritis, cystoid macular oedema; other complications include hypotony that may lead to phthisis bulbi.

NB In long-standing uveitis chronic breakdown of the blood aqueous barrier leads to persistent flare; AC cells are, therefore, a better guide than flare to disease activity.

Treatment

Refer to a tertiary referral centre for advice about specific immunosuppression if (1) complications are present at onset, or (2) if the disease is active after 2yrs of topical treatment. Management of complex cases is optimized in tertiary centres with joint clinics between a paediatric rheumatologist and specialist ophthalmologist.

- *Of uveitis*: treatment options include topical steroid eye drops mydriatics, sub-Tenon injections of steroids, orbital floor injections, occasionally systemic steroids and increasingly with weekly methotrexate. Ciclosporin. mycophenolate and anti-TNF agents (infliximab, adalimumab) may also be considered.
- *Of ↑IOP*: initially topical therapy, but up to 2/3 may require surgery (commonly an augmented trabeculectomy or a tube procedure).
- *Of cataract*: aim to defer until the eye has been quiet for a minimum of 3mths, although weigh against the risk of amblyopia in younger children; there is considerable debate over surgery, including whether to implant a lens or leave aphakic.
- *Of band keratopathy*: chelation with EDTA or excimer phototherapeutic keratectomy.

Other causes of uveitis in children

For clinical features, investigation, and treatment of these conditions see Uveitis (📖 pp.333–414).

Table 18.32 Uveitis in children

Anterior	JIA	📖 p.376
	HLA-B27 associated (e.g. psoriasis, ankylosing spondylitis, inflammatory bowel disease)	📖 p.370
	Kawasaki disease	📖 p.374
	TINU	📖 p.374
	Idiopathic	📖 p.368
	Tarantula hairs	
Intermediate	Idiopathic/pars planitis	📖 p.378
	Toxocara	📖 p.408
	Lyme disease	📖 p.404
	Inflammatory bowel disease	📖 p.370
Posterior	Toxoplasma	📖 p.406
	Toxocara	📖 p.408
	Congenital syphilis	📖 p.404
	TB	📖 p.400
	HIV associated (e.g. CMV retinitis)	📖 p.398
	Sarcoidosis	📖 p.382
	Behçet's disease	📖 p.386
Vasculitis	Leukaemia	📖 p.380
	Cat scratch disease	📖 p.380
	Systemic vasculitis, e.g. SLE	📖 p.380
	Herpes group, e.g. HSV	📖 p.394
	HIV related, e.g. CMV	📖 p.398

Treatment

While there are many similarities to adult disease, it should be noted that:
- *Children are still growing*: systemic steroids reduce growth rate and final height; topical steroids may have systemic side-effects.
- *Children are smaller*: all treatments should be appropriately titrated to body size/weight.
- *Children have longer to live*: they are at higher risk of delayed complications, e.g. post-immunosuppression malignancies.

Glaucoma in children: assessment

The childhood glaucomas are a significant cause of blindness in children but may be missed, being both rare and insidious. Unfortunately, the terms congenital, infantile, and juvenile are often used incorrectly and interchangeably rendering the nomenclature confusing. Classifying childhood glaucoma by aetiology may, therefore, be more useful.

Causes

Primary (syn. primary congenital glaucoma, trabeculodysgenesis)

In this rare syndrome (1/10 000 live births) angle dysgenesis causes reduced aqueous outflow. It is usually sporadic, but 10% are familial. Genes identified include GLC3A (Ch2p) and GLC3B (Ch1p), which result in autosomal recessive disease.

Secondary

Anterior segment dysgenesis (see 🕮 p.724)

Developmental abnormalities of the anterior segment result in a spectrum of anterior segment anomalies, including Axenfeld, Rieger, and Peter's anomalies, and associated abnormalities of the drainage angle. Glaucoma occurs in about 50%.

Aniridia

In aniridia (syn. iridotrabeculodysgenesis) the iris tissue is abnormal or absent, and is associated with glaucoma in up to 75%.

Lens/surgery related

Surgery for congenital cataracts is associated with glaucoma in up to 40% being highest for early total lensectomy.

Posterior segment developmental abnormalities

Persistent fetal vasculature syndrome and retinopathy of prematurity may cause glaucoma by a secondary angle closure mechanism.

Tumour related

Tumours may cause ↑IOP by reduced aqueous outflow (mechanical, clogging of trabecular meshwork by cellular debris, secondary haemorrhage or lead to rubeotic glaucoma). Tumours may be anterior (e.g. juvenile xanthogranuloma, medulloepithelioma), posterior (e.g. retinoblastoma), or systemic (e.g. leukaemia).

Phakomatoses

Sturge–Weber syndrome is associated with ipsilateral glaucoma in up to 50%, being highest where the naevus flammeus involves both upper and lower lid. Neurofibromatosis also carries an increased risk, particularly in the presence of an ipsilateral neurofibroma.

Connective tissue disease

Marfan syndrome, homocystinuria and Weill–Marchesani are associated with glaucoma. This may arise due to abnormal trabecular meshwork or lens block.

Uveitis

Chronic uveitis of childhood (e.g. associated with JIA) may result in secondary glaucoma. This is usually of relatively late onset.

Clinical features

- Watering eye(s), photophobia, blepharospasm, enlarged eye(s), cloudy cornea.
- ↑IOP, corneal oedema, enlargement of cornea/globe (buphthalmos, if onset <4yrs of age), breaks in Descemet's membrane (Haab's striae).

Additional features

These may indicate the underlying cause of glaucoma:

- *Ophthalmic*: posterior embryotoxon, leukoma, anterior iris strands, iris hypoplasia, aniridia, iris cyst/tumour, iritis, Lisch nodules (NF-1), cataract, ectopia lentis, aphakia, persistent fetal vasculature, ciliary body tumours, retinal masses.
- *Systemic*: naevus flammeus (Sturge–Weber syndrome), neurofibromas (NF-1 or 2), Marfanoid habitus (Marfan syndrome, homocystinuria), brachydactyly (Weill–Marchesani syndrome), abnormal dentition and umbilical hernia or failure of periumbilical skin involution (Rieger syndrome).

Intraocular pressure and central corneal thickness

Be aware that CCT variability has a clinically significant effect on IOP measurement in about half of paediatric glaucoma cases. A higher CCT or thicker cornea (e.g. aphakic glaucoma, aniridia, and microcornea) will lead to overestimating the IOP, i.e. the measured IOP will be higher than the actual IOP. In contrast a lower CCT or thinner cornea (e.g. keratoconus, keratoglobus) will lead to underestimating the actual IOP.

Glaucoma in children: treatment

Titrate treatment according to IOP (interpreted in the light of the CCT, see Ocularhypertension 🕮 p.306), worsening disc appearance, and increasing corneal diameter. In older children perimetry is also a valuable tool.

Medical treatment

Medical treatment is often unsatisfactory but may be useful while awaiting surgery. Alpha-2 agonist (brimonidine) causes CNS depression in children and is contraindicated. Systemic carbonic anhydrase inhibitors can sometimes cause decreased energy levels.

Surgical treatment

Preferred surgical technique depends on the type and severity of glaucoma. *Options include:*

- *Goniotomy*: incision of the uveal trabecular meshwork under gonioscopic view allows iris root to fall back and presumed to open the drainage angle
- *Trabeculotomy*: cannulation of Schlemm's canal *ab externo* and disruption of internal wall of canal and trabecular meshwork using trabeculotome.
- *Trabeculectomy*: forms a new drainage channel from AC to subconjunctival space; may be augmented by antimetabolites.
- *Aqueous shunting procedures ('tubes')*: silicone tube flows from AC via valve to episcleral explant.

Table 18.33 Summary of surgical treatments in paediatric glaucoma

Procedure	Indications	Advantages/disadvantages
Goniotomy and/or trabeculotomy	Congenital glaucoma due to trabeculodysgenesis especially good results (>90% IOP control at 5yrs). Clear cornea needed for goniotomy (unless endoscopic viewing)	Low rate serious complication Anatomical route of aqueous maintained Possible in small eyes with difficult access
Augmented trabeculectomy	Refractory glaucoma Consider especially in aniridia, uveitis, Sturge–Weber syndrome	*Bleb-related complications (failure, blebitis, leak, hypotony, endophthalmitis)* *Numerous postoperative procedures impractical in children*
Aqueous shunting procedure	Refractory glaucoma Consider especially in aphakic glaucoma	Less postoperative procedures *Initial hypotony* *Explant related complications (tube migration, plate extrusion, strabismus)*
Cyclodestructive laser	Failure of surgical treatment When glaucoma surgery contra-indicated due to co-morbidities	Minimal postoperative management *Hypotony, phthisis, inflammation, retinal detachment*

Retinopathy of prematurity (1)

Retinopathy of prematurity was first reported in 1942. By the 1950s it was the leading cause of childhood blindness. At this point tight oxygen control was introduced, with a dramatic fall in ROP, but a significant rise in neonatal death and neurological disability. Oxygen delivery is now a compromise between these factors.

Risk factors

- Low gestational age (<32wks).
- Low birth-weight (<1501g).
- High or variable oxygen tension.

Classification

Stages

These are defined by the International Classification of ROP revisited (ICROP):[1]

- *Stage 1*: demarcation line: flat white line separating vascular from avascular zones.
- *Stage 2*: ridge: line becomes elevated, thickened, may become pinkish with neovascular tufts ('popcorn') posterior to ridge.
- *Stage 3*: extraretinal fibrovascular proliferation: vascular tissue grows from the posterior margin on to the retina or into the vitreous.
- *Stage 4*: subtotal retinal detachment: extrafoveal (4A) or foveal (4B).
- *Stage 5*: total retinal detachment.

Plus and pre-plus disease

- *Plus disease*: there is significant venous dilatation and arteriolar tortuosity (compared with a standard photograph[1]) of the posterior retinal vessels in two or more quadrants.
- *Pre-plus disease*: there is more venous dilatation and arteriolar tortuosity than normal but insufficient to be defined as plus disease.

Location

- *Zone I*: circle centred on the disc, with radius twice the distance from the centre of the disc to the fovea.
- *Zone II*: ring centred on the disc, extending from zone 1 to ora nasally and equator temporally.
- *Zone III*: remaining temporal crescent.

Extent

Measured in clock-hours.

Threshold disease

- Originally an estimate of when progression and regression were equally likely, and so used as the level when treatment is indicated.
- Threshold disease is defined as stage 3 ROP with plus disease in zones I or II and of 5 continuous or 8 non-continuous clock-hours.

Prethreshold disease

The Early Treatment in ROP (ETROP) trial[2] suggested a benefit in treating some cases of ROP that are not yet at 'threshold'.

Prethreshold disease (type 1):
- Zone I, any stage ROP with plus disease.
- Zone I, Stage 3 ROP with or without plus disease.
- Zone II, Stage 2, or 3 ROP with plus disease.

Prethreshold disease (Type 2):
- Zone I, Stage 1, or 2 ROP without plus disease.
- Zone II, Stage 3 ROP without plus disease.

Fig. 18.1 ROP zones and examples of classification.

1. International Committee for the Classification of Retinopathy of Prematurity. The International Classification of Retinopathy of prematurity revisited. *Arch Ophthalmol* 2005;**123**:991–9.

2. Good WV. Early Treatment for Retinopathy of Prematurity Cooperative Group. Final results of the Early Treatment for Retinopathy of Prematurity (ETROP) randomized trial. *Trans Am Ophthalmol Soc* 2004;**102**:233–48.

Retinopathy of prematurity (2)

Screening

Indirect ophthalmoscopy with a 28D lens permits a wide field of view. Dilate in advance (cyclopentolate 0.5% + phenylephrine 2.5%; 2–3 doses; 1h before the examination), consider a lid speculum and scleral indentation as needed, and beware of the positions of all tubes/lines that may be vulnerable to a clumsy ophthalmologist.

Table 18.34 Summary of UK ROP screening guidelines[1]

Screening inclusion criteria	
All babies born at <31wks gestational age (i.e. up to 30wks and 6d) or <1251g birthweight.	*Must* be screened
All babies born at <32wks gestational age (i.e. up to 31wks and 6d) or <1501g birthweight.	*Should* be screened (less evidence but considered good practice)
First screening examination[2]	
Babies born <27wks gestational age	First exam to be at 30–31wks postmenstrual age
Babies born between 27 and 32wks gestational age	First exam to be at 4–5wks postnatal age
Babies born >32wks gestational age but <1501g birthweight	First exam to be at 4–5wks postnatal age
Frequency of screening	
If vessels end in zone I or posterior zone II, *or* any plus or pre-plus disease *or* any stage 3 disease (any zone)	Screen at least weekly
All other circumstances where termination criteria not reached	Screen at least fortnightly
Termination of screening	
In babies with no ROP:	
Vascularization has extended into zone III	Termination of screening (usually after 36 completed wks postmenstrual age)
In babies with ROP not requiring treatment:	
Two successive examinations showing any of: • Lack of increase in severity. • Partial resolution progressing towards complete resolution. • Change in colour in the ridge from salmon pink to white. • Transgression of vessels through the demarcation line. • Commencement of the process of replacement of active ROP lesions by scar tissue.	Termination of screening[3]

Treatment

Treatment has traditionally been recommended for threshold disease and worse; however, recent evidence suggests that 'high-risk' prethreshold disease may also benefit.

Cryotherapy has been used for over 30yrs but has largely been replaced by laser photocoagulation, which is more portable, better tolerated, and more effective for posterior disease. Photocoagulation should be with a trans-pupillary diode laser to give nearly confluent burns (half to one burn-width separation) to the whole avascular retina.

Vitreoretinal surgery aims to repair or prevent progression of ROP associated retinal detachment (stages 4A, 4B, and 5). Unfortunately, results are generally disappointing.

Table 18.35 Summary of UK ROP treatment guidelines[1]

Treatment criteria	
• Zone I, any ROP with plus disease. *or*	Treat
• Zone I, stage 3 without plus disease. *or*	
• Zone II, stage 3 with plus disease.	
• Zone II, stage 2 with plus disease.	Consider treating
Timing of treatment	
• Aggressive ROP	Treat as soon as possible (and <48h)
• All other ROP requiring treatment.	Treat within 48–72h
Technique	
Trans-pupillary diode laser to give near-confluent (0.5–1 burn-width) laser burn spacing to the entire avascular retina.[4]	
Post-treatment follow-up	
• First examination	5–7d post treatment
• Subsequent examination(s)	Initially at least weekly looking for signs of ↓activity and regression; Then as clinically indicated
Re-treatment	
• Failure of ROP to regress	10–14d post initial treatment

1. Guideline for the Screening and Treatment of Retinopathy of Prematurity 2008 (RCPCH, RCOphth, BAPN, BLISS) www.rcophth.ac.uk/.

2. First screening exam should occur prior to discharge.

3. Any stage 3 disease may require long-term follow-up as clinically indicated.

4. Where this is not possible, then treatment with cryotherapy or argon laser by an ophthalmologist experienced in these techniques is preferable to a delay in treatment.

Other retinal disorders

Retinopathy of prematurity-like syndromes

Familial exudative vitreoretinopathy

This rare condition usually shows autosomal dominant inheritance (Ch11q). Clinical features include abrupt cessation of peripheral retinal vessels at the equator (more marked temporally) and vitreous bands in the periphery. Complications include fibrovascular proliferation, macular ectopia, retinal detachment (akin to ROP), and subretinal exudation (akin to Coats' disease).

Incontinentia pigmenti (Bloch–Sulzberger syndrome)

This rare condition shows X-linked dominant inheritance being lethal in utero for male embryos. Clinical features include abnormal peripheral vasculature, gliosis, tractional retinal detachment, and systemic features, such as abnormal teeth, cutaneous pigment whorls and CNS anomalies.

Retinal dysplasia

A number of conditions are associated with more extensive retinal abnormalities, probably arising as a result of abnormal development involving the inner wall of the optic cup. Clinical features include extensive retinal folds, retinal detachments, retinal haemorrhages, vitreous haemorrhages, retrolental grey mass, and phthisis bulbi. Associated syndromes include Patau's syndrome, Edward syndrome (see Chromosomal syndromes 📖 p.728), Norrie's disease (retinal dysplasia, deafness, ↓IQ), and Walker–Warburg syndrome (retinal dysplasia, muscular dystrophy, Dandy–Walker malformation).

Other retinochoroidal disorders

Many stationary and progressive disorders of photoreceptors, RPE, choroid and retinal vasculature present in childhood. They are discussed elsewhere: RP (📖 p.508), congenital stationary night blindness (📖 p.510), macular dystrophies (📖 pp.512–515), choroidal dystrophies (📖 p.516), hereditary vitreoretinal degenerations (📖 p.436), albinism (📖 p.518), and Coats' disease (📖 p.504).

Developmental abnormalities: craniofacial and globe

Congenital craniofacial abnormalities

Congenital craniofacial abnormalities may have a profound effect on the developing orbit and globe. They may be divided into craniosynostosis, clefting defects and hemifacial microsomia. They are all rare.

Craniosynostosis

Craniosynostosis arises from premature fusion of the cranial sutures. It occurs in about 1 in 4000 live births. The clinical appearance and severity depends on the extent of premature suture fusion. The typical appearance is of a tall broad skull with frontal bossing and proptosis. If severe, compression of the enlarging brain results in ↑ICP.

Craniosynostosis may be isolated or part of a syndrome such as Crouzon or Apert syndrome. Crouzon and Apert syndromes are clinically distinct but both arise from mutations in the gene encoding the fibroblast growth factor receptor-2 (Ch10q26).

- *Apert syndrome*: autosomal dominant or sporadic, occurring in 1 in 100 000 births. Clinical features include craniosynostosis, syndactyly, broad distal phalanx of great thumb/toe, mental handicap; hypertelorism, proptosis, strabismus, keratoconus, ectopia lentis, glaucoma, and optic atrophy.
- *Crouzon syndrome*: autosomal dominant or sporadic, occurring in 1 in 50 000 births. Clinical features include craniosynostosis, maxillary hypoplasia, prognathism, hooked nose; proptosis, strabismus, micro/megalocornea, iris coloboma, cataract, ectopia lentis, and glaucoma.

Clefting defects

A number of defects have been ascribed to 'clefting' or failure of development of the branchial arches. This may result in hypertelorism or syndromes such as Treacher Collins syndrome.

Treacher Collins syndrome (mandibulofacial dysostosis): autosomal dominant; mutation in the 'treacle gene' TCOF1 (Ch5q32). Clinical features include antimongoloid palpebral fissures, lower lid colobomas, dermoids, mandibular hypoplasia, zygoma hypoplasia, choanal atresia.

Hemifacial microsomia

This is a relatively common birth defect (1 in 5600 live births; Ch14q32) involving first and second branchial arches. A spectrum of severity is seen varying from mild facial asymmetry with an extra auricular tag to more severe hemifacial hypoplasia and associated systemic features, as seen in Goldenhar syndrome.

Goldenhar syndrome: part of the spectrum of hemifacial microsomia; accessory auricle, limbal dermoid, hypoplasia of face, vertebral anomaly. corneal hyposthesia. Duane syndrome. iris and upper eyelid coloboma.

Nasolacrimal duct

Cannulation of the nasolacrimal cord may be delayed distally resulting in congenital obstruction. More commonly there is simply an imperforate mucus membrane at the valve of Hasna which disappears within the first year of life.

Overall 90% spontaneously resolve by 1yr of age. In those that persist a 'syringe and probe' carries a 90% success rate. Where blockage is sufficient to prevent the passage of the probe a DCR is usually required.

> **Box 18.1 Outline of 'syringe and probe' for congenital nasolacrimal obstruction**
>
> - Anaesthesia (usually GA).
> - Introduce nasolacrimal cannula into the lower or upper canaliculus.
> - Inject fluorescein stained saline solution to confirm nasolacrimal obstruction.
> - Pull the lower lid laterally and introduce probe into the inferior punctum and then medially to the sac.
> - Turn the probe 90° so as to direct it inferiorly down the nasolacrimal duct to perforate membrane.
> - Repeat syringing to confirm patency of nasolacrimal duct with recovery of fluorescein from the nose.

Anophthalmia and microphthalmia

Anophthalmia is the absence of an eye within the orbit. It may be divided into primary anophthalmia (complete failure of any ocular tissue to develop), secondary anophthalmia (partial development which then halts leaving a very small microphthalmic eye) and degenerative anophthalmia (partially developed eye regresses).

As normal development of the orbit and lids depend on the presence of the globe, early treatment with conformers and expanders is important, and continues until the face has fully developed.

Initially, clear conformers are used (until age 2yrs) as they have to be replaced every few weeks. Subsequently, they may be replaced by painted prostheses. Special conformers are available for microphthalmic eyes in which some limited vision is preserved; these improve cosmesis without obstructing vision. Surgery also has a role in reducing orbital asymmetry. A multidisciplinary approach is needed, including among others, a paediatric ophthalmologist, orbital surgeon, and orbital prosthesist.

Hamartomas and choristomas

Hamartomas (congenital tumours of tissues normal to that location) include the common capillary haemangioma. These bright red tumours usually appear before 2mths of age, reach full size by 1yr, and involute by 6yr. When located on the lid they may obscure the visual axis or cause astigmatism resulting in amblyopia. In these cases treatment may be indicated.

Choristomas (congenital tumours of tissues abnormal to that location) include dermoids that probably represent surface ectoderm trapped at lines of embryonic closure and suture lines. These are most commonly located on the superotemporal orbital rim, but may extend deceptively far posteriorly.

Developmental abnormalities: anterior segment

Axenfield-Rieger group

Anterior segment dysgenesis results in a spectrum of abnormalities of variable severity often complicated by glaucoma.. The Axenfield–Rieger group tend to have autosomal dominant inheritance. Based on their original descriptions, a posterior embryotoxon with anterior iris strands is known as Axenfield's anomaly, whereas more extensive iris involvement is known as Rieger anomaly.

Rieger anomaly may be associated with systemic abnormalities (teeth small and fewer than normal, maxillary hypoplasia), when it is known as Rieger's syndrome.

Peter's anomaly

This is a congenital corneal opacity (leukoma) associated with a posterior corneal defect (posterior stroma, Descemet's membrane and endothelium). It may be associated with anterior iris strands, lens-corneal strands and glaucoma. It is usually sporadic. Early corneal surgery may permit some vision to develop.

Box 18.2 Anterior segment dysgenesis

Posterior embryotoxon
+ anterior iris strands   = Axenfield's anomaly
   + iris hypoplasia   = Rieger anomaly
     + systemic abnormalities = Rieger syndrome

Corneal opacity (leukoma)/posterior corneal = Peters anomaly
defect   of increasing
+ anterior iris strands   severity
   + lens/corneal touch

Aniridia

Aniridia is characterized by iris hypoplasia. It occurs in up to 1 in 64000 births, being autosomal dominant in two-thirds, sporadic in one-third and rarely autosomal recessive. The disease ranges from mild defects of anterior iris stroma only to almost complete absence of the iris.

Aniridia may be associated with peripheral corneal opacification, lens opacity/subluxation, optic nerve hypoplasia, foveal hypoplasia (actually dysgenesis as OCT shows the fovea to be abnormally thick due to preserved inner retinal layers) and glaucoma (see Glaucoma in children 📖 pp.712–714).

Aniridia usually arises from point mutations in the PAX6 gene (11p13). Some sporadic cases arise from an 11p13 microdeletion, which depending on extent, results in increased risk of Wilms' tumour (due to loss of the tumour suppressor gene, WT1) or the full WAGR syndrome (Wilms' tumour, aniridia, genitourinary abnormalities, ↓IQ, craniofacial dysmorphism). Sporadic aniridia confers a high relative risk (estimated at 67) for development of Wilms' tumour.[1]

Gillespie syndrome is a very rare autosomal recessive form of aniridia that is not associated with PAX6 mutations. Aniridia is partial and is associated with ataxia and ↓IQ.

Treatment for aniridia is directed by severity of iris hypoplasia and the extent of associated problems. Interventions include tinted CL, cataract surgery with artificial iris–lens diaphragms, keratoplasty, and medical/surgical therapy for glaucoma.

Iris coloboma

A coloboma is a defect resulting from failure of closure of an embryological fissure. When this occurs at the level of the iris, a typical inferonasal defect is seen. This may be associated with a posterior coloboma.

1. Gronskov K et al. Population-based risk estimates of Wilms tumor in sporadic aniridia. *Hum. Genet* 2001;**109**:11–18.

Developmental abnormalities: posterior segment

Vitreous

Abnormalities within the vitreal cavity include remnants of the hyaloid vascular system (Table 18.36), and abnormalities of the vitreous structure, e.g. type II collagen abnormalities resulting in Stickler syndrome.

Table 18.36 Hyaloid remnants

Glial remnant just posterior to lens	Mittendorf's dot
Glial remnant just anterior to disc	Bergmeister's papilla
Vascular remnant arising from disc	Persistent hyaloid artery
Vascular remnant and retrolental mass	Persistent fetal vasculature

Optic fissure

A coloboma is a defect resulting from failure of closure of an embryological fissure. Within the eye, defects may occur anywhere from disc to iris, and vary dramatically in size and severity. Colobomas may be blinding and may be associated with more extensive disease.

Optic nerve anomalies

These include optic disc pits, optic disc hypoplasia, coloboma, and morning glory anomaly (see Congenital optic disc ananalies p.600). Although disc pits are often isolated findings, more severe disc abnormalities are often associated with systemic pathology.

Retina

Premature cessation of peripheral retina vascularization may occur due to an inherited defect (familial exudative vitreoretinopathy, Ch11q) or acquired insult (retinopathy of prematurity). This results in fibrovascular proliferation, traction, exudation, and retinal detachment.

Retinal dysplasia may occur in isolation but is usually part of a syndrome such as Edward's, Patau's, Norrie's, Warburg's, or incontinentia pigmenti. Severe forms present with bilateral leucocoria and very poor vision.

Macular hypoplasia may occur in isolation or with syndromes such as albinism or aniridia. There is loss of the normal foveal reflex and in some cases loss of the avascular zone.

Chromosomal syndromes

Trisomy syndromes

Down syndrome

Down syndrome (trisomy 21) is the commonest autosomal trisomy, with an incidence of 1 in 650 live births. It is also the commonest genetic causes of learning difficulties. Most cases arise by non-disjunction (94%), some by translocation (5%), and rarely by mosaicism (1%). Mosaic cases usually have a milder phenotype.

Table 18.37 Clinical features of Down syndrome

Ocular	Mongoloid palpebral fissures, hypertelorism, epicanthic folds, ectropia, blepharoconjunctivitis
	Myopia, astigmatism
	Strabismus, nystagmus
	Keratoconus, Brushfield spots, cataracts
	Hypoplastic disc
Systemic	Short stature, macroglossia, flat nasal bridge, broad hands, single palmar crease, clinodactyly, 'sandal gap' toes, hypotonia
	Congenital heart disease (ASD, VSD), duodenal atresia, hypothyroidism, diabetes mellitus, ↑risk of leukaemia
	↓IQ and early Alzheimer's dementia

Edwards syndrome

Edwards syndrome (trisomy 18) is the second commonest autosomal trisomy at 1 in 8000 live births. Life expectancy is less than 1yr.

Table 18.38 Clinical features of Edwards syndrome

Ocular	Epicanthal folds, blepharophimosis, ptosis, hypertelorism
	Microphthalmos, corneal opacities, congenital glaucoma, cataracts
	Uveal colobomas
Systemic	Failure to thrive
	Small chin, low set ears, overlapping fingers, 'rocker bottom' feet
	Congenital heart defects, renal malformations

Patau syndrome

Patau syndrome (trisomy 13) is the third commonest autosomal trisomy at 1 in 14 000 live births. Life expectancy is less than 3mths.

Table 18.39 Clinical features of Patau syndrome

Ocular	Cyclopia, microphthalmos, colobomas
	Corneal opacities, cataracts, intraocular cartilage, retinal dysplasia, optic nerve hypoplasia;
Systemic	Failure to thrive
	Microcephaly, scalp defects, hernias, polydactyly
	Congenital heart defects, renal malformations, apnoeas

Deletion syndromes

Turner syndrome

Turner syndrome (XO) occurs in 1 in 2000 live female births. Only half are XO (also known as 45,X), with 15% being mosaics and the remainder having partial deletions or other abnormalities. The Turner's phenotype arises from X-linked genes that escape inactivation (e.g. the SHOX short stature homeobox gene).

Table 18.40 Clinical features of Turner syndrome

Ocular	Antimongoloid palpebral fissures, epicanthus, ptosis, hypertelorism
	Strabismus, convergence insufficiency
	Cataracts
	'Male' levels of X-linked recessive disease (e.g. red–green colour blindness)
Systemic	Neonatal lymphoedema of hands/feet
	Short stature, webbed neck, low posterior hairline, wide carrying angle, broad chest with apparent wide spaced nipples
	Congenital heart defects (notably coarctation of the aorta)
	Primary gonadal failure,
	Normal IQ, sensorineural deafness, delayed motor skills

Other deletion syndromes

Although microdeletions are probably fairly common, macrodeletions other than Turner's are rare. Syndromes with ophthalmic features include the cri-du-chat syndrome (5p-), DeGrouchy syndrome (18q-), and the 13q- deletion syndrome. Common features are hypertelorism and epicanthal folds. In addition in 13q- there is a significantly increased risk of retinoblastoma.

Metabolic and storage diseases (1)

Although individually these conditions are rare (or very rare), as a group they feature regularly in the paediatric clinic. The ophthalmologist has an important role both in the diagnostic process and in the ongoing management of affected patients.

Table 18.41 Disorders of carbohydrate metabolism

Syndrome	Deficiency	Ocular features	Systemic features
Galactosaemia	Galactose-1-phosphate uridyl transferase	Cataracts (oil droplet)	↓ IQ Failure to thrive
Galactokinase deficiency	Galactokinase	Cataracts	Normal
Mannosidosis	α-mannosidase	Cataracts (spoke-like)	↓ IQ MPS-like changes but clear corneas

All the above conditions are autosomal recessive.

Table 18.42 Disorders of amino acid metabolism

Homocystinuria (I–III)	Cystathionine synthetase (I)	Ectopia lentis Myopia Glaucoma	↓ IQ Marfanoid habitus Thromboses Fine, fair hair
Cystinosis	Lysosomal transport protein	Crystalline keratopathy	Renal failure Failure to thrive
Lowe syndrome	Unknown	Microphakia Cataracts Blue sclera AS dysgenesis Glaucoma	↓ IQ Failure to thrive Rickets (vitamin D-resistant)
Zellweger syndrome	Unknown	Flat brows ON hypoplasia Pigmentary retinopathy Glaucoma	Dysgenesis of brain, liver and kidneys Metabolic acidosis
Albinism	📖 p.518	📖 p.518	📖 p.518
Alkaptonuria	Homogentisic acid dioxygenase	Scleral darkening	Ochronosis Arthritis
Sulphite oxidase deficiency	Molybdenum cofactor	Spherophakia Ectopia lentis	Neurodegeneration LE <2yr
Tyrosinaemia (II)	Tyrosine transaminase	Herpetiform corneal ulcers	↓ IQ (some) Hyperkeratosis of palms/soles
Gyrate atrophy	Ornithine 5-aminotransferase	📖 p.516	📖 p.516

All the above conditions are autosomal recessive other than Lowe syndrome and ocular albinism which are X-linked. LE, life expectancy: ON, optic nerve.

Table 18.43 Disorders of lipid metabolism

Syndrome	Deficiency	Ocular features	Systemic features
Lipoproteins			
Abetalipo-proteinaemia	Triglyceride transfer protein	Cataract Pigmentary retinopathy	Spinocerebellar degeneration LE <50yr
Sphingolipids			
G_M1 gangliosidosis	β-galactosidase	Cloudy corneas Cherry red spot Optic atrophy	Neurodegeneration (types 1 and 2) Visceromegaly (1) LE 1 <4yr, LE 2 <40yr
Tay-Sachs	Hexosaminidase A	Cherry red spot Optic atrophy	Visceromegaly LE <3yr
Sandhoff's	Hexosaminidase A Hexosaminidase B	Cherry red spot Optic atrophy	Visceromegaly Neurodegeneration LE <3yr
Gaucher's disease (I–III)	β-glucosidase	Supranuclear gaze palsy (type IIIb)	Visceromegaly neurodegeneration LE I (old), II (2), III (15)
Niemann–Pick (type A)	Sphingomyelinase	Cherry red spot Optic atrophy	Visceromegaly Neurodegeneration LE <3yr
Fabry's disease	α-galactosidase	Vortex keratopathy Cataract Tortuous vessels	Angiokeratomas Painful episodes Renal failure Vascular disease LE = middle-age
Metachromatic leukodystrophy	Arylsulphatase-A	Optic atrophy Nystagmus	Neurodegeneration LE α type
Krabbe's disease	Galacto-cerebrosidase	Optic atrophy	Neurodegeneration LE α type
Farber's disease	Ceramidase	Macular pigmentation	Granulomas Arthopathy
Other			
Neuronal ceroid lipofuscinosis (Batten's)	Unknown	Macular discolouration RP-like changes Optic atrophy	Neurodegeneration LE α type
Refsum syndrome	Phytanic acid α-hydrolase	Pigmentary retinopathy	Neuropathy Ataxia Deafness Icthyosis

All the above conditions are autosomal recessive, other than Fabry's disease, which is X-linked.
LE: life expectancy.

Metabolic and storage diseases (2)

Table 18.44 Disorders of glycosaminoglycan metabolism (mucopolysaccharidoses)

Syndrome	Deficiency	Ocular features	Systemic features
MPSI (Hurler/Scheie/ Hurler–Scheie)	α-iduronidase	Cloudy corneas Pigmentary retinopathy Optic atrophy	Skeletal/ facialdysmorphism ↓ IQ Severity α type: H > H/S > S
MPSII (Hunter)	Iduronate sulphatase	Pigmentary retinopathy Optic atrophy	Variable ↓ IQ and dysmorphism
MPSIII (A–C) (Sanfillipo)	Heparan-N-sulphatase (A)	Pigmentary retinopathy Optic atrophy	Neurodegeneration Hyperactivity Mild dysmorphism
MPSIV (A-B) (Morquio)	Galactose-6-sulphatase (A)	Cloudy corneas	Skeletal dysplasia Normal facies/IQ
MPSVI (Maroteaux-Lamy)	N-acetyl-galactosamine-4-sulphatase	Cloudy corneas	Skeletal/facial dysmorphism Normal IQ
MPSVII (Sly)	β-glucuronidase	Cloudy corneas	Skeletal/facial dysmorphism ↓ IQ

All the above conditions are autosomal recessive other than Hunter's, which is X-linked.

Table 18.45 Disorders of mineral metabolism

Wilson's disease	Cu binding protein	Kayser–Fleischer ring Cataract	Neurodegeneration Ataxia
Menkes syndrome	Cu transport protein	Optic atrophy	Kinky hair Neurodegeneration Ataxia

The above conditions are autosomal recessive Cu, copper.

Table 18.46 Disorders of connective tissues

Syndrome	Deficiency	Ocular features	Systemic features
Marfan syndrome	Fibrillin	Ectopia lentis glaucoma Blue sclera Keratoconus	Long-limbed arachnodactyly High-arched palate aortic dissection
Osteogenesis imperfecta	Collagen I	Blue sclera Keratoconus	Brittle bones
Stickler syndrome	Collagen II	Myopia Liquefied vitreous Retinal detachments	Arthropathy Midfacial flattening Cleft palate
Ehlers–Danlos syndrome (>10 types)	Collagens I and III	Blue sclera Keratoconus Angioid streaks	Hyperflexible joints Hyperelastic skin Vascular bleeds
Pseudoxanthoma elasticum	Elastin fragility	Angioid streaks	'Chicken' skin GI bleeds
Weill–Marchesani syndrome		Ectopia lentis microspherophakia	Short stature brachydactyly ↓ IQ

Marfan, and Stickler are autosomal dominant; Weill–Marchesani is autosomal recessive; Ehlers–Danlos, pseudoxanthoma elasticum and osteogenesis imperfecta have dominant and recessive forms.

Phakomatoses

The phakomatoses are a group of conditions with neurological, ocular, and cutaneous features, and a tendency to develop tumours, usually of a hamartomatous type. There is considerable debate about which conditions to include, but neurofibromatosis, tuberous sclerosis, and von Hippel–Lindau syndrome are generally considered to be the archetypes.

Neurofibromatosis

Neuro fibromatosis-1 (NF-1) is the commonest of all the phakomatoses (prevalence 1/4000) and arises from mutations in the neurofibromin gene (Ch17q). Neuro fibromatosis-2 (NF-2) is much less common (1/40 000) and the gene has been located to Ch22q. Both are autosomal dominant but with variable expressivity.

Table 18.47 Features of neurofibromatosis-1

Ocular	Systemic
Optic n glioma	**Café-au-lait spots (≥6; each >0.5cm pre-puberty or**
Lisch nodules (≥2)	**>1.5cm post-puberty)**
	Axillary/inguinal freckling
Lid neurofibroma	**Neurofibromas (≥1 plexiform type or ≥2 any type)**
Choroidal naevi	**Characteristic bony lesion (sphenoid dysplasia, which may → pulsatile proptosis; long bone cortex thinning/dysplasia)**
Retinal astrocytoma	**First degree relative with NF-1**

Diagnosis requires two or more of the features in bold.

Table 18.48 Features of neurofibromatosis-2

Ocular	Systemic
Early-onset posterior subcapsular or cortical cataracts	Acoustic neuroma
	Meningioma
Combined hamartoma of the RPE and retina	Glioma
	Schwannoma
	First degree relative with NF-2

Definite NF-2: bilateral acoustic neuroma OR first degree relative with NF-2 AND either unilateral acoustic neuroma (at <30yrs) or two of the other diagnostic features.
Probable NF-2: unilateral acoustic neuroma (at <30yrs) AND one of the other diagnostic features; OR multiple meningiomas AND one of the other diagnostic features.

Tuberous sclerosis

Tuberous sclerosis (TS) has a prevalence of 1/6000. It arises from mutations in TSC1 (Ch9q) or TSC2 (Ch16p), which code for hamartin and tuberin respectively. It is autosomal dominant with variable expressivity; however, 50% of cases of TS are from new mutations.

Table 18.49 Features of tuberous sclerosis

Ocular	Systemic
Retinal astrocytoma	Adenoma sebaceum
	Ash leaf spots
	Shagreen patches
	Subungual fibromas
	Cerebral astrocytomas (with epilepsy and ↓IQ)
	Visceral hamartomas (e.g. renal angiomyolipoma, cardiac rhabdomyoma)
	Visceral cysts
	Pulmonary lymphangioleiomyomatosis

Von Hippel–Lindau syndrome

This rare condition arises from mutations in the *VHL* gene (Ch3p), which appears to be involved in vascular proliferation.

Table 18.50 Features of von Hippel–Lindau syndrome

Ocular	Systemic
Retinal capillary haemangioma	Haemangioblastoma of cerebellum, spinal cord or brainstem
	Renal cell carcinoma
	Phaeochromocytoma
	Islet cell carcinoma
	Epididymal cysts/adenomas
	Visceral cysts

Sturge–Weber and Wyburn–Mason syndrome

These rare syndromes of vascular abnormalities differ from the above 'true' phakomatoses in that they occur sporadically and the tumours (or AV malformations for Wyburn–Mason) are present from birth.

Table 18.51 Features of Sturge–Weber syndrome

Ocular	Systemic
Episcleral haemangioma	Naevus flammeus of the face (port-wine stain)
Ciliary body/iris haemangioma	
Choroidal haemangioma (diffuse)	CNS haemangioma
Glaucoma	

Table 18.52 Features of Wyburn–Mason syndrome

Ocular	Systemic
Retinal AVM	Cerebral/brain stem AVM
Orbital/periorbital AVM	

Refractive ophthamology

Related pages

Refractive error: introduction

Refractive error is a failure of the eye to focus light from an object on to the retina to form a clear image. It is a frequent cause of reduced visual function. If there is a refractive error when viewing a distant object the eye is described as ametropic. Ametropia can be divided into myopia (*syn* 'short-sightedness'), hypermetropia (*syn* hyperopia; 'long-sightedness') and astigmatism (Table 19.1). If there is no refractive error when viewing a distant object the eye is said to be emmetropic.

Epidemiology

It is estimated that refractive error affects about 1–2 billion people world-wide. The prevalence of different types of refractive error varies widely according to the population surveyed. For example, in army recruits myopia is estimated at about 10%. However, in the general population it may be as high as 40%, although three-quarters of this is low myopia (≤2D). Other factors include age, geographical location.

Definitions

Table 19.1 Summary of definitions

Term	Definition	Optical correction
Emmetropia	No refractive error when looking at a distant object	• Nil
Myopia	Light from distant object focuses in front of the retina	• Concave lens
Hypermetropia	Light from distant object focuses beyond the retina	• Convex lens
Astigmatism	Optical power of eye uneven across different meridians	• Toric lens
Presbyopia	Loss of normal accommodation with failure to focus on near objects	• Convex lens

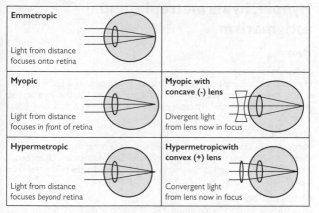

Fig. 19.1 Ray diagrams for myopia and hypermetropia and their refractive connection.

Myopia, hypermetropia, and astigmatism

Myopia

Definition

Myopia arises where light from a distance is brought to a focus in front of the retina either because the refracting power of the eye is too great (index myopia) or the anteroposterior diameter is too long (axial myopia).

Classification

Myopia may be classified according to the size of the refractive error; however, there is no universally accepted system. The American Optometric Association (AOA) definitions are: low (<−3D), moderate (−3 to −6D) or high (>−6D). Myopia may physiological or pathological.

Physiological myopia

Physiological myopia is common (20–40% population), is usually <2D and appears to be associated with increased time spent doing near work (usually reading) through teenage/early adulthood.

Pathological myopia (see Degentrative myopia 📖 p.182)

Pathological myopia is much less common (about 2% of the population) and is defined as enlargement of the eyeball with lengthening of the posterior segment. It is usually associated with much higher levels of myopia (>−6D).

Complications of pathological myopia

Choroidal and retinal degeneration, retinal detachment, staphyloma, open angle glaucoma.

Treatment

Treatment of myopia requires the provision of a concave lens external to the eye (either as spectacles or contact lenses (CLs) or a reduction in the refractive power of the eye itself (refractive surgery).

Hypermetropia

Definition

Hypermetropia arises where light from a distance is brought to a focus behind the retina either because the refracting power of the eye is too weak or the anteroposterior diameter is too short.

Classification

Hypermetropia may be classified according to the size of refractive error. The AOA definitions are: low (≤+2D), moderate (2–5D), and high (>5D). Hypermetropia may be classified as simple, pathological, or functional. In simple hypermetropia the structures and dimensions of the eye lie within normal limits, whereas in pathological hypermetropia the ocular anatomy is abnormal (e.g. developmental abnormality or other ocular pathology). Functional hypermetropia arises from failure of accommodation.

Complications

Accommodative esotropia, amblyopia (children), early-onset of presbyopia, angle-closure glaucoma, retinoschisis.

Treatment

Mild degrees of hypermetropia are often left untreated. Treatment of hypermetropia requires the provision of a convex lens external to the eye (spectacles or Contact lenses) or refractive surgery to increase in the refractive power of the eye.

Astigmatism

Definition

Astigmatism is where the refracting power of the eye is different in different meridians. It is defined in terms of its magnitude and direction. In the adult population up to 20% have astigmatism >1D.

Classification

Astigmatism may be regular (principal meridians 90° apart and so correctable by a toric lens) or irregular. Regular astigmatism may be 'with-the-rule' when the steepest meridian is at 90°, 'against-the-rule' when it is at 180°, or oblique where the principal meridians lie more than 20° from both 90 and 180°. Irregular astigmatism usually arises from an uneven corneal surface (e.g. scarring, keratoconus).

Treatment

Correction of astigmatism may be treated with spectacles using toric lenses (i.e. with different power in different meridians), CLs or refractive surgery. RGP CLs are particularly suited to the correction of astigmatism (including irregular astigmatism) as their rigidity allows the space between the lens and cornea to become filled by the tear film to form the 'lacrimal lens'. This effectively neutralizes corneal astigmatism. In contrast hydrogel CLs are less rigid and adopt the same shape as the cornea. Therefore, if a hydrogel CL is to be used to treat astigmatism, a toric design will be necessary. A certain degree of astigmatism may also be corrected as part of refractive surgery procedures.

Spectacles: types

Spectacles (*syn* glasses, eyeglasses) are the oldest and best established of all the refractive options.

Types of spectacles

Single vision

These are single prescription spectacles. Standard single vision spectacles are made up with the 'distance' prescription. 'Reading glasses' are single vision lenses made up with the 'reading' or near prescription and are one option in presbyopia.

- *Advantage*: simple, easily tolerated, economical.
- *Disadvantage*: presbyopes will not be able to perform distance or intermediate tasks with their reading glasses and will require multiple pairs to cope with viewing different tasks/distances.

Bifocal

These are corrective lenses with two distinct regions of differing optical power enabling refractive correction for two different focal distances in the same set of glasses; usually distance and reading, but may be intermediate, e.g. for VDU use.

- *Advantages*: more convenient—enables presbyopes to use one set of glasses for tasks at two focal distances.
- *Disadvantages*: reduces field of vision at each distance (defined by the compromise between the size of each segment); objects may appear to 'jump' when moving between segments; can be poor cosmetically; prismatic effects may be problematic for certain prescriptions.

Types of bifocal

Bifocal lenses are available in a number of designs. These include:

- *Round segment*: near vision region is a distinct small round segment. *Advantages*: excellent field of vision for distance; good cosmetically; good in terms of prismatic effects especially for plus powers where segment gives base down prism. *Disadvantages*: significant 'jump' when moving between segments.
- *D segment* (*syn* half-moon, flat-top): near vision region is a 'D' with the flat edge positioned superiorly. *Advantages*: good distance field; well-tolerated as little jump; little problem with prismatic effects. *Disadvantages*: relatively poor cosmetically.
- *C segment*: similar to D segment but with the flat edge positioned inferiorly. *Advantages*: good distance field; well-tolerated as little jump; little problem with prismatic effects; reasonable cosmetically.
- *Executive (or E line)*: the lens consists of a straight line segment. *Advantages*: no jump (optical centre of both portions is on dividing line); larger near field of vision. *Disadvantages*: cosmetically poor.
- *Franklin split bifocals*: these consist of two separate lenses mounted together; specially designed to incorporate prisms, especially if different amounts are required for distance and near. *Advantage*: large amounts of prisms can be incorporated and optical centras can be altered. *Disadvantage*: cosmetically poor.

Trifocals
- Similar to bifocals but contain three distinct optical regions, enabling three different focal distances (distance, intermediate, and near) in the same set of glasses. Occasionally used in the hospital eye service.

Progressive lenses
In progressive lenses (*syn* varifocal lenses) the positive refractive power gradually increases throughout the surface of the lens resulting in an intermediate corridor and a reading area at the bottom of the lens.
- *Advantages*: more convenient—enables presbyopes to use one set of glasses for tasks at multiple focal distances with minimal head adjustment; no 'jumping' of images; good cosmetically.
- *Disadvantages*: adaptation period required to adapt to peripheral distortion; more expensive; more distortion away from the optical axis; dependent on careful fitting (needs consideration of vertex distance, pantoscopic angle, and face form angle) to ensure correctly centred on the pupil.

Types of progressive lenses
There are a number of designs ranging from 'hard' to 'soft' based on how the optical components of the lens are blended together.
- *'Hard' progressive lenses*: designed to have minimal blur in the distance and near segments at the cost of a high degree of blur in the peripheral zones.
- *'Soft' progressive lenses*: the zone of peripheral blurring is less distinct but does encroach on the distance and near segments.
- *'Design by prescription' progressive lenses*: vary from hard to soft design within the same lens according to the different tolerance of hypermetropes and myopes to distortion in the near and distance segments.

Spectacles: materials

Lens material

Lenses may be made from glass, or various plastics (e.g. CR-39 or polycarbonate).

Glass

- Glass has the advantage of excellent optical properties, scratch resistance and has been used in spectacles (or their equivalent for about 700yrs).
- The commonest glass is ophthalmic Crown glass (refractive index 1.52) but alternative higher refractive index glasses are also available, e.g. flint glass (refractive index 1.62) may be used with crown glass in fused bifocals.

Plastics

- Plastics have the advantage of a higher refractive index and lower density than glass permitting thinner, lighter lenses. They are also safer if shattered.
- CR-39 is the preferred plastic for most applications as it has excellent optical properties, is more scratch resistance, and has low transmission of harmful UV light.
- Polycarbonate is mainly used for safety goggles as it is the most resistant to impact; its main disadvantage is reduced optical quality due to high light dispersion.

Coatings and tints

Surface coatings

Surface coatings may be used to provide scratch resistance, UV inhibition and anti-reflective properties (for cosmesis and to reduce glare).

Photochromic lenses

Photochromic lenses are lenses that darken on UV exposure. They may be useful for patients who are very sensitive to glare or are persistently photophobic (e.g. in retinites pigmentosa).

Glass photochromic lenses

- These depend on a UV-sensitive silver halide (usually silver chloride), which is scattered through the full thickness of the lens.
- *Advantage*: rapid reaction time; photochromic properties long-lasting.
- *Disadvantage*: yellowish tinge when 'clear'; solid tints so require multiple stock lenses and have uneven transmission and colour across lens according to thickness.

Plastic photochromic lenses

- These utilize a surface layer of an organic UV-sensitive compound (usually an oxazine or a naphthopyran).
- *Advantages*: surface layer so even transmission/colour across lens.
- *Disadvantages*: marginally slower reaction time; do not darken fully in hot weather; photochromic properties wane with time.

Spectacles: prescribing

For the principles and practice of refraction, see (📖 p.40–43). However, when filling in a prescription for spectacles make sure the following are noted:

General

- Record the prescription carefully and legibly and double check that you have transcribed it correctly.
- Ensure that the cylinder and axis are clearly stated and that + and − are clearly distinguishable.
- Ensure that the Reading Addition is clearly written for each eye.
- Record interpupillary distance and back vertex distance (especially if the prescription is ±5D in any meridian).

Specific

- If applicable record eligibility for any vouchers towards the expense of glasses (and inform patient) (see Eligibility for sight tests and optical vouchers, 📖 p.820).
- In young high myopes state if a high index lens is required.
- Record if a tint is clinically necessary especially in photophobic patients.
- If applicable, record if a small frame supplement is required for a young child or state any special frame requirements.
- Record if adaptation to the glasses is likely to be required or if the reading material needs to be held at a particular working distance.

Causes of spectacle intolerance

When a patient complains of 'eye-strain' they may mean refractive discomfort or asthenopia. It is most commonly seen after a recent change in refractive prescription. However, consider first:

Are the spectacles correct?

- Focimeter them to check that they match the prescription given to the patient.
- Check if the optical centres are correct, especially in high prescriptions with significant induced prismatic effect.
- In the case of progressive lenses the central fitting crosses of the progressive lens should coincide with the centre of the pupil.
- In the case of reading glasses, ensure that they are being used at the correct working distance.

Was the prescription correct?

- Without necessarily performing a full refraction it should be possible to quickly test VA and verify whether the prescription given was optimal/near optimal.

Was the prescription a significant change for the patient?

- In most cases, asthenopia is simply caused by a recent change in prescription. Look for:
- Significant change in axis or size of cylinder.
- Change of lens form.
- *Anisometropia*: the patient may not be coping with the difference between the two eyes and the treatment may need to be reduced.

- Overcorrection, especially of myopes who will end up permanently accommodating.
- Excessive near correction resulting in an uncomfortably near and narrow reading distance.
- Unsuitable bifocal or progressive lenses—consider occupation, requirements, and general faculties of the patient.

Is there a more serious problem?

Serious ocular pathology may present as a change in refraction (e.g. posterior segment tumour), or may cause ocular discomfort that the patient misinterprets as 'eye-strain'. A full ophthalmic examination may be required.

Contact lenses: outline

Contact lenses (CLs) are optical devices that rest on the surface of the cornea. They may be used for correction of refractive error, for a wide range of therapeutic applications, or for cosmesis.

Function

Refractive (or corrective) contact lenses

- This is the commonest application of CLs. Refractive designs include:
- Simple spherical lenses suitable for hypermetropia, myopia and mild astigmatism; can be used for presbyopia if one eye has a distance prescription and the other a near prescription (monovision).
- Toric lenses for more severe astigmatism.
- Bifocal and multifocal lenses for presbyopia.

Therapeutic contact lenses

Commonly called 'bandage' CLs, their range of applications is much wider than this implies.

Table 19.2 Applications of therapeutic contact lenses

Indication	Examples
Pain relief	Bullous keratopathy, band keratopathy, recurrent corneal erosion syndrome
Promotion of epithelial wound healing	Recurrent corneal erosion syndrome, persistent epithelial defect
Protection of ocular surface	Entropion, trichiatic lashes
Prevention of ocular dehydration	Dry eye (severe)
Maintain globe integrity	Threatened perforation or early leak
Maintain fornices	Stevens–Johnson syndrome, chemical burn
Therapeutic cosmesis	Severely scarred cornea, aniridia, phthisis, leucocoria
Drug delivery	Depot of high drug concentration (seldom used)

Cosmetic contact lenses:

In addition to their important 'therapeutic' role in improving cosmesis for a number of pathological conditions, cosmetic CLs are widely available for changing eye colour and for 'novelty' or theatrical use (e.g. cat-eyes, national flags, etc.).

Material

The ideal CL must not only have excellent optical properties but also be inert, well tolerated by the ocular surface, comfortable to wear, and have good oxygen transmissibility. Oxygen transmissibility (Dk/L) depends on oxygen permeability (Dk) and lens thickness (L). Oxygen permeability itself (Dk) depends on diffusion (D) and solubility (k). The different types of lenses are commonly classified according to their material, see pp.750–753).

Wearing schedule

Duration of wear: daily-wear vs extended wear

In daily wear there is a regular CL-free period. The lens is cleaned and disinfected (conventional CL) or discarded (disposable CL).

Extended wear has a role in certain patients (e.g. elderly aphakes, young babies) but is discouraged for the general population. The Dk values for soft hydrogels and many RGP materials are sufficient for daily wear but are inadequate for extended wear and result in corneal compromise. For those requiring extended wear certain silicone hydrogel lenses have been licensed for continuous wear of up to 30d.

Duration of lens: conventional vs disposable

Conventional lenses are usually replaced annually. They are more expensive (per lens), of superior optical quality but are more vulnerable to damage/loss due to their long life-span.

Disposable lenses are commonly replaced either daily or monthly. They are cheaper, of slightly poorer quality but are less likely to be damaged/lost during their life-span.

Lens notation

CL parameters are noted as follows: base curve (BC) or back optic zone radius (BOZR or r_o), total diameter (TD dia or $\varnothing_T$,) and power.

Contact lenses: hard and rigid gas permeable lenses

'Hard' lenses

Originally made of glass and later of PMMA, these have excellent optical properties but are minimally oxygen permeable (Dk = 0) so compromising epithelial metabolism with risk of 'overwear'.

Rigid gas permeable lenses

Made of complex polymers (which may include silicone, PMMA, and others), these lenses permit excellent diffusion of oxygen (D) with resultant good permeability (Dk from 15 to >100) and transmissibility (Dk/t where t = thickness of the lens). The main differences between RGP CLs relate to their wetting angle (a low value equates to good tear film spread and improved comfort), and their refractive index.

For refractive use they are usually 8.5–9.5mm in size ('corneal'). For therapeutic use both corneal and larger scleral (23mm) RGP lenses are used.

Rigid gas permeable lenses for refractive use

- *Indication*: most types of refractive error, including irregular astigmatism.
- *Design*: owing to their rigidity the space behind the RGP CLs becomes filled in by the 'lacrimal lens'. This effectively neutralizes corneal astigmatism, and makes them the treatment of choice for conditions where this is an issue (e.g. keratoconus). Toric lenses may be used for higher degrees of astigmatism; bifocal and multifocal designs for presbyopia; and tricurve designs for keratoconus.
- *Advantages*: excellent optical quality; good oxygen permeability; easy to handle (by patient); ↓risk of microbial keratitis.
- *Disadvantages*: moderate initial discomfort/FB sensation; require skilled fitting by CL practitioner (vs hydrogel CL).
- *Use of topical medication*: can safely use fluorescein; preservative-free treatments preferable, and preserved drops can be used but with caution.

Rigid gas permeable lenses for therapeutic use

- *Corneal RGP. Indications*: severe dry eye, exposure keratopathy, trichiasis. *Advantages and disadvantages and use of topical medication*: as for RGP lenses for refractive use.
- *Scleral RGP. Indications*: severe dry eye (provides good tear reservoir), exposure keratopathy, trichiasis, maintenance of fornices. *Advantages* (vs PMMA scleral lenses): better oxygen transmissibility; more easily fitted; more widely available. Use of topical medication: as for RGP lenses for refractive use.

PMMA scleral lenses

- *Indication*: may be useful in advanced keratoconus, severe irregular astigmatism, and some ocular surface disorders.
- *Design*: they are of 23–25mm in size, and are usually fenestrated in order to allow tear circulation. An impression is taken of the cornea and a specialist lens is hand-made. They are only available under the

hospital eye service in specialist centres, and in many areas have been largely replaced by RGP scleral lenses.
- *Advantages:* good optical properties.
- *Disadvantages:* minimally oxygen permeable; high risk of 'overwear'; require specialist fitting.
- Use of topical medication: can safely use fluorescein; preservative-free treatments preferable, but preserved drops can be used with caution.

Box 19.1 Inserting and removing RGP lenses: instructions to patients.[1]

Always wash hands before handling lenses, and inspect lens for any damage/foreign material prior to insertion.

Insertion
- Place lens on tip of index finger of dominant hand, concave side up.
- Place a couple of drops of a suitable wetting and soaking solution on to the lens.
- Look at the lens while you bring it towards the eye.
- Gently pull down lower lid (using remaining fingers of dominant hand) and lift upper lid (using fingers of non-dominant hand).
- Place lens on cornea.
- Look down for a couple of seconds while you release the lids.

Removal
- *Suction method:* a suction holder is applied directly to the lens, allowing it to be directly lifted off the eye. The lens can then be slid off the holder (avoid 'pulling' it off directly).
- *Blink method:* look straight ahead and open their eyes as wide as possible (so that upper lid is above lens); place a finger at the lateral margin of the lids and gently pull them laterally; blink firmly to displace the lens (catch it/ensure it will drop on to a suitable clean surface).

1. With only minor adjustment these same techniques can be used by the practitioner (or carer) to insert/remove RGP lenses.

Contact lenses: hydrogel lenses

Hydrogel (soft) lenses

Made of polymers of hydroxethyl methylacrylate, these absorb much more fluid (high water content) than the RGP lenses. In hydrogel lenses a higher water content results in greater solubility (k) and, therefore, better permeability (Dk from 10 to about 40). However, it also increases the minimum central thickness of the lens (t), thus the overall oxygen transmissibility (Dk/t) is fairly constant whatever the water content.

Hydrogel lenses for refractive use

- *Indication*: most types of refractive error.
- *Design*: hydrogel CLs do not vault over the cornea and thus there is no significant 'lacrimal lens' to neutralize corneal astigmatism. However, toric CLs can treat astigmatism provided the lens is stabilized (e.g. prism, thin zones).
- *Advantages*: comfortable, easy to fit, inexpensive.
- *Disadvantages*: less effective vs astigmatism; prone to spoilage; oxygen transmissibility not sufficient for overnight wear; optical quality may be less good than RGP lens.
- *Use of topical medication*: avoid fluorescein (will permanently stain); avoid preserved therapies except for very short-term use.

Hydrogel lenses for therapeutic use

- *Indication*: pain relief, promotion of wound healing, protection of ocular surface, maintenance of globe integrity.
- *Advantages*: wide range of sizes (13.5–20mm); comfortable, easy to fit.
- *Disadvantages*: oxygen transmissibility not sufficient for overnight wear.
- *Use of topical medication*: avoid fluorescein; avoid preserved therapies except for very short-term use.

Silicone hydrogel lenses

The new silicone hydrogel CLs combine some of the advantages of RGP materials with hydrogel lenses. Silicone hydrogel lenses are usually available 13.5–14.5mm diameter. They have a role in both refractive and therapeutic applications.

Silicone hydrogel lenses for refractive use:

- *Indication*: most types of refractive error.
- *Advantages*: excellent Dk values (up to 140) that permit longer wearing time.
- *Disadvantages*: higher rigidity, high wetting angle.
- *Use of topical medication*: avoid fluorescein (will permanently stain); avoid preserved therapies except for very short-term use.

Silicone hydrogel lenses for therapeutic use

- *Indication*: promotion of wound healing, pain relief, protection of ocular surface, maintenance of globe integrity.
- *Advantage*: lower Dk leads to ↓ risk of vascularization (vs hydrogel CL) (so use in keratoplasty patients).

- *Disadvantages*: less well tolerated in sensitive eyes due to higher rigidity, and high wetting angle; smaller range of sizes and powers available.
- *Use of topical medication*: avoid fluorescein; avoid preserved therapies except for very short-term use.

Table 19.3 Examples of hydrogel and silicone hydrogel lenses commonly used for therapeutic indications

Proclear	Hydrogel CL; very thin; drapes well on the cornea
Lunelle	Hydrogel CL; high water content; drapes well
Purevision	Silicone hydrogel CL; high Dk/t but stiffer than standard hydrogels
Night&Day	Silicone hydrogel CL; high Dk/t but stiffer than standard hydrogels
Acuvue Oasys	New generation silicone hydrogel CL; high Dk/t but less stiff than other silicone hydrogels

Box 19.2 Inserting and removing hydrogel lenses: instructions to patients.[1]

Always wash hands before handling lenses, and inspect lens for any damage/foreign material prior to insertion. Hold lenses with the tips of the thumb and index finger; fingernails can cause scratches.

Insertion
- Check that the lens is not 'inside-out': in the correct orientation the edges should curve slightly inwards, rather than outwards.
- Place lens on tip of index finger of dominant hand, concave side up.
- Look at the lens while you bring it towards the eye.
- Gently pull down lower lid (using remaining fingers of dominant hand) and lift upper lid (using fingers of non-dominant hand).
- Place lens on cornea.
- Look down for a couple of seconds while you release the lids.

Removal
- Use middle finger to pull down lower lid.
- Place index finger on lens.
- Look up and slide lens down on to inferior sclera.
- Lift the lens off between the tips of thumb and index finger.

1. With only minor adjustment these same techniques can be used by the practitioner (or carer) to insert/remove hydrogel lenses.)

Contact lenses: fitting

Refractive contact lenses

- Measure corneal curvature (keratometry), pupil diameter, vertical palpebral aperture, and corneal/visible iris diameter.
- Either:
  - predict the lens parameters required (from nomograms incorporating the above measurements and known refractive error) and order the lens on a 'sale-or-return' basis; or
  - use a trial lens set to determine the best fit.

Rigid gas permeable

Estimate contact lens parameters

The base curve is dictated by type of lens (consult specific manufacturer fitting guide), the flattest K reading and may be 'on K' (i.e. the same curvature), steeper than K or flatter than K. If 'on K' the lacrimal lens formed by the tear film is plano. If steeper or flatter it confers a plus or minus power of about 0.25D per 0.05mm difference of curvature.

The lens diameter may be influenced by the diameters of the cornea and pupil, and even lid position. A large lens may cause discomfort as it encroaches on the limbus and a small lens may cause flare if its edge impinges on the pupil.

The lens power is determined either by calculation (from the back vertex distance and spectacle correction) or by 'over-refraction' with a trial lens in place.

Assess fit after 20min

The CL should be centred either, with its lower edge >2mm above the lower lid but with its upper edge under the upper lid (lid attachment fit) or just below the upper lid (interpalpebral positioning). The lens should move 1–2mm with blinking and allow tear-flow under the cornea. Less movement implies too tight/steep; more implies too loose/flat.

Fluorescein is used to assess the fit. Good alignment results in shallow central clearance (little fluorescence seen) with intermediate touch (black ring) and free tear movement in the periphery (bright fluorescence). If too steep there is high central clearance (bright fluorescence); if too flat there is central touch (black).

Hydrogel (soft)

Estimate contact lens parameters

The base curve is estimated from the flattest K and adjusted according to type of lens (e.g. add 1mm for low water content lenses) and the individual patient.

The lens diameter should exceed the corneal diameter covering the limbus by ≥1mm. The lens power is calculated as above.

Assess fit after 20min

The CL should be comfortable, fully cover the cornea, be fairly centred, and should move 0.75–1mm with blinking (<0.5mm implies too tight/steep; ≥1.5mm probably too loose/flat).

Follow-up

Ensure that patients understand how to look after their lenses (including hygiene). Discuss potential complications (e.g. microbial keratitis), how they present and the need for lens removal and urgent review in such circumstances.

Follow-up should be fairly frequent initially but in long-standing uncomplicated CL wear may reduce to yearly.

Non-refractive contact lenses

Therapeutic ('bandage') and cosmetic CLs are plano (or even opaque). Hydrogel and silicone hydrogel CL for therapeutic use usually come in a few standard sizes and are fitted according to diameter/base curve. More skilled fitting is required for RGP therapeutic lenses (see CL: hard and RGP lenses 🔲 p. 750). PMMA lenses require a specialist fitting in a dedicated centre.

Contact lenses: complications

The majority of CL complications are associated with poor compliance with recommended CL practice.

Painful red eye in the contact lens wearer

First rule out microbial keratitis. Then consider alternative diagnoses.

Microbial keratitis (see Microbial keratitis, 📖 pp.194–197)
- White infiltrate ± epithelial defect, mucopurulent infiltrate, AC inflammation.
- *Ophthalmic emergency*: treat aggressively (see Microbial keratitis: Treatment 📖 pp.196–197). Consider pseudomonas and acanthamoeba (more commonly seen in CL wearers).

Sterile keratitis
- Small multiple anterior stromal infiltrates, usually non-staining; may be only mildly symptomatic.
- Differentiate from microbial keratitis.
- *Treatment*: Consider temporarily stopping (if severe) or reducing (if mild) CL wear; improve CL care, using preservative-free solutions or change to alternative CL.

Giant papillary conjunctivitis
- Itching + mucoid discharge in the presence of giant papillae of the upper lid.
- *Treatment*: Mast-cell stabilizer (e.g. sodium cromoglicate 4×/d).
- Consider temporarily stopping (if severe) or reducing (if mild) CL wear; improve CL care, using preservative-free solutions or change to alternative CL.

Tight lens syndrome
- Tight non-moving lens with anterior corneal oedema and AC reaction.
- *Treatment*: Remove lens; topical cycloplegic if severe AC reaction; replace with flatter lens when recovered.

Toxic keratopathy
- Disinfectant/enzyme inadvertently introduced into eye resulting in diffuse punctate epithelial erosions ± subepithelial infiltrates.
- *Treatment*: Remove lens; use preservative-free artificial tears; educate re CL care.

Preservative keratopathy
- Preservative (e.g. thiomersal) exposure with punctate epithelial erosions (may be superior limbic pattern) ± subepithelial infiltrates.
- *Treatment*: Remove lens; use preservative-free artificial tears.
- Educate re CL care and change to preservative-free cleaning solutions.

Tear film disturbance
- Poor blink response or ill-fitting lens resulting in punctate staining at 3 or 9 o'clock with interpalpebral hyperaemia.
- *Treatment*: Preservative-free artificial tears; check CL fit.

Painless red eye

Neovascularization

- Superficial neovascularization at 3 and 9 o'clock is common. It usually does not extend >2–3mm.
- *Treatment*: Remove lens; if severe consider a short course of topical steroid; replace with a lens with high oxygen permeability (Dk).

Other complications

- Other complications include abnormalities of the epithelium, including microcysts, endothelial polymegathism, loss of lens, and corneal abrasion.
- Optical effects include spectacle blur (their spectacle correction is transiently incorrect after CL wear), flexure (refractive change due to flexing of CL), visual flare (edge effect), accommodative effects (e.g. a myope has to accommodate more when switching from glasses to CL), and aberrations (spherical and chromatic).

Refractive surgery: introduction

The introduction of the excimer laser in the 1980s revolutionized refractive surgery.

Today, refractive surgery is more precise and reliable than ever, and patient's expectations are correspondingly extremely high. So it is even more important that patients have realistic expectations of what refractive surgery can and cannot do.

Should I have refractive surgery?

All patients should consider:

- Refractive surgery is permanent.
- Optical correction by refractive surgery may not improve their best possible vision. Although their vision without glasses/CLs is likely to be improved, they may still only achieve their best possible VA with glasses/CLs.
- There is a risk of permanently damaging their vision such that it will not be correctable with glasses/CLs.

In addition older patients should consider:

- Standard photorefractive surgery does not correct for presbyopia, thus myopes may be exchanging dependence on distance glasses for dependence on reading glasses. Surgical options to consider for presbyopia include: achieving monovision (one eye correct for distance, the other for near) via refractive surgery techniques, such as LASIK or conductive keratoplasty; refractive lens exchange with accommodating/multifocal IOLs. Emerging techniques include presbyopic/multifocal LASIK.
- If developing visually significant cataracts, early cataract surgery with correction by appropriate choice of IOL may be a better alternative.

Other pre-operative considerations

In their Standards for Laser Refractive Surgery, the Royal College of Ophthalmologists (UK)[1] have made recommendations on the information that should be provided to the patient considering laser refractive surgery. These include information on the range of refractive options available (whether or not they are available at the particular institution that they are attending), success/complication rates, qualifications of the surgeon, costs of procedures (including refund policies), follow-up arrangements (including emergencies), complaint procedures. In addition, the following factors, which are relevant to their long-term ophthalmic care, must be recorded and a copy provided to the patient:

- Pre-operative keratometry.
- Pre-operative pachymetry.
- Pre- and post-operative best corrected acuity.
- Pre- and post-operative intraocular pressure.
- Pre-operative and stabilized post-operative refraction.

---

1. www.rcophth.ac.uk/docs/publications/published-guidelines/Refractive_Surgery_Standards_Jan_2009.

Table 19.4 Outline of surgical refractive procedures

Procedure	Mechanism
CORNEAL	
Central	
PRK	Remove epithelium surgically, selectively ablate stroma with excimer laser, insert BCL
LASIK	Form partial thickness flap with microkeratome, selectively ablate stroma with excimer laser, replace flap
LASEK	Remove epithelium as sheet with alcohol, selectively ablate stroma with excimer laser, replace epithelial sheet, insert BCL
Epi-LASIK	Remove epithelium as sheet mechanically with epikeratome, selectively ablate stroma with excimer laser, replace epithelial sheet, insert BCL
IntraLASIK	Similar to LASIK except that the flap is created with femtosecond laser rather than a mechanical microkeratome
Keratomileusis	Remove partial thickness corneal button and reshape the button (keratomileusis) or corneal bed (*in situ* keratomileusis)
Epikeratophakia	Remove epithelium, perform annular keratectomy, suture on shaped donor lenticule of Bowman's layer/ anterior stroma
Keratophakia	Form partial thickness flap with microkeratome, place intrastromal donor lenticule of corneal stroma, replace flap
Intracorneal lens	Form partial thickness flap with microkeratome, place intrastromal synthetic lens (e.g. hydrogel), replace flap
Peripheral	
Radial keratotomy	Deep radial corneal incisions flatten central cornea
Laser thermokeratoplasty (LTK)	Laser shrinkage of peripheral stromal collagen in a radial pattern flattens periphery and steepens central cornea
Conductive keratoplasty	Similar to laser thermokeratoplasty but uses high radiofrequency currents rather than laser
Intracorneal ring	Thread synthetic ring into mid stromal tunnel
LENS	
Refractive lens exchange	Remove crystalline lens and replace with synthetic PCIOL (☐ Box 9.4)
Phakic intraocularlens	Leave crystalline lens intact and place synthetic IOL, which can be angle-supported, iris-fixated, or in the posterior chamber

Refractive surgery: PRK and LASIK

Photorefractive keratectomy

PRK has been widely practised since the 1980s, although it has been largely replaced by LASIK and LASEK. It is still quite commonly used for low refractive errors.

Indications

Good results for +3D to −6D and up to 4D of astigmatism.

Advantages

Advantages over LASIK: no issues of flap stability (important for military, contact sports), flap complications or epithelial ingrowth.

Method

Remove epithelium surgically, selectively ablate stroma with excimer laser, insert bandage CL.

Disadvantages

Postoperative pain, slow recovery, slow refractive stability, corneal haze.

Complications

Under/overcorrection, visual aberrations, corneal haze, corneal scarring, decentration, central corneal islands (elevations), microbial keratitis, recurrent erosions, dry eye syndrome.

Laser stromal in situ keratomilieusis

LASIK has become the predominant refractive operation since its introduction in the 1990s, in part due to its suitability for a wide range of refractive errors.

Indications

Good results for +4D to −8D and up to 4D astigmatism.

Advantages

Advantages over PRK: less painful, faster visual rehabilitation.

Method

Form partial thickness stromal flap with microkeratome, selectively ablate stroma with excimer laser, replace flap.

Disadvantages

Potential for serious complications such as flap complications and corneal ectasia, not suitable in thin corneas.

Complications

Diffuse lamellar keratitis
- Stage 1 white granular haze (2%); stage 2 'shifting sands' white infiltrate (0.5%); stage 3 white clumped central infiltrate (0.2%); stage 4 stromal melt (0.02%).
- Treat with intensive topical steroids and consider surgical flap lifting and irrigation.

Flap complications: incomplete flap (0.3%), buttonhole flap (0.1%), flap with cut-hinge (0.1%), thin flap, irregular flap, flap wrinkles or malposition (≥4%), lost flap.

- Treat lost flap as epithelial erosion (see Recurrent corneal erosion syndrome 📖 p.212); consider surgical repositioning of malpositioned flaps.

Other complications: under/overcorrection, visual aberrations, corneal haze, corneal scarring, central corneal islands, microbial keratitis, epithelial ingrowth (1.3%), keratectasia, dry eye syndrome.

Femtosecond laser-assisted LASIK

This procedure is essentially the same as standard LASIK but uses a femtosecond laser rather than a mechanical microkeratome to create the flap.

Refractive surgery: LASEK and other procedures

Laser subepithelial keratomilieusis

LASEK is similar to PRK but the epithelium is carefully removed and then replaced at the end of the procedure.

Indications
Similar to PRK.

Advantages
- *Advantages over PRK*: less painful, less haze, faster visual rehabilitation.
- *Advantages over LASIK*: no issues of flap-related complications.

Method
Remove epithelium as a sheet with 18–20% alcohol, selectively ablate stroma with excimer laser, replace epithelial sheet, insert bandage CL.

Disadvantages
Postoperative pain and slower visual recovery compared with LASIK.

Complications
Under/overcorrection, visual aberrations, corneal haze, epithelial defects, dry eye syndrome.

Epi-LASIK

This is a relatively new procedure that resembles LASEK but with the use of an epikeratome to mechanically remove the epithelium.

Indications
Similar to LASEK.

Advantages
Advantages over LASEK: avoidance of alcohol with better viability of epithelial cells.

Method
Remove epithelium as a sheet mechanically with epikeratome, selectively ablate stroma with excimer laser, replace epithelial sheet, insert bandage CL.

Complications
Under/overcorrection, corneal haze, visual aberrations, stromal penetration.

Thermokeratoplasty

In thermokeratoplasty local heat-induced shrinkage of corneal tissue results in corneal steepening. It may be used to treat mild degrees of hypermetropia.

Treatment is applied as a ring of spots generated by either holmium laser (laser thermokeratoplasty) or a heated wire (conductive thermokeratoplasty).

Radial keratotomy

One of the earliest surgical methods of treating myopia, this comprised shallow corneal incisions arranged in a radial manner. It is now mainly of historical interest.

Refractive surgery: efficacy and safety

A systematic review of photorefractive surgery conducted in 2005 by NICE (UK) considered the commonest photorefractive techniques: PRK, LASIK and LASEK (see Table 19.4). Considering studies from 2000 onwards they identified 16 randomized controlled trials comparing the procedures and 130 case series (40 for PRK, 26 for LASEK, and 64 for LASIK). The key findings of this review[1] and their subsequent recommendations[2] are summarized here:

Efficacy

Refractive outcome

Myopia

There were no significant differences in efficacy between the three procedures for myopia/myopic astigmatism:

- *With PRK*, a median of 69% were within 0.5D of target, and 89% within 1.0D.
- *With LASEK*, a median of 75% were within 0.5D of target, and a median of 92% within 1.0D.
- *With LASIK*, 77% were within 0.5D and 91% were within 1.0D.

Hypermetropia

Photorefractive surgery was less accurate in treating hypermetropia (vs myopia):

- With PRK and LASIK, 61% of eyes were within 0.5D of target, and 79% and 88% were within 1.0D for PRK and LASIK respectively.
- Success was greater for hypermetropia of <+3.50D.
- One randomized controlled trial found LASEK to be more accurate than PRK for hypermetropia.

Visual acuity outcome

Myopia

- With PRK, uncorrected VA at last follow-up was 70% ≥6/6 and 92% ≥6/12.
- With LASEK, uncorrected VA at last follow-up was 62% ≥6/6 and 92% ≥6/12.
- With LASIK, uncorrected VA at last follow-up was 64% ≥6/6 and 94% ≥6/12.
- Highly myopic eyes had significantly poorer outcomes. PRK achieved uncorrected VA ≥6/6 in 14% highly myopic eyes (>−6D) vs 76% in low/moderately myopic eyes; for LASIK this was 44% vs 81% respectively.

Hypermetropia

- With PRK, uncorrected VA at last follow-up was 59% ≥6/6 and 86% ≥6/12.
- With LASIK, uncorrected VA at last follow-up was 52% ≥6/6 and 96% ≥6/12.

Safety

Permanent visual loss

- In myopia, the median proportion of eyes with significant visual loss (≥2 Snellen lines of best spectacle-corrected VA) was 0.5% (0–20.5%) for

PRK, 0% (0–8.2%) for LASEK and 0.6% (0–3%) for LASIK. Patients with high myopia were more likely to have significant visual loss than those with moderate to low myopia.

- In hypermetropia (fewer studies), the rate was 7.0% for PRK and 3.5% for LASIK. Patients with hypermetropia of >+3.50 D were more at risk of significant visual loss.

Flap complications

- Flap complications in LASIK include incomplete/button-hole/cut-hinge flaps (0.5%) and epithelial in-growth (median of 1.3%). For LASEK, about 2% (range 0–19%) of treatments were converted to PRK due to flap complications.

Ectasia

Ectasia (a progressive structural corneal deformation resulting in refractive instability) was estimated to be about 0.4% after LASIK; however, it was suggested that improved case selection (i.e. identifying and excluding eyes with keratoconus) might reduce this rate. It was not reported after PRK or LASEK.

Other complications

Microbial keratitis after LASIK occurred in 0–0.16% of eyes. Significant corneal haze occurred with all procedures: 0–31% for PRK, 0–25% for LASEK, and 0–2% for LASIK.

Recommendations

NICE concluded that these procedures were safe and effective in appropriately selected patients. In addition, the clinician should:

- Ensure that patients understood the potential risks of the procedure so that they could weigh these risks against the alternatives of spectacles/ CLs.
- Audit clinical outcome.
- Receive adequate training before performing these techniques.

The Royal College of Ophthalmologists (UK) has produced standards for photorefractive surgery[3] and an assessment for certification of competence to practice (subject to annual appraisal and continuing professional development).[4]

1. www.nice.org.uk/ip320review/

2. www.nice.org.uk/Guidance/IPG164/Guidance/pdf/English/

3. www.rcophth.ac.uk/docs/publications/published-guidelines/Refractive_Surgery_Standards_ Jan_2009.pdf/

4. www.rcophth.ac.uk/exams/laser-refractive-surgery/

Aids to diagnosis

Acute red eye

Normal/near normal vision

Painful/discomfort

Diffuse superficial redness

- *Conjunctivitis*: infective, allergic, or chemical; gritty/itchy; watery, mucoid, mucopurulent, or purulent exudate; papillae or follicles.

Diffuse deep redness

- *Anterior scleritis*: severe pain; diffuse deep injection that does not blanch with vasoconstrictors (e.g. phenylephrine 10%), oedema; globe tender.

Circumlimbal redness

- *Keratitis*: photophobia watering, circumlimbal injection, corneal infiltrate ± epithelial defect ± AC activity.
- *Anterior uveitis*: photophobia, watering, keratic precipitates, AC activity, ± posterior synechiae.
- *Corneal FB*: appropriate history, FB sensation, visible FB.

Sectoral redness

- *Episcleritis*: mild discomfort; may be recurrent; sectoral (occasionally diffuse) redness which blanches with topical vasoconstrictor (e.g. phenylephrine 10%); globe non-tender.
- *Marginal keratitis*: photophobia, watering, marginal corneal infiltrate ± epithelial defect.

Painless

- *Subconjunctival haemorrhage*: well-defined confluent area of haemorrhage.

Reduced vision

Normal IOP

Abnormal corneosclera

- *Corneal abrasion*: photophobia, watering, sectoral/circumlimbal injection, epithelial defect.
- *Keratitis*: photophobia watering, circumlimbal injection, corneal infiltrate ± epithelial defect ± AC activity ± mucopurulent discharge.

Abnormal uvea
- *Anterior uveitis*: photophobia, watering, keratic precipitates, AC activity, ± posterior synechiae.
- *Endophthalmitis*: pain, floaters, watering, diffuse deep injection, inflammation (vitreous > AC), chorioretinitis.

↑ *IOP*
- *Acute glaucoma*: usually due to angle closure; photophobia, watering, corneal oedema, ± anterior segment/angle abnormalities such as rubeosis.
- *Hypertensive uveitis*: AC cells and flare ± corneal involvement; often due to herpes group of viruses.

Sudden/recent loss of vision

Painless

Few seconds duration

Unilateral

- *GCA:* usually age >55yrs, weight loss, fatigue, jaw/tongue claudication, pulseless/tender/thickened temporal artery, ↑ESR/CRP.
- *Papilloedema:* bilateral disc swelling, loss of SVP, peripapillary haemorrhages, features of raised ICP.
- *Impending central retinal vein occlusion:* dilated, tortuous retinal veins, haemorrhages.
- *Ocular ischaemic syndrome:* veins dilated and irregular but not tortuous, midperipheral haemorrhages; ± NVD, ↑IOP, carotid bruits.

Bilateral

- *Papilloedema:* see above.

Few minutes duration

Unilateral

- *Amaurosis fugax:* curtain across vision ± evidence of emboli, AF, carotid bruits.
- *GCA:* see above.

Bilateral

- Vertebrobasilar artery insufficiency: recurrent episodes ± ataxia, dysphasia, dysarthria, hemiparesis, hemisensory disturbance.

Up to 1h duration

- *Migraine:* fortification spectra, transient visual field defects, unilateral headache, nausea/vomiting, photophobia, aura, family history.

Persistent

Abnormal cornea

- *Hydrops:* acute corneal oedema associated with underlying disease, such as keratoconus.

Abnormal vitreous

- *Vitreous haemorrhage:* varies from microscopic level to completely obscuring the fundus.

Abnormal fundus

- *Central retinal artery occlusion:* RAPD, attenuated arterioles, pale fundus, cherry-red spot.
- *Central retinal vein occlusion:* dilated tortuous veins, haemorrhages in all four quadrants, ± CWS, RAPD; branch retinal vein occlusions may give symptomatic altitudinal defects particularly if on temporal arcade.
- *Rhegmatogenous retinal detachment:* flashes/floaters, tobacco dust, convex elevated retina with (multiple) break(s).
- *Exudative retinal detachment:* convex elevated retina with shifting fluid, no break; tractional: concave elevated retina with tractional membranes.
- *Intermediate uveitis:* floaters, vitritis, snow balls/banking ± macular oedema.

- *Posterior uveitis*: floaters, significantly reduced vision; vitritis, retinal/choroidal infiltrates, macular oedema, vascular sheathing/occlusion, haemorrhages.

Abnormal disc
- *Anterior ischaemic optic neuropathy*: RAPD, pale oedematous disc ± flame-shaped haemorrhages; may have altitudinal field defect; may be arteritic (with signs of GCA) or non-arteritic (usually sectoral).

Abnormal macula
- *Choroidal neovascular membrane*: distortion ± positive scotoma, drusen, subretinal membrane ± haemorrhage, exudate.
- *Central serous retinopathy*: colour desaturation, micropsia, serous detachment of neurosensory retina.

Normal fundus
- *Cortical blindness*: ± denial, small residual field; normal pupil reactions; abnormal CT/MRI head.
- *Functional*: inconsistent acuity between different tests and at different times, normal ophthalmic examination, normal electrodiagnostic tests.

Painful

Abnormal cornea
- *Acute angle closure glaucoma*: usually hypermetropic, haloes, frontal headache, vomiting; injected, corneal oedema, fixed semidilated pupil, shallow AC with closed angle, raised IOP.
- *Bullous keratopathy*: thickened, hazy cornea, stromal/subepithelial oedema, bullae, evidence of underlying pathology, e.g. ACIOL, Fuchs' endothelial dystrophy, etc.
- *Keratitis*: photophobia watering, circumlimbal injection, corneal infiltrate ± epithelial defect ± AC activity.

Abnormal disc
- *Optic neuritis*: usually age 18–45yrs, with retro-orbital pain especially on eye movement, RAPD, reduced colour vision, visual field defects, swollen disc ± peripapillary flame-shaped haemorrhages; may also be painless.

Abnormal uvea
- *Anterior uveitis*: anterior: pain, photophobia, mildly reduced vision, circumlimbal injection, AC cells and flare, keratic precipitates.

Normal fundus
- *Retrobulbar neuritis*: as for optic neuritis but with a normal disc; may also be painless.

Gradual loss of vision

Generalized

Abnormal cornea

- *Corneal dystrophies*: corneal clouding (deposition/oedema); usually bilateral but may be asymmetric; common types include Fuchs' endothelial dystrophy in the elderly and Reis–Buckler's dystrophy in young adults.
- *Keratoconus*: refractive error from progressive astigmatism; corneal oedema from acute hydrops; usually bilateral but may be asymmetric.

Abnormal lens

- *Cataract*: uni- or bilateral opacification of the lens; cloudy, misty; glare; commonest in the elderly.

Central

Abnormal macula

Macular disease usually leads to distortion ± microsia and early ↓VA; pupillary responses and colour vision are relatively preserved. Common causes include:

- *AMD*: very common bilateral disease of the elderly; the most common type are 'dry' changes that are associated with gradual patchy central loss.
- *Macular dystrophies*: group of diseases with specific patterns occurring in a younger age group; bilateral disease; may have family history, and genetic testing is sometimes possible.
- *Diabetic maculopathy*: ischaemia may lead to gradual ↓VA; oedema may lead to more acute distortion/↓VA; associated with other diabetic changes.
- *Cystoid macular oedema*: oedema resulting in distortion/↓VA may be associated with surgery, inflammation, or vascular disease.

Abnormal optic disc/nerve

Optic nerve disease usually leads to dimness and darkening of colours; although commonly central it may lead to peripheral or generalized loss of vision; pupillary responses, colour vision, and brightness testing are all reduced. Important causes include:

- *Compressive optic neuropathy*: progressive ↓VA, disc pallor ± pain, involvement of other local structures.
- *Leber's hereditary optic neuropathy*: severe sequential ↓VA over weeks/ months, telangiectatic vessels around disc (acutely); usually young adult males; family history.
- *Toxic or nutritional optic neuropathies*: slowly progressive symmetrical ↓VA with central scotomas; relevant nutritional, therapeutic or toxic history.
- *Inflammatory optic neuropathies*: associated with systemic disease (e.g. sarcoid, vasculitis, and syphilis); often very steroid-sensitive.
- *Chronic papilloedema*: sustained disc swelling due to raised ICP may cause permanent optic nerve dysfunction, including ↓VA and field defects, and optic disc pallor.

Peripheral or patchy

Abnormal choroid/retina

- *Posterior uveitis*: floaters, patchy loss of vision ± central distortion/↓VA from CMO; may include chorioretinitis, vitritis, retinal vasculitis.
- *RP*: bilateral concentric field loss, peripheral 'bone-spicule' pigmentation, retinal arteriole attenuation, and optic disc pallor.

Abnormal optic disc

- *Glaucoma*: asymptomatic peripheral field loss; usually bilateral but often asymmetric; characteristic cupping and other disc changes; often associated with ↑IOP.

The watery eye

Increased tear production

Basal increase
- *Increased parasympathetic drive*: from pro-secretory drugs (e.g. pilocarpine) or autonomic disturbance.

Reflex increase
- *Local irritants*: e.g. FBs, trichiasis.
- *Chronic ocular disease*: e.g. blepharitis, keratoconjunctivitis sicca.
- *Systemic disease*: e.g. thyroid eye disease.

Lacrimal pump failure

Lid tone
- *Lid laxity*: common involutional change in the elderly.
- *Orbicularis weakness*: associated with VIIn palsy.

Lid position
- *Ectropion*: most commonly an involutional change in the elderly but may also be cicatricial, mechanical, or congenital.

Decreased drainage

Punctal obstruction
- *Congenital*: punctal atresia.
- *Acquired*: punctal stenosis is most commonly idiopathic but may arise secondary to punctal eversion, post-HSV infection, or any scarring process (e.g. post-irradiation, trachoma, cicatricial conjunctivitis).

Canalicular obstruction
- *Acquired*: canalicular fibrosis is most commonly idiopathic but may arise secondary to HSV infection, chronic canaliculitis (usually actinomycosis), chronic dacrocystitis, cicatricial conjunctivitis, and 5-FU administration.

Nasolacrimal duct obstruction
- *Congenital*: delayed canalization.
- *Acquired*: stenosis is most commonly idiopathic but may arise secondary to trauma (nasal/orbital fracture), post-irradiation, Wegener's granulomatosis, tumours (e.g. nasopharyngeal carcinoma), and other nasal pathology (chronic inflammation/polyps).

Flashes and floaters

Flashes only

Retinal traction
Vitreo-retinal traction, proliferative diabetic retinopathy, sickle cell retinopathy, retinopathy of prematurity.

'Pseudoflashes'
Ocular
- *Photophobia*: discomfort commonly associated with anterior segment inflammation or retinal hypersensitivity.
- *Glare*: dazzle commonly associated with media opacities.
- *Haloes*: ring effect associated with corneal oedema and some media opacities.

CNS
- *Papilloedema*: transient, associated with straining or change in posture.
- *Migraine*: classic enlarging zig-zag fortification spectra moving central to peripheral, usually followed by headache.
- *Occipital lobe lesions* (tumours, AVMs): coloured shapes/blobs.
- *Other visual hallucinations*: bilateral severe visual loss may result in more complex visual hallucinations (Charles Bonnet syndrome).

Floaters only
- *PVD*: partial/complete Weiss ring overlying the optic disc ± visible posterior vitreous face.
- *Vitreous condensations*: degenerative changes within the vitreous lead to translucent opacities.
- *Vitreous haemorrhage*: red cells in the vitreous, varies from minor bleed ('spots' in vision, fundus easily visualized) to severe (severe ↓VA, no fundal view); may be followed by synchysis scintillans (golden particles that settle with gravity).
- *Vitritis*: white cells in the vitreous, may be bilateral and associated with features of intermediate or posterior uveitis.
- *Asteroid hyalosis*: small yellow–white particles that move with the vitreous (rather than settling with gravity), usually innocuous.
- *Amyloidosis*: sheet-like opacities, usually bilateral; most commonly seen with familial systemic amyloidosis.
- *Tumours* (e.g. choroidal melanoma, lymphoma): vitritis of inflammatory and/or tumour cells may be seen.

Flashes and floaters

- *PVD*: partial/complete Weiss ring overlying the optic disc ± visible posterior vitreous face.
- *Retinal tear*: usually U-shaped tear and pigment in the vitreous; may be associated with vitreous haemorrhage or retinal detachment.
- *Retinal detachment*: usually rhegmatogenous retinal detachment (associated with a tear) resulting in elevated retina with subretinal fluid.
- *Tumours*: visual phenomena include 'slow moving ball of light' and floaters secondary to tumour cells/inflammation associated with a choroidal or retinal mass.

Headache

Swollen optic discs

Bilateral

Serious/life-threatening headaches

- *Raised ICP*: worsening headache on lying flat, coughing/sneezing/Valsalva, visual obscurations, diplopia, disc swelling with loss of SVP, blind spot enlargement, VI n palsy. Causes include:
  - Cerebral tumour, idiopathic intracranial hypertension, venous sinus thrombosis, meningitis, encephalitis, brain abscess, congenital ventricular abnormalities, cerebral oedema.
  - Subarachnoid haemorrhage: 'thunderclap headache', meningism, altered consciousness.
- *Accelerated hypertension*: ↑↑BP, hypertensive retinopathy including CWS, haemorrhages, exudates.

Unilateral

Serious/life-threatening headaches

- *GCA*: usually age >55yrs; visual loss, scalp tenderness (± necrosis), jaw/tongue claudication, limb girdle pain/weakness, fevers, weight loss; non-pulsatile, tender, thickened temporal arteries; AION results in unilateral or less commonly bilateral disc swelling.

No optic disc swelling

Serious/life-threatening headaches

- *Raised ICP*: may occur in the presence of non-swollen discs (e.g. myopic discs, atrophic discs, anomalies of the optic nerve sheath).
- *GCA*: see above.
- *Pituitary adenoma*: endocrine dysfunction (amenorrhoea, galactorrhoea, infertility, acromegaly, Cushing's disease; optic atrophy; bitemporal field loss).
- *Pituitary apoplexy*: recent major hypotensive episode, e.g. surgery, postpartum haemorrhage; acute ↓VA, meningism, ± LOC.

Headache syndrome

- *Tension headache*: very common; tightness, bifrontal/biocciptal/band-like, may radiate to neck, headache-free intervals, no neurological/systemic features; this may be associated with *cervical spondylosis*.
- *Migraine*: common; prodrome, headache (usually hemicranial), nausea, photophobia, phonophobia; visual phenomena include scintillating visual aura (starts paracentral and expands as it moves peripherally), transient visual loss (unilateral or homonymous hemifield), or ophthalmoplegia.
- *Cluster headache*: sudden oculo-temporal pain, no prodrome, may have transient lacrimation, rhinorrhoea, and Horner syndrome.

Facial pain
- *Trigeminal neuralgia*: sudden stabbing pains in trigeminal branch distribution; precipitants include touch, cold, eating.
- *Ophthalmic shingles*: hyperaesthesia in acute phase followed by neuralgic-type pain.

Sinus pain
- *Acute sinusitis*: coryzal/URTI symptoms, tender over paranasal sinuses; proptosis, diplopia, or optic neuropathy warrant urgent exclusion of orbital involvement.

Ocular pain
- *Generalized*: includes acute angle closure glaucoma, anterior uveitis, keratitis, scleritis, ocular ischaemia.
- *Retrobulbar*: includes optic neuritis, orbital pathology (e.g. infection, infiltration, neoplasm, thyroid eye disease).
- *On eye movement*: includes optic neuritis.

Asthenopia (eye strain)
Usually worsens with reading/fatigue; ametropia (especially hypermetropia), astigmatism, anisometropia, decompensating phoria, convergence insufficiency, etc.

Diplopia

Monocular

Abnormal refraction

- *High ametropia, astigmatism, or edge effect* from corrective lenses: usually correctable with appropriate refraction; CLs may be more effective than glasses.

Abnormal cornea

- *Opacity*: associated with scarring (e.g. trauma, infection), oedema (e.g. ↑IOP, decompensation), deposition (e.g. corneal dystrophies).
- *Shape*: peripheral thinning associated with ectasias (e.g. keratoconus), peripheral ulcerative keratitis, and other marginal disease.

Abnormal lens

- *Opacity*: cataract.
- *Shape*: lenticonus.
- *Position*: subluxation of lens (ectopia lentis) or implant (especially if complicated surgery).

Abnormal iris

- *Defect*: polycoria due to trauma (e.g. IOFB), peripheral iridotomy (laser or surgical), or disease (e.g. ICE syndrome).

Normal examination

- *Not diplopia*: 'double vision' may be used by the patient to describe other visual anomalies (e.g. ghosting or blurring).
- *Functional*: this is a diagnosis of exclusion.

Binocular

Intermittent or variable

- *Decompensating phoria*: intermittent but usually predictable (e.g. when fatigued) with a constant pattern (e.g. only for distance, only horizontal); underlying phoria with variable/poor recovery.
- *Myasthenia gravis*: intermittent diplopia of variable orientation and severity, which worsens with fatigue; may be associated with ptosis generalized muscular fatigue.
- *Internuclear ophthalmoplegia*: diplopia may only be noticed during saccades when the adducting eye is slower to refixate.
- *GCA*: intermittent diplopia may occur due to ischaemia; may progress to become permanent.

Persistent

Neurogenic

In neurogenic lesions the diplopia is worst when looking in the direction of the paretic muscle(s); saccades are slowed in this direction; full sequelae will evolve with time. Forced duction test shows normal passive movements.

- *Horizontal only*: typically VIn palsy → underaction of LR → ipsilateral reduced abduction ± convergent.

- *Vertical/torsional only*: typically IVn palsy → underaction of SO with ipsilateral hypertropia, extorsion, and reduced depression in adducted position.
- *Mixed ± ptosis/pupillary abnormalities*: typically IIIn palsy → underaction of any/all of LPS, SR, MR, IR, IO, sphincter pupillae resulting in anything from single muscle involvement (rare) to complete ptosis obscuring a hypotropic divergent eye.
- *Complex*: unusual patterns may be due to brainstem lesions causing nuclear or supranuclear gaze palsies (often associated with other neurological signs), orbital pathology, or disorders of the neuromuscular junction (e.g. myasthenia gravis).

Mechanical

In mechanical lesions the diplopia is worst when looking away from the restricted muscle(s); signs of restriction may include IOP increase, globe retraction, and pain when looking away from the restricted muscle(s); ductions and versions are equally reduced but saccades are of normal speed; sequelae are limited to underaction of contralateral synergist. Forced duction test shows restriction of passive movements.

- *Congenital*: these rarely give rise to diplopia unless progressive or decompensating.
- *Acquired*: associated with inflammation (e.g. thyroid eye disease, myositis, idiopathic orbital inflammatory disease), trauma (orbital wall/floor fracture), or infiltration.

Anisocoria

Anisocoria greatest in bright light

This implies that the larger pupil is the abnormal one.

Abnormal iris appearance (slit-lamp examination)
Vermiform movements
- *Adie's pupil*: pupil initially dilated, later abnormally constricted; response to light is poor, response to near is initially poor, later tonic (exaggerated but slow), i.e. there is light–near dissociation; will constrict with 0.1% pilocarpine due to denervation hypersensitivity.

Structural damage
- *Iris trauma*: dilated pupil (often irregular) due to a torn sphincter with associated anterior segment damage (e.g. transillumination defects).
- *Iris inflammation*: dilated pupil (often irregular) due to sectoral iris atrophy (typically with herpes group of viruses) or stuck down by posterior synechiae.

Normal iris appearance
Constricts to pilocarpine 1%
- *Third nerve palsy*: dilated pupil associated with other features of a IIIn palsy (e.g. ptosis, oculomotor abnormality); will constrict with 1% pilocarpine.

Does not constrict to pilocarpine 1%
- *Pharmacological*: dilated pupil resulting from anticholinergic mydriatics, such as atropine (rather than adrenergics).
- *Iris ischaemia*: dilated pupil occurring after angle closure glaucoma or intraocular surgery (e.g. Urrets–Zavalia syndrome).

Anisocoria greatest in dim light

This implies that the smaller pupil is the abnormal one.

Abnormal iris appearance (slit-lamp examination)
Structural damage
- *Iris inflammation*: constricted pupil (may be irregular) stuck down by posterior synechiae.

Normal iris appearance
Dilates at normal speed in dim light
Both pupils dilate equally quickly when ambient light is dimmed.
- *Physiological anisocoria*: anisocoria is usually mild (≤1mm), and only marginally worse in dim rather than bright light; responses to light and near are normal; degree of anisocoria varies from day to day and may reverse; will dilate with 4% cocaine (cf. Horner syndrome).

Dilates in dim light but slowly (i.e. 'dilatation lag')
The smaller pupil is slower to dilate when ambient light is dimmed.
- *Horner syndrome*: constricted pupil, with mild ptosis; iris hypochromia suggests congenital or very long-standing lesion; confirm with 4% cocaine test (a Horner pupil will not dilate).

Dilates with hydroxyamphetamine 1%
  - Central or preganglionic Horner syndrome: constricted pupil, mild ptosis, facial anhydrosis; may have other features related to level of lesion (brainstem, spinal cord, lung apex, neck).

Does not dilate with hydroxyamphetamine 1%
  - Postganglionic Horner syndrome: constricted pupil, mild ptosis; may have other features related to level of lesion (neck, cavernous sinus, orbit).

Does not dilate in dim light
- Pharmacological: constricted pupil may be due to cholinergic miotics such as pilocarpine.

Nystagmus

Early onset

Horizontal jerk
- *Idiopathic congenital*: very early onset (usually by 2mths of age); worsens with fixation; improves within 'null zone' and on convergence; mild ↓VA.
- *Manifest latent*: fast phase towards fixing eye; worsens with occlusion of non-fixing eye, and with gaze towards fast phase; alternates if opposite eye takes up fixation; often associated with infantile esotropia.

Erratic
Sensory deprivation: erratic waveform ± roving eye movements; moderate/severe ↓VA due to ocular or anterior visual pathway disease.

Late onset

Conjugate
Present in primary position
Sustained
- *Peripheral vestibular*: conjugate horizontal jerk nystagmus, improves with fixation and with time since injury, worsens with gaze towards fast phase (Alexander's law) or change in head position.
- *Cerebellar/central vestibular/brainstem*: conjugate jerk nystagmus which does not improve with fixation; it may be horizontal, vertical, or torsional:
  - *Horizontal type*: e.g. lesions of the vestibular nuclei, the cerebellum, or their connections.
  - *Upbeat type*: usually cerebellar/lower brainstem lesions, e.g. demyelination, infarction, tumour, encephalitis, Wernicke syndrome.
  - *Downbeat type*: usually craniocervical junction lesions, e.g. Arnold–Chiari malformation, spinocerebellar degenerations, infarction, tumour, demyelination.

Periodic
- *Periodic alternating*: conjugate horizontal jerk nystagmus with waxing–waning nystagmus; 90s in each direction with a 10s 'null' period; usually associated with vestibulocerebellar lesions.

Present only in eccentric gaze
- *Gaze evoked*: conjugate horizontal jerk nystagmus on eccentric gaze with fast phase towards direction of gaze.
  - *Asymmetric type*: evoked nystagmus usually indicates failure of ipsilateral neural integrator/cerebellar dysfunction
  - *Symmetric type*: due to CNS depression (e.g. fatigue, alcohol, anticonvulsants, barbiturates) or structural pathology (e.g. brainstem, cerebellum)

Disconjugate
Unilateral
- *Internuclear ophthalmoplegia*: nystagmus of the abducting (and occasionally adducting) eye.
- *Superior oblique myokymia*: unilateral high-frequency low-amplitude torsional nystagmus.

Bilateral
- *See-saw nystagmus*: vertical and torsional components with one eye elevating and intorting while the other depresses and extorts; slow pendular or jerk waveform.
- *Acquired pendular nystagmus*: usually disconjugate with horizontal, vertical, and torsional components; may be associated with involuntary repetitive movement of palate, pharynx, and face.

Ophthalmic signs: external

The patient

Consider the patient as a whole. Simple observation of the patient provides a vast amount of additional information and should be practised in all cases.

Observe that the patient with juvenile cataracts and ↑IOP has severe facial eczema—they may not have thought to mention their topical corticosteroids when you asked about medication. Note the rheumatoid hands of the patient in whom you suspect scleritis. Such information will also help with management (e.g. they need assistance with topical medication). Further 'hands-on' systemic examination is directed according to clinical presentation.

Globe

Table 20.1 Ophthalmic signs: the globe

Sign	Causes
Proptosis	<ul><li>*Infection*: orbital cellulitis</li><li>*Inflammation*: thyroid eye disease, idiopathic orbital inflammatory disease, systemic vasculitis (e.g. Wegener's granulomatosis)</li><li>*Tumours*: capillary haemangioma, lymphangioma, optic nerve glioma, myeloid leukaemia, histiocytosis, dermoid cyst</li><li>*Vascular anomalies*: orbital varices, carotid–cavernous fistula</li><li>*Pseudoproptosis*: ipsilateral large globe or lid retraction; contralateral enophthalmos or ptosis; facial asymmetry</li></ul>
Enophthalmos	<ul><li>*Small globe*: microphthalmos, nanophthalmos, phthisis bulbi, orbital implant</li><li>*Soft tissue atrophy*: post-irradiation, scleroderma, cicatrizing tumours</li><li>*Bony defects*: orbital fractures, congenital orbital wall defects</li></ul>

Lymph nodes

Table 20.2 Ophthalmic signs: lymph nodes

Sign	Causes
Enlarged preauricular lymph node	<ul><li>*Infection*: viral conjunctivitis, chlamydial conjunctivitis, gonococcal conjunctivitis, Parinaud oculoglandular syndrome</li><li>*Infiltration*: lymphoma</li></ul>

Lids

Table 20.3 Ophthalmic signs: lids

Sign	Causes
Madarosis	• *Local*: cicatrizing conjunctivitis, iatrogenic (cryotherapy/radiotherapy/surgery) • *Systemic*: alopecia (patchy/totalis/universalis), psoriasis, hypothyroidism, leprosy
Poliosis	• *Local*: chronic lid margin disease • *Systemic*: sympathetic ophthalmia, Vogt–Koyanagi–Harada syndrome, Waardenburg syndrome
Lid lump	• *Anterior lamella*: external hordeolum, cyst of Moll, cyst of Zeis, xanthelasma, papilloma, seborrhoeic keratosis, keratoacanthoma, naevi, capillary haemangioma, actinic keratosis, basal cell carcinoma, squamous cell carcinoma, malignant melanoma, Kaposi's sarcoma • *Posterior lamella*: internal hordeolum, chalazion, pyogenic granuloma, sebaceous gland carcinoma
Ectropion	• Involutional, cicatricial, mechanical, paralytic (VIIn palsy), congenital
Entropion	• Involutional, cicatricial, congenital
Ptosis	• *True ptosis*: Involutional, neurogenic (IIIn palsy, Horner syndrome), myasthenic, myopathic (CPEO group), mechanical, congenital • *Pseudoptosis*: brow ptosis, dermatochalasis, microphthalmos, phthisis, prosthesis, enophthalmos, hypotropia, contralateral lid retraction
Lid retraction	• *Congenital*: Down syndrome, Duane syndrome • *Acquired*: thyroid eye disease, uraemia, VIIn palsy, IIIn misdirection, Marcus–Gunn syndrome, Parinaud syndrome, hydrocephalus, sympathomimetics, cicatrization, lid surgery, large/proptotic globe

Ophthalmic signs: anterior segment (1)

Conjunctiva

Table 20.4 Ophthalmic signs: conjunctiva

Sign	Causes
Hyperaemia	• *Generalized*: e.g. conjunctivitis, dry eye, drop/preservative allergy, CL wear, scleritis • *Localized*: e.g. episcleritis, scleritis, marginal keratitis, superior limbic keratitis, corneal abrasion, FB • *Circumcorneal*: e.g. anterior uveitis, keratitis
Discharge	• *Purulent*: bacterial conjunctivitis • *Mucopurulent*: bacterial or chlamydial conjunctivitis • *Mucoid*: vernal conjunctivitis, dry eye syndrome • *Watery*: viral or allergic conjunctivitis
Papillae	• Bacterial conjunctivitis, allergic conjunctivitis, blepharitis, floppy eyelid syndrome, superior limbic keratoconjunctivitis, CL
Giant papillae	• Vernal keratoconjunctivitis, CL-related giant papillary conjunctivitis, exposed suture, prosthesis, floppy eyelid syndrome
Follicles	• Viral conjunctivitis, chlamydial conjunctivitis, drop hypersensitivity, Parinaud oculoglandular syndrome
Pseudo-membrane	• Infective conjunctivitis (adenovirus, *Streptococcus pyogenes*, *Corynebacterium diphtheriae*, *Neisseria gonorrhoeae*), Stevens–Johnson syndrome, Graft-vs-host-disease, vernal conjunctivitis, ligneous conjunctivitis
Membrane	• Infective conjunctivitis (adenovirus, *Streptococcus pneumoniae*, *Staphylococcus aureus*, *Corynebacterium diphtheriae*), Stevens–Johnson syndrome, ligneous conjunctivitis
Cicatrization	• Trachoma, atopic keratoconjunctivitis, topical medication, chemical injury, ocular mucous membrane pemphigoid, erythema multiforme/Stevens–Johnson syndrome/TEN, other bullous disease (e.g. Linear IgA disease, epidermolysis bullosa), Sjögren syndrome, Graft-vs-host-disease
Haemorrhagic conjunctivitis	• Infective conjunctivitis (adenovirus, enterovirus 70, Coxsackie virus A24, *Streptococcus pneumoniae*, *Haemophilus aegyptius*)

Ophthalmic signs: anterior segment (2)

Episclera and sclera

Table 20.5 Ophthalmic signs: episclera and sclera

Sign	Causes
Injection	• *Superficial:* episcleritis • *Deep:* scleritis
Pigmentation	• *True:* naevus, melanocytoma, bilirubin (chronic liver disease), alkaptonuria, 'pigment spots' (at scleral perforations, e.g. nerve loop of Axenfield) • *Pseudo:* blue sclera
Blue sclera	• Osteogenesis imperfecta, keratoconus/keratoglobus, acquired scleral thinning (e.g. after necrotizing scleritis), connective tissue disorder (Marfan's, Ehlers–Danlos, pseudoxanthoma elasticum), other systemic syndromes (Turner's, Russell–Silver, incontinentia pigmenti)

Corneal iron lines (best seen on slit-lamp with cobalt blue light)

Table 20.6 Ophthalmic signs: corneal iron lines

Sign	Causes
Ferry's	• Trabeculectomy
Stocker's	• Pterygium
Hudson–Stahli	• Idiopathic with age (horizontal inferior 1/3 of cornea)
Fleischer	• Keratoconus (base of cone)

Cornea (other)

Table 20.7 Ophthalmic signs: cornea

Sign	Causes
Shape	
Thinning	• *Central:* Keratoconus, keratoglobus, posterior keratoconus, microbial keratitis • *Peripheral:* peripheral ulcerative keratitis, marginal keratitis, microbial keratitis, Mooren's ulcer, peullcid marginal degeneration, Terrien's marginal degeneration
Epithelial	
Punctate epithelial erosions	• *Superior:* vernal keratoconjunctivitis, superior limbic keratitis, floppy eyelid syndrome, poor CL fit • *Interpalpebral:* keratoconjunctivitis sicca, UV exposure, corneal anaesthesia • *Inferior:* blepharitis, exposure keratopathy, ectropion, poor Bell's phenomenon, rosacea, drop toxicity
Punctate epithelial keratitis	• Viral keratitis (adenovirus, HSV, molluscum contagiosum), Thygeson's superficial punctate keratitis
Epithelial oedema	• ↑IOP, postoperative, aphakic/pseudophakic bullous keratopathy, Fuchs' endothelial dystrophy, trauma, acute hydrops, herpetic keratitis, CL over wear, congenital corneal clouding
Corneal filaments	• Keratoconjunctivitis sicca, recurrent erosion syndrome, corneal anaesthesia, exposure keratopathy, HZO
Stromal	
Pannus	• Trachoma, tight CL, phlycten, herpetic keratitis, rosacea keratitis, chemical keratopathy, marginal keratitis, atopic/vernal keratoconjunctivitis, superior limbal keratoconjunctivitis, chronic keratoconjunctivitis of any cause
Stromal infiltrate	• *Sterile:* marginal keratitis, CL related • Infective: bacteria, fungi, viruses, protozoa
Stromal oedema	• Postoperative, keratoconus, Fuchs' endothelial dystrophy, disciform keratitis
Stromal deposits	• *Corneal dystrophies:* e.g. macular, granular, lattice, Avellino • *Systemic:* e.g. mucopolysaccharidoses (some), amyloidosis
Vogt's striae	• Keratoconus
Ghost vessels	• Interstitial keratitis (e.g. congenital syphilis, Cogan syndrome), other stromal keratitis (e.g. viral, parasitic)
Endothelial	
Descemet's folds	• Postoperative, IOP, disciform keratitis, congenital syphilis
Descemet's breaks	• Birth trauma, keratoconus/kerataglobus (hydrops), infantile glaucoma (Haab's striae)
Guttata	• *Peripheral:* Hassell–Henle bodies (physiological in the elderly) • *Central:* Fuch's endothelial dystrophy
Pigment on endothelium	• Pigment dispersion syndrome (Krukenberg spindle), postoperative, trauma
Keratic precipitates	• *Anterior uveitis:* e.g. idiopathic, HLA-B27, Fuchs heterochromic uveitis, sarcoidosis, associated with keratitis (e.g. herpetic disciform, microbial, marginal)

Ophthalmic signs: anterior segment (3)

Anterior chamber

Table 20.8 Ophthalmic signs: anterior chamber

Sign	Causes
↑IOP	• *Chronic with open angle:* e.g. primary open angle, normal tension, pseudoexfoliation, pigment dispersion, steroid-induced, angle-recession, intraocular tumour • *Chronic with closed angle:* e.g. chronic primary angle closure, neovascular, inflammatory, ICE syndrome, epithelial downgrowth, phacomorphic, aqueous misdirection • *Acute with open angle:* e.g. inflammatory, steroid-induced, Posner–Schlossman, pigment dispersion, red cell, ghost cell, phacolytic, lens particle, intraocular tumour • *Acute with closed angle:* e.g. primary angle closure, neovascular, inflammatory, ICE syndrome, epithelial downgrowth, phacomorphic, lens dislocation, aqueous misdirection
AC leucocytes	• *Corneal:* keratitis, FB, trauma, abrasion, chemical injury • *Intraocular:* anterior uveitis, endophthalmitis, tumour necrosis
Hypopyon	• *Corneal:* severe microbial keratitis • *Intraocular:* severe anterior uveitis, endophthalmitis, tumour necrosis
Hyphaema	• *Trauma:* blunt or penetrating • *Surgery:* trabeculectomy, iris manipulation procedures • *Spontaneous:* iris/angle neovascularization, haematological disease, tumour (e.g. juvenile xanthogranuloma), IOL erosion of iris
Pigment in AC and angle	• Idiopathic (↑ with age), pigment dispersion syndrome, pseudoexfoliation syndrome (Sampaolesi pigment line), intraocular surgery
Blood in Schlemm's canal	• Sturge–Weber syndrome, carotid–cavernous fistula, SVC obstruction, hypotony

Iris/ciliary body

Table 20.9 Ophthalmic signs: iris and ciliary body

Sign	Causes
Iris mass	• *Pigmented:* e.g. iris melanoma, naevus, ICE syndrome, adenoma, ciliary body tumours • *Non-pigmented:* e.g. amelanotic iris melanoma, iris cyst, iris granulomas, IOFB, juvenile xanthogranuloma, leiomyoma, ciliary body tumours, iris metastasis
Rubeosis	• Retinal vein occlusion (usually ischaemic CRVO), proliferative diabetic retinopathy, ocular ischaemic syndrome, CRAO, posterior segment tumours, long-standing retinal detachment, sickle cell or other ischaemic retinopathy
Heterochromia	• *Hypochromic:* congenital Horner syndrome, Fuchs' heterochromic cyclitis (the affected eye is bluer), uveitis, trauma/surgery, Waardenberg syndrome • *Hyperchromic:* drugs (e.g. latanaprost), siderosis (e.g. IOFB), oculodermal melanocytosis, diffuse iris naevus or melanoma, other intraocular tumours
Trans-illumination defects	• *Diffuse:* albinism, post-angle-closure, Fuchs' heterochromic cyclitis • *Peripupillary:* pseudoexfoliation syndrome • *Mid-peripheral spoke-like:* pigment dispersion syndrome • *Sectoral:* trauma, post-surgery/laser, herpes simplex/zoster, ICE syndrome, iridoschisis
Leucocoria	• Cataract, retinoblastoma, persistent fetal vasculature syndrome, inflammatory cyclitic membrane, Coats disease, ROP, Toxocara, incontinentia pigmenti, familial exudative vitreoretinopathy, retinal dysplasia (e.g. Norries' disease, Patau syndrome, Edward syndrome)
Corectopia	• Iris melanoma, iris naevus, ciliary body tumour, ICE syndrome, posterior polymorphous dystrophy, surgery (e.g. complicated cataract surgery, trabeculectomy), anterior segment dysgenesis, coloboma,
Ciliary body mass	• *Pigmented:* e.g. melanoma, metastasis, adenoma • *Non-pigmented:* e.g. cyst, uveal effusion syndrome, medulloepithelioma, leiomyoma, metastases

Ophthalmic signs: anterior segment (4)

Pupil function

Table 20.10 Ophthalmic signs: pupil function

Sign	Causes
RAPD	• Asymmetric optic nerve disease (e.g. AION, optic neuritis, asymmetric glaucoma, compressive optic neuropathy, etc.) or severe asymmetric retinal disease (e.g. CRAO, CRVO, extensive retinal detachment, etc.)
Anisocoria	• *Abnormal mydriasis:* Adie's pupil, iris trauma, iris inflammation, IIIn palsy, pharmacological, ischaemia • *Abnormal miosis:* physiological, Horner, pharmacological, iris inflammation
Light-near dissociation	• *Unilateral:* afferent defect (optic nerve pathology), efferent defect (aberrant regeneration of IIIn) • *Bilateral:* Parinaud syndrome, Argyll Robertson pupils, diabetes, amyloidosis, alcohol, myotonic dystrophy, encephalitis

Lens

Table 20.11 Ophthalmic signs: lens

Sign	Causes
Cataract	• *Sutural:* congenital, traumatic, metabolic (Fabry's disease, Mannosidosis), depositional (copper, gold, silver, iron, chlorpromazine) • *Nuclear:* congenital, age-related • *Lamellar:* congenital/infantile (inherited, rubella, diabetes, galactosaemia, hypocalcaemia) • *Coronary:* sporadic, inherited • *Cortical:* age-related • *Subcapsular:* age-related, diabetes, corticosteroids, uveitis, radiation • *Polar:* congenital • *Diffuse:* congenital, age-related
Abnormal size	• *Microphakia:* Lowe syndrome • *Microspherophakia:* familial microspherophakia, Peters anomaly, Marfan syndrome, Weill–Marchesani syndrome, hyperlysinaemia, Alport syndrome, congenital rubella
Abnormal shape	• Coloboma, anterior lenticonus (Alport syndrome), posterior lenticonus (sporadic, familial, Lowe syndrome), lentiglobus
Ectopia lentis	• *Congenital:* familial ectopia lentis, Marfan syndrome, Weill–Marchesani syndrome, homocystinuria, familial microspherophakia, hyperlysinaemia, sulphite oxidase deficiency, Stickler syndrome, Sturge–Weber syndrome, Crouzon syndrome, Ehlers–Danlos syndrome, aniridia • *Acquired:* pseudoexfoliation, trauma, high myopia, hypermature cataract, buphthalmos, ciliary body tumour
Superficial opacities	• Pseudoexfoliation, Vossius ring (trauma), Glaucomflecken (subcapsular opacities from acute angle closure glaucoma)

Ophthalmic signs: posterior segment (1)

Fundus (chorioretinal)

Table 20.12 Ophthalmic signs: fundus (chorioretinal)

Sign	Causes
Choroid	
Choroidal mass	• *Pigmented:* e.g. naevus, CHRPE, melanocytoma, metastasis, BDUMP syndrome
	• *Non-pigmented:* e.g. choroidal granuloma, choroidal detachment, choroidal neovascular membrane, haematoma (subretinal/sub-RPE/suprachoroidal), choroidal osteoma, choroidal haemangioma, posterior scleritis, metastasis
Choroidal folds	• Idiopathic, hypermetropia, retrobulbar mass, posterior scleritis, uveitis, idiopathic orbital inflammatory disease, thyroid eye disease, choroidal mass, hypotony, papilloedema
Choroidal detachment	• *Effusion:* hypotony, extensive PRP, extensive cryotherapy, posterior uveitis, uveal effusion syndrome
	• *Haemorrhage:* intra-operative, trauma, spontaneous
Retina	
Tractional retinal detachment	• ROP, sickle-cell retinopathy, proliferative diabetic retinopathy, proliferative vitreoretinopathy (e.g. trauma/IOFB, intraocular surgery, retinal breaks), vitreomacular traction syndrome, incontinentia pigmenti, retinal dysplasia
Exudative retinal detachment	• *Congenital:* nanophthalmos, uveal effusion syndrome, familial exudative vitreoretinopathy, disc coloboma/pit
	• *Vascular:* CNV, Coats disease, central serous retinopathy, vasculitis, accelerated hypertension, pre-eclampsia
	• Choroidal tumours
	• *Inflammatory:* posterior uveitis (e.g. VKH), posterior scleritis, orbital cellulitis, postoperative inflammation, idiopathic orbital inflammatory disease
General	
White dots	• *Idiopathic white dot syndromes:* PIC, POHS, MEWDS, APMPPE, serpiginous choroidopathy, birdshot retinochoroidopathy, multifocal choroiditis with panuveitis
	• *Infective (chorio)retinitis:* syphilis, toxoplasma, tuberculosis, candida, HSV
	• *Inflammatory (chorio)retinitis:* sarcoidosis, sympathetic ophthalmia, VKH

Fundus (vascular)

Table 20.13 Ophthalmic signs: fundus (vascular)

Sign	Causes
Hard exudates	• Diabetic retinopathy, choroidal neovascular membrane, macroaneurysm, accelerated hypertension, neuroretinitis, retinal telangiectasias
Cotton-wool spots	• Diabetic retinopathy, B/CRVO, ocular ischaemic syndrome, hypertension, HIV retinopathy, vasculitis
Retinal telangiectasias	• Coats' disease, Leber's miliary aneurysms, idiopathic juxtafoveal telangiectasia, ROP, RP, diabetic retinopathy, sickle retinopathy, radiation retinopathy, hypogammaglobulinaemia, Eales disease, C/BRVO
Arterial emboli	• Carotid artery disease, atrial thrombus, atrial myxoma, infective endocarditis, fat embolus (long-bone fracture), talc embolus (IV drug abuser), amniotic fluid embolus
Roth's spots	• Septic emboli, leukaemia, myeloma, HIV retinopathy
Vasculitis	• Idiopathic retinal vasculitis, intermediate or posterior uveitis (idiopathic), sarcoidosis, MS, Behçet's disease, SLE, toxoplasmosis, tuberculosis, HSV, VZV, CMV, ARN, Wegener's granulomatosis, polyarteritis nodosa, Takayasu's arteritis, Whipple's disease, Lyme disease
Arteritis	• ARN (HSV, VZV); less commonly in other vasculitides

Ophthalmic signs: posterior segment (2)

Macula

Table 20.14 Ophthalmic signs: macula

Sign	Causes
Cystoid macular oedema	• *Postoperative:* cataract/corneal/vitreoretinal surgery • *Postprocedure:* cryotherapy, peripheral iridotomy, panretinal photocoagulation • *Inflammatory:* uveitis (posterior > intermediate > anterior), scleritis • *Vascular:* retinal vein obstruction, diabetic maculopathy, ocular ischaemia, choroidal neovascular membrane, retinal telangiectasia, hypertensive retinopathy, radiation retinopathy • *Medication:* adrenaline, latanoprost • *Other:* vitreomacular traction syndrome, RP, autosomal dominant CMO, tumours of the choroid/retina
Macular hole	• Idiopathic, trauma, CMO, epiretinal membrane, vitreomacular traction syndrome, RRD, laser injury, myopia, hypertension, proliferative diabetic retinopathy
Epiretinal membrane	• Idiopathic, retinal detachment surgery, cryotherapy, photocoagulation, trauma (blunt or penetrating), posterior uveitis, persistent vitreous haemorrhage, retinal vascular disease (e.g. BRVO)
Choroidal neovascular membrane	• *Degenerative:* AMD, pathological myopia, angioid streaks • *Trauma:* choroidal rupture, laser • *Inflammation:* sarcoidosis, toxoplasmosis, POHS, PIC, multifocal choroiditis, serpiginous choroidopathy, bird-shot retinochoroidopathy, VKH • *Dystrophies:* Best's disease • *Other:* idiopathic, chorioretinal scar (any cause), tumour
Central serous detachment	• Central serous retinopathy, optic disc pit, CNV, posterior uveitis (e.g. VKH), accelerated hypertension; see also exudative retinal detachment
Bull's eye maculopathy	• *Drug:* chloroquine group, clofazimine • *Macular dystrophies:* cone dystrophy, cone-rod dystrophy, Stargardt's • *Neurological:* Batten's disease
Cherry red spot	• *Systemic:* Tay–Sachs disease, Sandhoff disease, GM1 gangliosidoses, Niemann–Pick disease, sialidosis, metachromatic leucodystrophy, • *Ocular:* CRAO
Foveal schisis	• X-linked juvenile retinoschisis

Optic disc

Table 20.15 Ophthalmic signs: optic disc

Sign	Causes
Pallor	*Congenital:* Kjer's, Behr's, or Wolfram's optic atrophy
	Acquired: compression (optic nerve or chiasm), glaucoma, ischaemia, toxins, poor nutrition, inflammation, infection, LHON, trauma, severe retinal disease, post-papilloedema
Apparent swelling	*Pseudo:* drusen, tilted, hypermetropic, myelinated
	True: ↑ICP (usually bilateral) or local causes (may be unilateral), e.g. inflammation, ischaemia, LHON, infiltration, tumour
Pit	*Congenital*
	Acquired: glaucoma

Ophthalmic signs: visual field

Normal		Temporal 90° Inferior 70° Nasal 60° Superior 50°
Arcuate		**Optic neuropathy 2' to:** Glaucoma Ischaemia (AION) Papilloedema (late)
Altitudinal		**Optic neuropathy 2' to:** Ischaemia (AION) Glaucoma **Vascular** Hemispheric RVO/ RAO
Enlarged blind-spot		**Optic neuropathy** (especially peripapillary axons)
Central		**Macular pathology** **Optic neuropathy** (especially central axons)
Centrocaecal		**Optic neuropathy** (central and peripapillary axons)
Bitemporal hemianopia	Worse superiorly → inferior lesion; worse inferiorly → superior lesion	**Chiasmal compression** (respect midline) **Pseudochiasmal defects** (may not respect mid-line): Tilted optic discs Bilateral retinoschisis Toxicity (chloroquine) Sector RP
Junctional scotoma		**Prechiasmal/optic nerve lesion,** e.g. compressive

Fig. 20.1 Visual field defects.

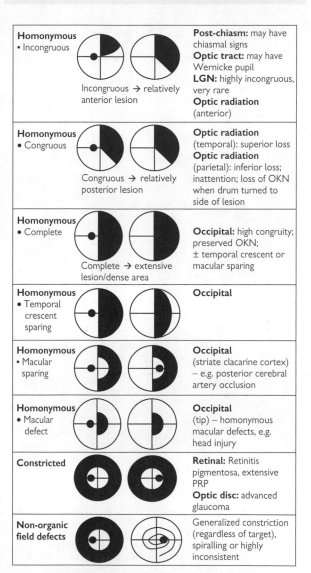

Homonymous • Incongruous	Incongruous → relatively anterior lesion	**Post-chiasm:** may have chiasmal signs **Optic tract:** may have Wernicke pupil **LGN:** highly incongruous, very rare **Optic radiation** (anterior)
Homonymous • Congruous	Congruous → relatively posterior lesion	**Optic radiation** (temporal): superior loss **Optic radiation** (parietal): inferior loss; inattention; loss of OKN when drum turned to side of lesion
Homonymous • Complete	Complete → extensive lesion/dense area	**Occipital:** high congruity; preserved OKN; ± temporal crescent or macular sparing
Homonymous • Temporal crescent sparing		**Occipital**
Homonymous • Macular sparing		**Occipital** (striate clacarine cortex) – e.g. posterior cerebral artery occlusion
Homonymous • Macular defect		**Occipital** (tip) – homonymous macular defects, e.g. head injury
Constricted		**Retinal:** Retinitis pigmentosa, extensive PRP **Optic disc:** advanced glaucoma
Non-organic field defects		Generalized constriction (regardless of target), spiralling or highly inconsistent

Fig. 20.1 Visual field defects (*continued*).

Vision in context

Low vision: taking a history

About 2.5% of the UK population have some degree of visual impairment that is not correctable by refraction. Of these up to two-thirds are thought to have sufficiently severe sight loss to qualify for visual impairment registration. However, even among those attending ophthalmology units up to half of those eligible are not actually registered.[1] There is concern that this may reflect a wider problem of access to support and services. It is probable that many of these people never seek help. However, even those who get to an ophthalmologist may only be rewarded with a diagnosis of an incurable eye disease for which 'nothing can be done'.

In these circumstances those involved in eye-care must be aware of 'what *can* be done' to optimize the patient's remaining vision and how best to advise and assist the patient. This is often best co-ordinated in a dedicated Low Vision clinic, ideally with access to specialist nurses, optometrists, rehabilitation workers, counsellors, and social services.

Definition

The UK Low Vision Services Consensus Group defines low vision as impairment of visual function that causes restriction to everyday life and that cannot be corrected by conventional spectacles, contact lenses, or medical intervention. This should not be confused with the WHO definition of low vision, which is VA<6/18, but ≥3/60 in the better eye with best possible correction; the WHO define <3/60 as blindness.

History

General—what are their concerns?

People are extremely variable. For some the priority will be to continue to solve the crossword, others will be afraid of social isolation. Sometimes this will also reveal misunderstandings about their condition.

Specific—consider the following:

Reading

Is reading an issue for them? If so, what do they want to read: what size print and in what context (i.e. at home or out-and-about). This will affect the type of optical devices used.

Television

If this is an issue for them, consider size of television, viewing distance, and whether colour or black-and-white (higher contrast).

Activities of daily living and recreation

Are they managing to look after themselves (± dependants)? What about shopping, cooking, and hygiene? Can they still manage the telephone or do they risk becoming isolated? Can they still do their hobbies?

Medication

Can they manage their tablets, instil drops and measure their injections?

Mobility

Do they manage to get around? Do they have access to public transport or lifts from family or friends? Mobility training can help them navigate and continue to use public transport with confidence.

Work and financial support
Have they got the help they need to continue working if they wish to? What resources are available to them in terms of equipment or personal assistance? Do they know how to access any benefits that they are entitled to?

Psychosocial
Are they coping emotionally with their visual impairment? Do they have access to local support groups? Would they benefit from talking to a counsellor?

Visual phenomena
Are they troubled by glare? Glare that worsens vision under bright conditions (effectively reducing contrast) is known as disability glare. Glare that is uncomfortable without necessarily affecting vision is known as 'discomfort glare'. Do they find it difficult changing between bright and dark conditions and vice versa? Problems with adaptation to light and dark is common in AMD, RP and advanced glaucoma.

Visual hallucinations
Ask specifically whether they are being troubled by 'seeing things that aren't real'. Charles Bonnet syndrome (visual hallucinations in people with severe sight loss) is relatively common, but patients frequently conceal it for fear of being thought to be mentally ill. Discussing and rationalizing the syndrome (e.g. 'your brain is filling in the gaps in your vision') can be very reassuring. The visual hallucinations fall into two broad types: abstract (patterns, lines, etc.) or life-like (people, animals, etc.). The images may be black and white or in colour, may be distorted and of the incorrect size (e.g. images of tiny people). In most cases it resolves within 12–18mths.[2]

1. Barry RJ, Muray Pl. Unregistered visual impairment: is registration a failing system. *Br J Ophthalmol* 2005;**89**: 995–8.

2. Ffytche DH. Visual hallucinations and the Charles Bonnet Syndrome. *Curr Psychiatry Rep* 2005;**7**: 168–79.

Further reading

Sinclair A, Ryan B. *Low vision: the essential guide for ophthalmologists.* The Guide Dogs for the Blind Association, 2008.

Low vision: assessing visual function

Visual function is more than just distance acuity. Do not overlook the effect of reduced contrast sensitivity or a constricted visual field.

Visual acuity: distance

Where possible use a LogMAR chart rather than a Snellen chart. In addition to the usual advantages of LogMAR over Snellen (*see* Assessment of version: acuity(2) 📖 p.6), the fact that there are five letters on every row (including the top row) avoids the 'one-chance only' scenario characteristic of the 6/60 line on a Snellen chart, and is somewhat less discouraging for the patient. If the top line cannot be read at the test distance, bring the chart nearer: don't just go straight to count fingers. The jump from 6/60 to counting fingers (CF) is a huge difference in functional terms.

Visual acuity: near

Previously, most reading charts were aimed at the normally sighted (albeit presbyopic) population with ranges of N5–N48. For low vision assessment it may be helpful to have a wider range such as the Bailey–Lovie near chart that runs from N2.5 to N80.

Contrast sensitivity

While not commonly used in the general ophthalmic clinic, measuring contrast sensitivity (e.g. with a Pelli–Robson chart) is an important part of assessing visual function in someone with low vision. It can explain an apparent discrepancy between reasonable acuity in the high-contrast clinic setting and poor functional vision in a dimly lit home; loss of contrast sensitivity is also associated with increased falls in the elderly.

Visual fields

Day-to-day function is greatly affected by the quality of your visual field, even in the presence of 6/6 central vision. Mobility is particularly affected by inferior/central field defects. Reading is also affected by central defects, but also by both right hemianopic defects (they can't jump to the next word) and left hemianopic defects (they can't find the next line). Specific reading techniques may be helpful in these cases (Box 21.1). If a patient is being referred for mobility assessment and training, it is helpful if the rehabilitation officer can be provided with a copy of the visual field plot.

Box 21.1 Reading strategies for patients with a hemianopic field defect*

Defect	Problem	Strategy
Left hemianopia	Can't find the start of the line	Keep thumb/marker at the start of the line as a marker to return to
Right hemianopia	Can't find the next word	Learn to skip beyond the next word so that the target word falls within the field of vision
		Try reading with the text rotated up to 90° so that the whole line falls within the field of vision

*The advice depends on direction of reading—a left to right reading direction is assumed here.

Low vision: doing something useful (1)

General

Optimize lighting conditions (e.g. brighter bulbs, more lights around the house, good reading light). Improve contrast where possible.

Make sure information is provided in a suitable format: written (should be in a clear typeface of minimum 14-point font size), audio, or electronic.

Equipment

Refraction (near and distance) should be optimized. In addition consider:

Optical devices (near)

- *Reading glasses*: these should be optimized, although they are often not sufficient on their own. Up to +4.00D is usually well tolerated but beyond this the reading distance is uncomfortably short. Higher reading additions may require a prism to assist convergence.
- *Hand magnifiers*: these are usually practical and inexpensive, but are limited by a small field of view (especially for the higher powers).
- *Stand magnifiers*: these have the advantage of keeping both hands free and keeping the working distance constant, but are less transportable.
- *Illuminated magnifiers*: these improve contrast (provided that the batteries are charged), but are generally bulkier.
- *Reading telescopes*: these may be useful for specific near work as they have a greater working distance than reading glasses of an equivalent magnification. However, they are expensive and are poor cosmetically.
- *Closed-circuit television*: excellent magnification with high contrast can be achieved with a television camera directed down on to a reading plinth and viewed on the adjacent screen. However, it is expensive, not portable, and generally superseded by computer/scanner technology.

Optical devices (distance)

- *Distance telescopes*: can be useful for specific tasks, although generally they are limited by the small field of view. They may be spectacle mounted (useful for static tasks, e.g. watching television, theatre, music, sport, etc.) or hand-held (used as required, e.g. bus number, signs, etc.).

Computers

Personal computers (either with enlarged text or speech facility) have made a spectacular difference to the lives of many visually impaired people. They provide an easy method of writing, 'reading' (with scanner and optical character recognition) and instant 'letter' communication by email. Web-based facilities also increase access to shopping, entertainment, and support.

Other devices

Other devices include
- talking watches/clocks
- writing guides
- typoscopes (black card with a slit used as a reading window; reduces glare)
- liquid-level indicators (prevent overfilling cups, baths)

- tactile controls on domestic appliances (either as standard or as 'bump-ons')
- large button telephones
- talking scales.

Entertainment
In addition to the improved accessibility of computers, consider:
- modified games (e.g. large playing cards)
- audio description DVDs or videos
- talking books/newspapers (available as mp3, audio CD and other formats)
- modified sports equipment.

Mobility
Mobility training can help people navigate and continue to use public transport with confidence; a mobility officer will tailor the training to the needs (type of transport/required routes) to that individual. Mobility may be assisted by the use of a cane (Box 21.2), guide dog (relatively uncommon), or a sighted guide. The use of a cane or of a guide dog require training.

Box 21.2 Types of cane (or 'white stick')

Type	Features	Purpose
Symbol cane	Small, lightweight, collapsible	Advises others that the bearer has visual impairment
Guide cane	Longer, more robust	Can be used to detect change in contour, e.g. steps
		Advises others that the bearer has visual impairment
Long cane	Long with a roller-ball tip	Used to sweep the path ahead to detect obstacles
		Advises others that the bearer has visual impairment
White walking stick	White, standard walking aid	Used as a walking aid (like a normal walking stick)
		Advises others that the bearer has visual impairment

Support
Ensure that they have access to support from social services and local support groups, and that they know how to get help in case of need.

Registration (see visual impairment regotration p.812)
If they are eligible but are not yet registered ensure that the purpose of registration is explained and that it is offered to them.

Low vision: doing something useful (2)

Benefits

Check that they are aware of what benefits they are entitled to, and know where to get help or further information, e.g. social services, and local and national support groups.

Box 21.3 Benefits available in the UK for those registered visually impaired

Tax relief and allowances

For blind and partially sighted people

- *Disability living allowance (DLA, if <65yrs)/attendance allowance (AA, if >65yrs):* for help with personal care and mobility; depends on level of disability.
- *Additional income support (if <60yrs)/pension credit (if >60yrs):* to top up low income.
- *Working tax credit:* if disabled and working ≥16h/wk but on low income.
- *Incapacity benefit:* for people of working age unable to work.
- *Council tax reduction.*

Additional benefits for those receiving DLA or AA:

- Additional housing benefit.
- Council tax benefit.
- Exemption from non-dependants deduction from Income Support, Pension Credit, Housing Benefit, and Council Tax Benefit (only applies to those on AA or middle/highest rate DLA).

Additional benefits for blind people only:

- Blind person's income tax allowance.

Other

For blind and partially-sighted people

- Community care services and local council assistance: home care, mobility training, counselling, equipment, home modification.
- Free NHS sight test.
- Free NHS prescriptions: depends on age and income.
- Low vision aids.
- Additional equipment/assistance/travel costs to make it possible to work.
- Free postage on 'articles for the blind', e.g. talking books.
- Railcard and other travel concessions.
- Exemption from BT directory enquiries.

Additional benefits for blind people only

- 50% reduction in television licence fee.
- Car parking concessions (blue badge scheme): also available to partially sighted people if they have mobility problems.
- Free loan of radios, cassette/CD players, and TV sound receivers.
- Help with telephone installation charges and line rental.

The exact benefits change according to governmental initiative; social services are available to provide up-to-the-minute advice for the patient.

Visual impairment registration (1)

Registration of visual impairment has traditionally had three roles: to formally recognize an individual's sight loss; to identify those patients eligible for assistance due to their disability; and to help eye services, social services, and government know the extent and distribution of visual impairment in the community. The National Assistance Act (NAA)1948 formalized this process and led to the BD8 form that has been in use in England and Wales for about 50yrs. Equivalent forms elsewhere include the BP1 form in Scotland and the A655 in Northern Ireland.

However, a recent review showed that for many people the registration process actually excluded or delayed access to services. More than half of those eligible choose not to be registered, and many are unhappy about being registered blind when they have (and are expected to continue to have) residual vision. In response to this the BD8 system has been replaced by a scheme that separates formal registration from the referral for needs assessment. The new form—the Certificate of Vision Impairment (CVI)—is now supported by the Referral of Vision Impairment (RVI) and the Low Vision Leaflet (LVL) both of which can be used to notify Social Services of a persons needs without requiring full registration. Among other changes the CVI replaces the category 'blind' with 'severely sight impaired or blind'.

Eligibility

Sight impaired/partially sighted

This is not legally defined. It is summarized by the Department of Health (UK)[1] as:

- VA 3/60–6/60 with normal visual field *or*
- VA 6/60–6/24 with moderate contraction of the visual field, media opacities or aphakia.
- VA 6/18 or better but with severe field loss. This may be either a large defect such as hemianopia or marked contraction of the visual field such as in RP or advanced glaucoma.

Severely sight impaired/blind

This is legally defined (NAA 1948) as 'so blind that they cannot do any work for which eyesight is essential'. This is conventionally regarded as:

- VA ≤3/60 *or*
- VA 3/60–6/60 with a very contracted visual field *or*
- VA 6/60 or better with a very contracted visual field, especially where there is significant inferior field loss; homonymous or bitemporal hemianopia are specifically excluded unless the central VA is worse than 6/18.

Table 21.1 Registration for blindness April 1999–March 2000 in England and Wales[1]

Age	Leading causes of blindness
0–15	1st Disorders of the visual cortex (15.9%)
	2nd Congenital ocular anomalies (13.4%)
	3rd Hereditary retinal disorders (13.1%)
16–64	1st Diabetic retinopathy (17.7%)
	2nd Hereditary retinal disorders (15.8%)
	3rd Degeneration of the macula and posterior pole (7.7%)
All ages	1st Degeneration of the macula and posterior pole (57.2%)
	2nd Glaucoma (10.9%)
	3rd Diabetic retinopathy (5.9%)

1. Bunce C, Wormald R. Causes of blind certifications in England and Wales: April 1999–March 2000. *Eye* 2008;**22**:905–11.

Visual impairment registration (2)

For the hospital eye service

Certificate of Vision Impairment

This replaces the BD8 (and the short-lived CVI2003) as the declaration of eligibility for registration.

- *Part 1*: contains (1) patient's consent to be registered, and (2) consultant ophthalmologist's confirmation of eligibility for registration (sight impaired vs severely sight impaired).
- *Part 2*: contains (1) contact details of patient, GP, local social services; (2) visual function (acuity and field); (3) diagnosis (with ICD10 codes).
- *Part 3*: contains (1) relevant social factors (e.g. lives alone, other disability, etc.); (2) urgency of contact required; (3) ethnic origin; and (4) preferred communication format.
- *Explanatory notes*: (1) patient information about the certificate; (2) summary of consent; (3) information about driving.

In signing the form the patient consents to the information within the form being passed: (1) to their local council, GP and Primary Care Trust for referral, assessment and registration purposes, and (2) to the Royal College of Ophthalmologists on behalf of Moorfields Eye Hospital and the Department of Health for epidemiological research and analysis.

Referral of vision impairment

This notifies social services of the patient's situation, requests an assessment for them, and how urgently this is required. It should be completed by Ophthalmic Clinic Staff with the consent of the patient. It does not result in registration.

For optometrists

Low vision leaflet

These should be provided by optometrists to any person in whom they identify sight impairment. It not only provides the patient with contact details for support, and local and national resources, but it also includes a form that can be filled in by the patient enabling them to 'self-refer' to social services. Social services will then carry out an assessment of their needs and advise them on what resources are available to them. It does not result in registration.

Box 21.4 Relevant documents available from the Department of Health (UK) website

- Certificate of vision impairment (CVI).
- Referral of Vision Impairment (RVI).
- Low Vision Leaflet (LVL).
- Explanatory notes for consultant ophthalmologists and hospital eye clinic staff.
- The identification, referral, and registration of sight loss: action for social services departments and optometrists, and explanatory notes.

1. http://www.dh.gov.uk/en/Healthcare/Primarycare/Optical/DH_4074843

Driving standards

Evidence that visual impairment alone causes accidents is surprisingly scarce. The strictness of driving standards varies internationally, in part affected by the density of traffic and driving conditions. In some parts of the USA partially sighted people may drive during daylight hours within a specified radius of their home.

In the UK any driver who has a condition that either already affects their fitness to drive or might do so in the future (e.g. glaucoma) must notify the DVLA unless anticipated to be of <3mths duration. The following driving standards are enforced by the DVLA:

Visual acuity

Group 1 drivers (car and light vehicles)
- Must be able to read in good light either the old (pre-September 2001) format number plate at 20.5m or the new (post-September 2001) format number plate at 20m.

This is a legal requirement, and corresponds roughly to 6/10 Snellen acuity.

Group 2 drivers (large goods and passenger carrying vehicles)
- At least 6/9 in the better eye AND
- At least 6/12 in the worse eye AND
- Uncorrected acuity in each eye must be at least 3/60.

Some drivers who fail these requirements may be permitted to drive under 'grandfather rights', which take into account the date of licensing. The licence holder needs to contact the DVLA who will require a certificate of recent driving experience and confirmation of no eyesight related road accidents in the previous 10yrs.

Visual fields

The preferred method of testing is now the Esterman program on the Humphrey analyser. For those patients who cannot use an automated perimeter, Goldmann testing is acceptable in exceptional circumstances. Bitemporal hemianopia may require monocular Esterman testing to ensure that there is adequate input from both hemifields in at least one eye to prevent dissociation (hemifield slip). A maximum of 20% false positives and of three attempts for each test is allowed.

Group 1 drivers
- At least 120' on the horizontal (Goldmann III4e setting or equivalent) AND:
- No significant defect in the binocular field encroaching within 20' of fixation above or below the horizontal meridian. 'Insignificant' central defects (equivalent to the normal blind spot in a monocular field) comprise:
  - Scattered single missed points.
  - A single cluster of 2 or 3 missed points.

Where a patient has fully adapted to a static, long-standing defect the DVLA may consider them as an 'exceptional case' and perform a practical driving assessment.

Group 2 drivers
- Full binocular field of vision.
- No missed points in the central 20'.

Other

These patients should inform the DVLA of their condition.

Monocularity

Patients may drive (Group 1 vehicles only) when clinically advised that they have adapted to the disability and they satisfy the usual VA requirements and have a normal monocular visual field.

Diplopia

Patients with uncorrected diplopia must not drive. Driving may be resumed if controlled; patching is acceptable subject to the above constraints on monocularity. Very rarely DVLA may permit someone to drive despite uncorrected diplopia if it is stable (>6mths).

Blepharospasm

Patients with severe blepharospasm must not drive. Patients with mild, successfully treated, blepharospasm may drive subject to consultant approval.

All drivers

If the patient fails to reach these standards they must not drive and have a legal requirement to notify the DVLA. Failure to comply is a criminal offence and can result in a fine of up to £1000.

Further details are available at www.dvla.gov.uk

Racing licenses

For racing in the UK

The MSA requires a best corrected VA of 6/6 (both eyes together) and a visual field of 120' horizontally without significant defect within 20' above or below the horizontal meridian.

For international racing

The FIA requires a best corrected VA of at least 9/10 in each eye or 8/10 in one eye and 10/10 in the other, normal colour vision, normal stereopsis and a visual field of 120' horizontally without significant defect within 20' above or below the horizontal meridian.

Professional standards

Pilots (civil aviation authority)

Class 1 pilots (commercial: aeroplane and helicopter)[1]

Visual acuity
- *Distance*: at least 6/9 in each eye and 6/6 with both eyes together (best corrected).
- *Near*: at least N5 at 30–50cm and N14 at 100cm (best corrected).

Refractive error and correction
- Refractive error less than +5.0D or –6.0D, astigmatism less than 2.0D and anisometropia less than 2.0D.
- Contact lenses may be used if they can be reliably used for >8h/d.
- *Refractive surgery*: stability of refraction must be demonstrated; usually unable to fly for 3mths post-LASIK and 1yr after other procedures; pre-operative refractive error may still be a bar to qualification.

Colour
- Satisfactory Ishihara testing; if fails this then must pass Lantern test.

Other
- Normal visual fields.
- No diplopia.
- Heterophoria less than 8 Δ exo, 10 Δ eso, or 2 Δ vertical at 6m and less than 12 Δ exo, 6 Δ eso, or 1 Δ vertical at 33cm: excess of this will require further assessment by a CAA ophthalmologist.
- No ophthalmic or adnexal disease.

Class 2 pilots (private: aeroplane and helicopter)[2]

Visual acuity
- *Distance*: at least 6/12 in each eye and 6/6 with both eyes together (best corrected); amblyopes with 6/18 in one eye may be permitted to fly provided the other eye is at least 6/6 uncorrected.
- *Near*: at least N5 at 30–50cm and N14 at 100cm (best corrected).

Refractive error and correction
- Refractive error less than +5.0D or –8.0D (in the most ametropic meridian), astigmatism <3D and anisometropia <3.0D; under some circumstances stable myopia in the range –5 to –8.0D may be acceptable.
- Contact lenses may be used if they can be reliably used for >8h/d.
- *Refractive surgery*: stability of refraction must be demonstrated; usually unable to fly for 3mths post-LASIK and 1yr after other procedures; pre-operative refractive error may still be a bar to qualification.

Colour
- Satisfactory Ishihara testing; if fails this then must pass Holmes Wright Lantern test or be restricted to day-time flying.

Other
- Normal visual fields.
- No diplopia.
- Heterophoria will require further assessment by a CAA ophthalmologist.

- No ophthalmic or adnexal disease.

Further information is available at www.caa.co.uk.

Armed forces (UK)

It should be stressed that certain military sections have their own visual requirements. When applying for the armed forces, standards can be checked at the local forces careers advice centre.

Generic branches

VA of at least 6/60 uncorrected, where fundoscopy is normal and there is no pathological condition. Refraction should not exceed −7.00 or +8.00DS and 5.00D of cylinder. Colour perception and stereopsis is variable depending on branch or trade.

Aircrew

Pilots

Pilots should have a VA of at least 6/12 uncorrected, correctable to 6/6 and N5. Stereopsis should be a minimum of 120s of arc.

- *RAF:* refraction should not exceed Plano to +1.75DS and +0.75D cylinder.
- *Fleet Air Arm (Royal Navy):* refraction should not exceed −0.75 to +1.75DS, +1.25D cylinder.
- *Army:* refraction should not exceed −0.75 to +1.75DS, +0.75D cylinder

Navigators and observers

Navigators (RAF and Army) or observers (Royal Navy) must have a vision of at least 6/24 unaided, correctable to 6/6; refraction should not exceed −1.25 to +3.00DS and +1.25D cylinder.

1. Civial Aviation Authority www.caa.co.uk/docs/49/SRG_MED-JARClass1InitialVisStds[2189].pdf/
2. Civil Aviation Authority www.caa.co.uk/docs/49/SRG_MED_JARClass2InitialVisStds[538].pdf/

Eligibility for sight tests and optical vouchers in the NHS(UK)

In England, Wales, and Northern Ireland a patient is eligible for free sight tests if they are

- <16yrs old.
- ≤18yrs old and in full-time education.
- ≥60yrs old.
- ≥40yrs old AND diagnosed with glaucoma or been told by an ophthalmologist that they are at risk of glaucoma or have a parent/sibling/child who has been diagnosed with glaucoma.
- Diagnosed with diabetes.
- Registered as sight-impaired (partially sighted) or severely sight-impaired (blind).
- In need of complex lenses.
- Receiving their sight test through the hospital eye department.
- Receiving (or their partner is receiving) Income Support, Income-based Jobseeker's Allowance, or Pension Credit Guarantee Credit.
- Entitled to or named on a valid NHS Tax Credit Exemption Certificate.
- Named on a valid HC2 certificate.

In Scotland everybody is eligible for a free sight-test annually.

This is subject to governmental vagaries and so may change with little warning. Up-to-the-minute information is available on the Department of Health (UK) website on www.dh.gov.uk

Box 21.6 Eligibility for NHS(UK) optical vouchers

In England, Wales and Northern Ireland a patient is eligible for vouchers towards the costs of glasses or contact lenses if they are:

- <16yrs old.
- ≤18yrs old and in full-time education.
- Receiving (or their partner is receiving) Income Support, income-based Jobseeker's Allowance, or Pension Credit Guarantee Credit.
- Entitled to or named on a valid NHS Tax Credit Exemption Certificate.
- Named on a valid HC2 certificate.

Up-to-the-minute information is available on the Department of Health (UK) website on www.dh.gov.uk

Perioperative care

Pre-operative assessment (1)

Pre-operative assessment seeks to identify any factors that may put the patient (or staff) at additional risk. The following are a practical interpretation of the recommendations of the Royal College of Ophthalmologists and the Royal College of Anaesthetists.[1,2]

General

- *Day surgery vs in-patient*: check whether appropriate for day surgery (adequate support) or in-patient care.
- *Case-notes and test results*: ensure medical records and any relevant investigations (including biometry, scans, and blood tests) are available.
- *Alerts*: check for hazards (e.g. allergies, MRSA, blood-borne diseases, e.g. hepatitis, HIV) and ensure that these are communicated appropriately to the rest of the team.
- *Special requirements*: check for special requirements (e.g. interpreter).

Systemic

History

- *Age*.
- *Past medical history*: ask specifically about diabetes, hypertension, ischaemic heart disease, and any current problems such as smoking, alcohol intake, tuberculosis, asthma, COPD, epilepsy, reflux, hepatic, renal and thyroid disorders.
- *Past surgical history*: previous surgery, anaesthetics and adverse reactions.
- *Systemic review*: CVS (e.g. chest pain and precipitating events, MI, palpitations, (paroxysmal noeturnal dyspnoea PND)), RS (recent chest infection, asthma, exercise tolerance e.g. breathlessness at rest or on exertion, orthopnoea), CNS (pre existing neurological damage, CVA, fits), Renal (e.g. dialysis), psychological issues (e.g. alcohol, anxiety), ability to lie flat.
- *Family history* (including problems with anaesthesia).
- *Medication and allergies*.
- *Social history*, e.g. home care.

NB Any patients with significant anaesthetic risk factors or other concerns (e.g. syndromic patients or those with congenital disorders) should be discussed with the anaesthetist, especially if a general anaesthetic is being considered.

Examination

- *General*: build, weight, height, and body mass index.
- *CVS*: anaemia, cyanosis, oedema, pulse (rate + rhythm), BP, heart sounds, any murmurs.
- *RS*: clubbing, respiratory rate and chest expansion, tracheal position, (tracheostomy scars), auscultation (air entry, wheeze, crepitations), pulse oximetry saturation.
- *Musculoskeletal*: neck/jaw/dental/back problems (may affect intubation and surgical position).
- *CNS*: comprehension, cooperation, hearing, tremor, neurological deficits, other abnormal movements, and mobility.

Ophthalmic

The ophthalmic history and examination should identify any new developments as the clinic assessment which may postpone surgery or might modify the planned operation in any way.

Contraindications

Any identified risk factors should be treated pre-operatively. This may require postponement of surgery and either co-ordination with the patient's GP or referral to an appropriate specialist.

> **Box 22.1 Specific systemic contraindications to ophthalmic surgery**
>
> • Uncontrolled BP (>180/100mmHg)
> • Myocardial ischaemia (unstable angina or MI in the last 3mths)
> • CVA (cerebrovascular accidents, TIA) in the last 3mths
> • Uncontrolled hyperglycaemia, e.g. BM >15
> • Uncontrolled arrhythmias
> • High INR
> • Acute systemic illness

Investigations

Operations under local anaesthesia

Routine investigations are usually not required unless history and systemic examination suggest significant systemic disease that would be worthy of investigation in its own right. (e.g. coronary artery disease, diabetes, severe respiratory disease, anticoagulation).

Operations under general anaesthesia

It is common practice not to routinely investigate fit ASA I patients (American Society of Anesthiologists level I; see Table 22.4 □ p.827) under the age of 40yrs in whom a general history and examination is satisfactory.

Specific investigations

• *Haematological and biochemical profile* (e.g. FBC, U+E, glucose, etc.) tests are indicated for patients in whom abnormalities are likely, e.g. those with renal, hepatic, metabolic, endocrine dysfunction, or patients on concurrent medication with steroids, bronchodilators, diuretics, cardiac drugs, or those presenting with acute systemic illness.
• *ECG:* is not routinely required for patients under age of 50 unless presenting with history of heavy smoking, diabetes, hypertension, renal disorders, previous cardiac disease, or excessive alcohol intake. A baseline ECG for patients over 50 is recommended.
• *Specific investigations:* CXR, echocardiography, coagulation screen, liver and thyroid function tests, etc. are indicated according to patient's history/examination.
• *Sickle cell test:* indicated if African-Caribbean or Mediterranean origin.
• *Pacemaker check:* required in patients with pacemakers.

1. Royal College of Ophthalmologists and the Royal College of Anaesthetists: Local anaesthesia for intraocular surgery 2001. Available at: www.rcophth.ac.uk/docs/publications/published-guidelines

2. Royal College of Ophthalmologists and the Royal College of Anaesthetists: Cataract surgery guidelines 2004. Available at: www.rcophth.ac.uk/docs/publications/published-guidelines

Pre-operative assessment (2)

Pre-operative management

Patients for intraocular surgery: appropriate pre-operative drops.

Table 22.1 Common pre-operative drop regimens

Cataract surgery	Cyclopentolate 1% + phenylephrine 2.5% + diclofenac 0.1%.
Vitreoretinal surgery	Cyclopentolate 1% + phenylephrine 2.5% + diclofenac 0.1%.
Penetrating keratoplasty	Pilocarpine 2%

Patients for general anaesthetic: patients should be fasted for 6h after a solid meal (includes milk, tea, coffee) and 4h after **clear** fluids and chewing gum.

Patients with diabetes: normal (or near-normal regimen) can be continued in most patients having local anaesthesia; a sliding scale will be required in poorly controlled patients and insulin-requiring patients having GA (liaise with the anaesthetist).

Table 22.2 Example of insulin sliding scale

Blood sugar (BM)	<2	2.0–4.9	5.0–9.9	10.0–14.9	14.9–19.9	≥20.0
Insulin IV (U/h)	0 Give glucose	0	1.0	2.0	3.0	6.0 Call Dr

This is a guide for use where an alternative locally agreed protocol is not available. It applies to the use of a fast acting insulin such as Actrapid®. Adjust according to insulin requirements.

Patients with hypertension: continue antihypertensives (including day of surgery); postpone surgery if BP >180/100mmHg.

Patients with ischaemic heart disease: continue usual anti-anginal medication and ensure their usual prn medication (e.g. sublingual GTN) is available in theatre; postpone surgery if unstable angina or within 3mths of myocardial infarct.

Patients with valvular heart disease: antibiotic prophylaxis is not required for intraocular procedures.

Patients on aspirin/clopidogrel: continue for intraocular and strabismus surgery; for orbital and oculoplastic surgery it would ideally be discontinued for at least 1wk before surgery. However, this must be discussed with their GP/physician.

Patients on anticoagulants: ideally, the INR should be <3 for intraocular and strabismus surgery but <2 for orbital and oculoplastic surgery. <2.5 for sharp needle blocks, e.g. peribulbar and <3.5 for sub-Tenons. INR should ideally be checked on the day of surgery. If this is not compatible with their therapeutic target liaise with their haematologist who may consider putting the patient on heparin (either IV or SC) in the perioperative period.

Table 22.3 Target INR levels[1]

Prophylaxis of DVT	INR 2.0–2.5
DVT or PE treatment AF Cardioversion Dilated cardiomyopathy Mural thrombus Symptomatic inherited thrombophilia Paroxysmal nocturnal haemoglobinuria	INR 2.5
Recurrent DVT or PE Mechanical heart valve[2]	INR 3.5

1. See *BNF* and British Society for Haematology recommendations: Guidelines on Oral Anticoagulation (warfarin): third edition—2005 update. *Br J Haematol* 2005;**132**:277–85.

2. Some variation in target INR (usually 3–3.5) according to type and location of the valve

Table 22.4 ASA (American Society of Anesthesiologists) classification of fitness for anaesthesia[1]

ASA I	Fit and healthy patient
ASA II	Mild systemic disease; no functional limitation (e.g. mild controlled asthma; smoking)
ASA III	Severe systemic disease; definite functional limitation
ASA IV	Severe systemic disease that is a constant threat to life
ASA V	Moribund patient, not expected to survive for 24h with or without surgical intervention

Suffix E (e.g. ASAIIIE) denotes emergency surgery.

1. Excerpted from ASA Physical Status Classification System© 2008 of the American Society of Anesthesiologists. A copy of the full text can be obtained from ASA, 520N. Northwest Highway, Park Ridge, Illinois 60068-2573.

Ocular anaesthesia (1)

Each year over 200 000 intraocular operations are performed in the UK. During the 1990s there was a dramatic shift from general to local anaesthesia for the majority of cataract surgery, and more recently a further shift towards topical anaesthesia. Currently, a similar shift in practice is being seen from general to local anaesthesia for vitreoretinal surgery.

Topical anaesthesia

Indications

If being used for intraocular procedures, topical anaesthesia requires a cooperative patient + experienced surgeon + routine suitable operation (usually cataract surgery).

Method

Repeated pre-operative ± intraoperative anaesthetic drop (e.g. oxybuprocaine 0.4% or proxymetacaine 0.5%).

For cataract surgery consider supplementing with intracameral lidocaine (1% isotonic preservative-free) and an anaesthetic-soaked sponge in the inferior fornix (e.g. oxybuprocaine 0.4%).

Complications

Pain, eye movement, epithelial toxicity; in an uncooperative patient surgery may be hazardous increasing risk of operative complications.

Sub-Tenon's block

Indications

Useful where relatively complete anaesthesia of the globe and akinesia are desired but the patient is unsuitable for a sharp needle blocks (blephrospasm, high myopes, unknown biometry, deep set enophthalmic eye, scleral explants, epicanthal folds, INR >2.5). The patient must be sufficiently cooperative to keep head still during block and surgery.

Method

- Establish baseline monitoring (ECG, NIBP, SPO2) and venous access.
- Topical anaesthetic to conjunctiva (e.g. oxybuprocaine 0.4% or proxymetacaine 0.5%).
- Observe aseptic precautions.
- Ask patient to look in opposite direction to intended injection site (e.g. superotemporally).
- Open conjunctiva about 8mm from the limbus (inferonasally), dissect down to bare sclera with blunt curved scissors, insert sub-Tenon's cannula (19-gauge, 25mm, blunt, curved), and slide posteriorly along the globe.
- Inject 3–5ml of lidocaine 2% for short procedures (or 6–7ml levobupivacaine 0.75%) for longer ones. Hyaluronidase 15 units/ml improves the quality and speed of onset of the block.
- Apply oculocompression for 5min (optional).

Complications

Failure (backflow if wide track, leaks out if conjunctiva perforated twice), conjunctival chemosis, subconjunctival haemorrhage, vortex vein injury, raised IOP, globe trauma (due to scleral scars, redo retinal surgery, operator inexperience), extraocular muscles damage, retrobulbar haemorrhage. Deep posterior dissection and injections run the risk of central spread of local anaesthetic.

Peribulbar block

Indications
Relatively complete anaesthesia of the globe and akinesia desired; patient sufficiently cooperative to keep head still during surgery; anaesthetist/surgeon trained in the technique.

Method
The injection is made in the extraconal space. The traditional dual injection technique consisted of making an inferolateral and a medial injection. Inferolateral injections are generally hazardous as the technique involves the needle being directed parallel to the floor of the orbit and then posteromedially towards the globe. This poses a risk of penetrating injury particularly in axial myopes due to staphylomas that tend to occur posteroinferiorly. A single medial canthal injection is adequate in experienced hands.

Medial compartment block
- Establish baseline monitoring (ECG, NIBP, SPO2), and venous access.
- Topical anaesthetic to conjunctiva (e.g. oxybuprocaine 0.4% or proxymetacaine 0.5%).
- Ask patient to fix on a target directly ahead in primary gaze.
- A 25mm, 25-gauge, sharp bevel needle is inserted at the medial canthus and advanced directly posteriorly in the medial compartment until the hub is at level with the plane of iris.
- Following negative aspiration, inject a total of 6–10ml levobupivacaine 0.5–0.75%, and 2% lidocaine mix). Gentle ptosis of the upper lid is a good sign. Maintain the globe in the primary gaze and avoid tethering tests.
- Following injection apply ocular compression (30–40mmHg with a Honan balloon) for 5min.

NB Excessive pain, chemosis during injection, trickle of fluid into nasopharynx are warning signs of needle misplacement.

Complications
Excessive positive pressure (surgery may become hazardous), ptosis, diplopia, globe perforation (<0.1% but 0.7% if axial length >26mm if using inferolateral routes), oculocardiac reflex (0.03%), expulsive retrobulbar haemorrhage, medial orbital wall puncture, optic nerve injury, systemic neurological complications, acute ischaemic optic neuropathy, amaurosis fugax.

Retrobulbar block

Retrobulbar intraconal blocks are no longer used in modern practice due to high incidence of local and systemic complications.

Ocular anaesthesia (2)

General anaesthesia

Indications

Complete akinesia and deep anaesthesia required; patient unlikely to keep still (mental impairment, children/young adult, very anxious, uncontrolled tremor) or previous adverse reaction to local anaesthetic; globe trauma contraindicating local anaesthesia.

Method

The patient must be adequately fasted (e.g. 6h after solids, 4h after clear fluids) and all appropriate investigations performed (e.g. FBC, U+E, ECG where indicated). GA requires pre-operative assessment to identify and if possible minimize anaesthetic risk factors, premedication (sedation, amnesia, antiemesis), induction, intubation, maintenance, recovery, and postoperative analgesia. Adequate monitoring of the vital signs will be needed throughout.

Effect on intraocular pressure

Box 22.2 General anaesthesia and IOP

Cause	Effect on IOP
Propofol	↓
Ketamine	Usually ↑ (dose-dependent)
Depolarizing neuromuscular blocking agents (e.g. suxamethonium)	↑
Non-depolarizing neuromuscular blocking agents (e.g. vecuronium, rocuronium)	No effect
Volatile anaesthetic agents	↓
Airways manipulation (e.g. laryngoscopy, intubation, LMA insertion, extubation)	↑
Coughing/straining, venous congestion/head down posture	↑
Positive end-expiratory pressure ventilation	↑
Systemic hypotension	↓
Hypoventilation/hypercarbia/hypoxia/metabolic alkalosis	↑
Hyperventilation/hypocarbia/hyperoxia/metabolic acidosis	↓
Nitrous oxide in presence of intraocular gas (**NB** should be avoided)	↑

Complications
Complications may arise due to patient, drug, equipment, or operator-related factors. The comorbidities of the patients have important bearing on the physiological responses during GA. Emergency surgery carries risk of aspiration of gastric contents. Airways management problems may lead to hypoxia, hypercarbia, and other metabolic disturbances. Anaphylaxis and malignant hyperthermia are noteworthy drug-related issues. Patient awareness during anaesthesia is fortunately a rare phenomenon.

Treatment of anaphylaxis

Anaphylaxis is most commonly encountered by the ophthalmologist during an FFA clinic. It is an extreme form of type I hypersensitivity reaction. Severe anaphylaxis occurs in 1 of every 1900 FFAs. Fatal anaphylaxis occurs in 1 of every 220 000 FFAs. The clinical picture may vary from generalized oedema, angioedema, cutaneous reaction (erythema, rash, urticaria), bronchospasm to pulmonary oedema and cardiovascular collapse. Appropriate initial treatment should be instituted by the ophthalmic team while calling for emergency medical support.

First-line
↓
Check responsiveness+ call for help
↓
Secure airways
↓
Give 100% O_2
↓
Lie patient flat and elevate legs
↓
Give 0.5mg (0.5ml of 1:1000) adrenaline IM
This may be repeated if necessary every 5min
according to BP, pulse, and respiratory function
↓
Secure IV access
↓
Give 10mg chlorphenamine IV
↓

Meanwhile: Remove precipitant (where possible)
Monitor: Pulse, BP, respiratory function

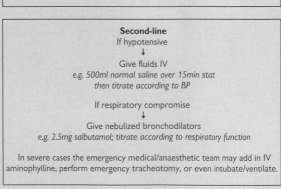

Second-line
If hypotensive
↓
Give fluids IV
e.g. 500ml normal saline over 15min stat
then titrate according to BP

If respiratory compromise
↓
Give nebulized bronchodilators
e.g. 2.5mg salbutamol; titrate according to respiratory function

In severe cases the emergency medical/anaesthetic team may add in IV aminophylline, perform emergency tracheotomy, or even intubate/ventilate.

Fig. 22.1 Management of anaphylaxis.

Needle-stick injuries

Needle-stick injuries are avoidable. Adopt safe practices for handling sharps including safe disposal. Needle-stick transmission rates from infected patients are estimated at about 0.5% for HIV, 10–15% for hepatitis C, and 20% for hepatitis B.

Immediate
↓
Encourage the injury to bleed and wash under running water; if body fluids splashed onto eyes irrigate them copiously
↓
Within 1 hour
↓
Report to the occupational health department (or Accident & Emergency department if out-of-hours)
↓
If high risk of HIV transmission start post-exposure prophylaxis
This should be started within 1h by the Occupational Health/A&E physician. See Box 22.3
↓
Store blood from the donor and the recipient.
Screening for hepatitis B and HIV where appropriate is generally arranged by the Occupational Health physician

This should be a 10ml clotted blood sample. State 'inoculation injury' on the microbiology request form. The donor's blood sample should not be taken by the recipient. The donor must be counseled before taking blood samples/testing for hepatitis/HIV.

Meanwhile:
Record 'donor' name, unit number and contact details
Inform head of department
Complete accident form(s)

Fig. 22.2 Management of needle-stick injury

Post-exposure prophylaxis where exposure to HIV

The Occupational Health/A&E physician will assess risk of HIV transmission based on patient history, nature of body fluid, and route of transmission. The decision of whether to start post-exposure prophylaxis is made according to risk. The following is common practice, but should be confirmed with local Occupational Health Department (for most recent guidelines):

High risk

This includes exposure to blood/high-risk body fluids (from a patient with known/suspected HIV) through sharps injury.

PEP drugs starting within 1h (e.g. zidovudine PO 250mg 2×/d + lamivudine PO 150mg 2×/d + indinavir PO 800mg 3×/d)

If donor is HIV positive (already known or discovered on testing):

- Continue PEP for 4wks.
- Test recipient for HIV seroconversion at 6wks, 3mths, and 6mths.
- Follow-up with occupational health.

If donor is found to be HIV negative

- Discontinue PEP.
- Test recipient for HIV seroconversion at 3mths and 6mths.
- Follow-up with occupational health.

Low risk

This applies to non-blood-stained low-risk material.

- PEP is not offered.

Hypoglycaemia

This is potentially fatal if left untreated. The causes are usually due to excessive utilization or underproduction of glucose. These include hepatic or adrenocortical insufficiency, excessive insulin and sulphonylurea activity, prolonged fasting, and excessive alcohol ingestion.

Clinical features

Clinical features usually appear at blood sugar levels below 2–3mmol/l, and symptoms range from confusion, restlessness, sweating, pallor, tachycardia, difficulty in speech, diplopia, convulsions, and coma.

NB In the absence of blood sugar levels hyperglycaemic coma may be indistinguishable from hypoglycaemia. If in doubt, do not delay treatment with dextrose. It will do little harm in hyperglycaemia and be potentially life-saving in hypoglycaemia.

Treatment

If patient is conscious

↓

Give glucose gel or
25mg glucose mixed in fruit-juice orally.

If patient is unconscious

(or unable to drink)

↓

Give bolus of 50ml of 50% glucose intravenously (IV)

↓

Commence 10% glucose infusion IV and
monitor blood sugar levels.

NB If IV access is not available glucagon 1mg IM may be given.

If persistent coma/suspected cerebral oedema:
- institute appropriate resuscitation therapy (ABC protocol);
- get immediate medical/anaesthetic help;
- maintain blood sugar at 5–7mmol/l;
- consider dexamethasone and mannitol.

Fig. 22.3 Management of hypoglycaemia

Management of severe local anaesthetic toxicity

Local anaesthesia administration. may rarely cause severe toxicity resulting in loss of consciousness, convulsions, and cardiovascular collapse. It may occur sometime after the actual local anaesthetic injection. Recovery may take up to an hour.

Clinical features

Loss of consciousness, cardiovascular collapse (± arrythmias), convulsions.

Treatment

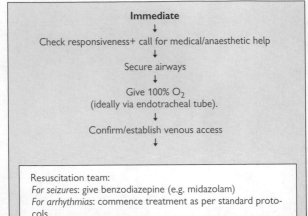

Immediate
↓
Check responsiveness+ call for medical/anaesthetic help
↓
Secure airways
↓
Give 100% O_2
(ideally via endotracheal tube).
↓
Confirm/establish venous access
↓

Resuscitation team:
For seizures: give benzodiazepine (e.g. midazolam)
For arrhythmias: commence treatment as per standard protocols
For resistant arrhythmias and cardiac arrest: continue CPR while using the following regimen using lipid emulsion, such as 20% intralipid®, until a stable circulatory state is achieved.

Fig. 22.4 Summary of the recommendations for management of severe local anaesthetic toxicity (the Association of Anaesthetists of Great Britain and Ireland)[1].

**For resistant arrhythmias/cardiac arrest
associated with local anaesthetic toxicity**

Follow algorithm until stable circulation achieved
↓
Administer 1.5ml/kg of intralipid® IV
(e.g. ≈100ml bolus for 70kg patient)
↓
Commence infusion at 0.25ml/kg/min
(e.g. 400ml over 20min)
↓
Repeat bolus injection at 5min
↓
Repeat bolus injection after further 5min
↓
Increase infusion to 0.5ml/kg/min after further 5min
(e.g. 400ml over 10min)
↓
Continue infusion until a stable circulation is achieved

NB Resuscitation should be continued throughout. Progression through the algorithm is only required until the point where a stable circulation is regained.

Fig. 22.5 Summary of recommendations for the management of cardiac arrest associated with severe local anaesthetic toxicity (The Association of Anaesthetists of Great Britain and Ireland).[1]

1. The Association of Anaesthetists of Great Britain and Ireland. Guidelines for the Management of Severe Local Anaesthetic Toxicity 2007. www.aagbi.org/publications/guidelines/docs/latoxicity07.pdf/

Basic and advanced life support

Adult basic life support algorithm

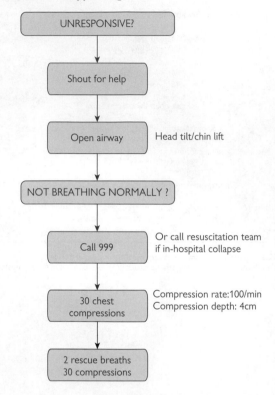

Fig. 22.6 Adult basic life support algorithm from the Resuscitation Guidelines 2005 published by Resuscitation Council (UK); reproduced with permission www.resus.org.uk

Basic life support and in-hospital collapse

The Resuscitation Council (UK) now include a separate protocol for in-hospital collapse (www.resus.org.uk/pages/inhralgo.pdf), which assumes the rapid availability of resuscitation equipment that is not always immediately available in the ophthalmology setting. The basic life support algorithm (above) for out-of-hospital arrest probably more accurately reflects the situation faced by the ophthalmologist when confronted with a collapsed patient in an outlying medical retina clinic, late on a Friday evening.

Adult advanced life support algorithm

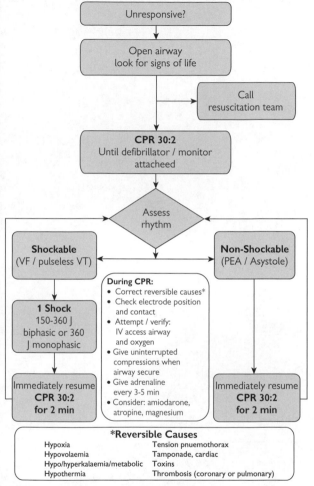

Fig. 22.7 Adult advanced life support algorithm from the Resuscitation Guidelines 2005 published by Resuscitation Council UK, reproduced with permission; www.resus.org.uk

Therapeutics

Principles and delivery of ocular drugs

All doses/frequencies of administration are those for a healthy adult. All medications should be checked against the *British National Formulary* or equivalent for licensed indications, side-effects, contraindications, interactions, and age- and weight-adjusted dosing.

When considering patients' medication it is important to check what they are actually taking rather than what you or anybody else think they are taking. Consider the issue of compliance, particularly when about to treat a suboptimal response with additional medications or more frequent regimens. For more invasive procedures (e.g. injections) formal consent should be taken.

Topical

Only about 1–10% of most topical agents are absorbed into the eye. Absorption is dependent on ocular contact time, drug concentration, and tissue permeability. Small lipophilic drugs pass through the cornea, whereas larger hydrophilic drugs are generally absorbed through conjunctiva and sclera. Topical agents may be in:

- *aqueous solution*: comfortable, no blurring but very short ocular contact time;
- *gel preparations*: mild blurring, longer contact time;
- *suspension*: longer ocular contact time, but bottle must be shaken and may get FB sensation; or
- *ointment*: liquefy at body temperature, longest ocular contact time, but blurs vision.

Technique

- Ensure that patients know how to instil any topical medication, and that they can physically manage it.
- If reliable self-administration is not possible ensure that there is somebody (even a district nurse) who can assist them.
- Consider ways of making it easier, e.g. lying flat, mirror positioning, or eye-drop dispensers. Smaller bottles and single use vials tend to be particularly difficult for the frail and elderly.
- Leave at least 5min between instilling topical medications.
- Keep the eye closed and put pressure over the lacrimal sac for 1–2min to try to increase ocular and reduce systemic absorption.

Medications

This includes most ophthalmic medication listed in Tables 23.1–23.26.

Subconjunctival injection

Technique

- Ensure adequate anaesthesia (e.g. a couple of drops of proxymetacaine 0.5%).
- Under direct vision (or slit-lamp or operating microscope) lift an area of conjunctiva to form a small bleb and slowly inject (sharp needle).

Medications

This route is most commonly used for post-operative injections of corticosteroids and antimicrobials, but may be used in acute anterior segment inflammation to deliver mydriatics and corticosteroids (e.g. mydricaine No2 with betamethasone 2–4mg).

Mydricaine no. 1 and no. 2

Mydricaine preparations are used to cause mydriasis and cycloplegia in severe anterior segment inflammation. Mydricaine no. 1 is for children, and mydricaine no. 2 (which is double-strength) is for adults.

Table 23.1 Subconjunctival mydriatic preparations

Drug	Dose	Active ingredients
Mydricaine No. 1	0.3ml	3mg procaine hydrochloride, 0.5mg atropine sulphate, and 0.06ml adrenaline solution (1 in 1000)
Mydricaine No. 2	0.3ml	6mg procaine hydrochloride, 1 mg atropine sulphate, and 0.12 ml adrenaline solution (1 in 1000).

These preparations are not commercially available but may be obtained from Special-Order Manufacturers (see BNF for list)

Other routes of delivery

More invasive routes of delivering ophthalmic drugs include: intracameral (📖 p.846), sub-Tenon's (📖 p.848), peribulbar/orbital floor (📖 p.848), intravitreal (📖 p.850) and systemic (mainly oral, intravascular, and intra-muscular).

Intracameral injections

Intracameral administration of drugs (i.e. into the AC) may be used during an operation either to facilitate the procedure itself or to reduce post-operative complications. Such drugs may be specifically injected using a blunt cannula via a paracentesis port, or may be added to the irrigation bottle (e.g. for phakemulsification surgery; unlicensed use).

Table 23.2 Intracameral preparations

Drug	Dose	Administration	Proprietary
Anaesthetic[1]			
Lidocaine 1%	0.3–0.5ml	Intracameral bolus	
Mydriatics[2]			
Adrenaline	1 in 1 000 000	In irrigation bottle, e.g. 0.5ml of 1 in 1000 adrenaline added to 500ml of irrigation solution	
Phenylephrine 2.5%[2]	0.25ml in 1ml BSS	Intracameral bolus	
Miotics			
Acetylcholine 1%	1–2ml	Intracameral bolus	Miochol-E®
Antibiotics			
Cefuroxime	1mg/0.1ml	Intracameral bolus	
Corticosteroids			
Triamcinolone acetonide[2]	4mg/0.1ml	Intracameral bolus	Kenalog®

With the exception of Miochol-E®, these drugs are not licensed for intracameral use.

1. Lidocaine also has mydriatic properties.

2. Gurbaxani et al (Eye 2007; **21**: 331-2) describe 0.25ml Minims® Phenylephrine in 1ml Balanced Salt Solution in cases of Idiopathic Floppy Iris Syndrome; however, the presence of sodium metabisulphite disodium edetate in the Minims® preparation is a concern regarding its intracameral use.

2. Triamcinolone acetonide is preserved and is not licensed for intraocular use. Some surgeons who do use it attempt to remove the triamcinolone from the preservative-containing solution by capturing it in a 5µm filter before resuspending it in balanced salt solution; others simply dilute the neat 40mg/ml solution in balanced salt solution.

Sub-Tenon's and peribulbar injections

In addition to their use in ocular anaesthesia (p.829), the sub-Tenon's and peribulbar routes may be used to deliver drugs such as corticosteroids to the posterior aspect of the globe.

Sub-Tenon's injection

Sub-Tenon's cannula technique

Method
- Topical anaesthetic to conjunctiva (e.g. proxymetacaine 0.5%).
- Wash hands and don sterile gloves.
- Instil 5% povidone iodine on to the ocular surface; drape (optional) and insert lid speculum (optional).
- Ask patient to look in opposite direction to intended injection site (e.g. inferonasally).
- Open conjunctiva about 8mm from the limbus (e.g. superotemporally), dissect down to bare sclera with blunt curved scissors, insert sub-Tenon's cannula (19-gauge, 25mm, blunt, curved), and slide posteriorly along the globe.
- Inject medication.
- Carefully withdraw cannula; forceps or a cotton-tipped applicator can be used to provide counter traction and to hold the conjunctival opening closed (which may help reduce regurgitation).

Advantage: relatively safe (blunt needle, appropriately curved for the shape of the globe).
Disadvantage: significant regurgitation of drug along the sub-Tenon's track may result in poor drug delivery.

Sharp-needle (Nozik[1]) technique
- *Method*: insertion and posterior advancement of a 26-gauge, 5/8-inch needle up to its hub through sub-Tenon's space.
- *Advantage*: less regurgitation and improved drug delivery.
- *Disadvantage*: ↑ risk of globe perforation.

Intravenous cannula technique[2]
- *Method*: insertion and posterior direction of a 22- or 23-gauge, 0.9/25mm IV cannula (made of polytetrafluoroethylene) through sub-Tenon's space.
- *Advantage*: relatively safe (blunt needle, flexible so moulds to shape of the globe), probably less regurgitation than with sub-Tenon's cannula.
- *Disadvantage*: can be difficult to direct the flexible cannula.

Medications

Although primarily used for ocular anaesthesia (e.g. lidocaine, bupivacine), these routes may be used for delivering corticosteroids (e.g. triamcinolone, methylprednisolone) in posterior segment inflammation, exudation, or macular oedema.

Box 23.1 Outline of intravenous cannula technique for sub-Tenon's injection

- enter the sub-Tenon's space by use of the trocar of a 22- or 23-gauge, 0.9/25mm IV cannula (made of polytetrafluoroethylene);
- advance the cannula (with the trocar still engaged and in the bevel up position) for about 3mm within the sub-Tenon's space;
- slightly withdraw the trocar (so sharp end no longer exposed) and continue to carefully advance the cannula for a further 3mm;
- completely withdraw the trocar and direct the cannula posteriorly for a further 12–15mm using gentle rotatory movements;
- attach the syringe to the cannula and inject medication.

Peribulbar injection

Method

Peribulbar injection is a sharp-needle technique that is used for delivering medication into the extraconal space. For delivery of local anaesthesia a medial compartment block via a medial canthal injection is preferred (see, Ocular anasthesia 📖 p.829). For delivery of medication such as corticosteroids the safer sub-Tenon's route is recommended. However, if the peribulbar route is used, an inferolateral injection is made with a 25-gauge, sharp bevel needle entering either through the lid or the conjunctiva and directed inferolateral to the globe, just above the orbital floor.

Table 23.3 Sub-Tenon and peribulbar corticosteroids

Drug	Dose	Proprietary
Triamcinolone acetonide	40mg	*Kenalog*®
Methylprednisolone	40mg	*Depo-Medrone*® *(suspension)*[1]

These are non-licensed uses of the commercial IM/intra-articular preparations of these corticosteroids.

1. Contains polyethylene glycol, myristyl-gamma-picolinium chloride.

1. Smith RE, Nozik RA. The nonspecific treatment of uveitis. In: Smith RE, Nozik RA (eds). *Uveitis: a clinical approach to diagnosis and management*, 2nd edn. Baltimore: Williams & Wilkins, 1989; 51–72.

2. Venkatesh *et al*. Posterior subtenon injection of corticosteroids using polytetrafluoroethylene (PTFE) intravenous cannula. *Clin Exp Ophthalmol* 2002;**30**:55–7.

Intravitreal injections

Principle

Intravitreal injections should be isotonic, should have a neutral pH and must not contain preservatives. Unfortunately, this is not always achievable with commercially available preparations.

Indications

- Intravitreal antimicrobials for endophthalmitis: usually performed immediately after a vitreous biopsy or core vitrectomy in theatre.
- Intravitreal triamcinolone or anti-VEGF therapies for CMO and various exudative posterior segment diseases; may be performed in theatre or a dedicated clean room.

Procedure

This outline summarizes the guidelines of the Royal College of Ophthalmologists).[1]

Setting

Intravitreal injections may be given in theatre or a dedicated clean room in outpatients that meets stringent conditions, such as being enclosed, free from interruptions, good illumination, washable floor, and non-particulate ceiling (i.e. dust free). In this context full gowning is not necessary but hands should be washed and sterile gloves worn. Below is a summary of the procedure for an intravitreal injection performed in isolation (i.e. not as part of a vitrectomy/biopsy for endophthalmitis).

Preparation

- Confirm consent and correct eye to be injected; measure IOP; ensure adequate dilation; instil topical anaesthesia.
- Set up equipment trolley and ensure all treatments (including post-injection antibiotics) are available.

Technique

- Wash hands and don sterile gloves.
- Instil 5% povidone iodine onto the ocular surface; clean periocular area with 10% povidone iodine; drape and insert lid speculum.
- Consider whether supplementation of anaesthesia is necessary: subconjunctival or sub-Tenon's (e.g. lidocaine 1%).
- Prepare syringe/needle/drug immediately before injection, and ensure any air in the syringe/needle is expelled before injection; maintain aseptic technique throughout.
- Note injection site: this should be 3.0–3.5mm (aphakic/pseudophakic) or 3.5–4mm (phakic) posterior to limbus, usually in the inferotemporal quadrant.
- Insert needle (27–30 gauge; 1/2–5/8inch long) perpendicularly, aiming towards the centre of the globe.
- Inject volume of anti-VEGF indicated for intravitreal use (usually not in excess of 0.1ml); carefully remove needle; a sterile cotton-tipped applicator can be used as counter pressure and to prevent any reflux.
- Instil topical antibiotic (e.g. chloramphenicol 0.5%); for immediate post-injection use a preservative-free preparation is recommended.

Post injection
- Test gross VA.
- Check for central retinal artery patency (may not be necessary if acuity satisfactory).
- Check injection site (at the slit-lamp) and IOP.
- Topical antibiotics (e.g. chloramphenicol 0.5% 4×/d) for ≥3d.

Medications

Table 23.4 Intravitreal antimicrobials

Drug	Dose	Reconstituted to
Antibacterial		
Vancomycin	1–2mg	0.1ml
Amikacin	400mcg	0.1ml
Ceftazidime	2mg	0.1ml
Antifungal		
Amphotericin	5–10mcg	0.1ml
Antiviral		
Ganciclovir	2–4mg	0.1ml
Foscarnet	1.2–2.4mg	0.1ml

Table 23.5 Intravitreal corticosteroid

Drug	Dose	Reconstituted to
Triamcinolone acetate[1]	2–4mg	0.05–0.1ml

1. Triamcinolone acetonide is preserved and is not licensed for intraocular use. Some surgeons who do use it attempt to remove the triamcinolone from the preservative-containing solution by capturing it in a 5μm filter before resuspending it in balanced salt solution; others simply dilute the neat 40mg/ml solution in balanced salt solution.

Table 23.6 Intravitreal anti-VEGF therapies (licensed for intraocular use)

Drug	Dose
Ranibizumab[1]	0.5mg/0.05ml
Pegaptanib	0.3mg/0.09ml

1. **NB** The vial for ranibizumab is 2.3mg/0.23ml.

1. Amaoku W RCOphth Intravitreal Injections Procedure Guideline www.rcophth.ac.uk/docs/publications/published-guidelines/IntravitrealInjectionsJuly2006.pdf

Topical antimicrobials

Table 23.7 Antibacterials

Generic	Forms	Pres-free	Frequency	Proprietary
Chloramphenicol	G 0.5%	Minims®	G: see below[1]	Chloromycetin Redidrops® Minims® Chloramphenicol
	Oc 1%	Oc	Oc: 3–4×/d	Chloromycetin® Ophthalmic Ointment
Ciprofloxacin	G 0.3% Oc 0.3%	Oc	See below[1,2]	Ciloxan®
Fusidic acid	Gel 1%	No	2×/d	Fucithalmic®
Gentamicin	G 0.3% G 0.3%,1.4–1.5% (SOM)	Available (SOM)	See below[1]	Genticin®
Levofloxacin	G 0.5%	Unit dose	See below[1]	Oftaquix® Oftaquix® Unit Dose
Neomycin	G 0.5% Oc 0.5%	No	See below[1]	Neosporin® (Neomycin/ gramicidin/ polymyxin B sulphate)
Ofloxacin	G 0.3%	No	See below[1]	Exocin®
Polymyxin B sulphate	Combination only Oc 10 000u/g	Oc	See below[1]	Polyfax® (PBS/ bacitracin)
Propamidine isetionate	G 0.1% Oc 0.15%	Golden Eye Ointment	G: 4×/d Oc: 1–2×/d	Brolene® Golden Eye®

1. *Frequency:* BNF recommends for antibacterial eye drops that they are administered at least every 2h then reduce frequency as infection is controlled and continue for 48h after healing; for ointments BNF recommends that they are used at night (with drops used during the day) or 3–4×/d if used alone.

2. *Ciloxan:* for corneal ulcer BNF recommends that if drops used that they are administered throughout day and night, day 1 being applied every 15min for 6h then every 30min, day 2 being applied every hour, days 3–14 being applied every 4h (max. duration of treatment 21d); if ointment used it should be administered throughout day and night; 1.25cm ointment being applied every 1–2h for 2d then every 4h for next 12d.

SOM: some preparations may only be available from Special-Order Manufacturers (see BNF for list).

Table 23.8 Antifungals

Generic	Forms	Frequency
Amphotericin	G 0.15%	≤q 1h initially for fungal keratitis reducing as infection is controlled (see Fungalkeratitis: Treatment 📖 p.202)
Clotrimazole	G 1%	
Econazole	G 1%	
Miconazole	G 1%	
Natamycin	G 5%	

SOM: some preparations may only be available from Special-Order Manufacturers (see *BNF* for list).

Table 23.9 Antivirals

Generic	Forms	Pres-free	Frequency	Proprietary
Aciclovir	Oc 3%	Oc	5×/d until healed then 5×/d for 3d1	*Zovirax*
Trifluoridine[2]	G 1%	SOM	9×/d	

1. *Frequency*: BNF recommends continuing at 5×/d for at least 3d after healing for aciclovir.
2. Trifluoridine (*syn* trifluorothymidine) is commonly used in the USA but is not commercially available in the UK. Viroptic®, the brand available in the USA is not available in preservative-free form but trifluorothymidine eye drops made by special-order manufacturers (SOM) are available as preservative free.

Topical anti-inflammatory agents

Corticosteroids

Table 23.10 Corticosteroids

Generic	Forms	Preservative free	Frequency	Proprietary
Betamethasone	G 0.1% Oc 0.1%	Oc	See below[1]	Betnesol® (g/oc) Vista-Methasone® (g)
Dexamethasone base	G 0.1%	No	See below[1]	Maxidex®
Dexamethasone sodium phosphate	G 0.1%	Minims®	See below[1]	Minims® Dexamethasone
Fluorometholone	G 0.1%	No	See below[1]	FML®
Hydrocortisone acetate	G 1% Oc 0.5%, 1%, 2.5%	Oc	See below[1]	
Loteprednol	G 0.5%	No	See below[1]	Lotemax®
Prednisolone sodium phosphate	G 0.5% G 0.05%, 0.1%, 0.3% (SOM)	Minims®	See below[1]	Predsol®
Prednisolone acetate	G 1%	No	See below[1]	Pred Forte®
Rimexolone	G 1%	No	See below[1]	Vexol®

1. *Frequency:* potency and frequency of corticosteroids should be titrated against degree of inflammation in order to achieve control while minimizing side-effects.

2. SOM: some preparations may only be available from Special-Order Manufacturers (see *BNF* for list).

Table 23.11 Corticosteroid/antibiotic combinations

Corticosteroid	Antibiotic	Forms	Frequency	Proprietary
Betamethasone 0.1%	Neomycin 0.5%	G or Oc	≤6×/d	Betnesol N® (g/oc) Vista-Methasone N® (g)
Dexamethasone base 0.1%	Neomycin 0.35% Polymyxin B sulphate 6000u/ml	G or Oc[1]	≤6×/d	Maxitrol®
	Tobramycin 0.3%	G	≤6×/d	Tobradex®
Dexamethasone sodium metasulpho-benzoate 0.05%	Framycetin 0.5% Gramicidin 0.005%	G	≤4×/d	Sofradex®
Prednisolone sodium phosphate 0.5%	Neomycin 0.5%	G	≤6×/d	Predsol-N®

1. Unlike most ointments Maxitrol® oc is preserved (with parabenzoates).

Table 23.12 Antihistamines and other anti-allergic agents

Generic	Forms	Preservative free	Frequency	Proprietary
Anti-histamine[1]				
Antazoline sulphate	G	No	2–3×/d	*Otrivine-Antistin*®
Azelastine hydrochloride	G	No	2–4×/d up to 6wks	*Optilast*®
Epinastine hydrochloride	G	No	2×/d up to 8wks	*Relestat*®
Emedastine	G	No	2×/d	*Emadine*®
Ketotifen	G	No	2×/d	*Zaditen*®
Olopatadine	G	No	2×/d up to 4mths	*Opatanol*®
Mast cell stabilizers				
Lodoxamide	G	No	4×/d	*Alomide*®
Nedocromil sodium	G	No	2–4×/d	*Rapitil*®
Sodium cromoglicate	G	Available[2]	4×/d	*Opticrom*® and others

1. Some of these antihistamine preparations also have mast cell stabilizing properties.
2. Preservative-free sodium cromoglicate available on named-patient basis.

Table 23.13 Other anti-inflammatory agents (NSAID type)

Generic	Forms	Pres-free	Frequency	Proprietary
Diclofenac sodium	G 0.1%	SDU	1–4×/d	*Voltarol Ophtha*® *Voltarol*® *Ophtha multi*
Flurbiprofen sodium	G 0.03% (only as SDU)	SDU	1–4×/d	*Ocufen*®
Ketorolac	G 0.5%	No	3×/d	*Acular*®

Topical glaucoma medications

Beta-blockers

Table 23.14 β-blockers

Generic	Forms	Pres-free	Frequency	Proprietary
Betaxolol hydrochloride	G 0.25%	Suspension single dose	2×/d	Betoptic® Suspension Betoptic® Suspension Single Dose
	G 0.5%	No	2×/d	Betoptic®
Carteolol hydrochloride	G 1 or 2%	No	2×/d	Teoptic®
Levobunolol hydrochloride	G 0.5%	Unit dose	1–2×/d	Betagan® Betagan® Unit Dose
Metipranolol	G 0.1% (only as Minims®)	Minims®	2×/d	Minims® Metipranolol
Timolol maleate	G 0.25% or 0.5%	Unit dose	2×/d	Timoptol® Timoptol® unit dose
	Gel 0.1%	No	1×/d	Nyogel®
	Gel 0.25% or 0.5%	No	1×/d	Timoptol-LA®

Prostaglandin analogues and related drugs

Table 23.15 Prostaglandin analogues and related drugs

Generic	Forms	Pres-free	Frequency	Proprietary
Bimatoprost	G 300mcg/ml 0.03%	No	1×/d (nocte)	Lumigan®
Latanoprost	G 50mcg/ml 0.005%	No	1×/d (nocte)	Xalatan®
Travoprost	G 40mcg/ml 0.004%	No	1×/d (nocte)	Travatan®

Miotics

Table 23.16 Miotics

Generic	Forms	Pres-free	Frequency	Proprietary
Pilocarpine	G 0.5, 1, 2, 3, or 4%	Minims® (2%)	≤4×/d	Minims® Pilocarpine Nitrate
	Gel 4%		1×/d	Pilogel®

Sympathomimetics

Table 23.17 Sympathomimetics

Generic	Forms	Preservative free	Frequency	Proprietary
Apraclonidine	G 0.5%	No	3×/d for <1mth	*Iopidine® 0.5%*
	G 1%	Yes	Pre-/post-YAG laser	*Iopidine® 1%*
Brimonidine tartrate	G 0.2%	No	2×/d	*Alphagan®*
Dipivefrine hydrochloride	G 0.1%	No	2×/d	*Propine®*

Carbonic anhydrase inhibitors

Table 23.18 Carbonic anhydrase inhibitors

Generic	Forms	Pres-free	Frequency	Proprietary
Brinzolamide	G 1%	No	2–3×/d	*Azopt®*
Dorzolamide	G 2%	Unit dose	3×/d or 2×/d if with β-blocker	*Trusopt®* *Trusopt® unit dose*

Combination drops

Table 23.19 Combinations with timolol

Generic	Forms	Preservative free	Frequency	Proprietary
Timolol + bimatoprost	G timolol 0.5% bimatoprost 0.03%	No	1×/d	*Ganfort®*
Timolol + brimonidine	G timolol 0.5% brimonidine 0.2%	No	2×/d	*Combigan®*
Timolol + dorzolamide	G timolol 0.5% dorzolamide 2%	Unit dose	2×/d	*Cosopt®* *Cosopt® unit dose*
Timolol + latanoprost	G timolol 0.5% latanoprost 0.005%	No	1×/d	*Xalacom®*
Timolol + travoprost	G timolol 0.5% travoprost 0.04%	No	1×/d	*Duotrav®*

Topical mydriatics

Mydriatics

Table 23.20 Mydriatics and cycloplegics

Generic	Forms	Pres-free	Frequency	Proprietary
Antimuscarinic				
Atropine sulphate	G 0.5% or 1% Oc 1%	Minims® (1%) Oc	Single–1×/d	Minims® Atropine Sulphate
Cyclopentolate hydrochloride	G 0.5% or 1%	Minims®	Single–3×/d	Mydrilate® Minims® Cyclopentolate Hydrochloride
Homatropine hydrobromide	G 1%	No	Single–4×/d	
Tropicamide	G 0.5% or 1%	Minims® (0.5% or 1%)	Single	Mydriacyl® Minims® Tropicamide
Sympathomimetic				
Phenylephrine	G 10%	Minims® (2.5% or 10%)	Single–3×/d	Minims® Phenylephrine Hydrochloride

Topical anaesthetics

Table 23.21 Anaesthetics

Generic	Forms	Pres-free	Frequency	Proprietary
Oxybuprocaine hydrochloride[1]	Minims® 0.4%	Yes	Single	*Minims® Oxybuprocaine hydrochloride*
Proxymetacaine hydrochloride	Minims® 0.5%	Yes	Single	*Minims® Proxymetacaine*
Tetracaine hydrochloride	Minims® 0.5% or 1%	Yes	Single	*Minims® Tetracaine Hydrochloride*
Combinations with fluorescein				
Proxymetacaine and fluorescein	Minims® P (0.5%) + F (0.25%)	Yes	Single	*Minims® Proxymetacaine and Fluorescein*
Lidocaine and fluorescein	Minims® L (4%) + F (0.25%)	Yes	Single	*Minims® Lidocaine and Fluorescein*

1. Oxybuprocaine hydrochloride was previously known as benoxinate.

Topical tear replacement

Artificial tears and astringents

Table 23.22 Artificial tears

Generic	Forms	Pres-free	Frequency	Proprietary
Low viscosity				
Hypromellose	G 0.3%, 0.5%, or 1%	Artelac® SDU	As required, e.g. hourly	Isopto Plain® Isopto Alkaline® Tears Naturale® Artelac® SDU
Hydroxy-ethylcellulose	Minims® 0.44%	Yes	As required, e.g. hourly	Minims® Artificial Tears
Polyvinyl alcohol	G 1.4%	Liquifilm® PF	As required, e.g. hourly	Sno tears® Liquifilm® Liquifilm PF
Sodium chloride	G 0.9% Minims® 0.9%	Minims®	As required	Minims® Saline
Medium viscosity				
Carbomer 980	Gel 0.2%	Viscotears PF®	≥4×/d	GelTears® Liposic® Viscotears PF®
Carbomer 974P	Gel 0.25%	No		Liquivisc®
Carmellose	G 0.5% or 1%	Yes	≥4×/d	Celluvisc®
High viscosity				
Liquid paraffin	Oc 30% or 42.5%	Yes	Nocte	Lubri-tears® Lacri-Lube®
Yellow soft paraffin	Oc 80%	Yes	Nocte	Simple eye ointment

Table 23.23 Mucolytics and astringents

Generic	Forms	Preservative free	Frequency	Proprietary
Acetylcysteine	G 5%	No	3–4×/d	Ilube®
Zinc sulphate	G 0.25%	No	3–4×/d	

Table 23.24 Hyaluronic acid preparations

Proprietary	Forms	Preservative free	Frequency
Clinitas Soothe™	G 0.4%	SDU	2–4×/d or prn
Oxyal™	G 0.1%	Preservative free in the eye[1]	prn
Vismed®	G 0.18%	SDU	prn
Vismed multi®	G 0.18%	No[2]	prn

1. Oxyal is preserved in the bottle but this biodegrades on contact with the eye, making it a non-preserved solution in the eye. This makes it suitable for people who are usually sensitive to preservatives.

2. Vismed multi is pres-free; the container is designed to prevent ingress of air (and micro-organisms) allowing the pres-free solution to be used for up to 3mths.

Systemic medication: antimicrobials

Table 22.26 is a summary of systemic antimicrobials commonly used in ophthalmology and discussed elsewhere in the text. It is not intended to be exhaustive; consult the *BNF* or other local formulary for details of dosing, contraindications, side-effects and a wider range of alternative therapeutic agents.

Table 23.25 Selected systemic antibacterial medications

Drug	Dose	Route	Page
Penicillins			
Flucloxacillin	250–500mg 4×/d	PO/IV/IM	📖 p.526
Amoxicillin	250–500mg 4×/d 500mg–1g 4×/d	PO IV	
Co-amoxiclav	250–500mg amoxicillin 3×/d 1g 3–4×/d	PO IV	📖 p.156
Cephalosporins			
Cefotaxime	1–2g 2–4×/d	IV/IM	
Ceftazidime	2g 3×/d	IV	
Cefuroxime	750mg 3–4×/d	IV/IM	📖 p.526
Tetracyclines			
Doxycycline	200mg stat then 100mg 1×/d	PO	📖 p.234
Oxytetracycline	250mg 4×/d	PO	📖 p.234
Quinolones			
Ciprofloxacin	500–750mg 2×/d 200–400mg 2×/d	PO IV	📖 p.196
Ofloxacin	200–400mg 2×/d 200–400mg 2×/d	PO IV	📖 p.196
Macrolides			
Azithromycin	1g stat	PO	📖 p.168
Erythromycin	500mg 2×/d	PO	📖 p.234
Other			
Metronidazole	200–400mg 3×/d 500mg 3×/d	PO IV	📖 p.526
Vancomycin	1g 2×/d	IV	

Antibiotic prescribing is being modified in the light of challenges such as *Clostridium difficile* and methicillin-resistant *Staphylococcus aureus* (MRSA). In the UK this has led to a nationwide drive to reduce the use of cephalosporins and quinolones.

Table 23.26 Selected systemic antiviral medications

Drug	Dose	Route	Page
Anti-HSV/VZV			
Aciclovir	800mg 5×/d (for HZO[1]) 5–10mg/kg 3×/d	PO IV	📖 p.208
Valaciclovir	1g 3×/d (for HZO[1])	PO	📖 p.208
Famciclovir	250mg 3×/d or 750mg 1×/d	PO	📖 p.208
Anti-CMV			
Ganciclovir	5mg/kg 2×/d	IV	📖 p.398
Valganciclovir	900mg 2×/d (induction) 900mg 1×/d (maintenance)	PO	📖 p.398
Cidofovir	5mg/kg every 1wk (induction) every 2wks (maintenance)	IV	📖 p.398
Foscarnet	60mg/kg 3×/d (induction) 60–120mg/kg (maintenance)	IV	📖 p.398

1. Doses given for aciclovir, valaciclovir, and famciclovir are for treatment of herpes zoster ophthalmicus (HZO) and should be given for 7d. In ARN aciclovir is usually given IV at 10mg/kg 3×/d 2wks before reverting to the oral dose for 6–12wks.

Table 23.27 Selected systemic antifungal medications

Drug	Dose	Route	Page
Polyene			
Amphotericin	1–3mg/kg/d for liposomal preparations; less for Fungizone®	IV	📖 p.202
Fluorinated pyrimidines			
Flucytosine	50mg/kg × 4/d; adjust as per blood level monitoring	IV	📖 p.202
Triazoles			
Itraconazole	100–200mg 1×/d 200mg 2×/d for 2d then ↓ to 200mg 1×/d	PO IV	📖 p.202
Fluconazole	50–200mg 1×/d	PO	📖 p.202
Voriconazole	400mg 2×/d for 2 doses then 200mg 2×/d (can ↑ to 300mg 2×/d)	PO	📖 p.202
	6mg/kg 2×/d for 2 doses then 4mg/kg 2×/d	IV	📖 p.202

Systemic medication: glaucoma

Systemic medication may be required to lower IOP in the acute setting (e.g. acute angle closure glaucoma) or if topical treatment alone has failed. It is also commonly used prophylactically post-procedure (e.g. acetazolamide after cataract surgery).

Acetazolamide may also be used in the treatment of raised ICP secondary to idiopathic intracranial hypertension, altitude sickness and epilepsy.

Table 23.28 Systemic glaucoma medications

Drug	Dose	Route	Contraindications	Side-effects
Acetazolamide	0.25–1g/day in divided doses or 1×/d for SR preparation	IV/PO	Sulphonamide allergy, salt imbalance, renal impairment, hepatic impairment	Nausea Vomiting Diarrhoea Paraesthesia Rashes Polyuria Hypokalaemia Salt imbalance Mood changes Blood disorders
Mannitol 20%	1–2g/kg over 45min single dose	IV	Cardiac failure	Fluid overload Fever
Glycerol	1g/kg in 50% lemon juice single dose	PO	Diabetes mellitus	Hyperglycaemia

Systemic corticosteroids: general

Indications and mechanism

In severe ophthalmic inflammation systemic corticosteroids may be required. Corticosteroids are anti-inflammatory but at higher doses are immunosuppressive. The immunosuppressive role of corticosteroids is via inhibition of nuclear factor-κB (NF-KB) transcription factor signalling, thus blocking the production of interleukin-2 and other pro-inflammatory cytokines.

Routes of administration (systemic)

- *Oral*: the preferred corticosteroid is usually prednisolone. This may be started at 1mg/kg and then titrated down as inflammation is controlled and/or steroid-sparing agents are added. Two forms are available: enteric and non-enteric coated. Absorption of the enteric-coated form may be less predictable. Corticosteroids are best taken in the morning (coincides with physiological morning cortisol peak).
- *IV*: the preferred corticosteroid is usually methylprednisolone. This may be given as a single 500–1000mg dose or 'pulsed', e.g. three doses of 500–1000mg on consecutive or alternate days given in a 100ml of normal saline over a minimum of 1h.

Efficacy

> ### Box 23.2 Corticosteroids: equivalent anti-inflammatory doses
>
> Prednisolone 5mg is equivalent to:
> - Dexamethasone   750mcg
> - Betamethasone   750mcg
> - Methylprednisolone 4mg
> - Triamcinolone   4mg
> - Hydrocortisone   20mg

Contra-indications

Systemic infection (unless covered with appropriate antibiotic(s)).

Monitoring

Pre-treatment

Owing to the profound effects of corticosteroids a short pre-treatment review is advised. This includes selected medical history (varicella status, TB status, pre-existing diabetes/impaired glucose tolerance, hypertension) and examination (weight, BP, glucose). If there is any possibility of tuberculosis a CXR should be performed.

During treatment

- BP, weight, glucose every 3mths.
- Lipids every 1yr.
- Bone density (DXA scan) if steroid course >3mths; repeated scans may be needed for monitoring bone density in at-risk individuals.

Side-effects

Table 23.29 Corticosteroid side-effects (selected)

Endocrine	Adrenal suppression (risk of Addisonian crisis with withdrawal), Cushing syndrome, weight gain, moon-face
Gastrointestinal	Nausea, indigestion, peptic ulcer, pancreatitis
Musculoskeletal	Myopathy, osteopenia, osteoporosis, avascular necrosis
Skin	Atrophy, bruising, striae, acne, hirsutism
Haematological	Leucocytosis, immunosuppression
Biochemical	Fluid/electrolyte disturbance
Psychiatric	Mood disturbance (high or low), insomnia, psychosis
Neurological	↑ICP, papilloedema, worsening of epilepsy
Cardiovascular	Myocardial rupture after recent MI
Ophthalmic	↑IOP, posterior subcapsular cataracts, worsening of infection (e.g. viral or fungal keratitis)

Systemic corticosteroids: prophylaxis

Avoiding side-effects

Prophylaxis of corticosteroid-induced osteoporosis

Consider prophylaxis (e.g. a bisphosphonate such as alendronic acid) if treating with the equivalent of ≥7.5mg prednisolone per day for ≥3mths as indicated in Table 23.30:

Table 23.30 Summary of the joint recommendations of the Royal College of Physicians, National Osteoporosis Society, and the Bone and Tooth Society for corticosteroid use of ≥3mths duration

	Fracture history	DXA scan	
Age >65yrs			Investigate[1] + Give prophylaxis
Age <65yrs	Previous fragility fracture		Investigate[1] + Give prophylaxis
	No previous fragility fracture	T below −1.5 SD	Give prophylaxis
		T between −1.5 and 0	Repeat DXA in 1–3yrs
		T above 0 SD	No repeat unless very high dose

www.rcplondon.ac.uk/pubs/books/glucocorticoid/

1. Investigations advised include: FBC, ESR, bone, and liver function tests, creatinine, TSH, and other specialist investigations (e.g. isotope bone scan) as indicated.

Dual X-ray absorptiometry scans compare the bone density of the lower spine and hip against normal (i.e. healthy young adult). The difference is calculated in standard deviations to give the T score:

Table 23.31 Bone densitometry scores

T score	Condition
0 to −1 SD	Normal
−1 to −2.5 SD	Osteopenia
Below—2.5 SD	Osteoporosis

Prophylaxis of gastrointestinal side-effects

Consider prophylaxis (e.g. an H_2 antagonist such as ranitidine 150mg 2×/d) if at risk, i.e. higher doses of corticosteroid, history of gastrointestinal disease, co-administration of NSAIDs (avoid if possible).

Withdrawal of corticosteroids

For most patients having short courses (<10d) of doses ≤40mg/d prednisolone (or equivalent) no tapering is necessary. However, where there is a risk of adrenal suppression (Box 23.3) tapering is required in which the dose is reduced fairly rapidly to physiological levels (equivalent to 7.5mg prednisolone/d) and thereafter reduced more gradually. One suggested tapering approach is given in Box 23.4.

Box 23.3 Increased risk of adrenal suppression due to corticosteroid administration

- The daily dose has been >40mg/d prednisolone (or equivalent)
- The duration has been >3wks
- The frequency has been >1×/d
- There have been other courses recently or long-term steroid administration within the last year

Box 23.4 Tapering schedule recommended by the Consensus Panel on Immunosuppression for Ocular Disease

- *Over 40mg/d*: reduce by 10mg/d every 1–2wks
- *40–20mg/d*: reduce by 5mg/d every 1–2wks
- *20–10mg/d*: reduce by 2.5mg/d every 1–2wks
- *10–0mg/d*: reduce by 1–2.5mg/d every 1–4wks

Am J Ophthalmol 2000;**130**:492–513.

Antimetabolites, calcineurin inhibitors, and cytotoxics

Indications and mechanism

Although corticosteroids are usually the drug of choice in severe systemic or ocular inflammation, other immunosuppressants have an important role either as second-line agents in unresponsive cases or in permitting reduction/withdrawal of corticosteroids to minimize their side-effects.

Table 23.32 Immunosuppressants and their mechanisms[1]

Drug	Dose	Route	Mechanism
Antimetabolites			
Azathioprine	1–3mg/kg	PO	Inhibits purine metabolism
Methotrexate	7.5–20mg/wk	PO/IM/SC	Inhibits dihydrofolate reductase
Mycophenolate mofetil	CellCept® 1g 2×/d Myfortic® 720mg 2×/d	PO	Inhibits purine metabolism
Calcineurin inhibitors			
Ciclosporin	2–5mg/kg/d	PO	*Inhibit calcineurin/NF-AT transcription factor → ↓ IL-2 + other cytokines*
Sirolimus	Adjusted according to blood levels	PO	*Inhibit mTOR pathway → ↓ IL-2 + other cytokines*
Tacrolimus[2]	100–200mcg/kg/d	PO	*Inhibit calcineurin/ NF-AT transcription factor l d IL-2 + other cytokines*
Cytotoxics			
Chlorambucil	100–200mcg/kg/d	PO	*Alkylating agent: DNA cross-linking blocks cell replication*
Cyclophosphamide	2–3mg/kg/d	PO/IV	*Alkylating agent: DNA cross-linking blocks cell replication*

IL, interleukin.

1. NB Many of these immunosuppressants are unlicensed for use in ophthalmology.

2. Recommended dose for tacrolimus in uveitis is 100–150mcg/kg/d, administered in 2 single doses; however, full dose not usually tolerated at outset; therefore, start at 50% of the calculated dose and increase slowly over few weeks to the full dose. In very resistant cases an increase to 200mcg/kg/d and/or the additional use of an other immunosuppressive agent (antimetabolite/alkylating agent) must be considered.

Cautions

These immunosuppressive agents should only be administered by someone with appropriate experience in their use (normally a general physician, rheumatologist, or immunologist) and with adequate monitoring. Patient education is essential. This will include the potential side-effects, necessary precautions (e.g. contraception during and for a period after taking most of these agents), and warning symptoms that would require urgent medical review (e.g. features suggestive of infection, especially sore throat).

Table 23.33 Immunosuppressants and their side-effects

Drug	Side-effects (selected)	Suggested monitoring
Antimetabolites		
Azathioprine	Bone marrow suppression GI upset	Pre-treatment: check TPMT levels (low levels increase risk of bone marrow suppression)
	Secondary malignancies Alopecia	FBC stat, weekly for 4–8wks then at least every 3mths
Methotrexate	Hepatotoxicity Bone marrow suppression GI upset	FBC, U+E, LFT stat, weekly until dose stable, then every 2–3mths Commonly folate (1mg/d or 5mg/wk) is given concurrently but not the same day as methotrexate
Mycophenolate mofetil	Bone marrow suppression GI upset Secondary malignancies	FBC stat, weekly for 4wks, then fortnightly for 8wks, then monthly for first year
Transcription factor inhibitors		
Ciclosporin	Nephrotoxicity Hypertension Hepatotoxicity Gingival hyperplasia Hypertrichosis	U+E, LFT, BP stat, fortnightly for 4wks then every 4–6wks
Sirolimus	Hyperlipidaemia Nephrotoxicity Hepatotoxicity	Sirolimus levels, U+E, LFT, Lipids weekly for 4wks then every 2–4wks or as directed
Tacrolimus	Nephrotoxicity Hypertension Neurotoxicity Hepatotoxicity	U+E, LFT, BP stat, fortnightly for 4wks then every 4–6wks
Cytotoxics		
Chlorambucil	Bone marrow suppression Hepatotoxicity Sterility	Intensive specialist supervision required; includes FBC (+differential), LFT weekly for 4wks then every 2–4wks
Cyclophosphamide	Bone marrow suppression Haemorrhagic cystitis GI upset Sterility	Intensive specialist supervision required; includes FBC (+differential), LFT weekly for 4wks then every 2–4wks

Biologics

The successful use of anti-TNF therapy in RA ushered in the age of biologics. These are monoclonal antibodies or other recombinant proteins that are used in a targeted manner to modulate biological systems.

Nomenclature of monoclonal antibodies

The rationale to naming monoclonal antibodies is as follows:

Prefix: can be anything but should ensure that the whole name is distinct.

Infix relating to target: e.g. -lim- for immune system, -tu- for miscellaneous tumour.

Infix relating to source: e.g. -u- for human, -o- for mouse, -xi- for chimeric and -zu- for humanized.

Suffix: the class of medicine, i.e. mab for all monoclonal antibodies.

Examples

- Ada-lim-u-mab is a fully human monoclonal antibody with an immune system target.
- Ri-tu-xi-mab is a chimeric monoclonal antibody with a tumour target (originally developed for use against B-cell non-Hodgkin lymphoma).

Mechanism

Table 23.34 Selected biologics and their mechanisms[1]

Drug	Dose	Route	Mechanism
TNFα inhibitors			
Adalimumab	40mg every 2wks	SC	Anti-TNFα: fully human monoclonal antibody against TNFα
Etanercept	25mg twice per wk	SC	Anti-TNFα: Fc fusion protein, which binds extracellular TNF-α
Infliximab	3–5mg/kg every 4–8 wks	IV	Anti-TNFα: chimeric monoclonal antibody against TNF-α
Interleukin receptor antagonists			
Anakinra	100mg/d	SC	Anti-IL1R: recombinant version of IL1 receptor antagonist (IL1RA)
Daclizumab	1mg/kg every 4wks	IV	Anti-IL2R: humanized monoclonal antibody against the IL2 receptor
Anti-B cell			
Rituximab	1g repeated 2wks later	IV	Anti-CD20: chimeric monoclonal antibody against CD20 (B cells)
Interferons			
Interferon-α[2]	Depends on preparation	SC/IV	Antiviral and anti-tumour: decreases NK cell activity

1. NB Many of these immunosuppressants are unlicensed for use in ophthalmology.

2. Interferons—in uveitis type 1 interferons, are used, i.e. interferon-α2a, sometimes interferon-α2b. In MS interferon-β may be used.

Cautions

Biologics should only be administered by someone with appropriate experience in their use (normally a general physician, rheumatologist, or immunologist) and with adequate monitoring. Patient education is essential. This will include the potential side-effects, necessary precautions (e.g. contraception during and for a period after taking most of these agents), and warning symptoms that would require urgent medical review (e.g. features suggestive of infection, especially sore throat).

Table 23.35 Selected biologics and their side-effects

Drug	Side-effects (selected)	Suggested monitoring
TNF-α inhibitors		
Adalimumab	TB and hepatitis B reactivation Severe infections	Pre-treatment: rule out TB infection (may be latent) FBC (+differential), U+E, LFT stat, fortnightly for 4wks then every 4–6wks
Etanercept	Hypersensitivity reactions TB and hepatitis B reactivation Severe infections	Pre-treatment: rule out TB infection (may be latent) FBC (+differential), U+E, LFT stat, fortnightly for 4wks then every 4–6wks
Infliximab	Human antichimeric antibodies serum sickness TB and hepatitis B reactivation Anaphylaxis Severe infections	Pre-treatment: rule out TB infection (may be latent) FBC (+differential), U+E, LFT stat, fortnightly for 4wks then every 4–6wks
Interleukin receptor antagonists		
Anakinra	Injection-site reaction Neutropenia Severe infections (esp. in asthma)	FBC (+differential) stat, monthly for 6mths then every 3mths
Daclizumab	Hypersensitivity reactions Hypertension Severe infections	Monitor for infection
Anti-B cell		
Rituximab	Severe infusion reactions(incl. dyspnoea, hypoxia, bronchospasm) Cytokine release syndrome Cardiac dysfunction (incl. arrest, hypotension, angina, arrhythmias) TB reactivation PML	Cardiac monitoring during infusion and resuscitation facilities must be available FBC (+differential), U+E stat, then weekly for 4wks, then every 4–6wks
Interferons		
Interferon-α	Leucopenia Depression TB reactivation Flu-like symptoms Nephrotoxicity Hepatotoxicity	FBC (+differential), U+E, LFT stat, fortnightly for 4wks then every 4–6wks Regular review of mental state

Evidence-based ophthalmology

Study design (1)

More than 2 million research papers are published every year. Faced with an impossible reading-list, how should you pick out and critically appraise those that will change your practice, and inform future clinical guidelines? The skills of critical appraisal enable you to systematically examine research to assess its validity and usefulness. Apply the same critical thinking to your own work: others will.

Study designs

Systematic reviews and meta-analyses

Systematic review: a retrospective review of relevant primary studies (i.e. original data-gathering studies) meeting pre-specified tests of quality and relevance. Many such reviews have been conducted under the auspices of the Cochrane collaboration, an organization dedicated to the preparation of such reviews to help better inform decisions about healthcare. (The Cochrane Collaboration has been at the forefront of the movement to an evidence-based approach to medicine. *See* www.cochrane.org/)

Meta-analysis: a mathematical analysis of the combined results of two or more primary studies of similar design.

Experimental studies

Randomized controlled trial: a prospective study in which participants are randomly allocated to groups comparing the intervention(s) with the control (e.g. placebo, standard treatment or no treatment.). Bias is reduced by masking: in single-masked trials the participants are unaware of whether they are in the 'treatment' or the 'control' group; in double-masked trials the participants and the investigators are unaware of who is in which group until after the recording (and sometimes the analysis) of all data. (For obvious reasons the synonymous term 'blinded' is generally avoided in ophthalmic research.)

Observational studies

Cohort study: a prospective (or sometimes retrospective) study in which a group of individuals are identified at the outset (e.g. by the presence of a disease, exposure to an environmental factor, etc.) and monitored to see outcome over time. This is usually against a control group, although some information on natural history can be obtained without. These studies may be useful in identifying disease risk factors, natural history, and prognosis. For retrospective cohort studies the group of individuals must be identified as they would have been had the observer been there at the time (i.e. not with knowledge of the outcome cf. *case–control study*).

Case–control study: a retrospective study in which a group of individuals with outcome of interest (e.g. sympathetic ophlhalmia after vitreoretinal surgery) are compared with a suitable control group; this type of study can be useful for rare conditions.

Cross-sectional survey: a single time-point survey in a defined population observing possible relationships between factors of interest and the disease.

Case series: a description of a series of cases, often describing intervention and outcome, without a control group.

Levels of evidence

Table 24.1 Levels of evidence (SIGN classification)

Level	Evidence
1	**Evidence from meta-analyses, systematic reviews of randomized controlled trials or randomized controlled trails.** Further classified as: 1++ (high quality with very low risk of bias), 1+ (well conducted with low risk of bias) and 1– (high risk of bias)
2	**Evidence from case–control or cohort studies** (including systematic reviews of case control or cohort studies). Further classified as: 2++ (very low risk of confounding, bias or chance and high probability that the relationship is causal) 2+ (low risk of confounding, bias or chance, and moderate probability that the relationship is causal) 2– (high risk of confounding, bias or chance, and significant risk that the relationship is not causal)
3	**Evidence from non-analytic studies (case reports/series)**
4	**Evidence from expert opinion**

Adapted from Scottish Intercollegiate Network. SIGN 50: A Guideline Developer's Handbook, Edinburgh 2001; www.sign.ac.uk; Harbour *et al. BMJ* 2001;**323**:334–6.

Study design (2)

Hypothesis testing and power calculations

Most studies are not simply descriptive, but seek to detect clinically important associations between variables (e.g. IOP and progression of glaucoma) or the effects of interventions (e.g. differences between treatments A and B in their reduction of IOP). Integral to the design of such studies is a clear definition of the hypothesis and a calculation of the statistical power of the study.

The null and the alternative hypotheses

The null hypothesis is the default. It states that there is no effect or association of interest. For example, in a study of a new treatment for AMD, the null hypothesis might be that there is no difference between treatment vs placebo in the extent of visual loss at 6mths. The alternative hypothesis is that the null hypothesis is false, i.e. that there *is* an effect or association of interest. In the example shown this might be that the extent of visual loss from AMD is significantly less in the group receiving treatment.

Power calculations

Study design should include a calculation of the statistical power of the study. This is its ability to detect an effect of a specified size. Technically, this can be defined as the probability that the appropriate statistical test will reject a false null hypothesis (known as a type II error). Generally, a power of ≥80% is considered acceptable in study design. Statistical power depends on:

- Statistical significance level required (i.e. p value; conventionally $p<0.05$).
- Size of the effect (difference) being looked for.
- Sensitivity of the data: this includes sample size and data reliability.

It should be noted that as most of these variables will already be determined, the main role of power calculations is to estimate how many participants will need to be recruited to have a ≥80% chance of finding an effect.

Power calculations are also sometimes used retrospectively in studies where no effect has been found to see whether this is likely to be due to inadequate powering of the study (i.e. a type II error).

Box 24.1 Hypotheses and type I and type II errors

Null hypothesis: there is no effect or association of interest.

Alternative hypothesis: the null hypothesis is false, i.e. there exists an effect or association.

Type I error: false positive, i.e. the null hypothesis is incorrectly rejected (statistical significance falsely claimed).

Type II error: false negative, i.e. the null hypothesis is incorrectly accepted (statistical insignificance falsely accepted).

Critical appraisal

Questions to ask of a research paper

1. Is it worth reading at all?

● Does it ask a clear question?
● Was an appropriate method used to answer the question?

Unless the answer is 'yes' to both these points, it is probably not worth carrying on.

2. What type of study is it?

Your appraisal of the validity of a paper will depend on the study design (see Study design 🕮 p.878). Specific questions to ask are:

Systematic review and meta-analysis

Would the search strategy have identified all relevant papers? Were studies assessed for quality? If data are combined, was this appropriate?

Randomized controlled study

Were patients satisfactorily allocated/randomized between groups? What was the level of masking/blinding (participants ± investigators ± data analysts)? Were both groups treated in the same way (apart from the intervention)? Was there a high 'loss-to-follow-up rate' and could this have affected the results? Was the study sufficiently powered (i.e. did it recruit enough patients to reduce the likelihood of a type II error (Box 24.1)?

Cohort study

Was there a control group and was it appropriate? How were patients selected and would they be typical of the defined cohort? Has the 'exposure' under consideration and the outcomes been accurately measured? Have any important confounding factors been overlooked? Was there a high 'loss-to-follow-up rate' and could the lost participants be atypical of the group (e.g. important to know about 'loss-to-follow-up' due to death)? Was the study sufficiently powered and of long enough duration to pick up important events which are uncommon or have a long lag-time?

Case–control study

Were the 'controls' appropriate matches for the cases? Is the assessment of the 'exposure' under consideration based on recall or records, and how reliable is this likely to be? Have any important confounding factors been overlooked?

3. What are the main results, and are they statistically and clinically significant?

A statistically significant difference is of little interest unless it reflects a change that is meaningful in clinical terms. In a comparison of ocular hypotensives, a difference in mean IOP reduction of 0.3mmHg at one particular time-point may be statistically significant, but most unlikely to translate into clinical benefit.

4. Are there other factors that need to be considered?

What other outcomes were reported or should be estimated? This is likely to include side-effects, quality of life, costs, etc?

5. Are the conclusions of this study locally applicable?

Is the study scenario similar enough to your local situation (e.g. population demographics, potential availability of intervention) to make these results applicable to the patients you see?

6. Should we change our practice?

In the final analysis, will the intervention overall benefit your patients (consider side-effects, quality of life, etc.)? You may also have to consider the cost–benefit profile in terms of its affordability to either the patient or the health service, depending on local/national health economics.

Clinical guidelines

Aims

Clinical guidelines usually aim to achieve the following:
- summarize the available evidence for the management of a particular clinical scenario;
- provide evidence-based recommendations for best management;
- provide expert consensus recommendations for good practice where evidence is lacking.

Process

The process of guideline development includes:
- the identification of the clinical questions;
- a systematic literature search directed towards answering these questions;
- selection of evidence according to previously determined inclusion criteria;
- critical appraisal of the included papers (see Critical appraisal □ p.882);
- formulation of recommendations (graded according to strength of evidence); and, if necessary
- a consensus process to agree 'good practice' in those areas where there is insufficient evidence.

Strength of recommendations

This is based on critical appraisal of the available evidence (see Critical appraisal □ p.882). There are a number of grading systems that help identify the level of evidence on which any recommendations is based (Table 24.2).

Table 24.2 Strength of recommendations (SIGN grading system)

Recommendation	Evidence
A	At least one meta-analysis, systematic review, or randomized controlled trial rated as 1++, and directly applicable to the target population; or
	A systematic review of randomized controlled trials or a body of evidence consisting principally of studies rated as 1+, directly applicable to the target population, and demonstrating overall consistency of results
B	A body of evidence including studies rated as 2++, directly applicable to the target population, and demonstrating overall consistency of results; or
	Extrapolated evidence from studies rated as 1++ or 1+
C	A body of evidence including studies rated as 2+, directly applicable to the target population and demonstrating overall consistency of results; or
	Extrapolated evidence from studies rated as 2++
D	Evidence level 3 or 4; or
	Extrapolated evidence from studies rated as 2+

This table should be read in conjunction with Table 24.1.

Scottish Intercollegiate Network. SIGN 50: A Guideline Developer's Handbook, Edinburgh 2001; www.sign.ac.uk; Harbour et al. BMJ 2001;**323**:334–6

Healthcare economics

The economic analysis of evidence-based is vital in a world where resources within most healthcare systems are limited. Sometimes termed 'value-based medicine', the application of these analytical tools seeks to quantify the value of an intervention in terms of its benefit in relation to its cost.

Aims

Puts a value on each intervention in relation to its cost; may help to direct allocation of resources.

Tools

Cost-minimization analysis

This simply considers which option costs less. It makes the assumption that there is no significant difference in benefit between the two interventions (or that any such difference does not matter). It is therefore very limited.

Cost–benefit analysis

This considers an intervention in terms of economic cost vs 'money saved'. For example, the cost of a cataract operation vs the saving of preventing blindness (work productivity, avoidance of disability costs/social care/healthcare).

Cost-effectiveness analysis[1]

This considers an intervention in terms of the cost to achieve a particular endpoint, e.g. to attain a VA of ≥6/12.

Cost-utility analysis[1]

This considers an intervention in terms of its benefit on length and quality of life. The benefit in terms of length of life is estimated from the literature. Quality of life can either be estimated from questionnaires such as the National Eye Institute Visual Functioning Questionnaire-25 (VFQ-25), or by utility analysis (Box 24.2). This provides an estimate of the number of Quality Adjusted Life Years (QALYs) gained by the intervention. This is then compared with the cost associated with the intervention to give the cost-utility analysis, measured in cost/QALY gained (e.g. £/QALY).

Based on these techniques it has been estimated that:
- laser therapy for threshold ROP costs about $781/QALY gained
- initial cataract surgery costs about $2141/QALY gained
- PDT for neovascular ARMD (6/60 initial VA) costs about $184 423/ QALY gained.[2]

Box 24.2 Utility analysis

If a year of life lived in perfect health = 1 QALY, what is the value of a year of life with impaired vision? Utility analysis tries to put numbers on this by a variety of methods:

Time trade-off technique:

Ask the patient:

(1) how many more years do you expect to live?

(2) how many of your remaining years of your life would you trade to have perfect health (or perfect vision)?

Utility value = 1 − (years traded/years of life expected)

Examples

Using this technique utility scores for vision have been estimated as follows:[2]

VA 6/6 (permanent and bilateral) 1.0

VA 6/12 (in the better eye) 0.8

VA 6/60 (in the better eye) 0.66

VA CF (in the better eye) 0.52

VA HM (in the better eye) 0.35

VA NPL (bilateral) 0.26

Thus according to these estimates 1yr of life with bilateral NPL has a value of 0.26 QALYs. Note that this value is derived from judgements made by the patient rather than by their ophthalmologist.

Other utility estimation techniques:

Other methods include the standard gamble and the willingness-to-pay techniques.

1. Some health economists do not distinguish between cost-effectiveness analysis and cost-utility analysis.

2. Brown MM *et al.* Healthcare economic analyses and value-based medicine. *Surv Ophthalmol* 2003;**48**:204–23.

Investigations

The process of clinical assessment—comprising history, examination, and investigation—is directed towards reaching a diagnosis. During this process we acquire a wealth of clinical data that we process, often subconsciously, to narrow down the diagnosis. The usefulness of each symptom, sign, and investigation in predicting a particular diagnosis can be described statistically by its sensitivity, specificity, positive predictive value, and negative predictive value.

Sensitivity and specificity are performance measures of a particular test, whereas positive and negative predictive values give the post-test probabilities of disease/health and so are affected by disease prevalence (i.e. the proportion of the population with that condition).

Sensitivity and specificity

Sensitivity
This is the 'pick-up', or how good a test is at being positive in disease (true positive—see Table 24.3). This is the number of people in whom the test correctly predicts disease as a proportion of the number of people who do have the disease, i.e.

Sensitivity = true positive/(true positive + false negative).

Specificity
This is how good the test is at being negative in the healthy (true negative—see Table 24.3). This is the number of people in whom the test correctly predicts no disease as a proportion of the number of people who do not have the disease, i.e.

Specificity = true negative/(false positive + true negative).

Positive and negative predictive values

Positive predictive value (PPV)
This indicates what proportion of people with a positive test do in fact have the disease. It is helpful in interpreting the significance of a positive test result. It is, however, affected by the prevalence of a particular condition. A test with a high PPV will be useful for confirming a particular condition.

Positive predictive value = true positive/(true positive + false positive)

Negative predictive value (NPV)
This indicates what proportion of people with a negative test are in fact free from the disease. Like the PPV it will be affected by disease prevalence. A test with a high NPV will be useful for ruling out a particular condition.

Negative predictive value = true negative/(true negative + false negative)

Table 24.3 Sensitivity and specificity depend on the rate of true positives and true negatives in their respective populations

Test result	Patients have disease	Patients do not have disease
Test is positive	True +	False +
Test is negative	False −	True −

Statistical terms

Populations and samples

Population: the defined group of interest.
Sample: a selected number of that population who are studied.

Types of statistics

Descriptive statistics

Technique of describing the sample by the use of a typical value (e.g. the median) and its distribution (e.g. the interquartile range).

Inferential statistics

Technique of using statistical analysis of the sample to make inferences about a particular parameter in the population. This includes hypothesis testing and estimation.

Hypothesis testing

Considers whether there is an effect or an association of interest. For example, consider the clinical question 'which of two treatments A or B is more effective at lowering IOP?' The null hypothesis would state that there is no difference in IOP reduction in the two groups, whereas the alternative hypothesis would state that the null hypothesis was false, i.e. that there was a statistically significant difference. Conventionally, a difference is considered significant if the probability of it arising by chance is less than 5% (i.e. $p < 0.05$).

Estimation

What magnitude of effect would be expected in the actual population? Estimation predicts from statistical analysis of the sample the size of the effect to be expected in the population, usually expressed as a 95% confidence interval. This is the range within which there is a 95% probability that the actual effect observed in the population will lie.

Types of variables

The main division is between categorical and numerical variables. The type of variable will dictate which statistical tests are appropriate to the data set.

- *Categorical variables*: variables that have values that can be distinguished from each other, but that are qualitative rather than quantitative. Examples include gender and race.
- *Numerical variables*: quantitative variables that can be measured numerically or to which numbers can be meaningfully assigned. They can be further divided into:
  - *discrete*: variable can only take certain values (e.g. number of patients)
  - *continuous*: variable can be measured on a continuous scale (e.g. IOP, duration of operation).

Frequency distribution

Frequency distributions may be normal or skewed. The type of distribution will dictate which statistical tests are appropriate to the data set.

Normal distribution

Many biological variables (e.g. height) have a 'bell-shaped' or normal (*syn* Gaussian) distribution. These can be described in terms of a mean and standard deviation. If uncertain as to whether a data set is normally distributed, this can be tested, e.g. with the Kolmogorov–Smirnoff test.

Skewed distribution

Some variables (e.g. IOP) have an asymmetric distribution, in which a few very high or very low values result in the distribution being skewed positively or negatively (respectively). Distributions that are not normally distributed are better described in terms of median and interquartile range rather than in terms of mean and standard deviation.

Independent vs dependent data

If samples are unrelated to each other, they are said to be independent. If samples are related to each other (e.g. VA pre- and post-intervention) then they are described as being dependent If only two groups of samples are being considered, independent and dependent data are commonly described as 'unpaired' and 'paired' respectively. The independence of the samples will dictate which statistical tests are appropriate for a given data set.

Statistical tests

The types of statistical tests undertaken will be dictated by the nature of the data: type of variable (categorical, numerical), its distribution (normal or skewed), and whether the samples are independent or dependent.

Statistical tests for categorical data

Categorical data can be conveniently described by a contingency table (Table 24.4). Hypothesis testing is with either chi-squared (χ^2) or Fisher's Exact test.

Chi-squared test

Commonly used test for categorical data, it compares observed and expected frequencies of mutually exclusive events. Actual numbers not percentages should be used; all expected values should be >1 and 80% should be >5.

Yates' correction helps adjust for smaller sample sizes, and should generally be used for all chi-squared tests.

Fisher's Exact test

Similar to the chi-squared test but more robust for small sample sizes. It should be used when the above conditions cannot be met.

Table 24.4 Example of categorical data that can be described in a 2×2 contingency table

		Outcome	
		Anatomical closure of macular hole	
		Success	Failure
Intervention	Vitrectomy with platelets	a	b
	Vitrectomy alone	c	d

Having constructed a 2×2 contingency table, the possible association of the use of platelets with improved surgical success can be tested by the chi-squared or Fisher's Exact tests.

Statistical tests for continuous data

Test selection will depend on the distribution of the data, whether values in the two data sets are paired, and whether testing for a difference (or lack of) between groups or testing for correlation between the groups.

Parametric tests: assume that the data are normally distributed (see Stastical terms 📖 p.890).

Non-parametric tests: make no assumptions about the distribution of the data, sometimes termed 'distribution free'.

It is important to use a test appropriate to the number of groups being considered. For example, one cannot sequentially apply the *t*-test to multiple groups to look for 'any' significant difference; applying such a test in this way greatly increases the chance of erroneously finding a 'statistically significant' difference (i.e. a type I error).

Table 24.5 Common statistical tests used for continuous data

	Parametric	Non-parametric
Tests on two groups		
Paired data	Paired t-test	Wilcoxon test
Unpaired data	Unpaired t-test	Mann–Whitney U test
Correlation	Pearson's test	Spearman's rank test
Tests on more than two groups		
Dependent data	Repeated measures ANOVA	Friedman test
Independent data	One-way ANOVA	Kruskal–Wallis test

Linear and logistic regression

Linear regression

Linear regression builds a model that describes the relationship between one or more independent (or predictor) variables and a single continuous dependent (or outcome) variable. At its simplest it describes the relationship between the dependent variable (y) and the independent variable (x) as a linear equation, $y = a + bx$, where a and b are constants.

- Simple linear regression determines the best equation to predict Y from a single variable, X; both variables must be continuous.
- Multiple linear regression finds the equation that best predicts Y from multiple independent variables. You would consider this approach when there are several independent (predictor) variables (e.g. X_1, X_2, X_3) and a single continuous dependent variable (e.g. Y); predictor variables may be continuous or categorical.

Logistic regression

Logistic regression quantifies the association between a risk factor (or treatment) and a disease (or any event), after adjusting for other variables. Whereas in multiple linear regression it is the value of the continuous variable (e.g. IOP) that can be predicted from two or more predictor variables (e.g. age, gender, time of day), in logistic regression it is the probability of obtaining one of the outcomes (e.g. the chance of being alive 1yr after phakoemulsification) that can be predicted.

Statistical issues relating to two eyes

The two-eye problem

The classical 'two-eye' problem is that observations from left and right eyes will tend to be correlated. If data from both eyes are pooled this will violate an important assumption of hypothesis testing, namely, that these are independent observations. However, dealing with this issue is problematic. For conditions that are equally likely to affect either eye, analyses based on either right or left eyes, or on a randomly selected eye are statistically equivalent. If information has been collected on both eyes then half of the data will be unused. In addition, bias may be introduced if there is non-random selection of the eye for inclusion in the analysis. This would also apply to the choice of the first eye with disease, better/worse eye, or operated eye.

Averaging results from right and left eyes also results in a loss of information, and would not be appropriate for studies that operate at the ocular level, e.g. the impact of topical treatment, or ocular surgery.

Solutions to the two-eye problem

In dealing with the two-eye problem, it is important to take account of between eye correlation by calculating the kappa statistic. If there is little or no correlation between eyes the kappa statistic will be close to zero. If the kappa statistic is greater than about 0.3 then between eye correlation is likely to be an important problem.

Statistical techniques exist that can utilize all available data while allowing for the correlation. In some circumstances a good study design would be to use the fellow eye as the 'control' (paired comparison).[1]

---

1. Murdoch IE, Morris SS, Cousens SN. People and eyes: statistical approaches in ophthalmology. *Br J Ophthalmol* 1998;**82**:971–3

Risks, odds, and number needed to treat

Absolute and relative risk

Absolute risk describes the likelihood of an event occurring in one particular group. Relative risk (or risk ratio) compares the likelihood of an event occurring in two groups. A relative risk of 1 means that there is no difference between the two groups. Relative risk is the preferred method of expressing likelihood in randomized controlled trials and cohort studies.

- Relative risk = $\dfrac{\text{risk of event on treatment}}{\text{risk of event in control group}}$ = $\dfrac{a/(a \pm b)}{c/(c+d)}$

Table 24.6 Risk table

		Outcome	
		Event occurs	No event
Intervention	Treatment group	a	b
	Control group	c	d

NB The 'event' may be beneficial (e.g. surgical success) or harmful (e.g. drug side-effect).

Odds ratio

The odds ratio compares the odds of an event occurring in two groups. An odds ratio of 1 means that there is no difference between the two groups. Odds ratios are the preferred method of expressing likelihood in case–control studies and retrospective studies.

- Odds ratio = $\dfrac{\text{odds of event on treatment}}{\text{odds of event in control group}}$ = $\dfrac{a/b}{c/d}$

Number needed to treat

Number needed to treat (NNT) or number needed to harm (NNH) describes the number of people that must be treated in order for one beneficial (or harmful) event to occur. It is derived from the absolute risk reduction (ARR).

- ARR = risk of event in control group – risk of event on treatment
  = $c/(c + d) - a(a + b)$
- NNT = 1/ARR

Miscellaneous

Eponymous syndromes

Aarskog syndrome X-linked; megalocornea, hypertelorism, antimongoloid palpebral fissures; short stature, syndactyly.

Aicardi syndrome Probably X-linked lethal to males; corpus callosal agenesis and other CNS abnormalities, infantile spasms, mental retardation, vertebral and rib malformations; chorioretinal lacunar defects, colobomas.

Albright syndrome Disorder of G-proteins resulting in polyostotic fibrous dysplasia (of bone), endocrine abnormalities (including precocious puberty) and café-au-lait spots; orbital involvement may cause proptosis, sinus mucoceles, and compressive optic neuropathy..

Alagille syndrome Autosomal dominant (Ch20); posterior embryotoxon, optic disc drusen, pale fundi, hypertelorism; intrahepatic bile duct hypoplasia, butterfly vertebrae, congenital heart disease.

Alport syndrome Disorder of type IV collagen; X-linked dominant but autosomal inheritance described; anterior lenticonus, anterior polar and cortical cataracts, fleck retina; sensorineural deafness, nephritis.

Alström–Olsen syndrome Autosomal recessive; cone-rod dystrophy with features of RP, posterior subcapsular cataracts; diabetes mellitus, sensorineural deafness, nephropathy, obesity, acanthosis nigricans.

Anderson–Fabry disease See Fabry's disease.

Apert syndrome Autosomal dominant or sporadic; gene encoding the fibroblast growth factor receptor-2 (Ch10q26); craniosynostosis, syndactyly, broad distal phalanx of great thumb/toe, mental handicap; hypertelorism, proptosis, strabismus, keratoconus, ectopia lentis, congenital glaucoma, optic atrophy.

Arnold–Chiari malformation Congenital herniation of the cerebellum/brainstem through the foramen magnum may cause hydrocephalus, cerebellar signs (e.g. nystagmus, ataxia) and may be associated with syringomyelia.

Bardet–Biedl and Laurence–Moon syndromes Autosomal recessive overlapping conditions; RP with early macular involvement; polydactyly, hypogonadism, obesity, microcephaly, nephropathy, ↓IQ.

Batten disease (neuronal ceroid lipofuscinosis) Autosomal recessive metabolic disorder resulting in neurodegeneration. *Juvenile form*: bull's eye maculopathy, pigmentary retinopathy, optic atrophy, epilepsy, life expectancy <25yrs.

Bassen–Kornzweig (abetalipoproteinaemia) Autosomal recessive deficiency of triglyceride transfer protein; RP, cataract; spinocerebellar degeneration, steatorrhoea, acanthosis (of erythrocytes).

Bloch–Sulzberger syndrome (incontinentia pigmenti) X-linked dominant, lethal to males; abnormal peripheral retinal vasculature, gliosis, tractional retinal detachment; abnormal teeth, cutaneous pigment whorls and CNS anomalies.

Bourneville disease (tuberous sclerosis) Autosomal dominant (Ch9q TSC1 and Ch16p TSC2) phakomatosis with neurocutaneous features and retinal astrocytomas.

Brown syndrome Mechanical restriction syndrome attributed to the superior oblique tendon sheath.

Caffrey disease Hyperplasia of subperiosteal bone and proptosis.

Cogan syndrome Idiopathic, probably autoimmune; interstitial keratitis, sensorineural deafness, tinnitus, vertigo, systemic vasculitis (including life-threatening aortitis).

Crouzon syndrome Autosomal dominant or sporadic; gene encoding the fibroblast growth factor receptor-2 (Ch10q26); craniosynostosis, maxillary hypoplasia, prognathism, hooked nose; proptosis, strabismus, micro/mega-locornea, iris coloboma, cataract, ectopia lentis, glaucoma.

De Morsier syndrome Optic nerve hypoplasia; midline brain abnormalities, including absent septum pellucidum and corpus callosal hypo/aplasia.

Down syndrome Trisomy 21; 1 in 650 live births; blepharitis, keratoconus, cataracts; musculoskeletal abnormalities, congenital heart disease, ↓IQ.

Duane syndrome Aberrant coinnervation of LR and MR resulting in horizontal gaze anomalies.

Edwards syndrome Trisomy 18; 1 in 8000 live births; microphthalmos, glaucoma, cataracts; failure to thrive, congenital heart disease; life expectancy <1yr.

Fabry disease X-linked; α-galactosidase A deficiency results in glycosphingolipid accumulation; vortex keratopathy, cataracts (posterior cortical and granular), conjunctival and retinal telangiectasia; peripheral neuropathy with painful 'Fabry crises', renal failure, angiokeratoma corporis diffusum, lymphoedema.

Foster Kennedy syndrome Ipsilateral optic atrophy due to compressive optic neuropathy with contralateral disc selling from ↑ICP.

Foville syndrome Lesion of lateral pons resulting in ipsilateral facial paresis, horizontal gaze palsy (towards side of lesion) and a contralateral hemiparesis.

Friedreich ataxia Autosomal recessive; triplet repeat expansion (GAA) of non-coding region of the frataxin gene (Ch9); degeneration of spinocerebellar tracts (ataxia, dysarthria, nystagmus), corticospinal tracts (weakness, extensor plantars), posterior columns (proprioception) and peripheral neuropathy (with absent tendon reflexes), pes cavus.

Gardner syndrome Variant of familial adenomatous polyposis (autosomal dominant) with bone cysts, hamartomas, and soft tissue tumours; atypical CHRPE.

Gaucher disease Autosomal recessive; β-glucosidase deficiency; visceromegaly (type I) or neurodegeneration (type II or III); supranuclear palsy (type IIIb).

Gerstmann syndrome Dominant parietal lobe lesion resulting in finger agnosia, right/left confusion, dysgraphia, acalculia; may be associated with failure of ipsilateral pursuit movements.

Gillespie syndrome Variant of aniridia (PAX-6 mutation) with mental retardation and cerebellar ataxia.

Goldenhar syndrome Part of the spectrum of hemifacial microsomia; accessory auricle, limbal dermoid, hypoplasia of face, vertebral anomaly. corneal hyposthesia. Duane's syndrome. iris and upper eyelid coloboma.

Goldman–Favre disease Autosomal recessive; optically empty vitreous, retinoschisis, macular changes, peripheral pigmentary retinopathy.

Gorlin syndrome Autosomal dominant (tumour suppressor gene PATCHED; Ch9q); multiple basal cell carcinomas, jaw cysts, skeletal abnormalities, ectopic calcification (e.g. falx cerebri); hypertelorism, prominent supraorbital ridges.

Gradenigo syndrome VIn palsy and pain in Vn distribution due to lesion at the apex of the petrous temporal bone; this may be related to chronic middle ear infection.

Gronblad–Strandberg syndrome angioid streaks with pseudoxanthoma elasticum.

Hallermann–Streiff–Francois syndrome micropthalmos, cataract, hypotrichosis, blue sclera; dyscephaly, short stature.

Heerfordt syndrome (uveoparotid fever) presentation of sarcoidosis with fever, parotid enlargement, uveitis.

Hermansky–Pudlak syndrome type II oculocutaneous albinism with platelet dysfunction, pulmonary fibrosis, granulomatous colitis.

Kasabach–Merritt syndrome giant haemangioma with localized intra-vascular coagulation causing low platelets and fibrinogen.

Kearns–Sayre syndrome Mitochondrial inheritance; CPEO, pigmentary retinopathy (granular pigmentation, peripapillary atrophy) and heart block; usually presents before 20yrs.

Laurence–Moon syndrome Grouped with Bardet–Biedl syndrome but no obesity or polydactyly.

Leber congenital amaurosis Autosomal recessive; blind from birth, eye-poking (oculo-digital sign), hypermetropia, sluggish or paradoxical pupillary reflexes, macular dysplasia but fairly normal fundal appearance.

Leber hereditary optic neuropathy Mitochondrial inheritance; rapid sequential visual loss in 20–30s due to optic neuropathy.

Löfgren syndrome presentation of sarcoidosis with fever, erythema nodosum, bihilar lymphadenopathy.

Louis-Bar syndrome (ataxia telangiectasia) Autosomal recessive (Ch11q, ATM gene); conjunctival telangiectasia, progressive oculomotor apraxia; cerebellar ataxia, ↓IQ, immunodeficiency.

Lowe syndrome (oculocerebrorenal syndrome) X-linked disorder of amino acid metabolism; congenital cataract, microspherophakia, blue sclera, anterior segment dysgenesis, glaucoma; ↓IQ, hypotonia, vitamin D resistant rickets.

Maffuci syndrome Multiple haemangiomas and enchondromas (which may cause limb deformities), with risk of malignant transformation.

Marfan syndrome Autosomal dominant (Ch15, fibrillin); ectopia lentis, retinal detachment, glaucoma, axial myopia; arachnodactyly, long-limbed, aortic dissection.

Meckel–Gruber syndrome Autosomal recessive; coloboma; micro-cephaly, occipital encephalocele, cleft lip/palate, polydactyly, polycystic kidney disease.

Menke disease X-linked recessive deficiency of copper transport protein; optic atrophy, retinal dystrophy; wiry hair, ataxia, neurodegeneration.

Mikulicz syndrome infiltrative swelling of salivary and lacrimal glands.

Millard–Gubler syndrome lesion of the facial colliculus (dorsal pons) resulting in ipsilateral VIn and VIIn palsies, ± contralateral hemiparesis.

Miller–Fisher syndrome Variant of Guillain–Barré syndrome character-ized by acute external ophthalmoplegia, ataxia, and areflexia.

Moebius syndrome Congenital facial paresis with ipsilateral abducens palsy. Other cranial nerves may be affected.

Niemann–Pick disease Autosomal recessive; deficiency of sphingomyelinase; type A is infantile onset with visceromegaly, neurodegeneration and cherry red spot; type B juvenile onset with visceromegaly, rarely cherry red spot; type C has variable onset, vertical supranuclear gaze palsy, ataxia and neurodegeneration.

Norrie disease X-linked; retinal dysplasia, retinal detachment, leucocoria, vitreous haemorrhage, cataract, phthisis; ↓IQ, deafness.

Oguchi disease Autosomal recessive; non-progressive nyctalopia (CSNB), pseudotapetal reflex which normalizes with dark adaptation (Mizuo phenomenon).

Parinaud syndrome Lesion of dorsal midbrain resulting in light-near dissociation, supranuclear upgaze palsy, convergence retraction nystagmus and failure of convergence and accommodation.

Patau syndrome Trisomy 13; 1 in 14 000 live births; cyclopia, colobomas, retinal dysplasia; microcephaly; life expectancy <3mths.

Raymond syndrome Lesion of the corticospinal tract in the ventral pons resulting in VIn palsy and contralateral hemiparesis.

Refsum disease Autosomal recessive; deficiency of phytanic acid α-hydrolase results in accumulation of phytanic acid; pigmentary retinopathy, optic atrophy; ichthyosis, deafness, cardiomyopathy, ataxia.

Riley–Day syndrome (familial dysautonomia) autosomal recessive; commoner in Ashkenazi Jews; tear deficiency → keratoconjunctivitis sicca, commonly with ulceration, reduced corneal sensation; sensory neuropathy, autonomic dysfunction/crises.

Rubinstein–Taybi syndrome (otopalatodigital syndrome) Developmental abnormality; hypertelorism, colobomas; broad thumbs/big toes, maxillary/mandibular hypoplasia, hypertrichosis, ↓IQ.

Sandhoff disease Autosomal recessive (Ch5q, HEXB); GM2 gangliosidosis with deficiency of hexosominadase A and B; cherry red spot, optic atrophy; splenomegaly, neurodegeneration.

Sjögren syndrome Autoimmune condition affecting up to 4% of population; inflammation of lacrimal and salivary glands → dry eyes (may be severe and lead to cicatrization) and dry mouth; can be primary or secondary to conditions such as RA and SLE; diagnosis supported by anti-Ro (SS-A), anti-La (SS-B), and parotid gland ultrasound; labial gland biopsy or. ↑ risk of B-cell lymphoma.

Stargardt disease (and fundus flavimaculatus) Autosomal recessive (usually Ch1p, ABCA4); commonest of the macular dystrophies, with two clinical presentations: Stargardt's ('beaten-bronze' atrophy, yellowish flecks of the posterior pole, significant ↓VA) and fundus flavimaculatus (widespread pisciform flecks with relative preservation of vision).

Steele–Richardson–Olszewski (progressive supranuclear palsy) Neurodegenerative disease of the elderly; supranuclear vertical gaze; postural instability, parkinsonism, pseudobulbar palsy, and dementia.

Stickler syndrome (hereditary arthro-ophthalmopathy) Autosomal dominant (Ch12q, COL2A1); abnormality of type II collagen; high myopia, optically empty vitreous, retinal detachments, cataract, ectopia lentis, glaucoma; arthropathy, Pierre Robin sequence (micrognathia, high arched/cleft palate), sensorineural deafness, mitral valve prolapse.

Sturge–Weber syndrome Phakomatosis with port-wine stain of the face with ocular and CNS haemangiomas.

Tay–Sachs disease Autosomal recessive (Ch15q, HEXA); GM2 gangliosidosis with deficiency of hexosominadase A; cherry red spot, optic atrophy; neurodegeneration.

Treacher Collins syndrome (mandibulofacial dysostosis) Autosomal dominant; 'treacle gene' TCOF1 (Ch 5q32); clefting syndrome; antimongoloid palpebral fissures, lower lid colobomas, dermoids; mandibular hypoplasia, zygoma hypoplasia, choanal atresia.

Turcot syndrome Variant of familial adenomatous polyposis (autosomal dominant) with CNS neuroepithelial tumours especially medulloblastoma and glioma; atypical CHRPE.

Turner syndrome XO; 1 in 2000 live female births; antimongoloid palpebral fissures, cataracts, convergence insufficiency; short stature, wide carrying angle, low hair line, webbed neck, primary gonadal failure, congenital heart defects.

Vogt–Koyanagi–Harada syndrome Multisystem inflammatory disease; bilateral granulomatous panuveitis; vitiligo, alopecia, deafness, tinnitus, sterile meningoencephalitis and cranial neuropathies.

Von-Hippel Lindau Autosomal dominant (Ch3p, VHL gene); phakomatosis with retinal capillary haemangiomas, CNS haemangioblastomas, renal cell carcinomas and other tumours.

Waardenburg syndrome Autosomal dominant (PAX3); heterochromia, hypertelorism; white forelock, deafness.

Wallenberg syndrome (lateral medullary syndrome) Lesion of the lateral medulla (typically posterior inferior cerebellar artery occlusion) resulting in ipsilateral Horner syndrome, ipsilateral cerebellar signs, ipsilateral palatal paralysis, ipsilateral decreased facial sensation (pain and temperature), contralateral decreased somatic sensation (pain and temperature).

Walker–Warburg syndrome Autosomal recessive; retinal dysplasia; muscular dystrophy, Dandy–Walker malformation.

Weber syndrome Upper midbrain lesion causing ipsilateral oculomotor paralysis (with loss of reaction to light and accommodation) with contralateral hemiparesis.

Weill–Marchesani syndrome Autosomal recessive; ectopia lentis, microspherophakia, retinal detachment, anomalous angles; short stature, brachydactyly, ↓IQ.

Wildervanck syndrome Klippel–Feil malformation (short neck due to cervical vertebrae anomalies) with deafness and Duane's syndrome.

Wyburn–Mason syndrome Phakomatosis with arteriovenous malformations of retina, orbit, and CNS.

Zellweger syndrome (cerebrohepatorenal syndrome) Autosomal recessive; severe end of a spectrum of peroxisomal disorders which includes neonatal adrenoleukodystrophy and infantile Refsum's disease; cataract, optic nerve hypoplasia, pigmentary retinopathy, corneal clouding; high forehead, flat brows; life expectancy <1yr.

Publications of the Royal College of Ophthalmologists

The Royal College of Ophthalmologists publishes a number of helpful practitioner and patient-related resources that can be found at http://www.rcophth.ac.uk

Published guidelines

General
Standards for the Retrieval of Human Ocular Tissue used in Transplantation, Research and Training (2008).
A National Research Strategy for Ophthalmology (2002).
Guidelines—Declaration of Interests (2008).

Cornea
Standards for Laser Refractive Surgery (2009).

Glaucoma
Guidelines for the Management of Open Angle Glaucoma and Ocular Hypertension (2004).

Lens
Revised statement on N Acetyl Carnosine for Cataracts (August 2008).
Cataract Surgery Guidelines (2007).
Local Anaesthesia for Intraocular Surgery (with The Royal College of Anaesthetists) (2001).
Example of consent for cataract surgery—information for patients.

Medical retina
Guidelines for Ranibizumab—The Clinician's Guide to commencing, continuing and discontinuing treatment (2008).
The Intravitreal Use of Bevacizumab (Avastin) in AMD (2007).
Commissioning Contemporary AMD Services: a guide for commissioners and clinicians—version 3 (2007).
Updated Age Related Macular Degeneration Interim Guidelines (2007).
Guidelines for Intravitreal Injections Procedure (2006).
Guidelines for Diabetic Retinopathy (2005).
The Ocular Side effects of Vigabatrin (Sabril)—Information and Guidance for Screening (2008).
Ocular Side Effects of Topiramate—Frequently Asked Questions (2006).
Ocular Toxicity and Hydrochloroquine: Guidelines for Screening (2004).
Retinal Vein Occlusion (2004).

Paediatric
UK Retinopathy of Prematurity Guideline (2008).
Procedures for the Ophthalmologist who Suspects Child Abuse (2000).
Guidelines for the Management of Strabismus in Childhood (2000).
Juvenile Arthritis (2006).
Management of Amblyopia (2006).

Ophthalmic information

General

Age Related Macular Degeneration (AMD) Rapid Access Referral Form and Atlas (2007).
Quality Development Programme—guidance for clinical governance in ophthalmology (1999).
Registration and Rehabilitation of the Visually Handicapped (1994).
The Provision of Low Vision Care (1998).
Vision and Display Screen Equipment (1993).
Creutzfeldt-Jakob Disease (CJD) and Ophthalmology (2004).

Ophthalmic Services Guidance

Audit & Clinical Effectiveness (2008).
Commissioning Cataract Surgery (2005).
Complaints in Ophthalmology (2005).
Day Care and Inpatient Facilities (2008).
Decontamination (2008).
Endophthalmitis (2007).
Informatics (2006).
Management of Retinal Detachment (2005).
Ophthalmic Emergency Services (2006).
Ophthalmic Imaging (2006).
Ophthalmic Services for Children (2005).
Ophthalmic Services for Patients with Diabetes (2006).
Ophthalmic Primary Care (2005).
Ophthalmic Outpatient Department (2008).
Patient Safety in Ophthalmology (2005).
Pre-operative Assessment (2005).
Theatres (2008).
Workforce Planning (2005).

Visual standards

Definition of the Minimum Field of Vision (1994).
Visual Standards for Driving (2005).

Patient information

Excimer Laser Photorefractive Surgery
Information for Patients on Corneal Transplantation
Understanding Age-Related Macular Degeneration
Understanding Cataracts
Understanding Glaucoma
Understanding Nystagmus
Understanding Retinal Detachment
Understanding Retinitis Pigmentosa

Patient information (paediatric)

Congenital Cataracts
Congenital Glaucoma
Retinopathy of Prematurity
Information for Parents on Squints

Web resources for ophthalmologists (1)

Ophthalmic and related associations

Box 25.1

American Academy of Ophthalmology www.aao.org
Association for Research in Vision and Ophthalmology www.arvo.org
American Association for Pediatric Ophthalmology and Strabismus
www.aapos.org
American Society of Cataract and Refractive Surgery www.ascrs.org
British Association of Retinal Screeners www.eyescreening.org.uk
British Contact Lens Association www.bcla.org.uk
British and Eire Association of Vitreoretinal Surgeons www.beavrs2008.org
British Oculoplastic Surgery Society www.bopss.org
British Ophthalmic Anaesthesia Society www.boas.org
British and Irish Orthoptic Society www.orthoptics.org.uk
British Society for Refractive Surgery www.bsrs.org.uk
Club Jules Gonin www.clubjulesgonin.com
College of Optometrists www.college-optometrists.org
European Association for Vision and Eye Research www.ever.be
European Community University Professors of Ophthalmology www.eupo.eu
European Neuro-Ophthalmological Society www.eunosweb.org
European Society of Cataract and Refractive Surgeons www.escrs.org
European Society of Ophthalmic Plastic and Reconstructive Surgery
www.esoprs.com
European Society of Ophthalmology www.soevision.org/home
Institute of Ophthalmology www.ucl.ac.uk/ioo
International Council of Ophthalmology www.icoph.org
International Ocular Information Society www.iois.org
International Society for Clinical Electrophysiology of Vision www.iscev.org
International Society of Refractive Surgery www.isrs.org
International Uveitis Study Group www.iusg.net
Medical Contact Lens and Ocular Surface Association www.mclosa.org.uk
Midland Ophthalmological Society www.the-mos.org
Moorfields Eye Hospital www.moorfields.nhs.uk
North of England Ophthalmological Society www.neos.org.uk
Ocular Immunology and Uveitis Foundation www.uveitis.org
Ophthalmic Imaging Association www.oia.org.uk
ORBIS International www.orbis.org
Oxford Ophthalmological Congress www.oxford-ophthalmological-
congress.org.uk
Royal Society of Medicine—Ophthalmology Section
www.rsm.ac.uk/academ/smtophth.php
Scottish Ophthalmological Club www.s-o-c.org.uk
Trends in Ophthalmology www.trendsinophthalmology.com
United Kingdom and Ireland Society of Cataract and Refractive Surgeons
www.ukiscrs.org.uk
Yorkshire Retina Society www.yorkshireretinasociety.org.uk

Royal Medical Colleges (UK)

Box 25.2

The Royal College of Anaesthetists www.rcoa.ac.uk
The Royal College of General Practitioners www.rcgp.org.uk
The Royal College of Obstetricians and Gynaecologists www.rcog.org.uk
The Royal College of Ophthalmologists www.rcophth.ac.uk
The Royal College of Paediatrics and Child Health www.rcpch.ac.uk
The Royal College of Pathologists www.rcpath.ac.uk
The Royal College of Physicians www.rcplondon.ac.uk
The Royal College of Physicians of Edinburgh www.rcpe.ac.uk
The Royal College of Surgeons of Edinburgh www.rcsed.ac.uk
The Royal College of Physicians & Surgeons of Glasgow www.rcpsg.ac.uk
The Royal College of Psychiatrists www.rcpsych.ac.uk
The Royal College of Radiologists www.rcr.ac.uk
The Royal College of Surgeons of Edinburgh www.rcsed.ac.uk
The Royal College of Surgeons of England www.rcseng.ac.uk
The Royal College of Surgeons in Ireland www.rcsi.ie

Other professional bodies and defence organizations

Box 25.3

Academy of Medical Royal Colleges www.aomrc.org.uk
Association of Surgeons in Training www.asit.org
British Medical Association www.bma.org.uk
General Medical Council www.gmc-uk.org
Medical Defence Union www.the-mdu.com
Medical and Dental Defence Union of Scotland www.mddus.com
Medical Protection Society www.medicalprotection.org

Neither the authors nor OUP are responsible for the content of any of the websites listed.

Web resources for ophthalmologists (2)

Training and career issues

Box 25.4

BMJ Careers careers.bmj.com
British Medical Association www.bma.org.uk
Medical Ophthalmology Training
www.jrcptb.org.uk/Specialty/Pages/MedicalOphthalmology.aspx
Modernising Medical Careers www.mmc.nhs.uk
MMC Scotland www.mmc.scot.nhs.uk
MMC Wales www.mmcwales.org
MMC Northern Ireland www.nimdta.gov.uk/mmc
NHS Employers www.nhsemployers.org
NHS Jobs www.jobs.nhs.uk
Ophthalmic Plastic Surgery Training www.oculo-plastics.org.uk
Royal College of Ophthalmologists www.rcophth.ac.uk
ePortfolio portfolio.rcophth.ac.uk
OST Curriculum curriculum.rcophth.ac.uk
Postgraduate Medical Education and Training Board www.pmetb.org.uk
Remedy UK www.remedyUK.org

On-line learning and exam preparation

Box 25.5

AAO Ophthalmic News & Education Network one.aao.org
As Seen From Here—podcasts www.asseenfromhere.com
BMJ Learning learning.bmj.com
Eye Info www.eyeinfo.info
European Computer Driving Licence www.ecdl.com
NeuroLogic Exam library.med.utah.edu/neurologicexam
Neuro-Ophthalmology Virtual Education Library library.med.utah.edu/NOVEL
Ophthalmic Hyperguides www.ophthalmic.hyperguides.com
Richmond Eye RAPD Simulator www.richmondeye.com/apd.asp
RootAtlas videos www.rootatlas.com
Success in MRCOphth www.mrcophth.com
UC Davis Eye Simulator cim.ucdavis.edu/eyes
UKOphth Forums ukophth.freeforums.org

Ophthalmic courses

Box 25.6

Basic Sciences Course for Ophthalmologists bsc.visionresearch.org
Brighton Cornea Course www.brightoncorneacourse.co.uk
East Grinstead Cornea/Oculoplastics course www.corneaoculoplasticscourse.org
Edinburgh FOCUS foundation skills www.edinburgh-focus.com
Moorfields courses www.moorfields.nhs.uk/Healthprofessionals/Medicaleducation
NeuroPass—Neurology/Ophthalmology practical course www.neuroophth.co.uk
Oculus Course www.oculus-course.com
Opticus www.opticus.org.uk

Images for ophthalmology

Box 25.7

Atlas of Ophthalmology www.atlasophthalmology.com
Eye Atlas Online www.eyeatlas.com
Eyetext Image Database www.eyetext.net
Eye Web www.eyeweb.org/atlas.htm
Google Images images.google.com
National Eye Institute www.nei.nih.gov/photo
New York Digital Atlas www.nyee.edu/digital-atlas-of-ophthalmology.html
Ophthalmic Photographers Society www.opsweb.org
Red Atlas www.redatlas.org

Neither the authors nor OUP are responsible for the content of any of the websites listed.

Web resources for ophthalmologists (3)

Journals

> Box 25.8
>
> ### Ophthalmic
> *American Journal of Ophthalmology* www.ajo.com
> *Archives of Ophthalmology* www.archophthalmol.com
> *BMC Ophthalmology* www.biomedcentral.com/bmcophthalmol
> *British Journal of Ophthalmology* bjo.bmj.com
> *Clinical and Experimental Ophthalmology* www.blackwellpublishing.com/journal.asp?ref=1442-6404
> *Cornea* www.corneajrnl.com
> *Current Opinion In Ophthalmology* www.co-ophthalmology.com
> *Digital Journal Of Ophthalmology* www.djo.harvard.edu
> *European Journal of Ophthalmology* www.eur-j-ophthalmol.com
> *Eye* www.nature.com/eye
> *Eye News* www.pinpointmedical.com/showPublication.php?publication=eye-news
> *International Ophthalmology Clinics* www.internat-ophthalmology.com
> *Investigative Ophthalmology & Visual Science* www.iovs.org
> *Journal of the American Association for Pediatric Ophthalmology and Strabismus* www.jaapos.org
> *Journal of Cataract and Refractive Surgery* www.jcrsjournal.com
> *Journal of Glaucoma* www.glaucomajournal.com
> *Journal of Neuro-Ophthalmology* www.jneuro-ophthalmology.com
> *Ophthalmology* www.aaojournal.com
> *Retina* www.retinajournal.com
> *Review of Ophthalmology* www.revophth.com
>
> ### General
> *British Medical Journal* www.bmj.bmjournals.com
> *Nature* www.nature.com
> *New England Journal of Medicine* www.nejm.org
> *The Lancet* www.thelancet.com

Other medical resources

Box 25.9

PubMED and MEDLINE www.pubmed.com
Cochrane Eyes and Vision Group www.cochraneeyes.org
Clinical evidence www.clinicalevidence.com
Doctors net www.doctors.net.uk
Emedicine www.emedicine.com
EMBASE www.embase.com
ISI Web of Knowledge www.isiwebofknowledge.com
OVID www.ovid.com
Google Scholar scholar.google.com
Internet Ophthalmology www.ophthal.org
National Audit Office www.nao.org.uk
NHS National Electronic Library for Health www.library.nhs.uk
NHS Scotland elibrary www.elib.scot.nhs.uk
Department of Health www.dh.gov.uk
UK Statistics Authority www.statistics.gov.uk
National Institute for Health and Clinical Excellence www.nice.org.uk
Scottish Medicines Consortium www.scottishmedicines.org.uk
Centres for disease control and prevention www.cdc.gov
World Health Organization www.who.int

Charities/institutions supporting ophthalmic research

Box 25.10

Action Medical Research www.action.org.uk
British Council for the Prevention of Blindness www.bcpb.org
Fight for Sight www.fightforsight.org.uk
Guide Dogs for the Blind Association www.guidedogs.org.uk
International Agency for the Prevention of Blindness www.iapb.org
Medical Research Council www.mrc.ac.uk
National Eye Research Centre www.nerc.co.uk
Royal National Institute of Blind People www.rnib.org.uk
Sight Savers International www.sightsavers.org
Vision 2020 UK www.vision2020uk.org.uk
Wellcome Trust www.wellcome.ac.uk

Neither the authors nor OUP are responsible for the content of any of the websites listed.

Web resources for patients

Accessibility and information for patients

Box 25.11

Action for Blind People www.afbp.org
BBC Disability Site www.bbc.co.uk/ouch
Benefits of Blind Registration www.rnib.org.uk/xpedio/groups/public/documents/
PublicWebsite/public_regbens.hcsp
Blind Business Association Charitable Trust www.bbact.org.uk
British Blind Sport www.britishblindsport.org.uk
British Computer Association For The Blind www.bcau.org.uk
British Wireless for the Blind Fund www.blind.org.uk
Calibre Recorded Books for the Blind www.calibre.org.uk
Disability Alliance (disability rights) www.disablityyalliance.org
Disability Advice Network www.dialuk.info
Driver and Vehicle Licensing Agency (DVLA) www.dvla.gov.uk
Infosound www.infosound.org.uk
Job Ability (job site for disabled people) www.jobability.com
Royal National College for the Blind www.rncb.ac.uk
Sortit! (for teenagers with visual impairment) www.sortit.org.uk
Vitalise www.vitalise.org.uk
Wellchild Trust www.wellchild.org.uk
Royal Blind Society www.royalblindsociety.org
Specialist Holidays for the Visually Impaired:
Action for Blind People www.actionforblindpeople.org.uk/holidays/
Royal Blind Society www.royalblindsociety.org/holidays.htm
Traveleyes www.traveleyes.co.uk/
Vitalise www.vitalise.org.uk/Visually-Impaired-Holidays/Overview.aspx

Support groups for patients and their families

Box 25.12

Albinism Fellowship www.albinism.org.uk
Aniridia Network www.aniridia.org
Behçet's syndrome society www.behcets.org.uk
British Retinitis Pigmentosa Society www.brps.org.uk
British Sjögren's syndrome association www.bssa.uk.net
British Thyroid Foundation www.btf-thyroid.org
Children's Chronic Arthritis Association www.ccaa.org.uk
Childhood Eye Cancer Trust (Retinoblastoma) www.chect.org.uk
Deafblind UK www.deafblind.org.uk
International Glaucoma Association www.iga.org.uk
Keratoconus Self-help and Support Group www.keratoconus-group.org.uk
Look UK (families with visually impaired children) www.look-uk.org
Macular Disease Society www.maculardisease.org
Micro and Anophthalmic Children's Society (MACS) www.macs.org.uk
National Association of Local Societies for Visually Impaired People www.nalsvi.cswebsites.org
National Blind Childrens Society www.nbcs.org.uk
National Ankylosing Spondylitis Society www.nass.co.uk
National Rheumatoid Arthritis Society www.rheumatoid.org.uk
Nystagmus Network Information Site www.nystagmusnet.org
Sense (The National Deaf Blind and Rubella Association) www.sense.org.uk
Uveitis Information Group www.uveitis.net
See also RNIB website www.rnib.org.uk

Reference intervals

Haematology

FBC

Hb	13.0–18.0g/dL	♂
	11.5–16.5g/dL	♀
Hct	0.40–0.52	♂
	0.36–0.47	♀
RCC	$4.5–6.5 \times 10^{12}$/L	♂
	$3.8–5.8 \times 10^{12}$/L	♀
MCV	77–95fL	
MCH	27.0–32.0pg	
Reticulocytes	$50–100 \times 10^9$/L (0.5–2.5%)	
WCC	$4.0–11.0 \times 10^9$/L	
Neutrophils	$2.0–7.5 \times 10^9$/L	
Lymphocytes	$1.5–4.5 \times 10^9$/L	
Eosinophils	$0.04–0.4 \times 10^9$/L	
Basophils	$0.0–0.2 \times 10^9$/L	
Monocytes	$0.2–0.8 \times 10^9$/L	
Platelets	$150–400 \times 10^9$/L	
ESR	age/2	♂
	📖 p.588	
	(age +10)/2	♀

Haematinics

Serum B12	150–700ng/L
Serum folate	2.0–11.0µg/L
Red cell folate	160–640µg/L
Serum ferritin	15–300µg/L

Clotting

INR	0.8–1.2
PT	12–14s
APTT ratio	0.8–1.2
APTT	26.0–33.5s
Protein C	80–135u/dL
Protein S	80–135u/dL
Antithrombin III	80–120u/dL
APCR	2.12–4.0

Biochemistry

U+E and glucose

Sodium (Na)	135–145mmol/L
Potassium (K)	3.5–5.0mmol/L
Urea	3.0–6.5mmol/L

Creatinine	60–125µmol/L
Glucose (fasting)	3.5–5.5mmol/L
Glucose (random)	3.5–11.0mmol/L (normal/IGT)

LFTs and protein

Total protein	63–80g/L
Albumin	32–50g/L
Bilirubin	<17µmol/L
Alkaline phosphatase	100–300iu/L
ALT	5–2iu/L
AST	5–42iu/L
γGT	10–46iu/L

Bone

Calcium (total)	2.15–2.55mmol/L
Phosphate	0.7–1.5mmol/L

Lipids

Cholesterol	3.9–6.0mmol/L
Triglycerides	0.55–1.90mmol/L
ACE	12–71 (age ≥20); 5–87 (age <20)

Iron studies

Iron	14–33µmol/L
	11–28µmol/L
TIBC	45–75µmol/L

Hormones

TSH	0.35–5.5mU/L
Free T4	9–24pmol/L
Cortisol (morning)	450–700nmol/L
FSH	2–8u/L (luteal); >25u/L (menopausal)
LH	3–16u/L (luteal)
Prolactin	<450u/L
	<650u/L

Arterial blood gases

pH	7.35–7.45
PaO_2	>10.6kPa
$PaCO_2$	4.7–6.0kPa
BE	±2.0mmol/L

Immunology

IgG	5.3–16.5g/L
IgA	0.8–4.0g/L
IgM	0.5–2.0g/L
C3	0.9–2.1g/L
C4	0.12–0.53g/L
C1 esterase	0.11–0.36g/L
CH50	80–120%

CSF analysis	
Lymphocytes	<4/mL
Neutrophils	0/mL
Glucose	≥2/3 plasma level
Protein	<0.4g/L
Opening pressure	<20cmH$_2$O, or <25cmH$_2$O in the obese

For some tests (such as ACE level) there may be significant variation between labs as to what constitutes the 'normal' range. It is, therefore, important to check values against local standards.

Index

Adult basic life support algorithm

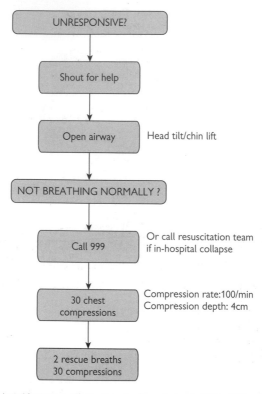

Adult basic life support algorithm from the Resuscitation Guidelines 2005 published by Resuscitation Council (UK), reproduced with permission; http://www.resus.org.uk